IMMUNOLOGY OF CLINICAL AND EXPERIMENTAL DIABETES

IMMUNOLOGY OF CLINICAL AND EXPERIMENTAL DIABETES

Edited by

Sudhir Gupta, M.D., F.R.C.P.(C), F.A.C.P.

Division of Basic and Clinical Immunology
University of California
Irvine, California

Library of Congress Cataloging in Publication Data

Main entry under title:

Immunology of clinical and experimental diabetes.

   Bibliography: p.
   Includes index.
   1. Diabetes—Immunological aspects. 2. Insulin resistance. 3. Diabetes—Animal
models. I. Gupta, Sudhir. [DNLM: 1. Diabetes mellitus, Experimental—Immunology.
2. Diabetes mellitus—Immunology. WK 810 I336]
RC660.I44   1984   616.4′62079   83-22974
ISBN-13: 978-1-4684-4561-9   e-ISBN-13: 978-1-4684-4559-6
DOI: 10.1007/978-1-4684-4559-6

©1984 Plenum Publishing Corporation
Softcover reprint of the hardcover 1st edition 1984

233 Spring Street, New York, N.Y. 10013

Plenum Medical Book Company is an imprint of Plenum Publishing Corporation

*To my wife Abha and our
daughter Ankmalika*

Contributors

M. Bajaj • Laboratory of Molecular Biology, Department of Crystallography, Birkbeck College, London WCIE 7HX, England

Clyde F. Barker • Department of Surgery, School of Medicine, University of Pennsylvania, Philadelphia, Pennsylvania 19104

David M. Brown • Departments of Pediatrics and Laboratory Medicine and Pathology, University of Minnesota School of Medicine, Minneapolis, Minnesota 55455

Peter Y. Chen • Section of Allergy–Immunology, Department of Medicine, Northwestern University Medical School, Chicago, Illinois 60611

Patricia L. Chinn • Department of Surgery, University of Minnesota Health Sciences Center, Minneapolis, Minnesota 55455

A. G. Cudworth† • Department of Diabetes and Immunogenetics, St.Bartholomew's Hospital Medical College, London, England

Gabriel Fernandes • Division of Clinical Immunology and Arthritis, Department of Medicine, University of Texas, San Antonio, San Antonio, Texas 78284

Leslie C. Grammer • Section of Allergy–Immunology, Department of Medicine, Northwestern University Medical School, Chicago, Illinois 60611

Sudhir Gupta • Division of Basic and Clinical Immunology, Department of Medicine, University of California, Irvine, Irvine, California 92717

Barry S. Handwerger • Rheumatology Research Unit, Departments of Medicine and Immunology, Mayo Clinic and Mayo Medical School, Rochester, Minnesota 55905

S. A. Huber • Department of Pathology, University of Vermont, Burlington, Vermont 05405

F. K. Jansen • Research Center, Klin-Midy, 34082 Montpellier Cedex, France.

C. Ronald Kahn • Joslin Diabetes Center, and Department of Medicine, Brigham and Women's Hospital, Harvard Medical School, Boston, Massachusetts 02115

Young Tai Kim • Division of Allergy and Immunology, Department of Medicine, Cornell University Medical College, New York, New York 10021

Dinesh Kumar • Division of Diabetes and Clinical Nutrition, University of Southern California School of Medicine, Los Angeles, California 90033

Åke Lernmark • Hagedorn Research Laboratory, DK-2820 Gentofte, Denmark

B. R. MacPherson • Department of Pathology, University of Vermont, Burlington, Vermont 05405

Dean Mann • Immunology Branch, National Cancer Institute, National Institutes of Health, Bethesda, Maryland 20205

Michael E. Miller • Department of Pediatrics, University of California at Davis, Sacramento, California 95817

Charles E. Moody, Jr. • Division of Geriatrics and Gerontology, Department of Medicine, Cornell University Medical College, New York, New York 10021

Charles E. Morrow • Department of Surgery, University of Minnesota Health Sciences Center, Minneapolis, Minnesota 55455

H. Müntefering • Institute of Pathology, University of Mainz, D-6500 Mainz, Federal Republic of Germany

Ali Naji • Department of Surgery, School of Medicine, University of Pennsylvania, Philadelphia, Pennsylvania 19104

Jørn Nerup • Steno Memorial Hospital, DK-2820 Gentofte, Denmark

Roy Patterson • Section of Allergy–Immunology, Department of Medicine, Northwestern University Medical School, Chicago, Illinois 60611

J. E. Pitts • Laboratory of Molecular Biology, Department of Crystallography, Birkbeck College, London WCIE 7HX, England

Alan S. Rosenthal • Merck, Sharp, and Dohme Research Laboratories, Rahway New Jersey 07065

Joanne Scott • Hagedorn Research Laboratory, DK-2820 Gentofte, Denmark

David E. R. Sutherland • Department of Surgery, University of Minnesota Health Sciences Center, Minneapolis, Minnesota 55455

Eva Wolf • Department of Diabetes and Immunogenetics, St. Bartholomew's Hospital Medical College, London, England

Preface

During the past 5 years, impressive progress has been made in understanding the etiopathogenesis of experimental and clinical diabetes. The rapid progress that has been made in the general field of immunology has made possible new understanding regarding the role of the immune system in the pathogenesis of diabetes. The other two areas in which recent progress has been made in the field of diabetes include genetics and the role of infectious agent(s) in the etiopathogenesis of diabetes. Because of these recent developments, a vast amount of data has been accumulated and published in a number of metabolic, endocrine, immunological, and general medicine journals. The purpose of this book is to consolidate all the available information and present it in its current state.

In the present volume, I strive to bring together relevant contributions from leaders in the fields of immunopathology, immunobiology, and genetics. The advancing understanding has in several instances reached the point of clinical application. This volume encompasses the entire scope of modern immunology of diabetes mellitus.

This volume has been divided into two major parts, Experimental Diabetes and Clinical Diabetes. In the Experimental part are included chapters dealing with the structure and functions of insulin and the immune response to insulin. Spontaneous and experimentally induced models of type I diabetes mellitus are presented. The role of virus(es) in the etiology of experimental diabetes and the influence of sex on experimental diabetes are discussed. The transplantation of pancreas and islets is reviewed in detail.

In the Clinical part the characteristics of insulin receptors and the relationship of antibodies to insulin receptors and insulin are discussed. Studies of genetic linkage and autoimmunity of human type I diabetes are reviewed. An extensive review of the role of virus(es) in the etiopathogenesis of type I diabetes mellitus is presented. The role of lymphocytes, at both cellular and molecular levels, in the pathogenesis of diabetes is discussed in detail. The phagocytic cell functions and the influence of metabolic abnormalities in diabetes mellitus on them are examined. The role of immune complexes in the pathogenesis of diabetes mellitus and their relationship to its complications, particularly vascular complications, are reviewed. A chapter is devoted to insulin hypersensitivity and its management.

It is hoped that this book will serve as a source of current literature on genetic, viral, and immunological aspects of experimental and human diabetes for immunologists, pathologists, endocrinologists, diabetologists, physicians, and pediatricians.

Sudhir Gupta

Irvine, California

Contents

II. CLINICAL DIABETES

13. Phagocytic Cell Functions in Diabetes Mellitus

14. Circulating Immune Complexes

*IMMUNOLOGY OF
CLINICAL AND
EXPERIMENTAL
DIABETES*

Experimental Diabetes

Structure and Function of Insulin

J. E. Pitts and M. Bajaj

I. INTRODUCTION

Knowledge of the conformation of insulin during its complex life cycle of biosynthesis, storage, receptor binding, and degradation may play an important part in the proper design of orally administered analogues, competitive inhibitors, and insulins with selectively enhanced biological activity.

The studies of different crystal forms have resulted in clinically useful long-acting preparations of insulin. The x-ray structure analysis of insulin (Adams *et al.*, 1969; Blundell *et al.*, 1972) allowed much of the past work on the biology and chemistry of insulin to be brought together and led the way for further chemical work to produce new insulin analogues with, for example, long half-lives and also improvement in yields from chemical synthesis by using a miniproinsulin. Studies into possible oral and superpotent insulins reflect the understanding gained from the analysis of the active site of the insulin molecule elucidated from studies of sequence variants, chemically modified insulins, and proinsulin. Further x-ray studies have defined the insulin structure in other crystal environments from species as distant as human and hagfish, while model-building studies based on the insulin fold have been applied to predict the structures of relaxin and insulinlike growth factors (Bedarkar *et al.*, 1977; Blundell *et al.*, 1978). The immunogenic region of insulin appears to be different from the receptor binding region and explains the lack of cross-reactivity of insulinlike growth factors and insulin with their respective antibodies.

In this chapter we will describe the structure of insulin and relate this to its functional determinants involved in correct synthesis and folding, storage, secretion, receptor binding, and rapid degradation of the molecule.

J. E. Pitts and M. Bajaj • Laboratory of Molecular Biology, Department of Crystallography, Birkbeck College, London WCIE 7HX, England.

II. THREE-DIMENSIONAL STRUCTURE OF INSULIN IN CRYSTALS

A. Crystal Forms

The crystallization of insulin may be complicated by the presence of impurities, low solubility, complex aggregation and required cofactors. The rhombohedral crystals of porcine insulin, which formed the basis of the first x-ray analysis, can co-crystallize with up to 5% of proinsulin and/or processing intermediates with some connecting peptide residues. The crystals are a two-phase system with approximately 40% solvent in the channels running through the crystals and must be kept wet for x-ray analysis. Table 1 gives some examples of different insulin crystal forms. Porcine insulin can be seen to crystallize in many different forms simply by altering the conditions of the buffer medium. Whereas sequence variants can be found to give rise to the same crystalline lattice, the optimal pH for crystal growth may differ. Even insulins with similar sequences may crystallize in different forms and so may require purification to homogeneity before crystallization. This occurs with the two polymorphic forms of rat and mouse insulin which differ within the B chain at positins B9 (Pro to Ser) and B29 (Lys to Met). Purification using ion exchange chromatography allows the monocomponent rat I insulin to form rhombohedral (R3) crystals and rat II insulin to give cubic ($P4_2 32$) crystals (Wood et al., 1978).

The method used to produce large single crystals of rhombohedral (R3) insulin involves dissolving insulin at approximately 5 mg/ml in acetate buffer at roughly pH 7 in the presence of zinc ions and acetone. Lowering the pH produces a slight turbidity which can be redissolved upon warming to 55°C. Slow cooling over 10–12 days in an insulated dewar allows large crystals to slowly form. The addition of anions at 1 M concentrations (e.g., Cl^-) produces the related four-zinc hexameric form (Harding et al., 1966). The addition of trace amounts of organic solvents such as m-cresol or phenol leads to a monoclinic crystal lattice, but remove the zinc and crystallization fails (Harding et al., 1966; Low and Chen, 1969). At acidic pH zinc binding does not occur and the highest aggregation state is dimeric which gives rise to an orthorhombic crystal form (Low and Berger, 1961).

Table 1. Examples of Different Crystal Forms of Insulin

Species (reference)	Space group	Association state
Porcine (Harding et al., 1966)	R3	2Zn Hexamer
Porcine (Harding et al., 1966)	R3	4Zn Hexamer
Porcine (Harding et al., 1966)	$I2_1 3$	Dimer
Porcine (Harding et al., 1966)	$P2_1$	Zn Hexamer
Porcine (Low and Berger, 1961)	$P2_1 2_1 2_1$	Dimer
Porcine–Protamine (Baker and Dodson, 1970)	$P2_1 2_1 2_1$	Hexamer
Porcine–Salmine (Simkin et al., 1970)	$P4_1 2_1 2$	Hexamer
Rat I (Wood, 1976)	R3	Zn Hexamer
Rat II (Wood, 1976)	$P4_2 32$	Zn Hexamer
Hagfish (Cutfield et al., 1974)	$P4_1 2_1 2$	Dimer
Turkey (Pitts, 1980)	$P2_1 2_1 2_1$	Dimer?

B. Insulin in Clinical Preparations

The two main problems with the control of diabetes by insulin involve the maintenance of the correct hormonal level for long periods and the avoidance of immunological reaction. The insulin preparations fall into three categories according to the length and strength of action. Soluble or regular insulin produces the strongest but shortest blood glucose lowering effects. Insulin crystals complexed with protamine/zinc or only zinc (ultralente) are the longest and weakest, and finally globin, isophane, and amorphous (semilente) are intermediate in both these respects. For severe diabetes soluble insulin should be given at frequent intervals. The original delivery method of injection for soluble insulin, perhaps six times a day, results in problems at the injecton site. The use of long-acting crystalline forms of insulin has allowed good control with only one or two injections a day.

The optimal method of control which would allow for the large fluctuations in sugar levels in response to a meal would be to monitor glucose levels and release insulin in response to changes in the plasma. Two methods have been attempted: one involves continuous artificial infusion of soluble insulin by various methods (Waldhausl, 1979), the second the transplantation of islet cells (Raskin, 1979). The first technique can lead to infection and the second to implant rejection but further research may soon solve the practical problems and allow these methods more widespread use clinically.

Immunological problems may arise by the production of antibodies against impurities in clinical insulin preparations or even to the insulin itself. Protamine insulin preparations can produce a reaction against the protamine component, which can be avoided by the use of ultralente insulin which has similar characteristics. Many insulin preparations contain impurities including proinsulin, intermediates of conversion of the prohormone, connecting peptide fragments, and traces of other pancreatic hormones. Bloom et al. (1978) have shown that many commercial insulins contain significant quantities of the pancreatic polypeptide hormone (PP), vasoactive intestinal peptide, somatostatin, and pancreatic glucagon. Thus the past use of porcine and bovine insulins containing both peptide contaminants and amino acid sequence differences to human insulin, (Table 2) has led to immunogenic reaction in some patients. In these cases the treatment with the fairly recent preparations of monocomponent insulins will often solve the problem. The ideal case would be to start all newly diagnosed young diabetic patients with human monocomponent insulin. The current research into genetic engineering has led to the production of human insulin for clinical trials produced from bacteria which may provide an economical source of human insulin (Gammeltoft, 1981; Keefer et al., 1981b; De Meyts et al., 1981). The recombinant human insulin has been crystallized in this laboratory (Fig. 1) and appears able to give rise to both the ultralente and lente forms which may be useful clinically.

C. The Structure of Insulin in Crystals

Insulin is a compact, globular protein which can self-associate via its two hydrophobic surfaces to form dimers and then zinc–insulin hexamers in the presence of zinc ions. The hexamers can aggregate to give rise to the porcine two-zinc insulin crystals which were studied to give the first detailed information of the conformation of insulin by

Table 2.   Amino Acid Sequences of Insulin

A chain	1	2	3	4	5	6	7	8	9	10	11	12	13	14
Porcine	(Gly)	(Ile)	Val	Glu	(Gln)	(Cys)	(Cys)	Thr	Ser	Ile	(Cys)	Ser	Leu	Tyr
Bovine								Ala		Val				
Human														
Rat I				Asp										
Rat II				Asp										
Guinea pig				Asp					Gly	Thr		Thr	Arg	His
Coypu				Asp					Asn				Arg	Asn
Chinchilla				Asp								Thr		
Casiragua				Asp					Asn				Arg	Asn
Porcupine				Asp					Gly	Val				
Cod				Asp				His	Arg	Pro		Asp	Ile	Phe
Angler fish								His	Arg	Pro		Asp	Ile	Phe
Hagfish								His	Lys	Arg			Ile	
Turkey								His	Asn	Thr				
Duck								Glu	Asn	Pro				
Rattlesnake								Glu	Asn	Thr				

B chain	−1	1	2	3	4	5	6	7	8	9	10	11	12	13	14
Porcine		Phe	Val	Asn	Gln	His	(Leu)	(Cys)	(Gly)	Ser	His	(Leu)	(Val)	Glu	Ala
Bovine															
Human															
Rat I				Lys						Pro					
Rat II				Lys											
Guinea pig				Ser	Arg						Asn				Thr
Coypu		Tyr		Ser		Arg					Gln			Asp	Thr
Chinchilla					Lys									Asp	
Casiragua		Tyr		Gly		Arg					Gln			Asp	Thr
Porcupine															
Cod	Met	Ala	Pro	Pro										Asp	
Angler fish	Val	Ala	Pro	Ala										Asp	
Hagfish		Arg	Thr	Thr	Gly					Lys	Asp			Asn	
Duck		Ala	Ala												
Turkey		Ala	Ala												
Rattlesnake		Ala	Pro			Arg									

*a*Empty spaces signify identity with the porcine sequence; circles indicate invariant residues.

x-ray analysis (Adams *et al.*, 1969; Blundell *et al.*, 1971). The equivalent dimers are related by a crystallographic threefold axis to form the hexamer with two zinc ions lying along the symmetry axis. The hexamer forms an oblate spheroid with a diameter of approximately 50 Å and about 34 Å thick, the B10 His of each protomer being coordinated to a zinc atom. The two protomers within each dimer are crystallographically independent molecules and are generally referred to as molecules I and II. However the Peking Insulin Structure Research Group (1974) define them as 2 and 1, respectively. Molecules I and II are similar in conformation but are not identical.

The insulin protomer has a compact hydrophobic core and interchain disulfide bridges which stabilize the molecule. The 21- amino-acid A chain contains two sections of imperfect helices running from A2 to A8 and from A13 to A20. Figure 2 shows schematically how they run antiparallel to each other, separated by the extended arm

A and B Chains from Various Species[a]

15	16	17	18	19	20	21	22
Gln	(Leu)	Glu	Asn	(Tyr)	(Cys)	(Asn)	
		Gln	Ser				
		Met	Ser			Asp	
		Leu	Thr				
		Gln					
Asp		Gln					
Asp		Gln					
Asn		Gln					
Asp		Gln					

15	16	17	18	19	20	21	22	23	24	25	26	27	28	29	30	31
(Leu)	Tyr	Leu	Val	(Cys)	Gly	Glu	Arg	(Gly)	(Phe)	Phe	Tyr	Thr	Pro	Lys	Ala	
															Thr	
															Ser	
														Met	Ser	
		Ser			Gln	Asp	Asp					Ile			Asp	
		Ser			Arg	His				Tyr	Arg	Pro	Asn	Asp	—	
						Asp								Met		
		Ser			Lys	His				Tyr	Arg	Pro	Ser	Glu	—	
						Asn	Asp									
						Asp										
						Asp										
		Ile	Ala			Val						Asp		Thr	Lys	Met
												Ser			Thr	
												Ser				
	Phe		Ile							Tyr		Ser		Arg	Ser	

(A9–A12) with an A6–A11 intrachain disulfide bridge. The resulting A-chain loop forms a planar U-turn which brings the N- and C-terminal residues into close proximity. The B chain (Fig. 3) has an extended region from B1 to B7 with a tight turn at Gly B8 followed by an α helix from B9 to B19 then a U-turn at B20–B23, leaving the rest of the chain in an extended form. Figure 4 shows the insulin molecule with amino acid sidechains completing the compact hydrophobic core of the molecule (Adams *et al.*, 1969; Blundell *et al.*, 1972).

High-resolution studies of porcine two-zinc insulin have been completed and refined (Dodson *et al.*, 1979; Sakabe *et al.*, 1978; Peking Insulin Structure Research Group, 1974). The structures of porcine four-zinc hexamers, and porcine and hagfish insulin dimers, indicate that one conformation occurs commonly in all crystal structures, that of molecule II (Dodson *et al.*, 1980a; Cutfield *et al.*, 1974, 1979; Bentley *et*

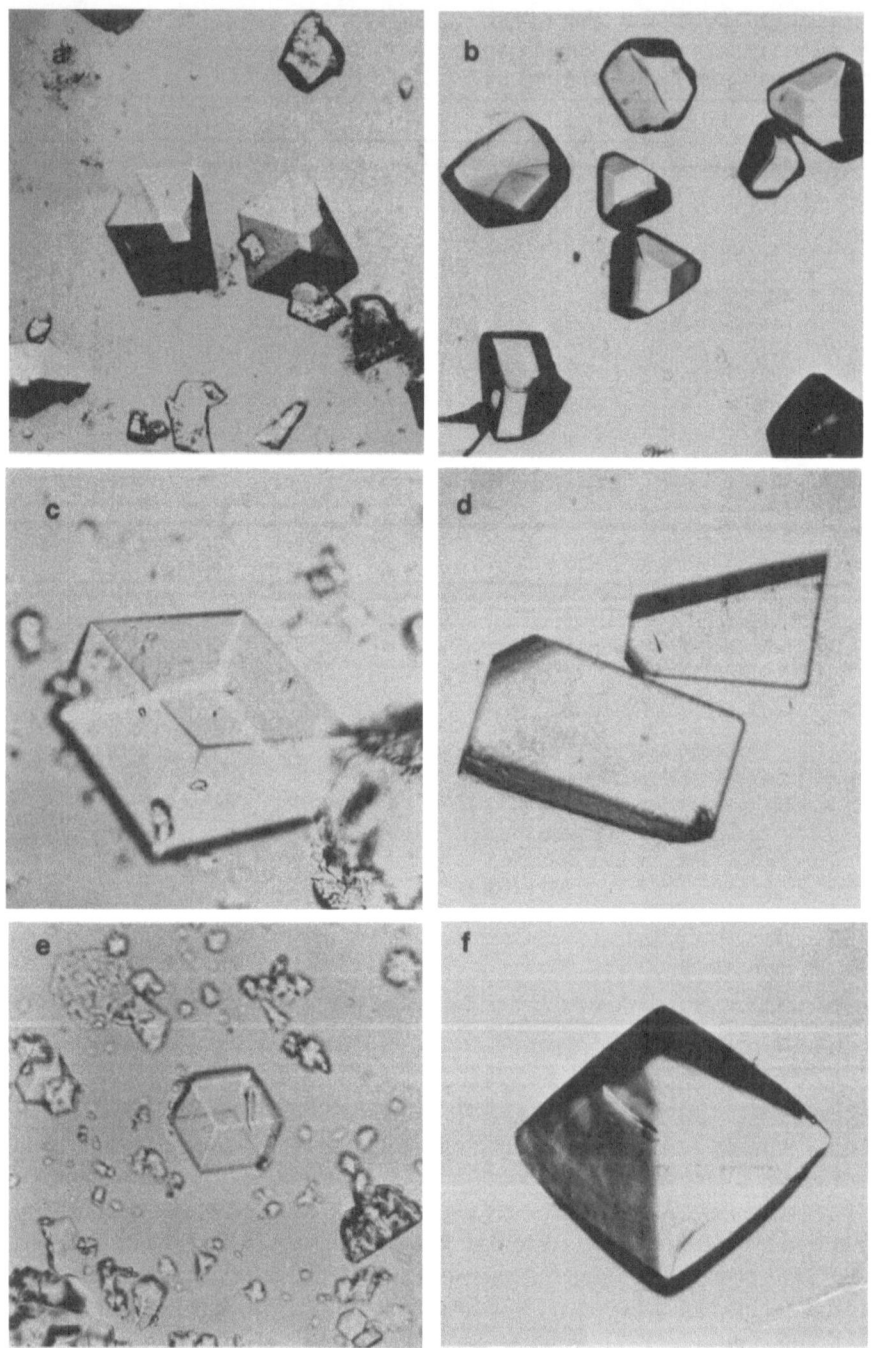

Figure 1. A selection of different crystal forms of insulin illustrating the variation in crystal morphology and symmetry. (a) Porcine insulin (R3). (b) Bovine insulin (R3). (c) Human insulin produced by genetic engineering in bacteria (R3). (d) Turkey insulin ($P2_12_12_1$). (e) Rat I insulin (R3). (f) Rat II insulin ($P4_232$).

al., 1976). The differences found in molecule I of porcine two-zinc insulin are probably due to crystal packing. The changes involve a rotation of the A1–A5 helical arm through 40° with movements of residues A6–A9 and B1–B8. Also there are altered conformations for B5 His and B25 Phe, with a large movement of the flexible B29 and B30 residues. In four-zinc hexamers a major conformational change occurs when B1–B8 rearranges to form an extension of the helix B9–B20. Thus conformational

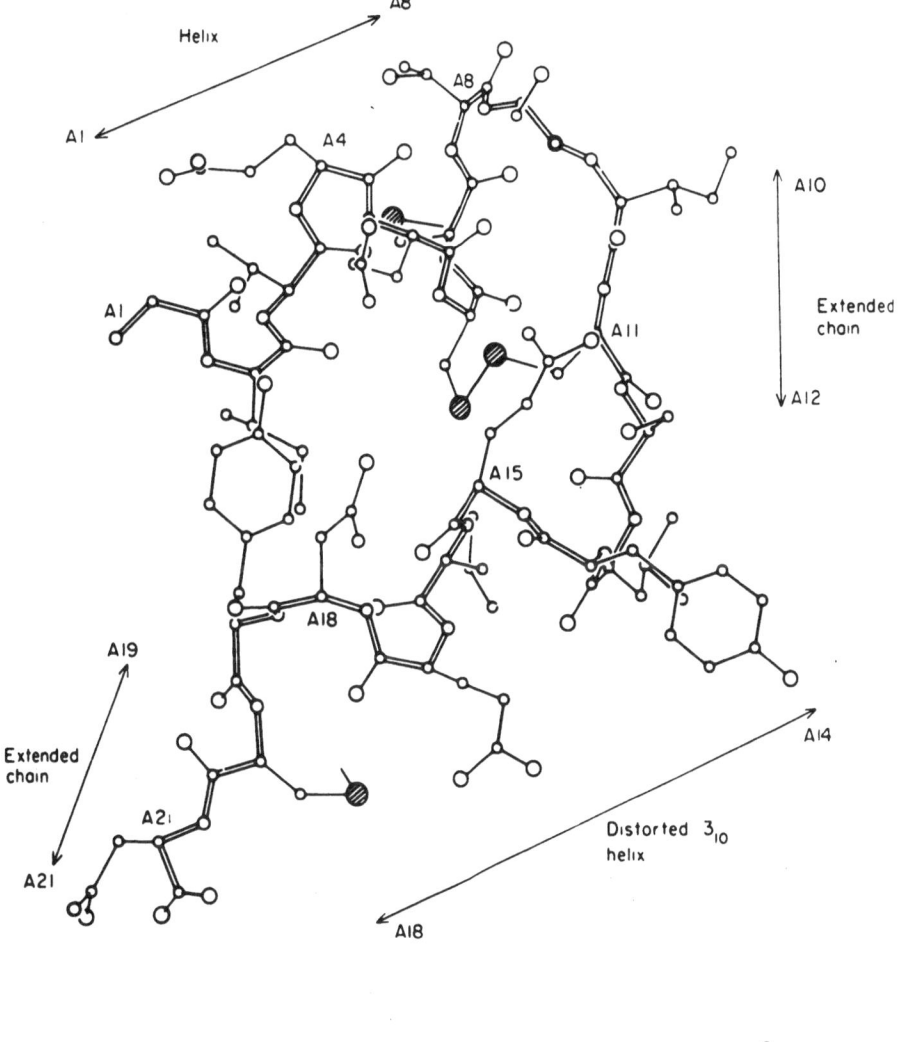

Figure 2. The secondary structural elements of the insulin A chain (reproduced from Blundell and Johnson, 1976).

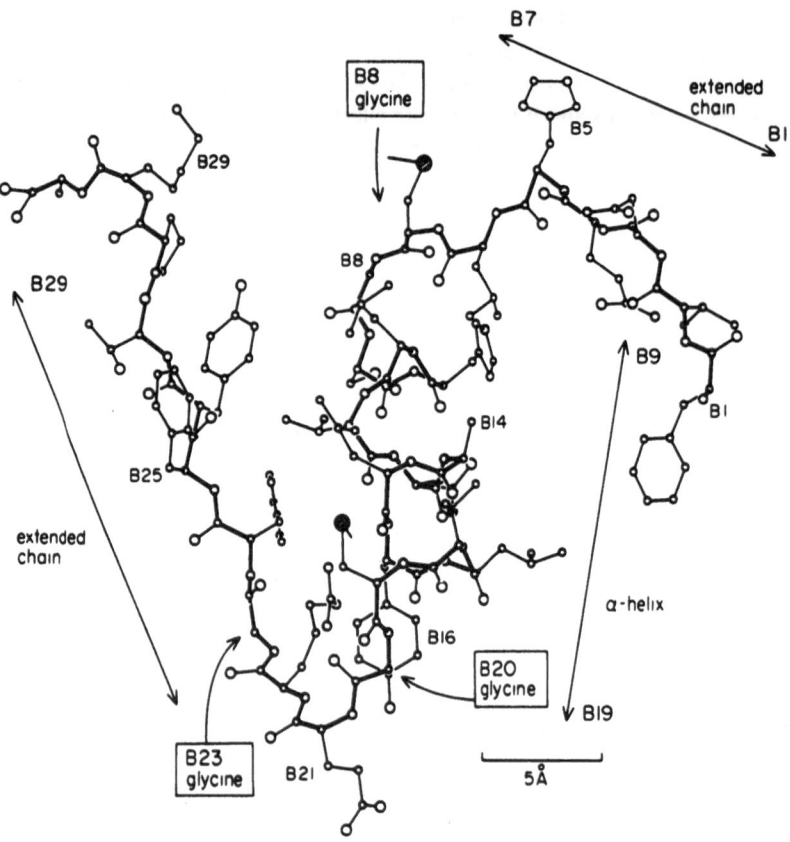

Figure 3.   The secondary structural elements of the insulin B chain (reproduced from Blundell and Johnson, 1976).

changes can be induced in the insulin molecule although it does have a preferred tertiary fold.

Many chemical modifications of insulin still allow crystal formation (Pullen *et al.*,
1975, 1976). The replacement of B1 Phe by Trp, the addition of groups to the A1 Gly
position such as glutamyl, thiazolidine, acetyl, and t-butoxy-carbonyl, or the deletion
of B1–B3 region still allows the modified insulin to crystallize isomorphously with
porcine insulin (Pullen *et al.*, 1976; Dockerill, 1978; Brandenburg *et al.*, 1980; Friesen
et al., 1977; Bedarkar, 1982). High-resolution x-ray studies on AO Glu insulin indicate small movements of the B24–B26 and A19 residues as well as movement of the
A1–A5 region already known to be affected by crystal-packing forces (Bedarkar,
1982). Crystals of A1–B29 diaminosuberic acid cross-linked insulin show very small
differences from native insulin (Dodson *et al.*, 1980b). Insulins with B chain deletions
have also provided crystals, for example B25–B30 des hexapeptide and B26–B30 des

pentapeptide insulin (Peking Insulin Structure Research Group, 1976a, b; Lu Zixian and Yu Ronghua, 1980; Cao *et al.*, 1981). The only superpotent insulin to have been studied by x-ray analysis is turkey insulin (Pitts, 1980), which has at least 250–300% higher potency than bovine insulin. The low-resolution studies indicate that the overall conformation is similar to porcine insulin suggesting that higher binding interactions occur once the insulin is bound to the receptor, rather than a gross change in the hormone's conformation.

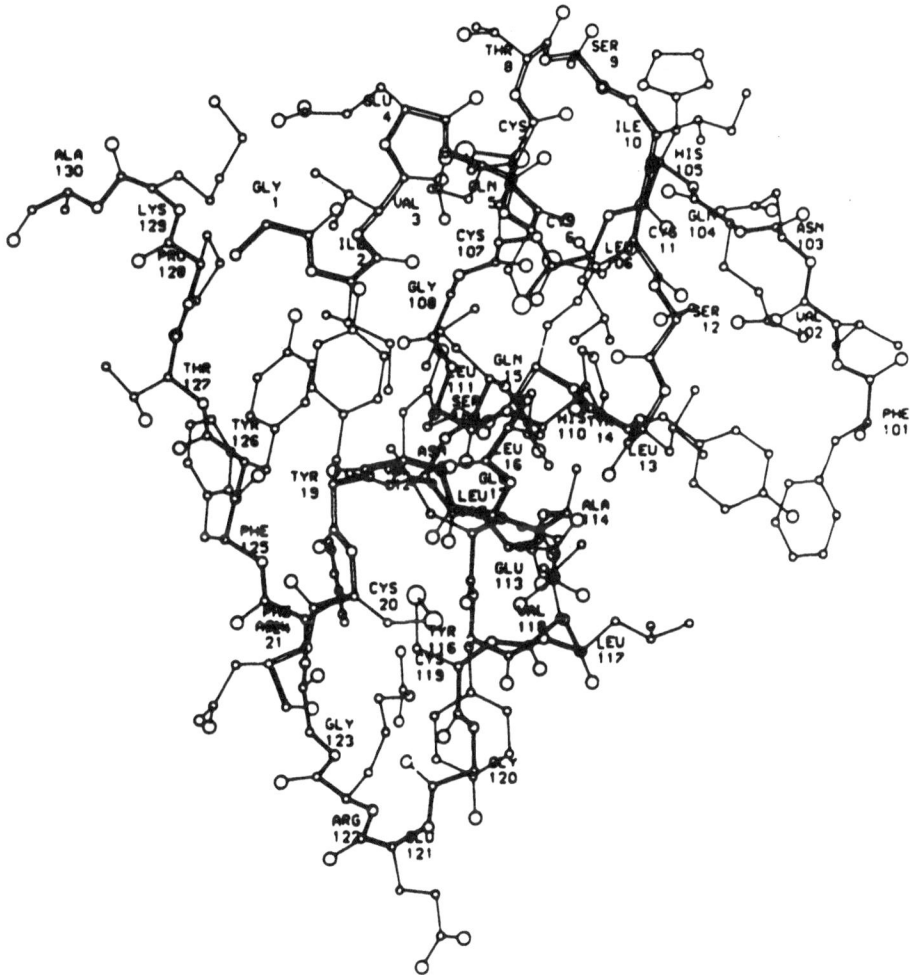

Figure 4. The complete tertiary structure of the insulin monomer viewed perpendicular to the threefold axis. The backbone of the A chain is represented by a double line and that of the B chain by a heavy line (reproduced from Blundell *et al.*, 1972).

III. INSULIN STRUCTURE IN SOLUTION

A. Bovine and Porcine Insulin

Many spectroscopic techniques have been applied to insulin including Raman spectra, nuclear magnetic resonance, electron spin resonance, and circular dichroism. These methods allow insulins which do not crystallize or are not available in large quantities to be studied and helps to answer the question "Does the insulin structure found in the wet crystal appear similar to that found in solution?"

Insulin has been studied and used as a model protein for many years due to its early purification and inherent "toughness." The use of crystalline powders of insulin in Raman spectroscopy resulted in a loss of order due to the local heating by the laser beam (Yu *et al.*, 1972a,b). The maintenance of two-zinc crystals in mother liquid with either D_2O or H_2O allowed the main-chain amide contributions to be recorded. The secondary structure contributions from the spectra agreed with that found in the x-ray analysis (Lippert *et al.*, 1976). The aggregation of protomers to dimers and zinc insulin hexamers must be remembered when interpreting solution studies that may involve these effects (Fig. 5). The change in α helix content recorded when the pH was varied from 7 to 2 may result from the dissociation of the hexamers to dimers in more acidic conditions. Comparisons of the insulin and proinsulin Raman spectra from the lyophilized form show great similarity (Yu *et al.*, 1972b).

The early studies using high-resolution proton nuclear magnetic resonance spectrometers were performed under conditions likely to disrupt the native conformation. At the more reasonable pH of 9 it was shown that for two-zinc hexamers, resonances could be assigned to methyl groups of Ile, Val, and Leu and to the aromatic protons of His, Tyr, and Phe (Williamson and Williams, 1979). The transformation from two-zinc to four-zinc insulin hexamers could also be followed in solution. Similarly conformational changes upon aggregation have been recorded by Bradbury and Brown (1977). Trifluoroacetylated (^{19}F) or carbamylated (^{13}C) insulin derivatives have given nuclear magnetic resonance measurements indicating asymmetric dimers in solution (Paselk and Levy, 1974; Led *et al.*, 1975) However, this may reflect only the alteration to the conformation of A1 Gly, which has a great influence on the aggregation and tertiary structure, with the change of the charge that occurs with the insertion of a probe at this position.

Electron spin resonance studies of Cu^{2+} substituted for Zn^{2+} in insulin hexamers showed line broadening, hyperfine splitting, and g-values in agreement with an octahedral complex with a tetragonal distortion (Brill and Venable, 1967). X-ray studies by Pallett and Wood (unpublished results, 1982) have confirmed these results. Further binding sites for copper have been indicated with lyophilized native and cross-linked insulin (Evans *et al.*, 1979) and by energy-dispersive analysis of x-rays on whole single crystals (Pitts, 1980).

Circular dichroism spectra using insulin were recorded as soon as the first instrument appeared (Beychok, 1966). Although small changes in the secondary structure can be detected, the self-association of insulin has caused some problems with interpretation of the spectra recorded (Ettinger and Timasheff, 1971). Restriction of movement of several aromatic side-chains occur during the beta-pleated sheet formation when

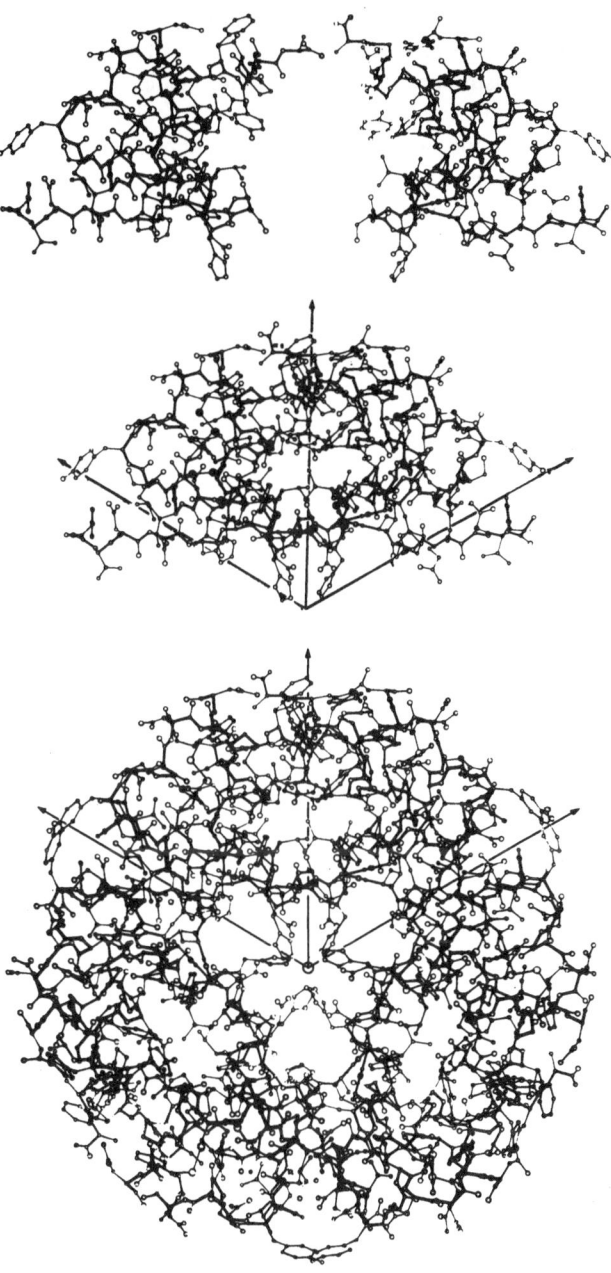

Figure 5. Insulin monomers (top) associated through hydrophobic interactions and as antiparallel β sheet to dimers (middle) and, in the presence of zinc, to two-zinc insulin hexamers (bottom). View along the crystallographic threefold axis (reproduced from Blundell *et al.*, 1972).

monomers aggregate to dimers. Further aggregation in the presence of zinc to hexamers produces large spectral changes in the near ultraviolet circular dichroism (Fig. 6). The circular dichroism spectrum in the far ultraviolet (Fig. 7) indicates a maintenance of secondary structure as the population of individual molecules increases, suggesting that the conformation of insulin does not rely upon aggregation for its stability. Recently Pocker and Biswas (1980) have attempted to record the circular dichroism spectra for very low insulin concentrations where monomers are predominant. The calculated spectra (Pocker and Biswas, 1981) indicate a great loss of secondary structure from dissociation of dimers to monomers. This result appears to disagree with the studies on the monomeric hystricomorph insulins which maintain the insulinlike secondary structure in the far ultraviolet (Horuk, 1980; Horuk *et al.*, 1980a).

B. Species Variants

The studies on insulin analogues with altered biological activity by circular dichroism have allowed some structure–function analysis without the detailed three-dimensional investigation from x-ray analysis (Goldman and Carpenter, 1974; Wood *et al.*, 1975). The x-ray analysis shows that two largely hydrophobic surfaces are buried when protomers form dimers and hexamers (Fig. 5). Dimerization involves the formation of an antiparallel pleated sheet between the B24–B26 regions of each protomer and hy-

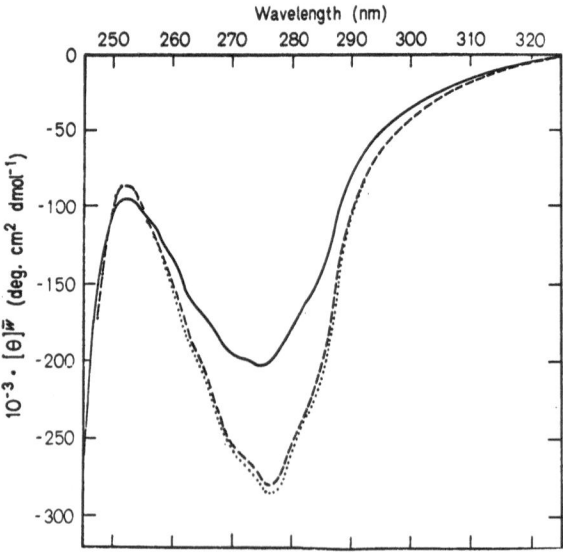

Figure 6.   Circular dichroism spectrum in the near ultraviolet of bovine insulin as a function of zinc concentration. Solid line, no zinc; dashed line, 0.33 atoms of zinc per insulin monomer; dotted line, 0.5 atoms of zinc per insulin monomer (reproduced from Wood, 1976).

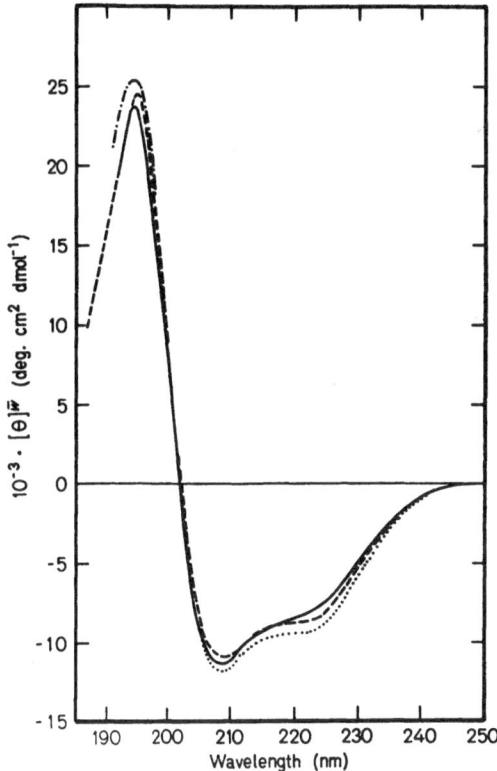

Figure 7. Circular dichroism spectrum in the far ultraviolet of bovine insulin as a function of concentration. Solid line, 3.5×10^{-6} M; dashed line, 3.5×10^{-5} M; dotted line, 3.5×10^{-4} M (reproduced from Wood, 1976).

drophobic interactions including B12 Val, B16 Tyr, B24 Phe, and B26 Tyr, and their equivalents. Although the different insulin crystal forms grown can contain either asymmetrical or symmetrical dimers, in solution it is likely that only the latter type with a pure twofold axis exists. The aggregation of dimers to give hexamers involves residues A13 Leu, A14 Tyr, B1 Phe, B14 Ala, and B17 Leu while each zinc ion is coordinated through the B10 His.

The superpotent turkey insulin appears to have a similar conformation to that found for bovine, porcine, human, and hagfish insulin as studied by x-ray and circular dichroism experiments (Pitts, 1980; Cao *et al.*, 1980). Turkey insulin undergoes dimer and zinc hexamer formation when observed by near ultraviolet circular dichroism during the addition of zinc and in rhombohedral R3 crystal formation. The far ultraviolet circular dichroism spectrum of turkey insulin is indistinguishable from the bovine measurement (Fig. 8), indicating a very similar secondary structure to mammalian in-

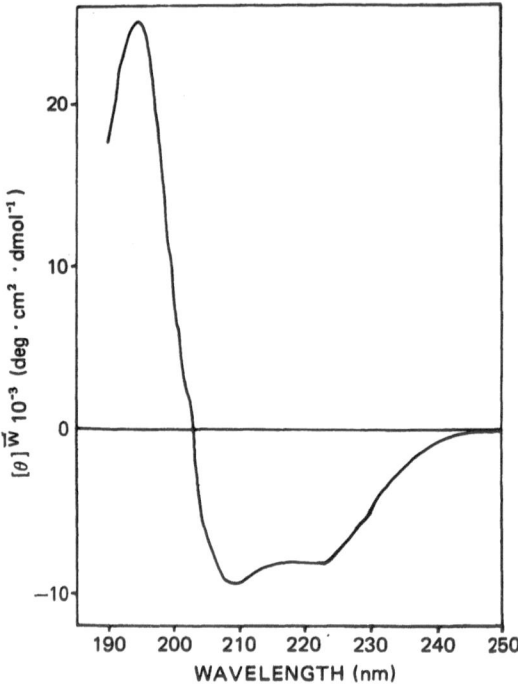

Figure 8.   Circular dichroism spectrum in the far ultraviolet of turkey insulin at 0.196 mg/ml (reproduced from Pitts, 1980).

sulins. The change of B1 Phe to Ala in turkey insulin does not alter the circular dichro-ism spectra. This agrees with the finding of Wollmer *et al.,* (1977) on des-B1 Phe insulin who reported that B1 Phe does not contribute to the tyrosyl circular dichroism of A14 Tyr upon hexamerization. Thus the superpotency has to be explained in other terms than gross conformational changes in the structure of the insulin.

Many fish insulins have been sequenced and they all appear to be able to form zinc insulin hexamers with the exception of the primitive vertebrate, the hagfish, which only forms dimers (Emdin and Falkmer, 1980). The changes at B10 from His to Asp and B1 Phe to Arg in hagfish may prevent higher aggregates forming although the sur-face involved remains hydrophobic with residues A13 Ile, A14 Tyr, B6 Leu, B14 Ala, B17 Ile, and B20 Gly. This implies that the requirement for the potential hexamerization surface to be hydrophobic occurred during evolution before the ability to produce zinc insulin hexamers.

A very useful group of insulin sequence variants is provided by the hystricomorph rodents. They include guinea pig, casiragua, coypu, chinchilla, and porcupine insulins and this group of low-biological-activity insulins contains a large variety of primary sequence changes (Wood *et al.,* 1975; Horuk *et al.,* 1979,1980a; Horuk, 1980). Chin-chilla insulin can form four-zinc insulin hexamers in a similar way to porcine insulin (Wood, 1976). Casiragua insulin can also adopt the insulin fold but it does not dimerize, mainly because of the effect of the B26 Arg substitution and the changes in conformation due to the B20 Lys change which is normally a Gly. Guinea pig and casiragua insulin have the amino acids required for dimerization, but the conformation is disrupted by the close proximity of B22 Asp to the terminal carboxylate of A21 resulting in a charge repulsion; since both carry a negative charge at neutral pH. The far ultraviolet circular dichroism spectrum indicates this change in conformation (Fig. 9) which can be partially reversed at low pH, with the neutralization of the negative charge, to give a more insulinlike conformation (Wood, 1976; Horuk et al., 1980a).

IV. INSULIN BIOSYNTHESIS

Insulin is synthesized in the B cell as preproinsulin with an N-terminal extension to the B chain of proinsulin (Table 3) of approximately 20 amino acids (Chan et al., 1976). The length and sequence of this extension varies in different species (Lomedico et al., 1977; Ullrich et al., 1977; Bell et al., 1979; Perler et al., 1980), although its function as a signal peptide involved with ribosome location and transport of preproinsulin into the endoplasmic reticulum is a commonly found requirement. The hydrophobicity of this presequence extension may help to cover the molecule during transmembrane movement. The removal of the preregion may or may not be required before the correct folding of the proinsulin molecule occurs.

Proinsulin is a single-chain polypeptide with positions A1 and B30 joined by a connecting peptide which varies between 20 and 35 residues depending on the species (Table 4; Fig. 10). It is the major molecular species during transport within the endo-

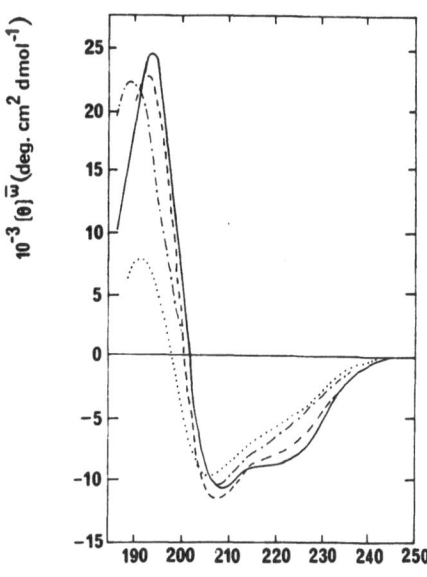

Figure 9. Combined circular dichroism in the far ultraviolet of bovine (———), chinchilla (- - -), guinea pig (. . . .) insulins (Wood, 1976) and casiragua (· - · - ·) insulin (Horuk, 1980). Insulin concentration 4×10^{-5} M, 0.025 M Tris buffer pH 7.8, zinc-free (reproduced from Horuk et al., 1980b).

$10^{-3} [\bar{\theta}]_{\lambda} (\text{deg. cm}^2 \text{ dmol}^{-1})$

wavelength (nm)

Table 3. *Comparison of Amino Acid Sequences of Preregions of Preproinsulin*[a]

Hagfish	Leu	—	—	Leu	Ala	Ala	—	Leu	—	Leu	Leu	Leu	—	—	Ala	—	Ala	—	—	Ala
Sea raven	Met	Leu	—	Leu	—	—	—	Leu	—	Leu	Leu	Leu	—	—	—	—	—	—	—	—
Angler fish	Ala	Leu	—	Leu	—	Phe	—	Leu	Leu	Val	Leu	Leu	Val	—	—	—	—	Ala	Val	
Bovine	—	Leu	—	—	Leu	—	Leu	Leu	Leu	—	Leu	—	—	—	—	—	—	Phe		
Rat I	Met	Ala	Leu	Trp	Ile	Arg	Phe	Leu	Pro	Leu	Leu	Ala	Leu	Leu	Ile	Leu	Trp	Glu	Pro	Arg	Ala	Pro	Ala	Gln	Ala	Phe
Rat II												Val						Lys								
Human		Met	Met									Ala		Gly			Gly	Asp							Ala	
Chicken		Ile	Ser									Val	Phe	Ser		Gly	Gly	Thr	Ser	Tyr						Ala

[a]Dashes signify unknown amino acids; spaces signify identity with rat I sequence. Reproduced from Perler *et al.*, 1980.

Table 4. *Alignment of Mammalian and Avian C Peptides from Sequencing the Preproinsulin Genes*[a]

	Glu	Val	Glu	Asp	Pro	Gln	Val	Pro	Gln	Val	Pro	Gln	Leu	Glu	Leu	Gly	Gly	Gly	Pro	Gly	Ala	Gly	Asp	Leu	Gln	Thr	Leu	Ala	Leu	Glu	Val	Ala	Arg	Gln
Rat I																																Gly	Ser	Leu
Rat II																				Gly														
Human		Ala			Leu			Gly			Val		Ser						Pro		Gly											Glu	Tyr	Gln
Chicken		Asp			Gln	Leu		Ser	Ser	Pro	—	Arg			Val				—	—	Pro	Phe	Gln	Gln							Glu	Tyr	—	Gln
Duck		Asp			Gln	Leu		Asn	Gly	Pro		His			Glu				—	—	Pro	Phe	Gln	His						Val	Glu	Tyr	—	Gln

[a]Dashes signify unknown amino acids; spaces signify identity with rat I sequence. Reproduced from Porter *et al.*, 1980.

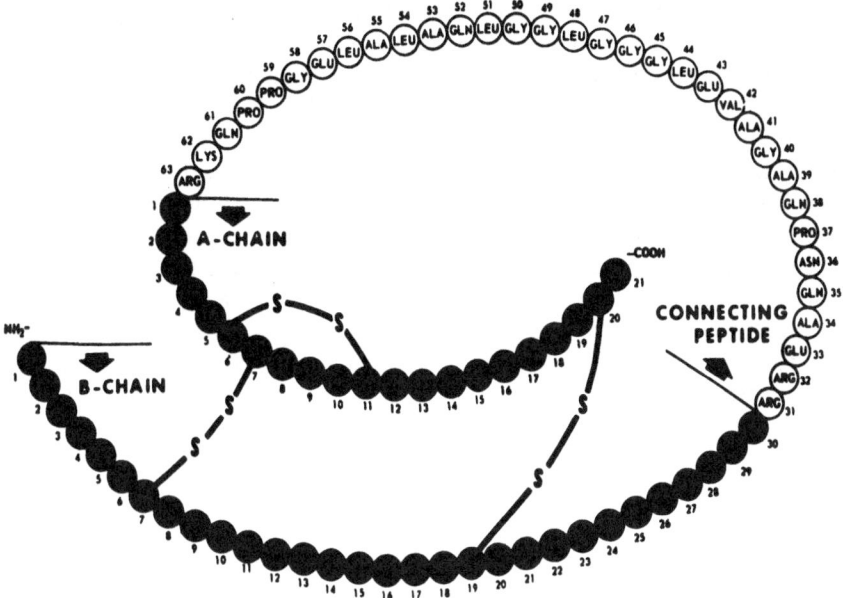

Figure 10. The primary structure of proinsulin with the A and B chains indicated by black circles and the connecting peptide by white circles (reproduced from Steiner *et al.*, 1969).

plasmic reticulum and Golgi before the storage granules are formed (Steiner *et al.*, 1969). The connecting peptide assists in directing the correct pairing of the disulfide bridges and formation of the insulin fold. Proinsulin can form dimers, and in the presence of zinc gives rise to hexamers which are more soluble at physiological pH than zinc–insulin hexamers (Fullerton *et al.*, 1970; Grant *et al.*, 1972). This may play an important role in keeping the prohormone soluble during transport to its storage location.

The recent work sequencing the DNA for the polymorphic forms of rat insulins shows an intervening region of 119 base pairs corresponding to the 5′ untranslated portion of the messenger RNA (Lomedico *et al.*, 1979; Bell *et al.*, 1980). The rat II gene also has within the connecting peptide coding region an inserted 499 base pair sequence. The human and chicken insulin genes have the extra insertion at the same position and thus resemble the rat II gene (Bell *et al.*, 1979; Perler *et al.*, 1980). The position of the intervening region is interesting in relation to the insulin folding units. The A and B chains of insulin would not maintain their conformations individually but together they form the single insulin domain. The folding and interactions involved in the combination of the A and B chains to give insulin may have been obligatory early in evolution. The division of the insulin gene may indicate that smaller polypeptides were once coded by the ancestral genes. The intervening sequence provides a mechanism for the variation of the connecting peptides from different species. Their high variability allows optimization of the control and direction of folding of the A and B chains. This would optimize the solubility during transport to the site of granulation and allow changes of specificity to enzymatic modification.

Although the connecting peptide directs correct folding it does not appear to have a preferred conformation when isolated (Vogt *et al.*, 1976). Studies in the ultracentrifuge (Markussen and Schiff, 1973) show that the axial ratio is large which is consistent with the ends of the connecting peptide linking the A1 and B30 resides of insulin, the latter two residues being only 10 Å apart. Although prediction studies suggest some helical structure within the connecting peptide (Snell and Smyth, 1975), spectroscopic evidence suggests a lack of any secondary structure for this region in proinsulin (Yu *et al.*, 1972b; Vogt *et al.*, 1976; Frank *et al.*, 1972a,b). The connecting peptide probably lies over the face of the molecule involving the A chain, B22 and B25 (Blundell *et al.*, 1972; Arquilla *et al.*, 1972; Snell and Smyth, 1975). The variation of the primary sequences of the connecting peptides from different species suggest variation of interactions and a lack of a common conformation (Fig. 11). This flexible arrangement over the surface is consistent with hexamer formation and antibody-binding studies (Arquilla *et al.*, 1978). The answer to the correct conformation of the connecting peptide may soon be provided by the x-ray studies currently underway on crystals of proinsulin in this laboratory (Wood *et al.*, unpublished results; Fig. 12).

V. INSULIN IN STORAGE GRANULES

After enzymatic conversion of proinsulin to insulin the hormone is stored in electron-dense, membrane-enclosed granules which are eventually released into the circulation

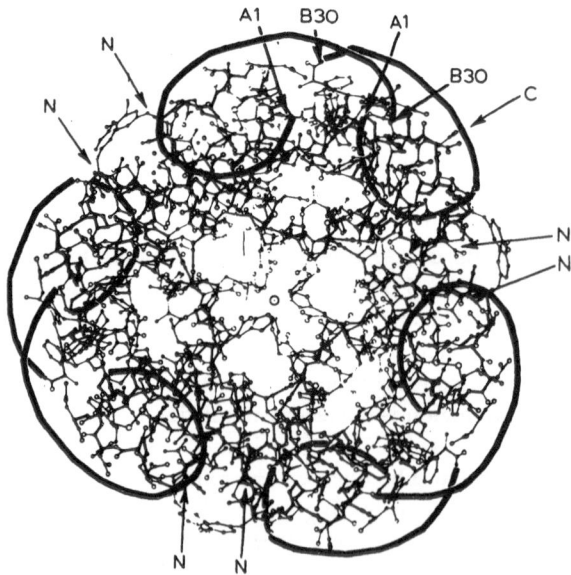

Figure 11. Diagrammatic representation of the accommodation of the proinsulin connecting peptide over the surface of the two-zinc insulin hexamer (reproduced from Blundell *et al.*, 1972).

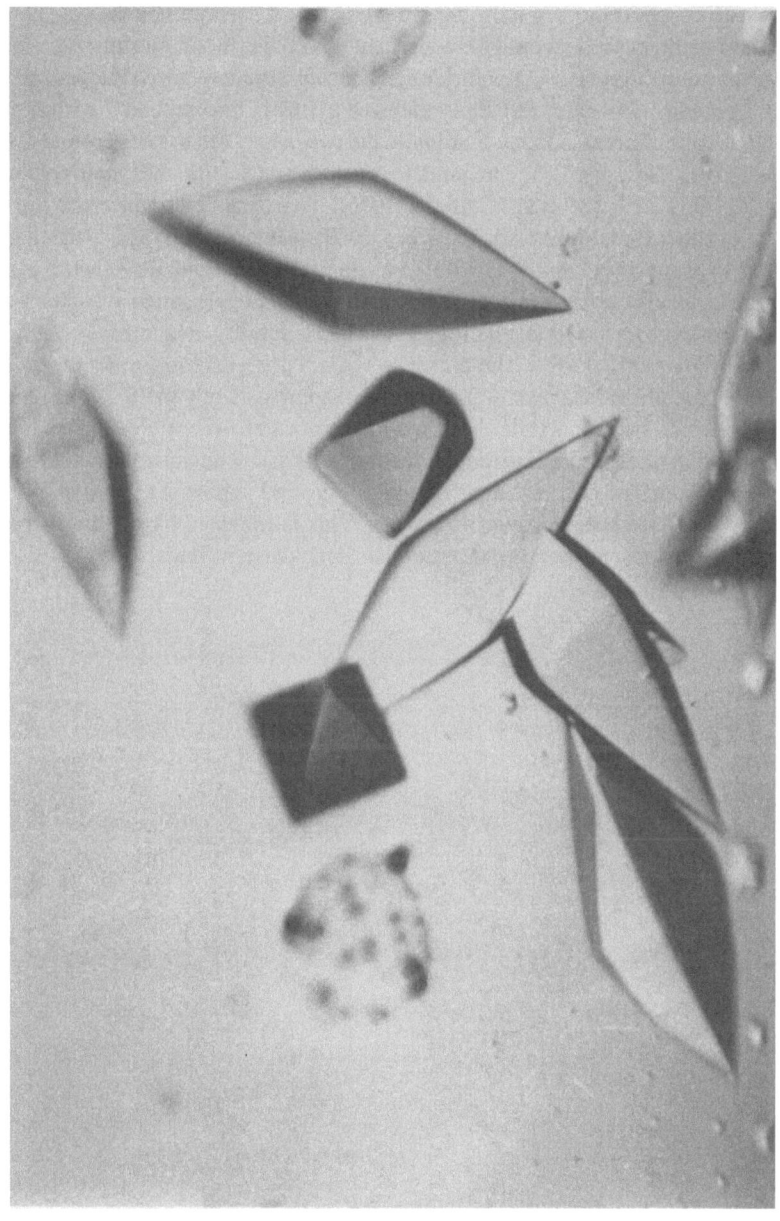

Figure 12. Crystals of the tetragonal form of proinsulin grown at acid pH (Wood, S. P., Pitts, J. E., Godley, G., Blundell, T. L., and Chance, R., unpublished results).

(Steiner *et al.*, 1972). The high zinc concentrations within the granules would allow the formation of hexamers and higher aggregates which then precipitate within the storage compartment. The type of zinc insulin hexamer present is open to conjecture as the pH and metal ion concentrations within the granules are not accurately known. The *in vitro* studies on insulin crystals would be consistent with the two-zinc insulin hexamer form in the absence of high (1.2 M) chloride ion concentrations required for four-zinc insulin crystal growth. However, the likely elevated pH from 6 to around 7 within the granules could result in increased zinc binding to the two-zinc form to sites around B13 Glu (Wood, 1976). Zinc at pH 7 can bind to sites on the insulin hexamer surface around B30, B1, B5, A17, and B21 (Cutfield, 1975). Two-zinc insulin hexamers also bind a variety of other metal ions (Adams *et al.*, 1969). More recently Ca^{2+} has been shown to bind to a site involving A17 Glu, A4 Glu, B29 Lys, and B30 carboxylate crosslinking three insulin hexamers together (Fig. 13). This aggregation of hexamers by calcium is most probably responsible for the reduced solubility at neutral pH leading to precipitation (Pitts *et al.*, 1980). The presence of Ca^{2+} may help to form and stabilize a crystal lattice at pH values distant from optimal: approximately pH 6.3 for human and porcine two-zinc insulin crystals. This may have occurred in species that exhibit crystal habits within their storage granules (Lange, 1973). The insulins which are known to be monomeric, for example, guinea pig and casiragua, cannot form hexamers and precipitate in a nonordered fashion. This is reflected by the absence of any crystalline inclusions in the storage granules from these rodents.

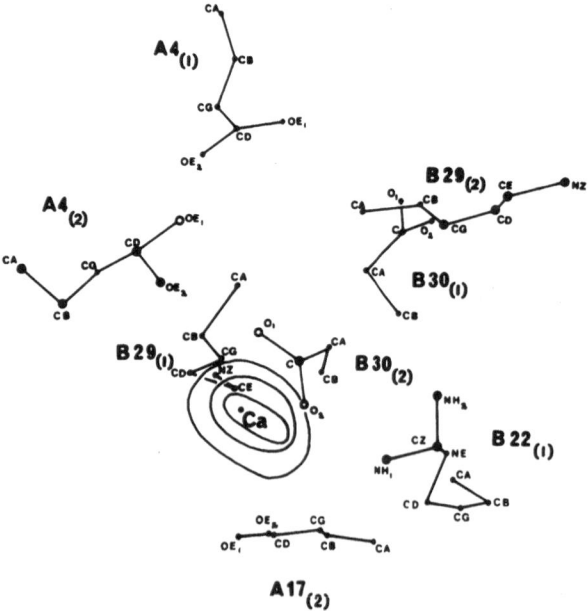

Figure 13. Schematic diagram of the calcium-binding site of porcine insulin (reproduced from Pitts *et al.*, 1980).

Mature insulin granules may contain crystalline inclusions which have regular repeats and sharp edges. Electron micrographs of rat granules show distinct cross-sections of square, diamond, and hexagonal shapes (Greider *et al.*, 1969; Watari, 1970). Similarly in the grass snake, regular structure is observed which may be cubic and show a 90- Å repeat. The polymorphic forms of rat I and II insulin give rise to different crystal forms in vitro (Wood *et al.*, 1978; Fig. 1). Both give zinc insulin hexamers, rat I forms rhombohedral (R3) crystals (Fig. 14), while rat II crystals are regular octahedra (P4$_2$32). Model building of the rat II form in Fig. 15 shows how

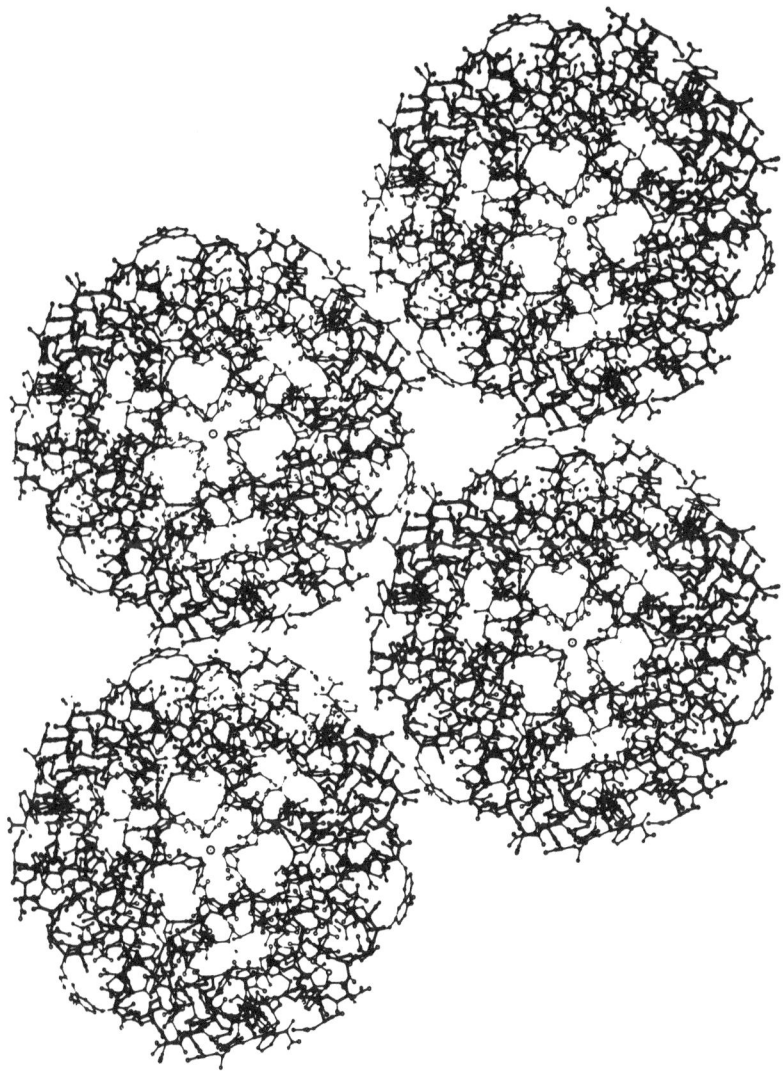

Figure 14.   Likely arrangement of hexamers when viewed down the crystallographic threefold axis of the R3 crystal form of rat I insulin (reproduced from Blundell *et al.*, 1972).

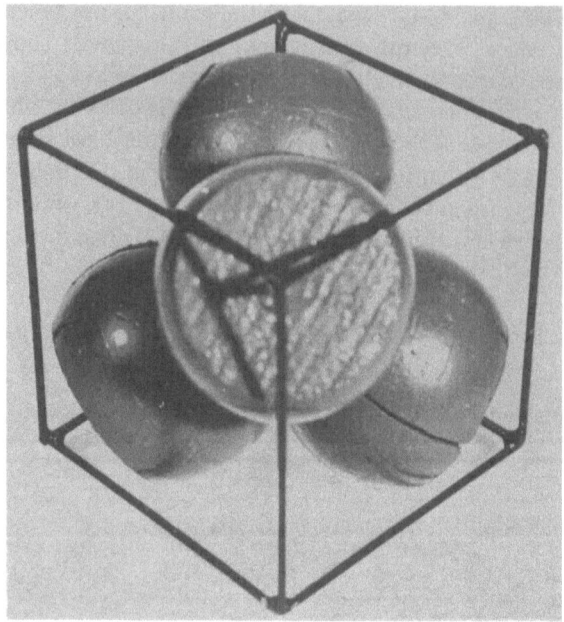

Figure 15.   Proposed packing model for rat II insulin hexamers in the space group P4$_2$32 (reproduced from Pitts *et al.*, 1980).

four-insulin hexamers could form the basic unit cell of the crystal (Wood *et al.*, 1978; Pitts *et al.*, 1980). The observation of hexagonal edges with 50-Å repeats could be explained by the rat I (R3) crystal form, while the other views with square and diamond shapes are consistent with the rat II (P4$_2$32) form.

Electron microscopy has shown that grass snake granules contain crystalline inclusions with cubic symmetry and repeats of 74 Å (Lange, 1971; Watari, 1974), close to the values found for the dimeric form I2$_1$3 grown in the laboratory with $a = 79$Å. Model building using insulin hexamers in P2$_1$3 with $a = 67$Å provides an arrangement which would also give rise to a 90-Å repeat (Pitts *et al.*, 1980). Figure 16 shows this arrangement of hexamers which would provide a stable storage form. Purified grass snake insulin has not been studied but a related snake insulin and a fish insulin give rhombic dodecahedral crystals of similar appearance to those seen in the grass snake storage granules (Cao *et al.*, 1980; Yunev *et al.*, 1976). Thus the properties of insulin exploited in an x-ray crystallography laboratory (aggregation and crystallization) may be fortuitous byproducts of the requirement for biological storage.

VI. EVOLUTIONARY DIFFERENCES IN INSULIN

A. Evolution of the Insulin Cell

The movement of the B cell from the alimentary canal into the islets during evolution has been followed in a review by Van Noorden and Falkmer (1980). Insulin, which belongs to the group of gastroenteropancreatic hormones, has been shown by immunochemistry and radioimmunological assay to have counterparts in lower vertebrates. These hormonelike materials, related to insulin, were found in many invertebrate species of both the protostomian and deuterostomian lines; for example, in the alimentary tract of molluscs (Plisetskaya *et al.*, 1978). In the next stage the cyclostomes, which include hagfish, have undergone a relocation of the B cells from the gut to a primitive islet organ. The holocephalan and elasmobranchian cartilaginous fish from the final links that result in a distinct pancreatic organ emptying via the common exit with the bile duct into the gut cavity.

Immunoreactive evidence for insulinlike material in the central nervous system has also been observed. Insulinlike activity in the blowfly has its origins in the median neurosecretory cells (Duve *et al.*, 1979). A molecule capable of decreasing hemolymph trehalose from the corpus cardiacum/corpus allatum of the hookworm also has a neurosecretory cell origin (Tager *et al.*, 1976). Insulinlike protein levels in rat brain extracts have been found to be higher than those found in the plasma (Havrankova *et al.*, 1978; Rosenzweig *et al.*, 1980). Comparison of the properties of this molecule and those of pancreatic insulin in response to radioimmunoassay, bioassay and radioreceptor assay suggest that the former material is genuine insulin or a very similar polypeptide and not a proinsulin or insulinlike growth factor. Studies on the genetically obese (ob/ob) diabetic mouse, which has elevated circulating insulin levels and reduced receptor numbers on fat, liver, and other tissues, have shown the levels of insulin and insulin receptors in the brain are unaltered compared to those found in normal

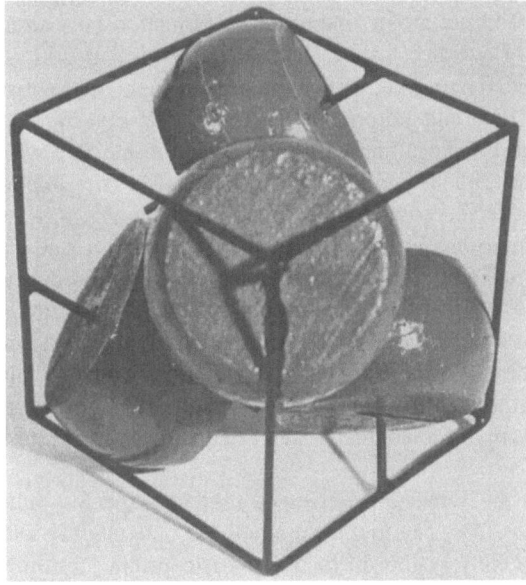

Figure 16. Proposed packing model for snake insulin hexamers in the space group $P2_13$ (reproduced from Pitts *et al.*, 1980).

mice (Havrankova *et al.*, 1978). Streptozotocin treatment of rats to make them hypoinsulinemic and diabetic indicates that insulin synthesis can occur locally in the brain and other nonpancreatic tissues, which makes the role of insulin in neurotransmission an interesting possibility. These results have been disputed by Eng and Yalow (1980), however further research is required to establish the possible synthesis of insulin in the mammalian central nervous system. An alternative explanation for the elevated levels of insulin could be the concentration of insulin bound to brain receptor sites after diffusion across the blood–brain barrier.

The wide distribution of insulin cells may be explained by a common origin for the embryonic neuroectoderm of nerve cells and insulin-producing cells in the programmed neuroendocrine cells of the ectoblast (Pearse, 1968). The replacement of a diffuse regulatory mechanism of the neuronal system may have been superceded by the concentration of endocrine cells in a specialized pancreatic organ. Insulin and insulinlike growth factors may have evolved from duplication of ancestral genes, possibly coding for neurotransmitters, which mutated through natural selection to produce a collection of homologous insulin molecules; insulinlike growth factors (IGF), and relaxin.

B. Variations in Insulin Sequences

The insulin sequences from many species (Table 2) have generally conserved residues required to form the insulin fold. The hydrophobic core and disulfide bridges of the monomer are invariant. The variation in residues occurs at various locations and the capacity to aggregate to dimers and hexamers has been retained with the exception of the hystricomorphs. High variation can be seen at the A8–A10 region and at B29–B30; these residues are not important in zinc hexamer formation but can alter both crystal form and solubility. This effect can be seen in the bovine insulin with the hexamer contacts involved at A10 being Val while porcine insulin has an Ile residue resulting in an altered crystal packing and morphology (Wood, 1976; Fig. 1). The change of B30 Ala in porcine insulin to Thr in human insulin does not interfere with crystal growth and both crystal forms are identical in appearance (Fig. 1). These changes in mammals have little effect on the receptor binding of the insulin.

One of the polymorphic forms shown by the rat contains a unique Pro at B9 for rat I insulin. The biological activities of both rat I and II are similar but rat I shows a very different zinc dependent change in the near ultraviolet circular dichroism (Wood *et al.*, 1978). The proline at B9 decreases the association constant for the production of zinc hexamers, although hexamers do form with sufficient zinc addition. The packing of the rat insulins in the different crystal forms shows that a change which appears to be selectively neutral in terms of biological activity may affect a different function, that of storage.

Table 2 shows the nonrandom changes found in species of fish. The region A8–A10 greatly varies from that in the mammals but only slightly within the group of fish as a whole. The conservation of histidine–basic–proline residues within the fish contrasts with the smaller, nonbasic, and occasionally hydrophobic A8–A10 region of the mammals. Differences are found in the A12–A15, A17 and B0, B1–B3 amino acids with an extra B31 residue in the hagfish. The variable residues form a surface which is in contact with a similar area during the formation of zinc hexamers from dimers. The loss of B10 His replaced with Asp in the jawless hagfish, together with the changes in the dimer/dimer interface, prevents zinc hexamer formation. Hagfish insulin produces only crystals containing dimers and the storage form must be quite different from mammalian species (Cutfield et al., 1974, 1979). The hagfish appears to not have the severe storage restraints and the complex enzyme-resistant storage form developed in higher animals. However cod insulin does form zinc insulin hexamers in the laboratory (Baker and Dodson, 1970) but the packing results in different molecular contacts producing an orthorhombic form. The altered nature of the crystal packing may have effects on granulation at the biological storage location.

The avian insulins show only a small number of changes. The turkey insulin has an altered A8–A10 region in common with duck insulin as well as changes at B1–B2 and B27. Turkey and chicken insulin have the same sequence and both can form zinc-insulin hexamers in crystals and in solution (Weitzel et al., 1969; Pitts, 1980; Cao et al., 1980). An interesting property of turkey insulin is its high receptor-binding affinity resulting in the only naturally occurring superpotent insulin known (Simon et al., 1974, 1977). The threefold increase in biological activity of turkey compared to bovine insulin has been proposed to be due to the substitution of A8 His (Pullen et al., 1976) and this has been confirmed by altering the human sequence with this residue and producing an A8 His human insulin analogue which is also superpotent (Marki et al., 1979).

Although hystricomorphs are mammals belonging to the suborder Rodentia, they have been grouped into a separate class because of their high rate of amino acid substitution and the considerable variation they exhibit in their primary structure. Early experiments by Moloney and Coval (1955) showed that the guinea pig produced high titers of antibodies when challenged with bovine insulin and this can be seen to be reflected by the large number of differences in the two insulins (Table 2). Both coypu and guinea pig insulins have replaced His at B10 with Gln and Asn, respectively. Changes in the residues B1, B3, B4, B14, B17, B20, A13, and A14 and loss of B10 His in coypu and guinea pig interferes with hexamerization. Chinchilla insulin with a B4 Lys may destabilize the two-zinc hexamers as indicated by the failure to crystallize in the usual form and instead produce four-zinc hexamers (Wood, 1976). The residue changes found in guinea pig and coypu make the surface more hydrophilic which makes the molecule more thermodynamically stable in the monomeric form in an aqueous environment. No crystalline inclusions have yet been reported for these two nondimerizing hystricomorph insulins in the B cell granule (Lange, 1973). The change of B22 Arg to Asp in guinea pig results in an ion pair repulsion with the B chain carboxy terminus which would disturb the insulin fold. This effect can be reversed by lowering the pH which results in a far ultraviolet circular dichroism spectrum similar to that of bovine insulin (Wood, 1976). Thus it appears that all insulins can achieve the insulin fold to a lesser or greater degree and this will depend on the other functional constraints placed upon the insulin molecule.

C. Proinsulin, Insulinlike Growth Factor, and Relaxin

Figure 17 shows a schematic diagram of the probable conformation of proinsulin and is based on immunological and spectroscopic data (see Section IV). The variation in connecting peptide sequences (Table 4) suggests that no one conformation has been con-

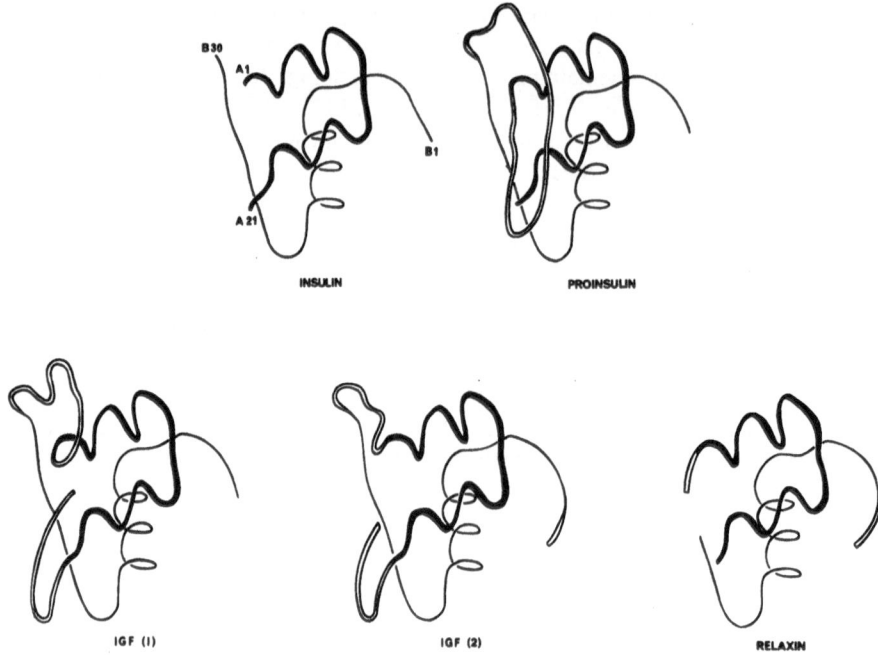

Figure 17. Schematic diagrams showing the three-dimensional structure of the insulin monomer based on the x-ray analysis of rhombohedral porcine two-zinc insulin crystals and proposed conformations based on model building for proinsulin, porcine relaxin, and insulinlike growth factors I and II (reproduced from Blundell and Humbel, 1980).

served between species for the bridging sequence during evolution. The connecting chain probably runs over the face of the molecule near the surface buried during dimer formation.

The incomplete removal of insulinlike activity in human serum using insulin antisera led to the characterization of two insulinlike growth factors: IGF I and II (Froesch *et al.*, 1976). The primary sequences are shown in Table 5 and these can be seen to have more structural similarity to proinsulin than to insulin (Rinderknecht and Humbel, 1978a,b). IGF I and II are single polypeptides with three intrachain disulfide bridges, the regions in common being limited to the A and B chain parts of proinsulin. The connecting peptide is shorter than the 35 amino acids found in human proinsulin, being only 12 residues for IGF I and 8 residues for IGF II. IGF I and II also have carboxy-terminal extensions of eight and six amino acids, respectively, this configuration does not occur in proinsulin. The similarity of proinsulin and IGF suggests a common ancestor with the divergence occurring before the appearance of the vertebrates. IGF I and II probably diverged at the appearance of the first mammals.

Model-building studies based on the insulin fold have been reported on IGF I and II (Fig. 18; Blundell *et al.*, 1978; Bedarkar, 1982). The residues Gly 7 (B8), 19 (B20), and 22 (B23) and the disulfide bridges allow the backbone of IGF I to form the insulin fold. Hydrophobic groups required to make the core of the globular structure are present; Leu 5 (B6), Leu 10 (B11), Val 11 (B12), Ala 13 (B14), Leu 14 (B15), Val 17

(B18), Phe 23 (B24), Ile 43 (A2), Val 44 (A3), Leu 57 (A16), and Tyr 60 (A19). The remaining residues occur on the surface and are mostly hydrophilic (Fig. 18). Residues 25–29 of IGF can be located in a similar position to the equivalent B26–B30 region of insulin. The connecting peptide sequence can be placed over the surface of the IGF containing two β-turns at 28–34 which results in the hydrophilic residues at 33–37 pointing into the solvent. The region 63–70 probably folds back onto the molecule bringing the carboxy-terminus into the region of Arg 21 (B22). A similar conformation for IGF II has also been produced and thus both IGF molecules appear to be able to mimic to some degree the insulin fold. The models suggested that IGF II with its shorter connecting peptide and its closer similarity to insulin may have a higher affinity for the insulin receptor than either proinsulin or IGF I and this has been confirmed experimentally (Zapf et al., 1978; Piron et al., 1980).

Relaxin, a polypeptide hormone from the corpus luteum which produces dilation of symphysis pubis prior to parturition, has also undergone model building (Bedarkar et al., 1977; Isaacs et al., 1978). Relaxin has an A and B chain linked by disulfide bridges but there is little sequence homology (Table 5). However model building shows that porcine relaxin may form a backbone conformation similar to insulin which lacks residues equivalent to A21 and the B chain C terminal end of insulin (Fig. 19). This would tend to destabilize the insulin fold but would still allow its formation. The hydrophobic core of relaxin contains close-packed side-chains but these differ in type from those involved in insulin. Further model building studies of sand tiger shark relaxin indicate a possible insulinlike structure with a sequence very different from that of porcine relaxin (Gowan et al., 1981). A comparative circular dichroism study by Schwabe and Harmon (1978) of insulin and relaxin shows that both molecules have essentially similar features, supporting the model-building studies.

The tertiary fold of insulin and relaxin may be similar (Fig. 17) but the residues on the surface are very different. Thus relaxin does not cross-react with insulin antibodies or appear to have any insulinlike activity. This raises the question of whether relaxin and insulin had a common ancestry and the resulting divergent evolution has left only approximately 20% sequence homology between the two structures. Blundell and Humbel (1980) have suggested that if there are only a few stable structures for small proteins then structural restrictions to retain secondary elements will be strongly conserved, that is, the capacity to fold in a certain way. Conformationally Gly is very versatile and allows bends to occur in the main polypeptide chain; thus the glycines at B8 and B20 are very important for correct folding. Similarly, disulfide bridge formation acts as a rigid constraint in maintaining the globular structure while changes in other residues, including core side-chains, may be explored. Whether an ancestral molecule diverged or the different hormones converged to the same stable tertiary structure is unclear, but only molecules with hormonal function have been shown to attain the insulin fold, which perhaps lends support to a divergent route.

VII. INSULIN RECEPTOR BINDING AND POTENCY

A. The Active Site of Insulin

The receptor-binding region of insulin was first proposed on the basis of the activity and receptor binding of different species of insulins and of chemically modified ana-

Table 5. Comparison of the Amino Acid Sequences of Insulin, Insulinlike Growth Factor, and Relaxin

A-chain

	-2	-1	1	2	3	4	5	6	7	8	9	10	11	12	13	14	15	16	17	18	19	20	21	22	23	24	25	26	27	28	29	30
Bovine insulin	—	—	Gly	Ile	Val	Glu	Gln	Cys	Cys	Ala	Ser	Val	Cys	Ser	Leu	Tyr	Gln	Leu	Glu	Asn	Tyr	Cys	Asn	—	—	—	—	—	—	—	—	—
IGF I	—	—	Gly	Ile	Val	Asp	Glu	Cys	Cys	Phe	Arg	Ser	Cys	Asp	Leu	Arg	Arg	Leu	Glu	Met	Tyr	Cys	Ala	Pro	Leu	Lys	Pro	Ala	Lys	Ser	Ala	—
IGF II	—	—	Gly	Ile	Val	Glu	Glu	Cys	Cys	Phe	Arg	Ser	Cys	Asp	Leu	Ala	Leu	Leu	Glu	Thr	Tyr	Cys	Ala	Thr	—	—	Pro	Ala	Lys	Ser	Glu	—
Porcine relaxin	Arg	Met	Thr	Leu	Ser	Glu	Lys	Cys	Cys	Glu	Val	Gly	Cys	Ile	Arg	Lys	Asp	Ile	Ala	Arg	Leu	Cys	—	—	—	—	—	—	—	—	—	—

B-chain

	-2	-1	1	2	3	4	5	6	7	8	9	10	11	12	13	14	15	16	17	18	19	20	21	22	23	24	25	26	27	28	29	30	31
Bovine insulin	—	—	Phe	Val	Asn	Gln	His	Leu	Cys	Gly	Ser	His	Leu	Val	Glu	Ala	Leu	Tyr	Leu	Val	Cys	Gly	Glu	Arg	Gly	Phe	Phe	Tyr	Thr	Pro	Lys	Ala	—
IGF I	—	—	—	Gly	Pro	Glu	Thr	Leu	Cys	Gly	Ala	Glu	Leu	Val	Asp	Ala	Leu	Gln	Phe	Val	Cys	Gly	Asp	Arg	Gly	Phe	Tyr	Phe	Asn	Lys	Pro	Thr	—
IGF II	Ala	Tyr	Arg	Pro	Ser	Glu	Thr	Leu	Cys	Gly	Gly	Glu	Leu	Val	Asp	Thr	Leu	Gln	Phe	Val	Cys	Gly	Asp	Arg	Gly	Phe	Tyr	Phe	Ser	Arg	Pro	Ala	—
Porcine relaxin	Ser	Thr	Asn	Asp	Phe	· Ile	Lys	Ala	Cys	Gly	Arg	Glu	Leu	Val	Arg	Leu	Trp	Val	Glu	Ile	Cys	Gly	Ser	Val	Trp								

C-chain

	1	2	3	4	5	6	7	8	9	10	11	12	13	14	15	16	17	18	19	20	21	22	23	24	25	26	27	28	29	30	31	32	33	34	35
Bovine	Arg	Arg	Glu	Val	Glu	Gly	Pro	Gln	Val	Gly	Ala	Leu	Glu	Leu	Ala	Gly	Gly	Pro	Gly	Ala	Gly	Gly	Leu	Glu	Gly	Pro	Pro	Gln	Lys	Arg	—	—	—	—	—
IGF I	—	—	—	—	—	—	—	—	—	—	—	—	Gly	Tyr	Gly	Ser	Ser	Ser	Arg	Arg	Ala	Pro	Gln	Thr	—	—	—	—	—	—	—	—	—	—	—
IGF II	—	—	—	—	—	—	—	—	—	—	—	—	Ser	Arg	Val	Ser	Arg	Arg	Ser	Arg	—	—	—	—	—	—	—	—	—	—	—	—	—	—	—

aDashes indicate the absence of an amino acid.

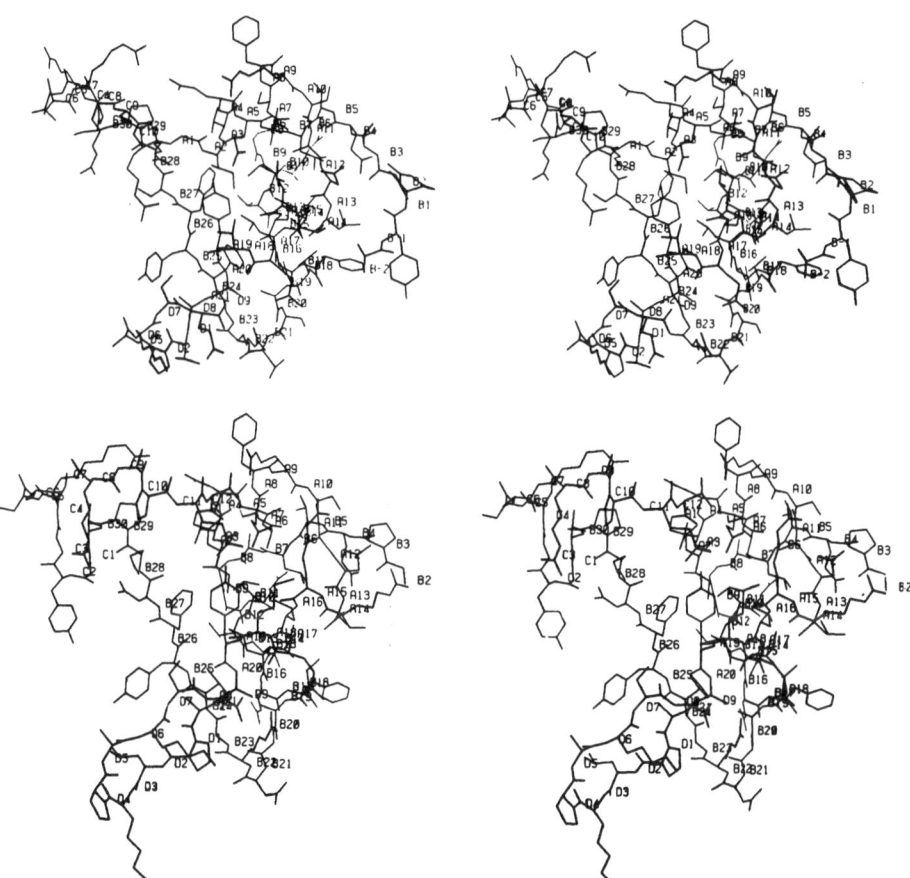

Figure 18. Stereo view of the proposed three-dimensional structure of IGF I (above) and II (below) (reproduced from Blundell *et al.*, 1978; Bedarkar *et al.*, 1981).

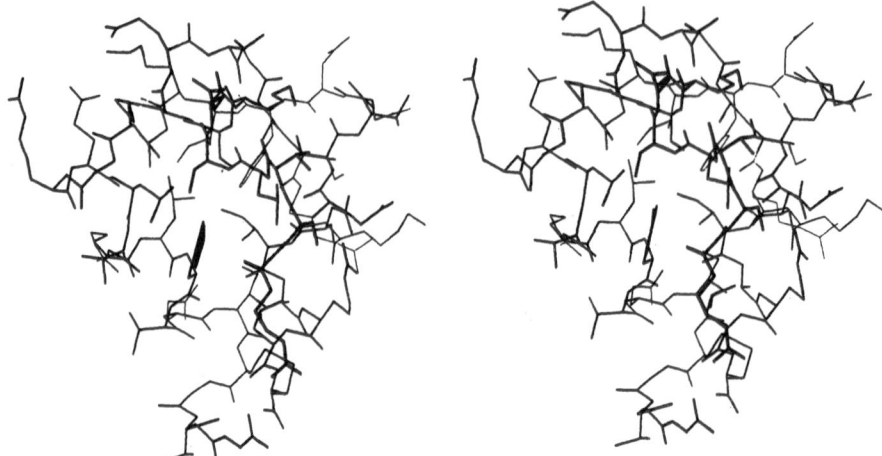

Figure 19.   Stereo view of the proposed three-dimensional structure of relaxin (reproduced from Bedarkar *et al.,* 1977).

logues (Blundell *et al.,* 1971, 1972). A large invariant surface region involved in dimerization was suggested to be involved in receptor-binding interactions (Fig. 20). Analysis of the thermodynamics of the interactions suggest that receptor binding involves largely hydrophobic interactions (Waelbroeck *et al.,* 1979; Waelbroeck, 1980). Heat capacity estimations suggest that the exclusion of solvent from a surface larger

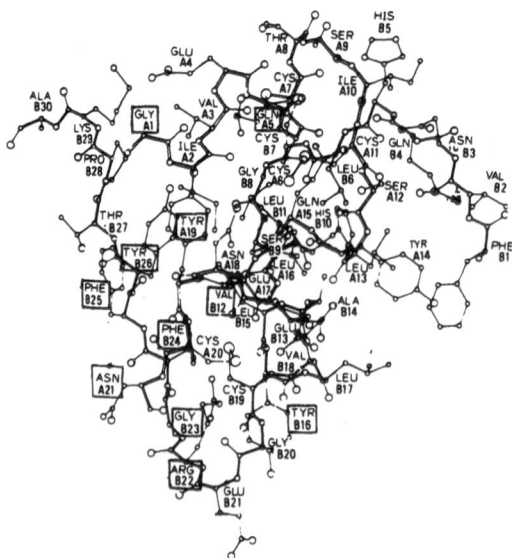

Figure 20.   The residues of the proposed receptor-binding region of insulin are indicated by a box enclosing the residue type and number (reproduced from Pullen *et al.,* 1976).

than that involved in dimerization occurs during the receptor-binding process. The change in pH optimum upon binding was used in the thermodynamic studies to help identify two ionizable groups; an α amino group (possibly A1 Gly) and an unprotonated carboxyl group. The active site consists of a central hydrophobic region (A19 Tyr, B12 Val, B16 Tyr, B24 Phe, B25 Phe, B26 Tyr) and polar side groups (A1 Gly, A4 Glu, A5 Gln, A21 Asn, B13 Glu, B21 Glu, B22 Arg) and on the periphery B9 Ser, B10 His, and B27 Thr (Fig. 21). Residue A8 His has been included to show that this large sidechain residue, which is found in the superpotent turkey insulin, is similarly located near the active site (Pitts, 1979).

The studies on chemically modified insulins have focused on residues which fall in the proposed receptor binding region. Changes to A1 Gly which modify the net charge and alter the conformation produce a loss of biological activity (Pullen *et al.*, 1976; Friesen *et al.*, 1977; Rosen *et al.*, 1979; 1980a, b). Increasing the size, while maintaining the charge of the A0 substituent, has little effect on the loss of receptor affinity. A discrepancy occurs when the A chain is extended by one to three basic amino acids (Rosen *et al.*, 1980a). The lipogenic potency in fat cells was 40% but the

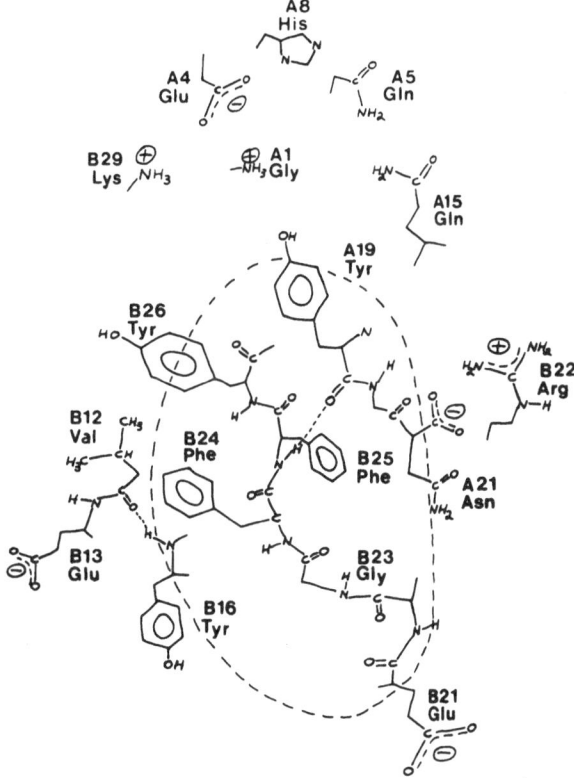

Figure 21. Diagrammatic representation of the amino acids on the insulin molecular surface which are probably involved in receptor binding. The A8 histidine found in superpotent avian insulins has been included to show the localization of this residue near the active area (modified from Blundell, 1979).

binding affinities to beef liver membranes ranged between 80 (A-1 Lys to A0 Arg) and 125% (A0 Arg_3-insulin). The long flexible extension containing three Arg residues of the latter may allow interaction with a receptor side-chain normally not accessible to native insulin. Although A1 Gly is not directly involved in dimer formation, analogues of this type, which have a reduced capacity to aggregate, also exhibit a reduced receptor-binding capacity. The A1 to B29 diamino suberic acid cross-linked insulin has been shown to dimerize in a similar fashion to native insulin but exhibits a lower biological and receptor-binding activity on fat cells of 5% (Dodson et al., 1980b). This apparent conflict may be a result of this more rigid cross-linked function interacting with the receptor. The requirement of the receptor-binding model proposed is that any reduction of dimerization will occur concurrently with a reduced receptor affinity but the reverse effect does not necessarily pertain. However restriction of conformational change upon receptor binding, as suggested by Dodson et al. (1980b), may explain the inhibition of biological activity by the A1 to B29 cross-link.

The other major region studied extensively which falls in the active site is B22–B27. Changes are seen in this region in the low-activity hystricomorph insulins from casiragua, guinea pig, and porcupine (Wood et al., 1975; Horuk et al., 1980a, b, c). Casiragua insulin has alterations at B25 Tyr and B26 Arg which would place a positive group in a usually hydrophobic and noncharge region and would interfere strongly with receptor interactions (Horuk, 1980; Horuk et al., 1980c; Blundell and Horuk, 1981). The effect of the B22 Arg to Asp change in guinea pig and porcupine insulin destabilizes the insulin fold and results in reduced dimerization and biolgocial potency (Wood, 1976; Horuk et al., 1980a).

Enzymatic cleavage has allowed removal and partial replacement of the end of the insulin B chain. Des octapeptide (des B23–30; Goldman and Carpenter, 1974; Canova-Davis and Carpenter, 1980), des heptapeptide (des B24–B30; Lu Zixian and Yu Ronghua, 1980) des hexapeptide (des B25–B30; Peking Insulin Research Group, 1973) and des pentapeptide (Gattner, 1975; Peking Insulin Structure Research Group, 1976a) have been reported and have shown that the B29–B30 region is dispensable but further stepwise removal of B26, B25, and B24 results in an increased loss of biological activity. A mutant human insulin with either a B24 or B25 Phe to Leu substitution has been reported by Tager et al. (1979). Synthesis of both B24 and B25 Leu insulins gave 10 and 1% activities, respectively, using iodoinsulin competition to human lymphocytes and rat adipocytes (Tager et al., 1980). The reported antagonistic activity for B24 Leu, when mixed with native insulin, was not reproducible in the laboratory of Diaconescu et al. (1982). The low receptor binding of B25 Leu which does not have large conformational changes implies an important role for B25 Phe in the binding process. Replacement of B24 and B25 with Ala results in large conformational alterations and results in the B24 analogue being less active.

Most insulin analogues studied exhibit both a single receptor-binding and biological response of equal magnitude suggesting that the active area of insulin contains the information for both the recognition and switching-on process. A few analogues have shown a variation in binding potency and biological response including hagfish, des alanine des asparagine, porcupine, and A0 Arg_3 insulin (Emdin et al., 1977; Pitts, 1980; Horuk et al., 1980a; Rosen et al., 1980a). The residues important in dimer formation and binding are confined to the same surface and it has been proposed that a dimer could bind to the receptor. This is unlikely because insulins that cannot form dimers are still able to produce a biological response. This has been reported for tetranitro-, casiragua, porcupine, and guinea pig insulins (Boesel and Carpenter, 1972; Wood, 1976; Horuk *et al.*, 1979, 1980a; Zimmerman *et al.*, 1972) which are full agonists with lower binding to receptors. Changes in the active site (Fig. 21) either of conformation or the type of side-chain will lead to reduced receptor affinity but may leave a full agonist activity intact. Similarly, gross conformational changes away from the porcine insulin structure which distort this area will result in reduced activity.

The proposal that the insulin receptor consists of an $(\alpha/\beta)_2$ complex linked by disulfide bridges in a manner not unlike an antibody has been made by Czech *et al.* (1981). The α receptor subunit with bound insulin has been shown to be more sensitive to tryptic digestion than the unoccupied receptor which is consistent with a conformational change of the receptor structure upon hormone binding (Pilch and Czech, 1980). The model for the receptor-binding process requires a complementary fit with close hydrophobic packing, charge interactions, and hydrogen bond formation. Some flexibility in the insulin molecule may be required for binding and may be reflected in the slight conformational differences seen in different crystal forms. The capacity of antireceptor antibodies to produce the insulin response makes the critical role of a covalently modified or degraded insulin unlikely (Kahn *et al.*, 1978).

B. The Active Site of Insulinlike Growth Factor

The model-building studies of IGF I and II indicate a surface region similar to the insulin active site which is both hydrophobic and accessible. This area on IGF II is less covered than IGF I and suggests that the former would have a higher insulin receptor affinity and in adipocytes this was found to be the case (Zapf *et al.*, 1978; Piron *et al.*, 1980). The binding of the insulinlike growth factors to the insulin receptor does not explain their growth-promoting effects which are 300 times that of insulin. The existence of specific receptors for IGF has been shown by the blockage with antireceptor antibodies for the insulin receptor (King *et al.*, 1980). Expansion of the insulin model for receptor binding involving an area complementary to both the insulin dimerizing surface and the A chain extensions may be important during growth factor receptor binding. King and Kahn (1981) have studied many insulins for receptor-binding, insulin activity, and growth-promoting capacity. Potent growth factors were found in the hystricomorph group although they have lower insulinlike potencies. This ability of the hystricomorph receptor to accommodate a greatly altered insulin may indicate that this receptor is involved mainly in mitogenic effects (Horuk *et al.*, 1980b, c; Lazarus *et al.*, 1980).

C. The Negative Cooperative Site of Insulin

The curvilinear Scatchard plots found for insulin receptor binding can be interpreted as either consisting of a mixed population of high- and low-affinity state receptors or as a negative cooperative interaction between a single class of receptor molecule (De Meyts *et al.*, 1976). The loss of affinity of receptor sites with the binding to other receptors due to an accelerated disoociation rate has been shown experimentally. De Meyts *et al.* (1978) have identified a region of the insulin molecule by using a kinetic assay for negative cooperativity which may trigger the site–site interactions between receptors. The change of B25 Phe to Leu results in a loss of the negative cooperativity (Keefer *et al.*, 1981a; Jonczyk *et al.*, 1981; Olefsky *et al.*, 1981). Removal of the end of the B chain in des octapeptide insulin or the A21 Asn, B30 Ala of insulin similarly abolishes this effect. The biological activity was also greatly reduced, which required that the concentrations of the noncooperative analogues be raised to compensate and ensure that the receptor pool was maintained under saturating conditions. A subsite involving these residues within the active site of insulin involving the hydrophobic central region B23–B26 and A21 was proposed as being important in the negative cooperative effect (De Meyts *et al.*, 1978). The observed cooperativity becomes reduced as the hormone concentration and dimer numbers increase, while in monomeric insulin, such as guinea pig, this effect has not been seen. The insulin protomer contains two aggregation sites; one is involved in dimerization which falls within the receptor-binding area, the other is involved in hexamer formation. The hexamer surface may possibly have a role in a "back-to-back" interaction when bound to the receptor, perhaps implicating the nonstandard dimer in negative cooperativity.

Similarly, insulinlike growth factors also have slightly reduced cooperativity at elevated concentrations (Piron *et al.*, 1980). The casiragua insulin and insulinlike growth factors have altered primary structures in the proposed cooperative site residues. The B25 and B26 residues suggested to be important for this phenomenon are Tyr and Arg in casiragua and Tyr and Phe in the insulinlike growth factor. Both these hormones exhibit negative cooperativity and indicate that aromatic residues in this part of the B chain promote this activity.

The loss of negative cooperativity observed in des alanine des asparagine insulin allows the accurate estimation of receptor numbers due to the linearity of the Scatchard plots. This effect may be useful in the studies of diabetes where reduced receptor numbers of poor binding capacities are suspected. Mapping of the topology of the receptor complex has been attempted using covalently linked insulin molecules (Piron *et al.*, 1980). These studies suggest the receptor complex consists of at least a tetramer and this is supported by the work of Kahn (1979). Using naturally occuring antibodies to the insulin receptor found in certain insulin-resistant diabetic patients, Kahn *et al.* (1978) found that the bivalent antibody bound to the receptor, blocked insulin binding, and mimicked insulin action. However, the monovalent antibody fragments, although they bind and block insulin binding, do not have any insulinlike activity. This could be overcome by crosslinking the monovalent antibody with a second antibody. The physiological significance of negative cooperativity may be as a role in desensitizing receptors when excess insulin is present although it is still not clear. However, the study of this effect has led to a greater insight into the mode of insulin/receptor interactions.

VIII. IMMUNOGENICITY AND THREE-DIMENSIONAL STRUCTURE

A. Antigenicity to Clinical Preparations

The first immunological problem with insulin treatment was that reported by Williams (1922) in response to impure porcine insulin and probably was due to noninsulin contaminants. Berson and Yalow (1957; 1959a, b) using radioactive-iodine-labeled insulin showed that the insulin could be dissociated from the antibody and the variable affinity suggested a heterogeneous antibody population. The production of these insulin-binding antibodies appear to result in few problems clinically and it has been even suggested that they may act in a buffering capacity producing a storage compartment in the plasma (Dixon *et al.*, 1975). However stable control relies greatly on correct B-cell function, although a change in regime from a high dose of beef insulin to a lower dose of pork insulin when a patient has antibodies with a higher affinity for the bovine material can cause clinical problems (Berson and Yalow, 1966; Devlin *et al.*, 1967). Many of the problems associated with antibody reactions to insulin preparations have been reduced with the advent of the monocomponent insulins (Schlichtkrull *et al.*, 1972; Yue and Turtle, 1975). The use of these preparations although desirable (Alberti and Nattrass, 1978) may still result in antigenic reaction as even insulin prepared from a particular species may produce antibodies when injected into that species (Lockwood and Prout, 1965; Deckert and Grundahl, 1970). A similar result with an impure preparation of human insulin has been reported (Deckert *et al.*, 1972). This suggests that the production process has rendered the insulin antigenic.

The likely natural storage form of insulin in the B cell of zinc–insulin hexamers undergoes rapid dissociation to dimers and monomers when released into the blood stream (Blundell *et al.*, 1971, 1972). Dimers of human, bovine, and porcine insulin predominate at concentrations over 10^{-7} mol/liter and thus injected insulin should completely dissolve in the blood where the insulin concentration is approximately three orders of magnitude lower. In the circulation the insulin is mainly monomeric and no insoluble or polymerized material should be left after injection. Long-term storage of highly purified insulin does result in nondissociable higher-molecular-weight material which becomes greater with elevation of temperature. The physical form of the administered insulin may have an influence on immunological response. Insulin is administered as a solution or as a suspension of crystals, the latter may be in the zinc–hexamer form or complexed with, for example, protamine. Upon injection, a high local concentration of insulin at 37°C results and this is likely to cause polymerization. This may last for extended periods with the crystalline preparations. The production of large amounts of insulin aggregates has even blocked the cannulae of infusion devices (Albisser *et al.*, 1980). The presence of insulin in aggregated forms, instead of the monomeric form, is likely to be antigenic and result in antibody production. The use of mixtures of beef and pork insulin has been shown to result in mice developing antibodies to porcine insulin when normally there are insufficient carrier determinants to this insulin (Keck, 1977). This suggests that it may be very important not to give porcine and bovine insulin mixtures to patients.

The use of species variants therapeutically has shown that resistance to bovine insulin may not result in a similar resistance to porcine insulin (Kurtz *et al.*, 1979). Resistance to porcine insulin can be lowered by using des alanine (B30) porcine insulin (Kumar, 1979); human insulin usually has a Thr at this position. The use of fish insulins has been suggested for resistant patients (Yalow and Berson, 1964) but this may introduce more problems than it solves. The clinical trials on human insulin produced by biotechnology may show that this new source of material avoids many of the problems associated with using species variants in the treatment of diabetics.

B. Antigenicity and the Conformation of Insulin

The immunological problems associated with the clinical treatment of diabetics related to insulin-binding antibodies can be divided into (1) variation of the primary structure of insulin, (2) altered conformation and spatial arrangement of antigenic determinants, (3) a combination of altered primary and tertiary structure, and (4) production of a new array of antigenic determinants, for example, cross-linking. The highly purified insulin preparations of insulin remove the problems associated with noninsulin contaminants and therefore only insulin binding antibodies will be discussed here.

The clinically useful insulins are bovine, porcine, and human. The variation in primary sequence invovles the changes of A8 Ala and A10 Val in bovine insulin to A8 Thr and A10 Ile in porcine and human insulin. Human insulin also has B30 Thr while the porcine and bovine materials have a B30 Ala. These alterations do not appear to alter the biological activity or the tertiary structure and suggest that, superficially, antibodies raised against bovine and porcine insulin in humans may contain some antibodies that recognize side-chain differences and not tertiary changes. However the problem is more complex because the form in which the insulin is given can have an effect on the hormone conformation. The tertiary structure of the free insulin monomer in solution can undergo conformational alteration within the different crystal forms. The long-lasting preparations may contain either two-zinc or four-zinc hexamers in the R3 microcrystals (Figs. 22 and 23). The change in the conformation of molecule I in the four-zinc hexamer with the induction of an extension of the α-helix along the B1–B6 regions which forms a part of the hexamer surface may cause antibody production di-

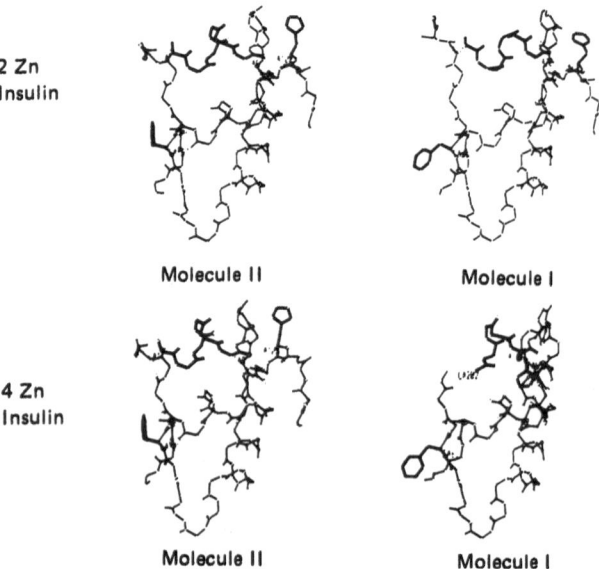

Figure 22.   The major conformational differences between molecules I and II in the two-zinc and four-zinc forms of porcine insulin (reproduced from Dodson *et al.*, 1980a).

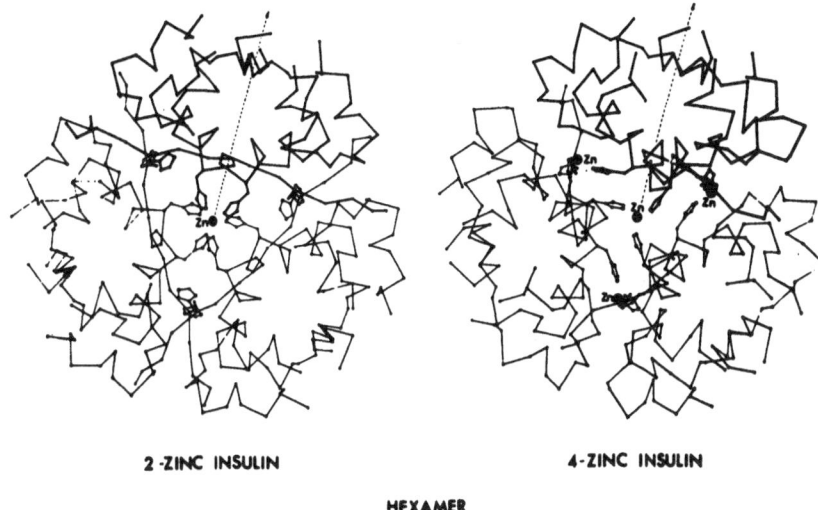

2 -ZINC INSULIN   4-ZINC INSULIN

HEXAMER

Figure 23.   Backbone structure of two-zinc and four-zinc insulin hexamers (reproduced from Bentley *et al.*, 1976).

rected to this part of the B chain. This idea is supported by the work of Arquilla *et al.* (1980) which indicated that a mixed antibody pool reacted differently to zinc insulin and nickel insulin. Nickel insulin cannot undergo the "two-zinc to four-zinc" transition and remains in the two-nickel form and therefore some of the antibodies probably bind to the altered conformation of the B-chain determinants (De Graaff *et al.*, 1981). An alternative possibility is that nickel may bind to the surface in a different manner to zinc and alter the antigenic properties of this material. Similarly the effect of protamine on the insulin conformation is unknown and the length of time these crystals are present may allow antibody production against conformational differences not normally found naturally. The soluble forms of insulin given clinically have varying amounts of polymer but these oligomers would be more flexible than the more stable and rigid hexameric form and less likely to induce large amounts of antibody. However aggregated forms of porcine insulin (ultralente), once they have induced insulin antibodies in human subjects and broken the tolerance, would then allow injections of neutral solutions of soluble insulin to act as a booster to the initial response (Brunfeldt and Deckert, 1964; Deckert and Grundahl, 1970).

Antibodies generated against insulin and proinsulin have given an insight into the tertiary relationships of the antigenic determinants of insulin. The work of Yagi *et al.* (1965) and Corcos and Ovary (1965) demonstrated that the majority of antigenic determinants on insulin were disrupted when pure A or B chain was reacted against insulin antiserum or when insulin was challenged with antisera to A or B chain. This suggests that the relative positions of the antigenic determinants on the insulin molecule require the A and B chains to be in a precise three-dimensional relationship. Arquilla *et al.* (1969, 1972, 1976, 1980) investigated this using enzymatically and chemically

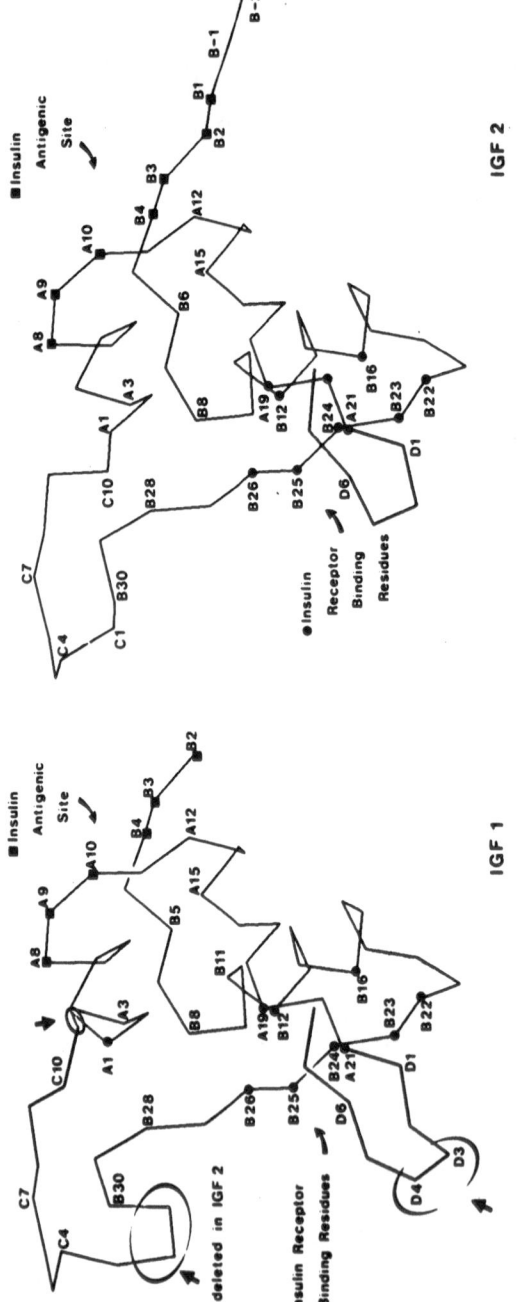

Figure 24. The tertiary fold of IGF I and II as predicted by model building. The numbering follows that for porcine insulin for the A and B chains with only carbons shown. The connecting peptide residues are prefixed with a C and the extension of the A chain with D (reproduced from Blundell and Wood, 1982).

modified forms of bovine insulin. The studies indicated that residues A1 Gly and B29 Lys would lie in close proximity and also that the aromatic residues of the A and B carboxyl terminals together would form a center rich in aromatic amino acids. They also noted a correlation of the loss of biological activity with a decrease in the intactness of the antigenic determinants which similarly correlated with a loss of the insulinlike fold by circular dichroism. The x-ray analysis confirmed these proposed tertiary relationships (Blundell *et al.*, 1972). Similarly the interference of the connecting peptide of proinsulin to antibodies that bind specifically surface residues of the A chain led to the proposal that this peptide chain lies in opposition to this solvent surface of the insulin molecule (Blundell *et al.*, 1972; Steiner *et al.*, 1974). This awaits confirmation by x-ray analysis.

The models proposed for IGF I and II based on model building using the insulin fold explain the lack of cross reactivity with antibodies raised against insulin (Blundell and Humbel, 1980). The immunogenic region of insulin seems to be different to the receptor-binding area and the former consists of the A8–A10 loop and residues B1–B10 (Blundell *et al.*, 1972; Walter *et al.*, 1979). Figure 24 indicates the altered

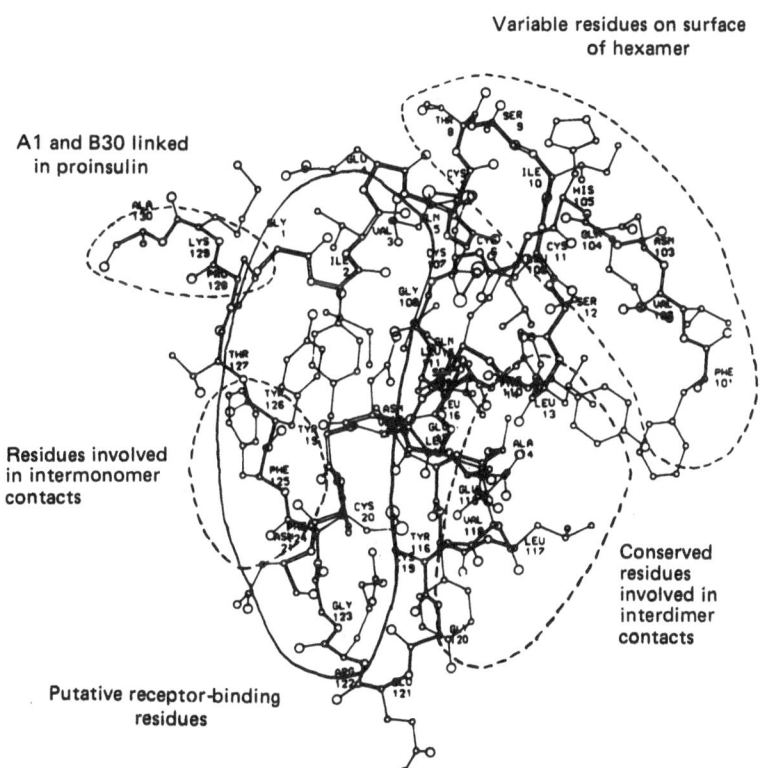

Figure 25. View of the insulin monomer indicating how the surface may be described in terms of various areas involved in activation from the prohormone, variable residues involved in antibody binding, binding to the receptor, and self-association (reproduced from Blundell and Wood, 1975).

conformation of this region in the insulinlike growth factors. Similarly for relaxin and insulin, although they share an insulinlike fold, the surfaces of the two molecules are very different and thus it is not surprising that no cross-reactivity has been seen with insulin antibodies nor has relaxin any binding to insulin receptors (Piron et al., 1980; Schwabe et al., 1978). The recognition of antigenic determinants is not directed to the overall insulin fold or the region required for biological activity as indicated by the studies on the insulinlike growth factors and relaxin. However the tertiary structure is a requirement for the presentation of the antigenic determinants in space in a manner which can easily be recognized by the antibody.

The understanding of the functional regions of insulin has been summarized in Figure 25. The B30 residue and the highly variable region with around the A8–A10 loop and B1–B10 form the important centers for immunological problems in clinical treatment using bovine and porcine insulins. The putative receptor-binding area lies close to the interface buried during dimer formation and contains the A21 Asn and the carboxyl end of the B chain proposed to be involved in the phenomenon of negative cooperativity. The conserved region which allows dimer/dimer contacts to form hexamers has importance in both biological storage and the production of the long-lasting preparations used clinically. The differentiation of the surface of the insulin molecule into the varied functions required the evolution of the stable globular structure of the insulin molecule which forms the basis for the molecular biology of the hormone.

REFERENCES

Adams, M. J., Blundell, T. L., Dodson, E. J., Dodson, G. G., Vijayan, M., Baker, E. N., Harding, M. M., Hodgkin, D. C., Rimmer, B. and Sheat, S., 1969, Structure of rhombohedreal 2-zinc insulin crystals, *Nature* **224**:491–495.

Alberti, K. G. M. M., and Nattrass, M., 1978, Highly purified insulins, *Diabetologia* **15**:77–80.

Albisser, A. M., Lougheed, W., Perlman, K., and Bahoric, A., 1980, Nonaggregating insulin solutions for longterm glucose control in experimental and human diabetes, *Diabetes* **28**:241–243.

Arquilla, E. R., Bromer, W. W., and Mercola, D., 1969, Immunology, conformation and biological activity of insulin, *Diabetes* **18**:193–205.

Arquilla, E. R., Miles, P. V., and Morris, J. W., 1972, Immunochemistry of insulin, in: *Handbook of Physiology* D. F. Steiner, and N. Freinkel, eds. vol. 1, pp. 159–173, Waverley Press, Baltimore.

Arquilla, E. R., Dorio, R. J., and Brugman, T. M., 1976, Structural studies of insulin and insulin derivatives using various immunologic indicators and antibody populations, *Diabetes* **25**:397–403.

Arquilla, E. R., Thiene, P ., Brugman, T. M., Ruess, W., and Sugiyama, R., 1978, Effects of zinc ion on the conformation of antigenic determinants on insulin, *Biochem. J.* **175**:289–297.

Arquilla, E. R., Kelso, J. M., Tamai, I. Y., and Roth, M. D., 1980, The induction of hyperglycaemia with insulin antibodies to B chain determinants in: *Insulin. Chemistry, Structure and Function of Insulin and Related Hormones* (D. Brandenburg, and A. Wollmer, eds.), pp. 593–601, Walter de Gruyter and Co., Berlin.

Baker, E. N., and Dodson, G., 1970, X-ray diffraction data on some crystalline varieties of insulin, *J. Mol. Biol.* **54**:605–609.

Bedarkar, S., 1982, Conformation and molecular biology of insulin and related growth factors. Ph.D. Thesis, University of London.

Bedarkar, S., Turnell, W. G., Blundell, T. L., and Schwabe, C., 1977, Relaxin has conformational homology with insulin, *Nature* **270**:449–451.

Bell, G. I., Swain, W. P., Pictet, R. L., Cordell, B., Goodman, H. M., and Rutter, W., 1979, Nucleotide sequence of a cDNA clone encoding human preproinsulin, *Nature* **282**:525–527.

Bell, G. I., Pictet, R. L., Rutter, W. J., Cordell, B., Tischer, E., and Goodman, H. M., 1980, Sequence of the human insulin gene, *Nature* **284**:26–32.

Bentley, G. A., Dodson, E. J., Dodson, G. G., Hodgkin, D. C., and Mercola, D. A., 1976, Structure of insulin in 4-Zn insulin, *Nature* **261**:166–168.

Berson, S. A., and Yalow, R. S., 1957, Studies with insulin-binding antibody, *Diabetes* **6**:402–405.

Berson, S. A., and Yalow, R. S., 1959a, Quantitative aspects of the reaction between insulin and insulin-binding antibody, *J. Clin. Invest.* **38**:1996–2016.

Berson, S. A., and Yalow, R. S., 1959b, Species-specificity of human anti-beef, pork insulin serum, *J. Clin. Invest.* **38**:2017–2025.

Berson, S. A., and Yalow, R. S., 1966, Insulin in blood and insulin antibodies, *Am. J. Med.* **40**:666–690.

Beychok, S., 1966, Circular dichroism of biological macromolecules, *Science* **154**:1288–1299.

Bloom, S. R., West, A. M., Polak, J. M., Barnes, A. J., and Adrian, T. E., 1978, Hormonal contaminants of insulin, in: *Gut Hormones* (S. R. Bloom, ed.), pp. 318–322, Churchill Livingstone, London.

Blundell, T. L., 1979, Conformation and molecular biology of polypeptide hormones. 1. Insulin, insulin-like growth factors and relaxin, *Trends Biochem. Sci.* **4**:51–53.

Blundell, T. L., and Horuk, R., 1981, A monomeric insulin from the casiragua: Model building using computer graphics, *Hoppe Seylers Z. Physiol. Chem.* **362**:727–737.

Blundell, T. L., and Humbel, R. E., 1980, Hormone families: Pancreatic hormones and homologous growth factors, *Nature* **287**:781–787.

Blundell, T. L., and Johnson, L. N., 1976, *Protein Crystallography*, Academic Press, London.

Blundell, T. L., and Wood, S. P., 1982, The conformation, flexibility and dynamics of polypeptide hormones. *Annu. Rev. Biochem.* **51**:123–154.

Blundell, T. L., Cutfield, J. F., Cutfield, S. M., Dodson, E. J., Dodson, G. G., Hodgkin, D. C., Mercola, D. A., and Vijayan, M., 1971, Atomic positions in rhombohedral 2-zinc insulin crystals *Nature* **231**:506–511.

Blundell, T. L., Dodson, G. G., Hodgkin, D., and Mercola, D., 1972, Insulin: The structure in the crystal and its reflection in chemistry and biology, *Adv. Protein Chem.* **26**:279–402.

Blundell, T. L., Bedarkar, S., Rinderknecht, E., and Humbel, R. E., 1978, Insulin-like growth factor: A model for tertiary structure accounting for immunoreactivity and receptor binding, *Proc. Natl. Acad. Sci. USA* **75**:180–184.

Boesel, A. W., and Carpenter, F. H., 1972, Preparation and properties of tetranitro (nitrotyrosine) insulin (bovine) *Fed. Proc. Fed. Am. Soc. Exp. Biol.* **31**:255–258.

Bradbury, J. H., and Brown, L. R., 1977, Nuclear magnetic resonance spectroscopic studies of the amino groups of insulin, *Eur. J. Biochem.* **76**:573–582.

Brandenburg, D., Lei Kejian, Wang Zhizhen, Dong Bei, Ru Binggen, and Zhu Shangquan, 1980, Preparations and properties of crystalline porcine and bovine (Trp) B1 insulin, *Sci. Sin.* **13**:1443–1452.

Brill, A. S., and Venable, J. H. Jr., 1967, electron paramagnetic resonance spectroscopy of protein single crystals. I. Experimental methods, in: *Proceedings of the 2nd Internatinal Conference of Magnetic Resonance in Biological Systems"* (A. Ehrenberg, B. Malmström, and T. Vänngard, eds.), Pergamon Press, Oxford, pp. 365–372.

Brunfeldt, K., and Deckert, T., 1964, Antibodies in the pig against pig insulin, *Acta Endocrinol.* **47**:366–367.

Canova-Davis, E., and Carpenter, F. H., 1980, Specific activation of the arginine carboxyl group of the B chain of bovine des-octapeptide-(B23-30)-insulin, in: *Insulin. Chemistry, Structure and Function of Insulin and Related Hormones* (D. Brandenburg, and A. Wollmer, eds.), pp. 107–115, Walter de Gruyter and Co., Berlin.

Cao, Q. P., Li, T., Peng, X., and Zhang, Y. S., 1980, Insulins from different species—chicken and snake. *Sci. Sin.* **23**:1309–1315.

Cao, Q. P., Cin, D. F., and Zhang, Y. S., 1981, Enzymatic synthesis of des-hexapeptide insulin, *Nature* **292**:774–775.

Chan, S. J., Keim, P., and Steiner, D. F., 1976, Cell-free synthesis of rat preproinsulins; characterization and partial amino acid sequence determination, *Proc. Natl. Acad. Sci. USA* **73**:1964–1968.

Corcos, J., and Ovary, A., 1965, Biological properties of guinea pig anti-insulin antibodies, *Proc. Soc. Exp. Biol. Med.* **119**:142–148.

Cutfield, S., 1975, X-ray studies of insulin. D. Phil Thesis, Oxford University.

Cutfield, J. F., Cutfield, S. M., Dodson, E. J., Dodson, G. G., and Sabesan, M. N., 1974, Low resolution crystal structure of hagfish insulin, *J. Mol. Biol.* **87**:23–30.

Cutfield, J. F., Cutfield, S. M., Dodson, E. J., Dodson, G. G., Emdin, S. F., and Reynolds, C. D., 1979, Structure and biological activity of hagfish insulin, *J. Mol. Biol.* **132**:85–100.

Czech, M P., Massague, J., and Pilch, P. F., 1981, The insulin receptor: Structural features. *Trends Biochem. Sci.* **8**:222–225.

Deckert, T., and Grundahl, E., 1970, The antigenicity of pig insulin, *Diabetologia* **6**:15–20.

Deckert T., Andersen, O. O., Grundahl, E., and Kerp, L., 1972, Iso-immunization of man by recrystallized human insulin, *Diabetologia* **8**:358–361.

De Graaff, R. A. G., Lewit-Bentley, A., and Tolley, S. P., 1981, Effects of destabilizing agents on the insulin hexamer structure, in: *Structural Studies on Molecules of Biological Interest* (G. Dodson, J. P. Glusker, and D. Sayre, eds.), pp. 547–556, Clarendon Press, Oxford.

De Meyts, P., Bianco, A. R., and Roth, J., 1976, Site–site interactions among insulin receptors. Characterization of the negative co-operativity, *J. Biol. Chem.* **251**:1877–1888.

De Meyts, P., Van Obberghen, E., Roth, J., Wollmer, A., and Brandenburg, D., 1978, Mapping of the residues responsible for the negative co-operativity of the receptor binding region of insulin, *Nature* **273**:504–509.

De Meyts, P., Halban, P., and Hepp, K. D., 1981, *In vitro* studies on biosynthetic human insulin: An overview, *Diabetes Care* **4**:144–146.

Devlin, J. G., Brien, T., and Stephenson, N., 1967, Relation between antibody and insulin dose, *Br. Med. J.* **I**:542–544.

Diaconescu, C., Saunders, D., Gattner, H. G., and Brandenburg, D., 1982, (Leu^{B24}) and(Leu^{B25}) insulins are not antagonists of lipogenesis in adipocytes, *Hoppe Seylers Z. Physiol. Chem.* **363(2)**:187–192.

Dixon, K., Exon, P. D., and Malins, J. M., 1975, Insulin antibodies and the control of diabetes, *Q. J. Med.* **44**:543–553.

Dockerill, S., 1978, Structure and function studies with insulin and glucagon, D. Phil Thesis, University of Sussex, U.K.

Dodson, E. J., Dodson, G. G., Hodgkin, D. C., and Reynolds, C. D., 1979, Structural relationships in the 2-zinc insulin hexamer, *Can. J. Biochem.* **57**:469–479.

Dodson, E. J., Dodson, G. G., Reynolds, C. D., and Vallely, D. C., 1980a, A comparison between the insulin molecules in 2- and 4-zinc insulin crystals, in: *Insulin. Chemistry, Structure and Function of Insulin and Related Hormones* (D. Brandenburg, and A. Wollmer, eds.), pp. 9–16,, Walter de Gruyter and Co., Berlin.

Dodson, G. G., Cutfield, S., Hoenjet, E., Wollmer, A., and Brandenburg, D., 1980b, Crystal structure, aggregation and biological potency of beef insulin cross-linked at A1 and B29 by diamino suberic acid, in: *Insulin. Chemistry, Structure and Function of Insulin and Related Hormones* (D. Brandenburg, and A. Wollmer, eds.), pp. 17–26, Walter de Gruyter and Co., Berlin.

Duve, H., Thorpe, A., and Lazarus, N., 1979, Isolation of material displaying insulin-like immunological and biological activity from the brain of the blowfly "Calliphora Vomitoria," *Biochem. J.* **184**:221–227.

Emdin, S. O., and Falkmer, S., 1980, On the molecular biology of hagfish insulin, in : *Insulin. Chemistry, Structure and Function of Insulin and Related Hormones* (D. Brandenburg, and A. Wollmer, eds.), pp. 683–691, Walter de Gruyter and Co., Berlin.

Emdin, S. O., Gammeltoft, S., and Gliemann, J., 1977, Degradation, receptor binding affinity and potency of insulin from the Atlantic hagfish (myxine glutinosa) determined in isolated rat fat cells, *J. Biol. Chem.* **252**:602–608.

Eng, J., and Yalow, R. S., 1980, Insulin recoverable from tissues, *Diabetes* **29**:105–109.

Ettinger, M. J., and Timasheff, S. N., 1971, Optical activity of insulin. I. On the nature of the circular dichroism bands, *Biochemistry* **10**:824–830.

Evans, J. C., Morgan, P. H., Mahbouba, M., and Smith, H. J., 1979, An electron paramagnetic resonance study of native and modified freeze-dried cupric insulin hexamer, *J. Inorg. Biochem.* **11**:129–137.

Frank, B. H., Veros, A. J., and Pekar, A. H., 1972a, Physical studies on proinsulin. A comparison of the titration behaviour of the tyrosine residues in insulin and proinsulin, *Biochemistry* **11**:4926–4931.

Frank, B. H., Pekar, A. H., and Veros, A. J., 1972b, Insulin and proinsulin conformation in solution, *Diabetes* **21**:486–491.

Friesen, H. J., Brandenburg, D., Diaconescu, C., Gattner, H.-G., Naithani, V. K., Nowak, J., Zahn, H., Dockerill, S., Wood, S. P., and Blundell, T. L., 1977, Structure-function relationships of insulin modified in the A1-region, in: *Proceedings, 5th American Peptide Symposium* (M. Goodman and J. Meienhofer, eds.), pp. 136–140. John Wiley, New York.

Froesch, E. R., Burgi, H., Muller, W. A., Humbel, R. E., Jakob, A., and Labhart, A., 1976, Nonsuppressible insulinlike activity of human serum: Purification, physicochemical and biological properties and its relations to total serum ILA, *Rec. Prog. Horm. Res.* **23**:565–616.

Fullerton, W. W., Potter, R., and Low, R. W., 1970, Proinsulin: Crystallization and preliminary x-ray diffraction studies, *Proc. Natl. Acad. Sci. USA* **66**:1213–1219.

Gammeltoft, S., 1981, Receptor binding of biosynthetic human insulin on isolated pig hepatocytes, *Diabetes Care* **4**:235–237.

Gattner, H. G., 1976, Darstellung-und Eigenschaften von despentapeptide (B26–B30)—Rinderinsulin. *Hoppe Seylers Z. Physiol. Chem.* **356**:1397–1404.

Goldman, J., and Carpenter, F. H., 1974, Zinc binding, circular dichroism and equilibrium sedimentation studies on insulin (bovine) and several of its derivatives, *Biochemistry* **13**:4566–4574.

Gowan, L., Reinig, J. W., Schwabe, C., Bedarkar, S., and Blundell, T. L., 1981, On the primary and tertiary structure of relaxin from the sand tiger shark, *FEBS Letts* **129**:80–82.

Grant, P. T., Coombs, T. L., and Frank, B. H., 1972, Differences in the nature of the interaction of insulin and proinsulin with zinc, *Biochem. J.* **126**:433–440.

Greider, M. H., Howell, S. L., and Lacy, P. E., 1969, Isolation and properties of secretory granules from rat islets of Langerhans, *J. Cell. Biol.* **41**:162–166.

Harding, M. M., Crowfoot Hodgkin, D., Kennedy, A. F., O'Connor, A., and Weitzmann, P. D. J., 1966, The crystal structure of insulin II. An investigation of rhombohedral zinc insulin crystals and a report of other crystalline forms, *J. Mol. Biol.* **16**:212–216.

Havrankova, J., Schmechel, D., Roth, J., and Brownstein, M., 1978, Identification of insulin in rat brain, *Proc. Natl. Acad. Sci. USA* **75**:5737–5741.

Horuk, R., 1980, A biophysical approach to the investigation of the properties of insulin and its receptor. D. Phil Thesis, Birkbeck College, University of London.

Horuk, R., Goodwin, P., O'Connor, K., Neville, R. W. J., Lazarus, N. R., and Stone, D., 1979, Evoluationary change in the insulin receptors of hystricomorph rodents, *Nature* **279**:439–440.

Horuk, R., Blundell, T. L., Lazarus, N. R., Neville, R. W. J., Stone, D., and Wollmer, A. 1980a, A monomeric insulin from the porcupine (hystrix cristata) an old world hystricomorph, *Nature* **286**:822–823.

Horuk, R., Wood, S. P., Blundell, T. L., Lazarus, N. R., and Neville, R. N. J., 1980b, The use of hystricomorph insulins in defining the insulin-receptor interactions. *Actual. Chim. Thera.* **7**:15–25.

Horuk, R., Wood, S. P., Blundell, T. L., Lazarus, N. R., Neville, R. W. J., Raper, J. H., and Wollmer, A., 1980c, Structure, self-association and potency of casiragua and guinea pig insulins: evidence that monomeric insulin can bind receptors, in *Hormones and Cell Regulation* (J. Dumont and J. Nunez, eds.), vol 4, pp. 123–139, Elsevier/North-Holland Biomedical Press, Amsterdam.

Isaacs, N., James, R., and Niall, H., 1978, Relaxin and its structural relationship to insulin, *Nature* **271**:278–281.

Jonczyk, A., Keefer, L. M., Naithani, V. K., Gattner, H. G., De Meyts, P., and Zahn, H., 1981, Preparation and biological properties of (Leu^{B24}, Leu ^{B25}) human insulin, *Hoppe Seylers Z. Physiol. Chem.* **362**:557–561.

Kahn, C. R., 1979, What is the molecular basis of the action of insulin? *Trends in Biochem.* **11**:N263–N265.

Kahn, C. R., Baird, K. L., Jarrett, D. B., and Flier, J. S., 1978, Direct demonstration that receptor crosslinking or aggregation is important in insulin action, *Proc. Natl. Acad. Sci. USA* **75**:4209–4213.

Keck, K., 1977, Ir gene control of carrier recognition: III Cooperative recognition of two or more carrier determinants on insulin of different species, *Eur. J. Immunol.* **7**:811–816.

Keefer, L. M., Piron, M. A., De Meyts, P., Gattner, H.-G., Diaconescu, C., Saunders, D., and Brandenburg, D., 1981a, Impaired negative cooperativity of the semisynthetic analogues human (Leu^{B24}) and (Leu^{B25}) insulins, *Biochem. Biophys. Res. Commun.* **100**:1229–1236.

Keefer, L. M., Piron, M. A., and De Meyts, P., 1981b, Receptor binding properties and biological activity *in vitro* of biosynthetic human insulin, *Diabetes Care* **4**:209–214.

King, G. L., and Kahn, C. R., 1981, Non-parallel evolution of metabolic and growth-promoting functions of insulin, *Nature* **292**:644–646.

King, G. L., Kahn, C. R., Rechler, M. M., and Nissley, P. S., 1980, Direct demonstration of separate receptors for growth and metabolic activities of insulin and MSA (an insulin-like growth factor) using antibodies to the insulin receptor, *J. Clin. Invest.* **66**:130–140.

Kumar, D., 1979, Immunoreactivity of insulin antibodies in insulin-treated diabetics: Significance of the beta-chain carboxy-terminal amino acid (B-30) of insulin, *Diabetes* **28**:994–1000.

Kurtz, A. B., Harrington, M. G., Matthews, J. A., and Nabarro, J. D. N., 1979, Factitious diabetes and antibody mediated resistance to beef insulin, *Diabetologia* **16**:65–67.

Lange, R. H., 1971, Crystalline B-granules: Rhombic dodecahedra (a=7.4nm), *Diabetologia* **7**:465–466.

Lange, R. H., 1973, Histochemistry of the Islets of Langerhans, in *Handbook of Histochemistry*, W. Graumann, and K. Neumann, eds. pp. 1–141, Fischer, Stuttgart.

Lazarus, N. R., O'Connor, K., Neville, R. W. J., Goodwin, P., Horuk, R., and Stone, D., 1980, Hystricomorph insulins and insulin receptors in: *Insulin. Chemistry, Structure and Function of Insulin and Related Hormones* (D. Brandenburg, and A. Wollmer, eds.), pp. 301–306, Walter de Gruyter and Co., Berlin.

Led, J. J., Grant, D. M., Horton, W. J., Sundby, F., and Vilhelmsen, K., 1975, Carbon-13 magnetic resonance study of structural and dynamical features in carbamylated insulins, *J. Am. Chem Soc.* **97**:5997–6007.

Lippert, J. L., Tyminski, D., and Desmeules, P. J., 1976, Determination of the secondary structure of proteins by laser Raman spectroscopy, *J. Amer. Chem. Soc.* **98**:7075–7080.

Lockwood, D. H., and Prout, T. E., 1965, Antigenicity of heterologous and homologous insulin, *Metabolism* **14**:530–538.

Lomedico, P. T., Chan, S. J., Steiner, D. F., and Saunders, G. F., 1977, Immunological and chemical characterization of bovine preproinsulin, *J. Biol. Chem.* **252**:7971–7978.

Lomedico, P. T., Rosenthal, N., Efstratiadis, A., Gilbert, W., Kdodner, R., and Tizard, R., 1979, The structure and evolution of the two nonallelic rat preproinsulin genes, *Cell* **18**:545–558.

Low, B. W., and Berger, J. E., 1961, Insulin-preliminary X-ray studies of citrate crystals, *Acta Cryst.* **14**:82.

Low, B. W., and Chen, C. C. H., 1969, Monoclinic insulin crystals, *J. Mol. Biol.* **43**:227–229.

Lu Zixian and Yu Ronghua, 1980, Preparation and crystallization of des (B-chain C-terminal) heptapeptide insulin. *Sci. Sin.* **13**:1592–1598.

Marki, F., De Gasparo, M., Eisler, K., Kamber, B., Riniker, B., Rittel, W., and Sieber, P., 1979, Synthesis and biological activity of seventeen analogues of human insulin, *Hoppe Seylers Z. Physiol. Chem.* **360**:1619–1632.

Markussen, J., and Schiff, H. E., 1973, Molecular parameters of C-peptide from bovine proinsulin, *Int. J. Pep. Protein Res.* **5**:69–72.

Moloney, P. J., and Coval, M., 1955, Antigenicity of insulin: Diabetes induced by specific antibodies. *Biochem. J.* **59**:179–185.

Olefsky, J. M., Green, A., Ciaraldi, T. P., Saekow, M., Rubenstein, A. H., and Tager, H. S., 1981, Relationship between negative cooperativity and insulin action, *Biochemistry* **20**:4488–4492.

Paselk, R. A., and Levy, D., 1974, Fluorine nuclear magnetic resonance studies of trifluoroacetyl-insulin derivatives. Effects of pH on conformation and aggregation, *Biochemistry* **13**:3340–3345.

Pearse, A. G. E., 1968, Common cytochemical and ultrastructural characteristics of cells producing polypeptide hormones (the APUD series) and their relevance to thyroid and ultimobranchial c cells and calcitonin, *Proc. R. Soc.* **B170**:71–80.

Peking Insulin Structure Research Group, 1973, Studies on the structure–function relationship of insulin. The relationship of the C-terminal peptide sequence of the B chain to the activity of insulin, *Sci. Sin.* **16**:61–70.

Peking Insulin Structure Research Group, 1974, Studies on the insulin crystal sructure: The molecule at 1.8Å resolution, *Sci. Sin.* **17**:752–777.

Peking Insulin Structure Research Group, 1976a, Structural studies on des-pentapeptide (B26-30) Insulin. I. The preparation and properties of des-pentapeptide insulin, *Sci. Sin.* **19**:351–357.

Peking Insulin Structure Research Group, 1976b, Structural studies on des-pentapeptide (B26-30) Insulin. II. Growth of crystals and preliminary crystallographic observations, *Sci. Sin.* **19**:358–361.

Perler, F., Efstratiadis, A., Lomedico, P., Gilbert, W., Kolodner, R., and Dodgson, J., 1980, The evolution of genes: the chicken preproinsulin gene, *Cell* **20**:555–566.

Pilch, P. F., and Czech, M. P., 1980, Hormone binding alters the conformation of the insulin receptor, *Science* **210**:1152–1153.

Piron, M. A., Michiels-Place, M., Waelbroeck, M., De Meyts, P., Schuttler, A., and Brandenburg, D., 1980, Structure–activity relationships of insulin-induced negative cooperativity among receptor sites, in: *Insulin. Chemistry, Structure and Function of Insulin and Related Hormones* (D. Brandenburg, and A. Wollmer, eds.), pp. 371–391, Walter de Gruyter and Co., Berlin.

Pitts, J. E., 1979, Active sites of insulin, in: *Diabetes 1979, Proceedings of the 10th Congress of the International Diabetes Federation,* (W. K. Waldhausl, ed.), pp. 88–91, Excerpta Medica, Amsterdam.

Pitts, J. E., 1980, Structure and function of pancreatic polypeptide hormones, D.Phil Thesis, University of Sussex, U.K.

Pitts, J. E., Wood, S. P., Horuk, R., Bedarkar, S., and Blundell, T. L., 1980, Pancreatic hormone storage granules: The role of metal ions and polypeptide oligomers, in: *Insulin. Chemistry, Structure and Function of Insulin and Related Hormones* (D. Brandenburg, and A. Wollmer, eds.), pp. 673–682, Walter de Gruyter and Co., Berlin.

Plisetskaya, E., Kazakov, V. K., Solbitskaya, L., and Leibson, L. G., 1978, Insulin producing cells in the gut of Freshwater bivalve molluscs, *Anodonta aygrea* and *Unio pictorum,* and the role of insulin in the regulation of their carbohydrate metabolism, *Gen. Comp. Endocrinol.* **35**:133–145.

Pocker, Y., and Biswas, S. B., 1980, Conformational dynamics of insulin in solution. Circular dichroic studies, *Biochemistry* **19**:5043–5049.

Pocker, Y., and Biswas, S. B., 1981, Self-association of insulin and the role of hydrophobic binding: A thermodynamic model of insulin dimerisation, *Biochemistry* **20**:4354–4361.

Pullen, R. A., Jenkins, J. A., Tickle, I. J., Wood, S. P., and Blundell, T. L., 1975, The relation of polypeptide hormone structure and flexibility to receptor binding: The relevance of X-ray studies on insulin, glucagon and human placental lactogen, *Mol. Cell. Biochem.* **8**:5–20.

Pullen, R. A., Lindsay, D. G., Wood, S. P., Tickle, I. J., Blundell, T. L., Wollmer, A., Krail, G., Brandenburg, D., Zahn, H., Gliemann, J., and Gammeltoft, S., 1976, Receptor-binding region of insulin, *Nature* **259**:369–373.

Raskin, P., 1979, Treatment of diabetes mellitus: The future, *Metabolism* **28**:780–796.

Rinderknecht, E., and Humbel, R. E., 1978a, The amino acid sequence of human insulin-like growth factor I and its structural homology with proinsulin, *J. Biol. Chem.* **253**:2769–2775.

Rinderknecht, E., and Humbel, R. E., 1978b, Primary structure of human insulin-like growth factor II, *FEBS Letts.* **89**:283–289.

Rosen, P., Ehrich, B., Junger, E., Bubenzer, H. J., and Kuhn, L., 1979, Binding and degradation of insulin by plasma membranes from bovine liver isolated by a large scale preparation, *Biochem. Biophys. Acta.* **587**:593–605.

Rosen, P., Simon, M., Reinauer, H., Brandenburg, D., Friesen, H. J., and Diaconescu, C., 1980a, A1-modified insulins: receptor binding and biological activity, in: *Insulin. Chemistry, Structure and Function of Insulin and Related Hormones* (D. Brandenburg, and A. Wollmer, eds.), pp. 403–408, Walter de Gruyter and Co., Berlin.

Rosen, P., Simon, M., Reinauer, H., Friesen, H. J., Diaconescu, C., an Brandenburg, D., 1980b, Binding of insulin to bovine liver plasma membrane: Use of insulin analogues modified at A1 residues, *Biochem. J.* **186**:945–951.

Rosenzweig, J. L., Havrankova, J., Lesniak, M. A., Brownstein, M., and Roth, J., 1980, Insulin is ubiquitous in extrapancreatic tissues of rats and humans, *Proc. Natl. Acad. Sci. USA* **77**:572–576.

Sakabe, N., Sakabe, K., and Sasaki, K., 1978, Insulin structure at 1.2Å resolution: Flexibility of local conformation and surrounding water molecules, in: *Proinsulin, Insulin, C-Peptide* (S. Baba, T. Kaneko, and N., Yanaihara, eds.), pp. 73–80, Excerpta Medical, Amsterdam.

Schlichtkrull, J., Brange, J., Christiansen, A. H., Hallund, O., Heding, L. G., and Jorgensen, K. H., 1972, Clinical aspects of insulin-antigenicity, *Diabetes* **21**:649–656.

Schwabe, C., and Harmon, S. J., 1978, A comparative circular dichroism study of relaxin and insulin, *Biochem Biophys. Res. Commun.* **84**:374–380.

Schwabe, C., Steinetz, B., Weiss, G., Segaloff, A., McDonald, K., O'Byrne, E., Hochman, J., Carriere, B., and Goldsmith, L., 1978, Relaxin, *Rec. Prog. Horm. Res.* **34**:123–211.

Simkin, R. D., Cole, S. A., Ozawa, H., Magdoff-Fairchild, B., Eggena, P., Rudko, A., and Low, B. W., 1970, Precipitation and crystallization of insulin in the presence of lysozyme and salmine, *Biochem. Biophys. Acta* **200**:385–394.

Simon, J., Freychet, P., and Rosselin, G., 1974, Chicken insulin—radioimmunological characterization and enhanced activity in rat fat cells and liver plasma membranes, *Endocrinology* **95**:1439–1449.

Simon, J., Freychet, P., Rosselin, G., and De Meyts, P., 1977, Enhanced binding affinity of chicken insulin in rat liver membranes and human lymphocytes: Relationship to the kinetic properties of the hormone-receptor interaction, *Endocrinology* **100**:115–121.

Snell, C. R., and Smyth, D. G., 1975, Proinsulin: A proposed 3-dimensional structure, *J. Biol. Chem.* **250**:6291–6295.

Steiner, D. F., Clark, J. L., Nolan, C., Rubenstein, A. H., Margoliash, E., Atne, B., and Oyer, P. E., 1969, Proinsulin and the biosynthesis of insulin, *Rec. Prog. Horm. Res.* **25**:207–282.

Steiner, D. F., Kemmler, W., Clark, J. L., Oyer, P. E., and Rubenstein, A. H., 1972, The biosynthesis of insulin, in: *Handbook of Physiology* (D. F. Steiner and N. Freinkel, eds.) Section 7, Endocrinology Volume 1, (Waverly Press, Baltimore, pp. 175–198.

Steiner, D., Wolfgang, K., Tager, H. S. and Peterson, J. D. (1974) Proteolytic processing in the biosynthesis of insulin and other proteins. *Fed. Proc.* **33**:2105–2115.

Tager, H. S.,Markese, J., Kramer, K. B., Spiers, R. P., and Childs, C. N., 1976, Glucagon-like and insulin-like hormones of the insect neurosecretory system, *Biochem. J.* **156**:515–520.

Tager, H., Given, B., Baldwin, D., Mako, M., Markese, J., Rubenstein, A., Olefsky, J., Kobayashi, M., Kolterman, O., and Poucher, R., 1979, A structurally abnormal insulin causing human diabetes, *Nature* **281**:122–125.

Tager, H., Thomas, N., Assoian, R., Rubenstein, A., Saekow, M., Olefsly, J., and Kaiser, E. T., 1980, Semisynthesis and biological activity of porcine (Leu B24) insulin and (Leu B25) insulin, *Proc. Natl. Acad. Sci. USA* **77**:3181–3185.

Ullrich, A., Shine, J., Chirgwin, J., Pictet, R., Tischer, E., Rutter, W. J., and Goodman, H. M., 1977, Rat insulin genes: construction of plasmids containing the coding sequences, *Science* **196**:1313–1319.

Van Noorden, S., and Falkmer, S., 1980, Gut-islet endocrinology—some evolutionary aspects. *Invest. Cell. Pathol.* **3**,:21–35.

Vogt, H. -P., Wollmer, A., Naithani, V. K., and Zahn, H., 1976, The conformational potential of porcine proinsulin C-peptide, *Hoppe Seylers Z. Physiol. Chem.* **357**:107–116.

Waelbroeck, M., 1980, Thermodynamic analysis of insulin binding to its membrane receptor. D. Phil Thesis, Université Catholique De Louvain, Belgium.

Waelbroeck, M., Van Obberghen, E., and De Meyts, P., 1979, Thermodynamics of the interaction of insulin with its receptor, *J. Biol. Chem.* **254**:7736–7740.

Waldhausl, W. K., 1969, Treatment of diabetes mellitus: pathophysiological aspects and state of the art, in: *Diabetes* (W. K. Waldhausl, ed.), pp. 10–22, Excerpta Medica, Amsterdam.

Walter, H., Humbel, R. E., and Schwander, J., 1979, Separate determination of the two components of NSILA-S (IGF I and II) by specific radio-immunoassays(RIAS), in: *International Congress Series No. 481; 10th Congress, International Diabetes Federation* (W. Waldhausl and K. G. M. M. Alberte, eds.), p. 248, Abstr. No. 465, Excerpta Medica, Amsterdam.

Watari, N., 1970, The correlative light and electron microscopy of the islets of Langerhans in the pancreas of some vertebrates, with special reference to the synthesis, storage and extrusion of the islet hormones, *Gunma Symp. Endocrinol.* **7**:125–150.

Watari, N., 1974, Three-dimensional structure of crystalline insulin granules in B-cells of pancreatic islets, in: *Proceedings of the 8th International Congress on Electron Microscopy*, Canberra, II, 434–435.

Weitzel, G., Oerlel, W., Rager, K., and Kemmler, W., 1969, Insulin. Vom-Truthuhn (Meleagris galloparo) Turkey insulin. *Hoppe Seylers Z. Physiol. Chem.* **350**:57–62.

Williams, J. R., 1922, A clinical study of the effects of insulin in severe diabetes, *J. Metabol. Res.* **2**:729–751.

Williamson, K. L., and Williams, R. J. P., 1979, Conformational analysis by nuclear magnetic resonance: Insulin, *Biochemistry* **18**:5966–5972.

Wollmer, A., Fleishhauer, J., Strassburger, W., Thiele, H., Brandenburg, D., Dodson, G., and Mercola, D., 1977, Sidechain mobility and the calculation of tyrolsyl circular dichroism of proteins. Implications of a test with insulin and des-B1-phenylalanine insulin, *Biophys. J.* **20**:233–243.

Wood, S. P., 1976, The structure and biology of insulin. D.Phil. thesis, University of Sussex, U. K.

Wood, S. P., Blundell, T. L., Wollmer, A., Lazarus, N. R., and Neville, R. W. J., 1975, The relation of conformation and association of insulin to receptor binding: X-ray and circular dichroism studies on bovine and hystricomorph insulins, *Eur. J. Biochem.* **55:**531–542.

Wood, S. P., Tickle, I. J., Blundell, T. L., Wollmer, A., and Steiner, D. F., 1978, Insulin polymorphism: Some physical and biological properties of rat insulins. *Arch. Biochem. Biophys.* **186:**175–183.

Yagi, Y., Maier, P., and Pressman, D., 1965, Antibodies against component polypeptide chains of bovine insulin, *Science* **147:**617–619.

Yalow, R. S., and Berson, S. A., 1964, Reactions of fish insulins to human insulin antiserum, *N. Engl. J. Med.* **270:**1171–1173.

Yu, N. -T., Liu, C. S., Culver, J., and O'Shea, D. C., 1972a, A preliminary Raman spectroscopic study of native zinc-insulin crystals, *Biochim. Biophys. Acta* **263:**1–6.

Yu, N. -T., Liu, C. S., and O'Shea, D. C., 1972b, Laser Ramam spectroscopy and the conformation of insulin and proinsulin, *J. Mol. Biol.* **70:**117–132.

Yue, D. K., and Turtle, J. R., 1975, Antigenicity of "monocomponent" pork insulin in diabetic subjects, *Diabetes* **24:**625–632.

Yunev, O. A., Dmitrenko, L. V., and Ostrovskii, D. I., 1976, Isolation, purification and crystallization of avian and fish insulins, in: *The Evolution of Pancreatic Islets.* (T. A. I. Grillo, L. G. Leibson and A. Epple, eds.) p. 335, Pergamon Press, Oxford.

Zapf, J., Schoenle, E. and Froesch, E. R. (1978) Insulin-like growth factors I and II: Some biological actions and receptor binding characteristics of two purified constituents of nonsuppressible insulin-like activity of human serum. *Eur. J. Biochem.* **87:**285–296.

Zimmerman, A. E., Kells, D. I. C. and Yip, C. C. (1972) Physical and biological properties of guinea pig insulin. *Biochem. Biophys. Res. Commun.* **46:**2127–2133.

2

Genetic Control of the Immune Response to Insulin in Man and Experimental Animals

Alan S. Rosenthal, Dean Mann, and C. Ronald Kahn

For most patients with juvenile-onset diabetes mellitus and many patients with maturity-onset diabetes mellitus, replacement therapy with insulin is required. Because commerical insulin is obtained by acid–ethanol extraction of animal pancreas, one is not surprised to find that after as little as 2 months many diabetic patients give indication of immunity to insulin. Although most such immune responses are not significant, a certain number of insulin-taking diabetics will present clinically with signs and symptoms of allergy. Obviously the exact form of these allergic reactions will depend on which pathway(s) in the immune system are dominant (Fig. 1). The various types of immune response which have been noted after insulin administration are listed in Table 1. A broad perspective on the basic and clinical aspects of immunity to insulin has been recently published (Keck and Erb, 1981). It is obvious that a desire to lessen the likelihood of such untoward immunological reactions as well as projected supply problems with a nonallergic form of human insulin by recombinant DNA technology (Rosenthal, 1981). This review will focus only on two aspects of the problem of insulin immunogenicity. The first will briefly describe studies of insulin as an antigen in experimental animals. The second and major portion of this report will consider HLA associations of the more common types of insulin immune responses in man.

Alan S. Rosenthal • Merck, Sharp, and Dohme Research Laboratories, Rahway, New Jersey 07065.   *Dean Mann* • Immunology Branch, National Cancer Institute, National Institutes of Health, Bethesda, Maryland 20205.   *C. Ronald Kahn* • Joslin Diabetes Center, and Department of Medicine, Brigham and Women's Hospital, Harvard Medical School, Boston, Massachusetts 021215.

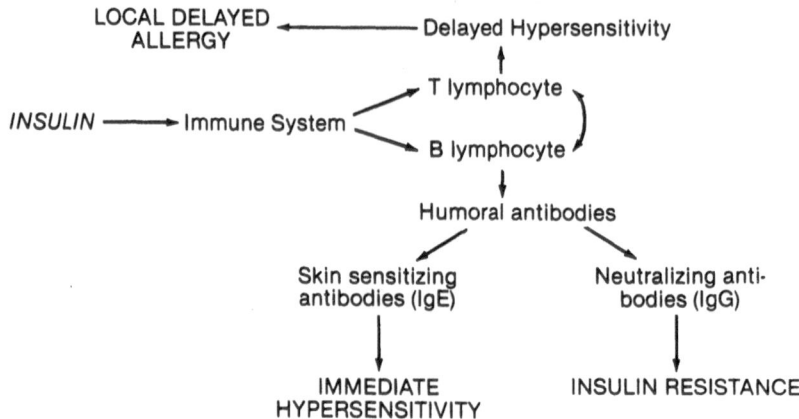

Figure 1. The immune response to insulin.

I. GENETIC CONTROL OF THE IMMUNE RESPONSE TO INSULIN IN GUINEA PIGS AND MICE

A. Guinea Pigs

The availability of well-characterized strains of inbred congenic mice and guinea pigs as well as knowledge of the chemical and physical structure of insulin makes it an ideal model for the study of the contribution of discrete molecular regions to its immunogenicity. Insulin is a small polypeptide hormone (mol.wt. 5750) of known primary, secondary, and tertiary structure (Blundell *et al.*, 1972). It consists of two polypeptide chains: the A chain is composed of 21 amino acid residues and the B chain has 30 residues. The chains are held together by two interchain disulfide bonds. When compared with the two mouse insulins, bovine insulin has six amino acid exchanges, occurring at positions A4, A8, A10, B9, B29, and B30 (Markussen, 1971; Bunzli *et al.*, 1972). Pork insulin differs from the two mouse insulins at four sequence positions: A4, B9, B29, and B30. Thus, insulin provides a precisely defined antigenic protein probe for studying the control of antigen recognition. The immune response to insulin in both mouse and guinea pig has been shown to be under major histocompatibility complex (*MHC*)-linked immune response (Ir) gene control. In both, a clear pattern of response has emerged distinguishing those regions of the molecule important in delayed-type hypersensitivity, a process dependent upon macrophage–T-cell interaction *in vivo* and *in vitro,* and those regions recognized by antibody of B cell. Extensive amino acid substitutions exist between guinea pig and beef and pork insulin. When guinea pigs are immunized to beef or pork insulin, T-cell responses can be measured *in vitro* by [³H]thymidine incorporation into lymphocyte DNA after addition of insulin or its peptides to the culture medium. In strain 2 guinea pigs this response has been shown to vary with the amino acid sequence of the A chain loop (8, 9, and 10 amino acid). Using synthetic peptide fragments of the B chain, T-cell response in strain 13 guinea

Table 1. Immunologic Reactions to Insulin

Cutaneous
  Local (limited to the injection site)
    Immediate: IgE-mediated
    Intermediate: ? Arthus reaction
    Delayed: T-cell-mediated
    Combinations of the above
  Lipoatrophy or lipohypertrophy: uncertain role of immune response

Systemic
  Urticaria and angioedema with or without shock
  Insulin resistance
  Serum sickness
  Purpura
    Thrombocytopenic
    Nonthrombocytopenic
  Arthus phenomenon with lupus erythematosus cells, eosinophilia, and hyperglobulinemia

Autoimmune insulin syndrome

pigs can be localized to a few amino acids around the histidine at the 10th residue of the B chain.

The data presented in Table 2 demonstrate that only a limited number of epitopes on a globular protein need be recognized for generation of cellular immunity. This study extends previous observations that denatured proteins can retain the ability to induce delayed hypersensitivity but lose antibody reactivity (Gell *et al.*, 1959) and more recently that denatured antigen can elicit specific helper cells (Ishizaka *et al.*, 1974). The pepotide sequence composed of the first 16 amino acids of the insulin B chain (Fig. 2) clearly contains all of the immunogenic information present in the native molecule as reflected in the generation of T-cell proliferation and in the expression of T-cell-helper activity. B(5–16) is as active as B(1–16) and contains all of the immunologically important determinants. Synthetic sequences of the region B(5–16)

Table 2.   Data Demonstrating That
Position 10 of Insulin B Chain Is Critical
for T-Cell Activation of Insulin-Immune
Strain 13 Guinea Pigs

Antigen (10 μg/ml)	Δcpm $\times 10^{-3}$
Beef insulin	63.4 ± 0.42[a]
B chain	50.0 ± 0.31
B(1–16)	54.4 ± 0.45
B(5–16)	41.0 ± 0.41
B(5–16)/Ala → Thr/[b]	49.9 ± 0.35
B(5–16)/His → Asn/[b]	3.2 ± 0.03
B(5–16)/Ala → Thr + His → Asn/[b,c]	1.6 ± 0.02

[a]Mean ± SEM of two experiments.
[b]Brackets indicate substitution(s) made from original sequence.
[c]Guinea pig sequence.

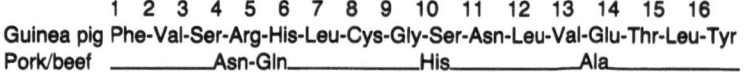

Figure 2. Amino acid sequence of N terminal 16 residues of insulin B chain.

having the amino acid sequences present in guinea pig insulin, or possessing on the B14 alanine of beef insulin but not the histidine 10th position, are not stimulatory. Using the (1–16) peptide, this reactivity was found to be reciprocal in that either peptide or whole molecule could be used as the immunogen. These observations support the concept that the T-cell responses to insulin with guinea pig are specific for a primary amino acid sequence on the antigen, and also emphasize the restricted nature of the T-cell recognition process.

All of the peptides that activate T cells contain a common amino acid variation at the 10th position. Ths histidine for asparagine exchange makes guinea pig insulin unique among mammalian insulins—being unable to form heximeres with zinc (Blundell *et al.*, 1972). Using a computer-generated space-filing model developed by Mr. Richard Feldman of the National Institutes of Health, we have located this residue as residing on the surface of the molecule. The other amino acid exchange (14th residue) within the B(5–16) peptide is not available on the surface of the molecule. If one considers variations from "self" to be a key in the recognition process, then the B–10 position assumes a critical role for T-cell activation. A single amino acid has recently been shown to be critical for immune response to another peptide: human fibrin peptide (Blundell *et al.*, 1972). However, the failure of peptide B(9–16) to induce T-cell proliferation emphasizes that the presence of this exchange alone is not sufficient for T-cell activation. Since a synthetic fragment consisting of B(1–4)–(9–16) also fails to activate insulin immune T cells, more thån fragment size is important. Possibly another residue(s) important for Ir gene product interaction is contained within the 5–9 region. A requirement for recognition of two specificities (one for Ir and another for T cell) within even such a limited peptide sequence as the 5th through 16th amino acid of the B chain is not inconsistent with recent hypotheses for the mechanism of Ir gene function (Benacerraf, 1978; Rosenthal, 1978).

While primary structure is of key importance in T-cell activation, the role of conformation in orienting an amino acid sequence for recognition should not be overlooked. For example, the B(5–13) peptide is the smallest found to stimulate insulin immune T cells; however, slightly larger peptides B(1–13) and B(5–16) are more powerful stimulators of T-cell proliferation. These additional residues may in some way sustain a propensity to reform the helix found in this region of the native molecule (Blundell *et al.*, 1972). Helical regions tend to be important sites of immunological determinants in at least two other proteins: nuclease (Sachs *et al.*, 1978) and cytochrome *c* (Corradin and Chiller, 1979). Though transient in solution, such conformation may be essential for activation on the cell surface. Reasonably, both recognition events taking place during antigen presentation and the physiochemical nature of the antigen are important in achieving maximum T-cell activation. Such a mechanism could conformationally approximate two nonsequential amino acids (e.g., B-5 and

B-10) to create a single topographical determinant for cytochrome *c* (Schwartz *et al.*, 1979). Currently, we are attempting to resolve the extent to which recognition of specific residues and conformational integrity is necessary for T-cell activation by the synthesis of pseudopeptide analogues.

The antibody specificity of the response to insulin and its fragments in inbred guinea pigs does not reflect the same characteristics as that of the T cell. Using radiolabeled species variants of insulin and isoelectrically focused sera, determinant specific antibody spectrotypes could not be detected in strain 2 sera (Thomas *et al.*, 1980). When we radiolabeled fragments for which strain 13 T cells are highly specific, we could not detect significant binding in either strain 2 or strain 13 serum with high antiinsulin titers (Barcinski *et al.*, 1977). Even though immunizing with the B(1–16) fragment will produce antibodies that bind the fragment, they did not appear to bind the native molecule. The determinants recognized by these antibodies are probably not available on the surface of the insulin molecule. These results may be somewhat analogous to the data obtained in mice hyperimmunized with nuclease in which the antibody titer in low responders reached the same level as seen in high responders. However, when these hyperimmune sera were examined for binding of the nuclear fragment (99–146), the pattern of response was similar to that noted in the primary (Sachs *et al.*, 1978), suggesting that the failure to find determinant restriction of antibody specificity in the guinea pig is due to the magnitude of the response in the primary. Thus, shared specificity between antibody and T cell could be present but not detectable because it represents such a small percent of the total antiinsulin response. This has been recently emphasized in H-2^b mice where hybridoma antibodies have been produced which bind the same A chain loop region seen by strain 2 guinea pig T cells (Loblay *et al.*, 1980). More importantly, the fragment studied here is quite small in comparison to the nuclease fragment which is about the same size as the whole insulin molecule. Nonetheless, in our present studies of insulin where the T-cell response is directed at a limited epitope, an antibody population with identical specificity to the T cell does not constitute a detectable portion of the antibody response.

B. Mice

The immune response of mice to insulin has also been studied by assaying T-cell proliferation (Rosenwasser *et al.*, 1979) and serum antibody titers (Keck, 1975a, b; Kapp and Shayer, 1978) and more recently by isoelectric focusing of immune sera (Kapp *et al.*, 1979). Mice possessing the H-2^d haplotype respond to pork insulin whereas mice possessing other H-2 haplotypes (*a, b, q, k, r, s, u, v, f*) do not. In contrast, mice of haplotypes H-2^d, H-2^b, and H-2^v all respond to beef insulin and mice of other H-2 haplotypes (*a, q, k, r, s, u*) do not.

The *I* region of the murine major histocompatibility complex (*MHC*) consists of a series of genes which control a diverse array of immunologic functions (Klein *et al.*, 1978; Meo *et al.*, 1973; Livnat *et al.*, 1973; Rosenthal and Shevach, 1973; Katz and Benacerraf, 1976). Genes located in the *I* region control immune responses (Ir gene) to various synthetic and natural portein antigens (Benacerraf and McDevitt, 1972), and they also encode for serologically detectable cell surface glycoproteins (Shreffler and David, 1974). Most studies directed at defining the relationship of *Ir* gene products and

Ia molecules have traditionally compared the immune responses of intra-H-2 recombinant strains which have subdivided the I region into at least five juxtaposed subregions; *A, B, J, E,* and *C* (Benacerraf and McDevitt, 1972; Klein *et al.,* 1978). However, because the number of genes contained within each region is uncertain, comparisons of allogeneic mouse strains must involve an unknown number of genetic differences.

Alternatively, the relationship of Ia molecules and *Ir* gene products can be approached by assessing the inhibition of immune responses by anti-Ia antisera (Schwartz *et al.,* 1976; Shevach *et al.,* 1972). Lerner *et al.,* (1980) showed that a monoclonal antibody directed against an Ia determinant could inhibit T-cell proliferation in an antigen-specific manner, thus suggesting that Ia-bearing molecules (the putative product of the *Ir* gene) were indeed the structures whose function was being inhibited, presumably at the macrophage (antigen-presenting-cell) surface. However, the possibility formally remains that *Ir* and *Ia* loci are distinct but closely linked in the genome and that the products of these putative two loci are also closely associated on the cell surface, such that anti-Ia antibodies sterically interfere with *Ir* gene function.

A new approach for the study of a single *IA* subregion gene has been made possible by discovery of the *IA* mutation, B6.C-H-2^{bm12} (McKenzie *et al.,* 1979; Hansen *et al.,* 1980). The *H-2^{bm12}* haplotype was first detected as a gain/loss mutation in skin graft studies using (B6 X BALB/c)F$_1$ mice. Breeding studies demonstrated that the mutation occurred in the *H-2* haplotype of the B6 mice, and the mutant haplotype was made homozygous and coisogeneic with B6, thus establishing the B6.C-H-2^{bm12} strain. Besides skin graft rejection, the *H-2^{bm12}* mutation also induces the mixed lymphocyte reaction and exhibits changes in the serologically detected Ia specificities (McKenzie *et al.,* 1979).

We investigated the *Ir* gene function of B6.C-H-2^{bm12} mice by comparing the T cell proliferation of B6.C-H-2^{bm12} and B6 mice with several soluble antigens, some of which are under *IA^b* gene control. B6.C-H-2^{bm12} mice, unlike their responder parent B6, have a selective immune response defect resulting in undetectable response upon immunization to beef insulin.

Immune responses to several soluble antigens were compared between B6.C-H-2^{bm12} mutant and wild-type B6 mice by using a lymph node T-cell proliferation assay. B6.C-H-2^{bm12} mice failed to respond to beef insulin whereas other *IA* gene-controlled responses, such as response to poly (*L*-Tyr, *L*-Glu)—poly (*DL*-Ala, *L*-Lys) and collagen, were indistinguishable between mutant and parent (Fig. 3). The responses to multideterminant antigens such as ovalbumin and purified protein derivative of tuberculin were also found to be comparable in B6.C-H-2^{bm12} and B6 mice, thus indicating that this mutation resulted in a selective loss of the ability to respond to a certain antigen(s), for example, beef insulin. Populations depleted of adherent cells were used to examine the mechanism by which Ia molecules mediate *Ir* gene control of antigen recognition. We found that the nonresponsiveness to beef insulin in the mutant mouse was the result of defective antigen presentation (Table 3). These findings taken together with other serologic and biochemical studies in the B6.C-H-2^{bm12} (Lin *et al.,* 1981) presented convincing genetic evidence for the direct association of the A$_\beta$ polypeptide chain of the Ia^b molecules with the expression of immune responsiveness

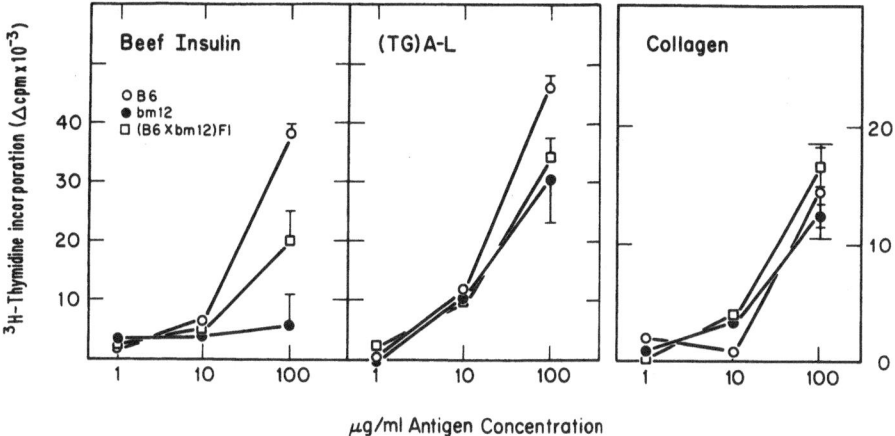

Figure 3. Mice were immunized with 50 μg beef insulin, 50 μg (TG)A-L, and 50 μg type II collagen in complete Freund's adjuvant in hind foot pads. Eleven days after immunization T cells from draining lymph nodes were collected and cultured in flat-bottom well microtiter plates at 3×10^5 cells/well with the same number of irradiated spleen cells from normal mice of appropriate strain. Antigens at different dilutions were added to triplicate wells. The cultures were incubated at 37°C, 5% CO^2 in air for 4 days. [³H]Thymidine was added 18–24 hours prior to harvesting. Δcpm was calculated by subtracting medium control from antigen stimulated cultures. Each experimental point represents the average of triplicate cultures.

to beef insulin. Study of the B6.C-H-2^{bm12} mouse should provide new insight into the cellular and molecular mechanisms by which *Ir* genes determine the nature of the immune response.

II. IMMUNITY TO INSULIN IN HUMANS

The human major histocompatibility complex (*MHC*) is in many respects homologous to the murine *MHC*. In both species this gene complex controls the expression of histocompatibility antigens, certain complement components, and the expression of

Table 3. Proliferative Response of (B6 × B6.C-H-2^{bm12})F_1 T Cells in the Presence of Antigen-Presenting Cells from F_1 Hybrid or Parental Strains[a]

| Source of spleen cells | Beef insulin (100 μg/ml) | [³H]Thymidine incorporation, Δcpm | | | Purified protein derivative (25 μg/ml) | Medium control, Δcmp |
		(TG)AL (100 μg/ml)	Collagen (100 μg/ml)	Ovalbumin (100 μg/ml)		
F_1	28,746	43,294	10,654	33,813	51,279	9,120
B6	38,527	39,458	8,213	33,184	50,045	5,362
B6.C-H-2^{bm12}	8,935	26,537	8,986	27,454	49,750	8,400

[a](B6 × B6.C-H-2^{bm12})F_1 mice were immunized with 50 μg each of beef insulin, (TG)AL, type II collagen, and ovalbumin in complete Freund's adjuvant. T-cell proliferation was measured as in Table 1. cmp was calculated by subtracting medium control from values for antigen-stimulated cultures. Each experimental point represents the mean of triplicate cultures.

antigens found preferentially on B lymphocytes and macrophages which are known as the Ia antigens in mice and the DR antigens in humans (McDevitt, 1980). While it is clear that the *Ir* gene controls immune response in mice, the definition of the genetic control of immune response in humans has been difficult. A number of factors may account for this difficulty. The *MHC* is a polymorphic gene complex. This polymorphism is compounded by the outbreeding which occurs in species such as humans. In addition, the immunogens that have been studied for association with the human *MHC* are generally complex structures having a variety of determinants which individually may be under separate genetic control.

In our attempts to define immune response genes in humans we decided to investigate patterns of immune response in diabetic patients receiving insulin. We rationalized that the diabetic population would have a rather restricted gene pool because of the known association of certain HLA antigens with diabetes, particularly of the type I variety. In addition, there has been adequate demonstration in animal studies as noted above that immune response to insulin was controlled by the major histocompatibility complex of other species. A potential advantage was that the therapeutic insulins are primarily beef and pork-derived and the biochemical structure of these insulins has been well studied. Table 4 shows the differences in the amino acid composition of beef and pork insulins. Amino acid differences exist between human and pork and beef insulins and consist of differences at positions 8 and 10 the A chain and the C terminal amino acid in the B chain. Pork insulin has the same amino acid composition in the A chain as the human insulin, however it differs in position 30 on the B chain. Beef insulin differs from human insulin at positions 8 and 10 on the A chain and has the same amino acid as pork at position 30 in the B chain. Thus, beef and pork insulins are potential immunogens and have relatively restricted differences to which the human could potentially respond immunologically.

The epidemiological variables in the diabetic population studied are shown in Table 5. One hundred ten diabetic patients who historically demonstrated some clinical manifestation of allergy to the administration of insulin were admitted to the Clinical Center of the National Institutes of Health. These patients were withdrawn from insulin at least 24 hr prior to the initiation of our studies. We also studied 29 insulin-receiving diabetics who had no demonstrable clinical allergies to insulin administration. The criteria for including the patients in the insulin-allergic group were that there were skin reactions at the site of the injection that could be characterized as immediate, intermediate, or delayed hypersensitivity reactions; the patients were resistant to insulin ther-

Table 4.   Difference in Amino Acids in Three Mammalian Insulins

| Insulin | A Chain (α loop) | | | B Chain |
	position 8	position 9	position 10	position 30
Human	Threonine	Serine	Isoleucine	Threonine
Porcine	Threonine	Serine	Isoleucine	Alanine
Bovine	Alanine	Serine	Valine	Alanine

Table 5. Epidemiological Variables in the Insulin-Receiving Diabetic

	Population studied		Mean age of onset diabetes[a]	Duration of insulin therapy prior to allergy month[a]	Mean age at time of study[b]
	Race	Number			
Insulin	Caucasian	91	36.8	2.73	52.08
allergic[c] diabetics	Black	19	36.5	2.04	
Insulin-non-	Caucasian	25	26.5	0	49.34
allergic diabetics	Black	4	43.9		

[a]Criteria for insulin allergy: immediate, intermediate delayed skin reaction at site of injection: resistance to therapy, generalized allergic reaction.
[b]No statistically significant differences between groups.
[c]Mean age of caucasians and blacks in each group.

apy; or the patients had a generalized or systemic reaction to insulin administration. The mean age of onset of diabetes in these groups ranged from 43.9 to 26.5 years and included patients who could be considered to be both Type I and Type II diabetics. Historically the mean duration of insulin therapy prior to the onset of an allergic manifestation to insulin administration was approximately 2 months. Full details of the epidemiological variables in the patients are reported elsewhere (Kahn et al., 1982).

In vivo and in vitro tests that might potentially assess the capability of an immune response were performed in these patients. Skin testing was carried out with beef insulin, pork insulin, pork single component, and protamine ($1\mu g/ml$). These antigens were injected intradermally (0.1 ml) and the skin test reactions read for erythema and induration at 1 hr, 16 hr, and 48 hr. Using these parameters, the positive reactions were classified as immediate, intermediate, or delayed skin test responses. Serum samples were obtained from each of the patients and measured for the capability to bind insulin. Sera that were demonstrated to bind insulin were used in competition assays to determine the relative affinity of the antibody to beef and pork insulins. Peripheral blood lymphocytes were obtained from the patients and the capability to respond in vitro to the therapeutic insulin components was measured. The details of the methodology are described elsewhere (Mann et al., in press). In brief, lymphocytes were incubated with 1 μg, 10 μg, or 100 μg of beef insulin, pork insulin, beef insulin containing the C peptide, pork insulin containing the C peptide, and protamine   triplicate culture. After 6 days [^{3}H]-thymidine incorporation was measured. Lymphocytes were obtained from the patients and typed for the HLA-A, B, C, and DR antigens by the standard techniques (Amos et al., 1976; Mann et al., 1975). Using the above-described techniques we were able to define 17 alloantigens controlled by the A locus, 31 alloantigens controlled by the B locus, 6 alloantigens controlled by the C locus, and 9 alloantigens controlled by the DR (w) locus.

Table 6 shows the frequency of skin test reactions in the insulin allergic diabetic patients. The percentage of individuals reacting to individual antigens as well as the type of skin test response to any of the antigens are tabulated. Eighty-four percent of the insulin-allergic diabetic population studied reacted to at least one of the four antigens. There was no difference in the percentage of positivity to any of the four antigens in the Caucasian and black populations. Table 7 shows the association of the HLA anti-

Table 6. Frequency of Skin Test Reactions in Insulin-Allergic
Diabetic Patients

		Percent all allergic diabetics	Percent allergic diabetics (N)	
			Caucasians	Blacks
Skin test antigen				
Beef insulin	Positive	80 (93)	80 (73)	80 (60)
	Negative	16 (18)	16 (14)	16 (4)
	No data	4 (5)	4 (4)	4 (1)
Pork insulin	Positive	79 (91)	79 (72)	76 (19)
	Negative	17 (20)	17 (15)	20 (5)
	No data	4 (5)	4 (4)	4 (4)
Pork single	Positive	54 (63)	55 (50)	52 (13)
	Negative	38 (44)	40 (36)	32 (8)
	No data	8 (9)	5 (5)	16 (4)
Protamine	Positive	39 (45)	39 (35)	56 (10)
	Negative	57 (66)	57 (52)	40 (14)
	No data	4 (5)	4 (4)	4 (1)
Type of skin test response				
Immediate	Positive	76 (88)	75 (68)	80 (20)
	Negative	22 (25)	22 (20)	20 (5)
	No data	2 (3)	3 (3)	0 (0)
Intermediate	Positive	38 (44)	40 (36)	32 (8)
	Negative	57 (66)	57 (53)	56 (14)
	No data	5 (6)	3 (3)	12 (3)
Delayed	Positive	43 (50)	44 (40)	40 (10)
	Negative	52 (60)	52 (47)	52 (13)
	No data	5 (6)	4 (4)	8 (2)
Skin test				
At least one	Positive	84 (97)	84 (76)	84 (21)
Four types above	Negative	13 (15)	12 (11)	16 (4)
All four	No data	3 (4)	4 (4)	0 (0)

gens with skin test response in diabetics who had historical allergic reactions to insulin. HLA-Aw23, Aw33, and Cw2 tended to be more frequent in those individuals who had either an immediate, intermediate, or delayed skin reaction to protamine. HLA-A3 appears to be negatively associated with the skin test response to protamine in that there was a greater number of individuals negative for this skin test response who were positive for the A3 antigen. HLA-Bw15 was also found more frequently in those individuals who were negative for a skin test reaction to beef insulin. When pork single-component insulin was used as a skin test antigen, HLA-Bw 35 and Cw5 tended to be associated with the negative skin test population while HLA-Cw2 tended to be positively associated with those individuals who had a positive skin test response. HLA-A28 and DR3 tended to show associations with an intermediate skin reaction to any of the four antigens tested. HLA-Bw35 was more frequently positive in persons who were negative for a delayed hypersensitivity reaction to any of the skin test antigens. The level of significance reported here was determined by Chi square analysis using the Fisher exact test (two tailed) with Yates correction. The p values are not corrected for the number of antigens that could be detected. The associations of HLA alloantigen with these different skin test responses can not therefore be considered to be highly significant. However, they do show trends in association with skin test responses to different skin test antigens.

Lymphocyte proliferation studies were performed using beef insulin, pork insulin, beef insulin with C peptide, pork insulin with C peptide, and protamine. Figure 4 illustrates types of responses seen in individual patients to four of the antigens tested, beef insulin, pork insulin, and protamine. The average counts per minute are plotted against the dose of antigen used in triplicate cultures. Figure 4A demonstrates the response to beef insulin alone with increasing [^{3}H]thymidine incorporation as the dose of insulin was itself increased. There were also individuals who had positive responses to both beef and pork insulin where the response to beef was greater than to pork. Figure 4B shows the dose-response curve in an individual who responded in this fashion. Figure 4C shows an equal response to both beef and pork insulin with increasing levels of response to both antigens as the dose of insulin was increased in the culture. Figure 4D demonstrates an individual patient's dose-response to the antigen protamine.

Table 8 summarizes the lymphocyte proliferation response to the therapeutic insulin components. The range of response to the antigens as well as the mean ratio plus or minus the standard mean are shown. In considering those who responded to beef insulin alone, 13 individuals had ratios of response ranging from 2.2 to 4.0 with a mean ratio of 2.4. The mean level of the ratio of response of those individuals who demonstrated higher responses to beef and pork was 7.3 with a range of 2.2 to 31.3. This result suggested an augmentation of the response by the recognition of the antigenic determinant conferred by amino acid differences in the A chain. There were 50 persons

Table 7. Association of HLA Antigens with Skin Test Response in Diabetics Allergic to Insulin

HLA antigen	Skin test antigen[a]	Type of skin response[b]	Number positive	Percent positive for HLA	Number negative	Percent positive for HLA	Significance
A3	D	1,2,3	45	13	65	35	$p < 0.05$
AW23	D	1,2,3	45	16	65	2	$p < 0.05$
AW33	D	1,2,3	45	13	65	2	$p < 0.05$
CW2	D	1,2,3	45	23	65	3	$p < 0.01$
BW15	A	1,2,3	93	5	18	28	$p < 0.05$
BW35	C	1,2,3	63	9	44	30	$p < 0.05$
CW2	C	1,2,3	63	18	44	2	$p < 0.05$
CW5	C	1,2,3	63	10	44	29	$p < 0.05$
A28	A,B,C,D	2	44	15	66	6	$p < 0.05$
DR3	A,B,C,D	2	44	36	64	17	$p < 0.05$
BW35	A,B,C,D	3	49	4	59	20	$p < 0.05$

[a]A, beef insulin; B, pork insulin; C, pork single-component insulin; D, protamine.
[b]1, immediate; 2, intermediate; 3, delayed.

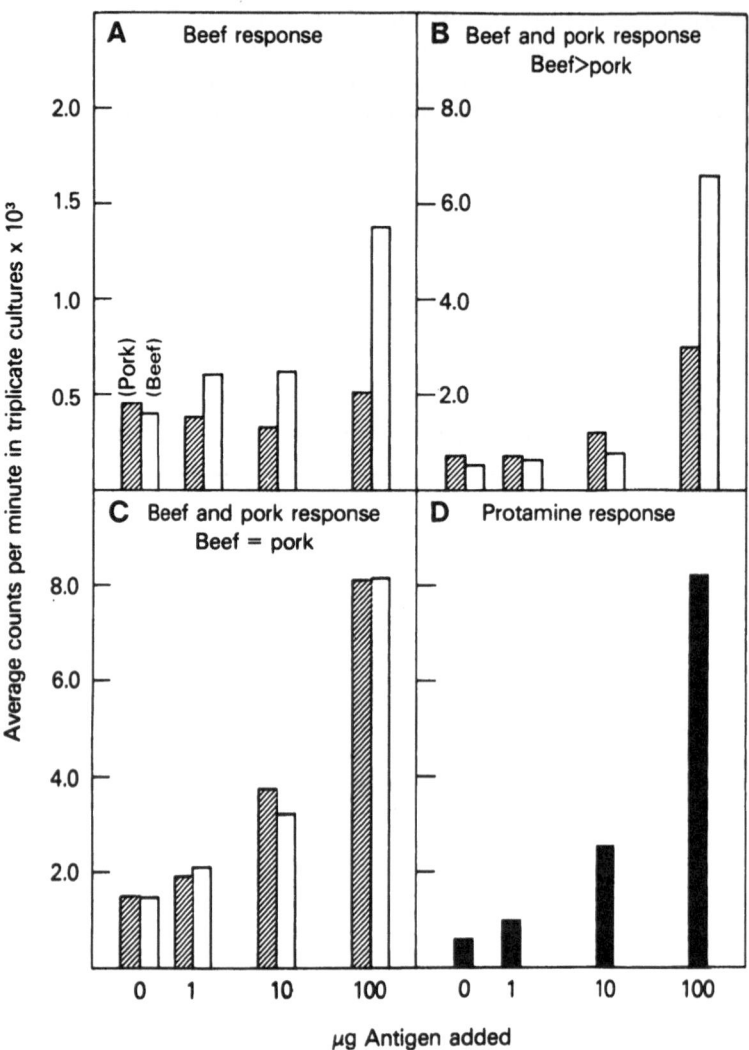

Figure 4. Response of lymphocytes (average cpms in triplicate cultures) from different individuals to increasing concentrations of beef and pork insulins and protacine.

whose lymphocytes responded equally to both pork and beef insulin (mean 4.55 ± 5.03). These individuals could be considered to be responders to the single C terminal amino acid difference in the B chain of these insulins and human insulin. There were groups who responded to the C peptide of both beef and pork insulins when response was observed to the insulin with the C peptide or where response to the antigens was greater than the ratio of response to the beef or pork insulin without the C peptide. Quite unexpectedly we found that 81 of the 137 patients tested had positive lymphocyte proliferation responses to protamine.

The responses observed to any of the above antigens were not limited to patients who had a history of insulin allergy. On a percentage basis there were equal numbers among the insulin-receiving diabetics with no history of insulin allergy and those with the positive history of an allergic reaction to insulin. The finding that groups within the diabetic population demonstrated unique responses to therapeutic insulin components suggests an element of genetic control.

The HLA alloantigenic phenotype was determined on the lymphocytes from the patients with diabetes receiving therapeutic insulin. The patients were grouped based on their response to antigen stimulation and the frequencies of each of the HLA alloantigen determinants calculated in the responder and non-responder groups. Table 9 shows the significant HLA associations found in the responder and nonresponder populations to each of the above antigens. The HLA-DR4 had a higher frequencey ($p < 0.0001$) in the group responding to beef insulin compared to the nonresponder population. HLA-DR5 was decreased in frequency ($p > 0.05$) in the responder population compared to the nonresponders. It would appear that a gene or genes associated with the HLA-DR4 antigen in the *MHC* recognize the amino acid differences in the A chain and effect positive proliferative responses. HLA-DR3 was increased in frequency in those who respond equally to beef and pork insulins. The frequency of this antigen was approximately 40% in the responder population compared to 70% in the nonresponder population and had a significance level of p equal to or less than 0.005.

These results suggest a regulatory control to the C terminal amino acid in the B chain by genes associated with HLA-DR3. Those individuals responding to beef proinsulin had increased frequencies of HLA-Bw4, Cw2, Cw5, DR2, and DR5. Levels of significance varied with the most striking association being that of the HLA-Cw5 antigen. The fact that the HLA-DR5 antigen was increased in the population of individuals responding to beef proinsulin and was decreased in frequency in those who re-

Table 8. Summary of Lymphocyte Proliferation Response to Beef Insulin, Beef and Pork Insulin, Beef Proinsulin, Pork Proinsulin, and Protamine

	Number	Range of response	Mean ratio ± SEM
Beef response	13	2.2– 4.0	2.9 ± 6.62
Beef > pork response	18	2.2– 31.3	7.3 ± 7.2
Beef nonresponse	106	0.5– 1.9	1.25 ± 0.33
Beef and pork response	50[a]	2.1– 28.6	4.55 ± 5.03
Beef and pork nonresponse	71	0.6– 1.9	1.31 ± 3.2
Beef proinsulin response	21	2.2– 7.2	3.05 ± 1.15
Beef proinsulin > beef response	16	2.0– 65.5	11.6 ± 15.5
Beef proinsulin nonresponse	100	0.5– 1.9	1.35 ± 0.33
Pork proinsulin response	24	2.3– 16.6	4.49 ± 2.95
Pork proinsulin > pork response .	23	1.6– 33.4	7.64 ± 8.32
Pork proinsulin nonresponse	90	0.6– 1.9	1.27 ± 0.32
Protamine response	81	2.2–263.4	14.8 ± 18.3
Protamine nonresponse	56	0.5– 1.9	1.35 ± 0.45

[a]Sixteen individuals who responded to beef and pork whose beef response was greater than pork are not included.

Table 9.   HLA Alloantigen Association with Lymphocyte Response to
Therapeutic Insulin Components

| | | Frequency | | |
	HLA antigen	Responders	Nonresponders	P value
		(N = 31)	(N = 106)	
Beef insulin	DR4	0.709	0.273	<0.001
(A chain)	DR5	0.064	0.245*	<0.05
		(N = 66)	(N = 71)	
Beef and pork insulin	DR3	0.393	0.169	<0.005
(B chain)				
		(N = 37)	(N = 100)	
Beef proinsulin	BW3	0.837	0.560	<0.008
	CW2	0.243	0.080	<0.02
	CW5	0.405	0.090	<0.001
	DR2	0.378	0.150	<0.008
	DR5	0.378	0.150	<0.008
		(N = 47)	(N = 90)	
Pork proinsulin	B7	0.148	0.300[a]	<0.05
	BW4	0.468	0.722[a]	<0.008
	DR2	0.320	0.156	<0.05
	DR3	0.148	0.367	<0.01
		(N = 81)	(N = 86)	
Protamine	A3	0.123	0.392[a]	<0.00
	BW6	0.765	0.928[a]	<0.025
	CW3	0.345	0.160	<0.025
	CW5	0.246	0.071	≤0.014
	DR7	0.358	0.089	<0.001

[a]Frequency higher in nonresponders.

sponded to beef insulin alone clearly separates these two populations and in turn gives further evidence that the genetic control of the immune response to these antigens is controlled by the *MHC*. In an assessment of HLA alloantigen in frequencies in the population of individuals having positive proliferative responses to pork proinsulin, HLA-DR2 was the antigen found to be increased. A decrease in frequency was seen with the B7 and Bw4 as well as HLA-DR3. There are two points of interest in this observation. In a normal population HLA-B7 is in linkage disequilibrium with HLA-DR2. The results suggest that this linkage group in and of itself does not carry the genes for immune response to this antigen. The second point to be made is that HLA-DR3 antigen is decreased in frequency in the nonresponder population to beef proinsulin and increased in frequency in individuals responding to beef and pork insulins. As with beef proinsulin, the results strongly indicate that these are genetically two different groups of individuals. Table 9 also documents the genetic control of a proliferative response to the protamine antigen. The most significant HLA association was with the HLA-DR7. HLA-Cw5 and Cw3 antigens were also increased in frequency in the responder population. HLA-A3 and Bw6 were more frequent in the nonresponder population than in the responder populations in this study. This is the first known documentation of genetic control of immune response to protamine. Protamine was also used to stimulate the peripheral blood lymphocytes from a normal control population (nondiabetic) and an increase in frequency of the HLA-DR7 antigen was found comparable to the frequency observed in the diabetic population (data not shown). One can conclude from these experiments that a gene or genes closely linked to the *HLA-DR7* gene is responsible for a primary response to protamine and that a known prior exposure to this protein is not necessary for demonstration of *in vitro* lymphocyte proliferative response.

The presence of antibody was measured in 101 of the patients studied. Total antigen-binding capacity of the serum and the titer of the serum that bound 50% of radiolabeled beef insulin was determined. Sixteen of the individuals had no demonstrable antibody production to insulin. In addition, antibody production was not limited to those who had a history of clinical allergic reactions to insulin therapy. The relative affinity of the antibody was measured to beef and pork insulins using a radiolabeled beef insulin and competition for binding with purified beef and pork insulins. A ratio of beef insulin binding to pork insulin binding was calculated and the individuals grouped into four categories. Sixteen individuals had high beef-to-pork binding ratios ranging from 100 to 1000. Fifty-three individuals had intermediate ratios of inhibition (range 5–99). Sixteen individuals had low ratios of inhibition ranging from 1 to 4 and 16 individuals had no demonstrable antibody production to beef or pork insulin. The frequency of HLA alloantigens was calculated in each of the four groups. Figure 5 shows the frequency distribution of the HLA alloantigens that differed significantly in the four groups of patients. The most striking finding is the relationship between DR2 and DR3 in the four groups studied. DR3 was found in 75% of the individuals who had no antibody reaction while DR2 was absent. In those individuals who had low ratios of beef insulin to pork-insulin-binding, DR3 was found in 50% and again DR2 was found to occur in none of the individuals with this ratio of bind. In those individuals with intermediate ratios of bind, DR3 and DR2 were approximately equal in frequency. DR2 was present in approximately 50% of the individuals who had high beef-insulin-binding antibody while DR3 was present in only 6% of these individuals. HLA-B8, which is in linkage disequilibrium with DR3, showed essentially the same distribution of frequency in the four groups as did the HLA-DR3 antigen. HLA-Cw5 was significantly increased in those individuals who had no demonstrable antibody to insulin compared to those who had low or intermediate levels of beef to pork ratios of inhibition. This antigen was found in 50% of those individuals who had high beef-to-pork ratios of inhibition. These results strongly suggest an association of the HLA-DR2 antigen with production of high-affinity antibody to beef insulin. Conversely, the result suggests that genes closely linked to the *HLA-DR 3* gene suppressed the production of antibody to insulin and particularly to the beef insulin molecule. The interesting distribution of frequency of the antigen HLA-Cw5 suggests that more than one gene may control the production of antibody to beef insulin. This antigen was found in relatively high frequency in those individuals who had no antibody production and in those who had high-affinity antibody to beef insulin. These results suggest a two-gene model for the recognition of the beef insulin antigen and subsequent production of antibody to this insulin. The presence of a gene or genes linked to or associated with the Cw5

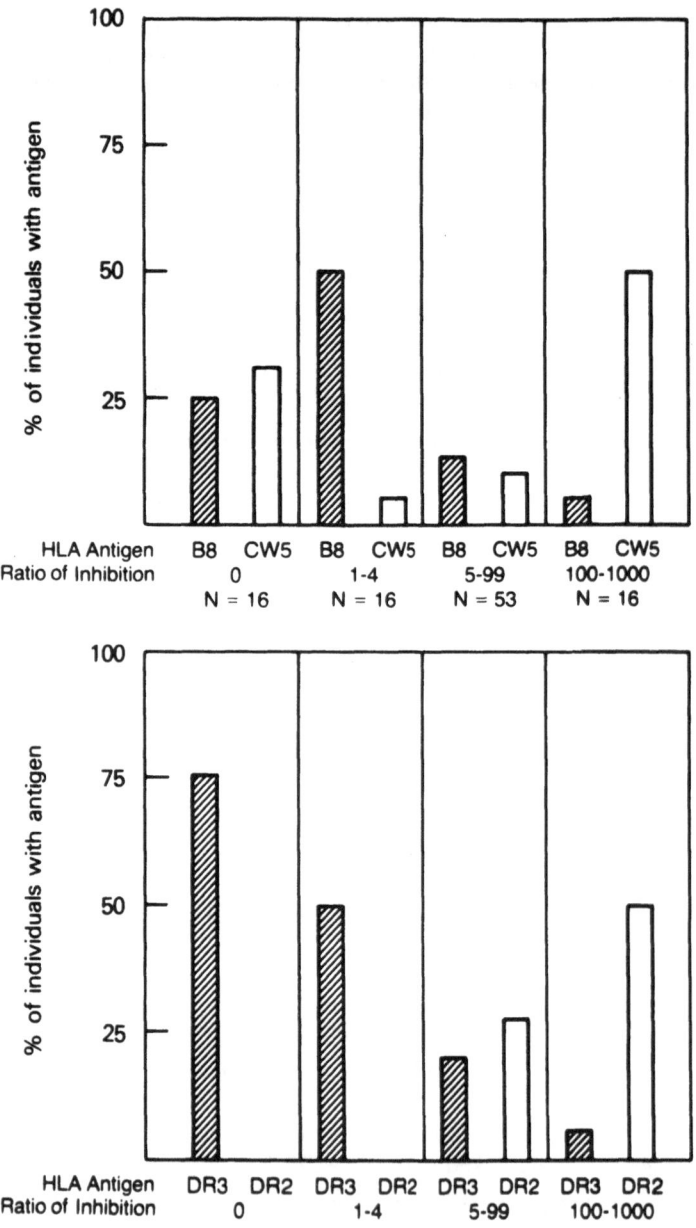

Figure 5. Frequency of HLA antigens in groups of patients with serum antibodies of increasing affinity to beef insulin (expressed as ratio of inhibition).

antigen is insufficient to allow recognition and subsequent immune response to the beef insulin. However, the combination of a gene or genes linked to *CW5* and those linked to *HLA-DR2* genes affects the production of high-affinity antibody to beef insulin.

Having measured a number of the parameters of immune response in humans to therapeutic insulin components, we compared these individual parameters with each other in an attempt to determine if there is an association of one measurement of immune response with another (Table 10). Limited associations were found. The titer of antibody to beef insulin was highly associated with the clinical history of the systemic reaction to insulin administration. Resistance to therapy was associated with both the antibody titer and the total antigen-binding capacity. Antibody production was negatively associated with any type of skin reaction with insulin administration. Lower levels of association were seen only with proliferation responses to pork insulin and protamine and a localized skin reaction.

The results of these studies clearly demonstrate that the immune response to insulin from the bovine and porcine species is under genetic control in humans. Genetic control is suggested by the observation that there are responders and nonresponders to beef and pork insulin in measurements of *in vitro* lymphocyte proliferation and also in production of antibody to the insulins. Furthermore, genes controlling the immune response appear to be located in the *MHC* by virtue of the association of the HLA alloantigens with the particular response seen. The results of these studies parallel those findings in other animal species, particularly mice and guinea pigs, which have demonstrated immune response genes in these species to beef insulin and pork insulin. The results strongly indicate that humans, like the mouse and guinea pig, can recognize the two amino acid differences in the loop of the A chain of beef insulin as well as the C terminal amino acid in the B chain of beef and pork insulin with subsequent immunological response. Bertrams and Gruneklee showed an association of humoral immune responsiveness to beef insulin in insulin-dependent (Type I) diabetic patients

Table 10. Comparison of the Association of the Historical Manifestation of Allergy to Insulin and In Vitro Parameters of Immune Response[a]

| | Association with lymphocyte proliferation response | | | ABC50 | Antigen-binding |
Clinical variable	Beef ratios	Pork ratios	Protamine ratio	(titer)	capacity
Systemic	NS	NS	NS	+++	NS
Resistance to therapy	NS	NS	NS	+++	+++
Skin reaction	NS	NS	NS	− − −	NS(−)
Immediate skin reaction	NS	NS	NS	NS	NS
Intermediate skin reaction	NS	NS	NS(−)	NS(−)	NS
Localized skin reaction	NS	NS(+)	+	NS	NS
Delayed reaction	NS	NS	NS	NS	NS

[a]Level of significance (nonparametric analysis): NS, $p > 0.05$; +, $p < 0.05$ (higher values in clinical positive group); ++, $p < 0.01$ (higher values in clinical positive group); +++, $p > 0.005$ (higher values in clinical positive group); −, $p < 0.05$ (lower values in clinical positive group); − −, $p < 0.01$ (lower values in clinical positive group); − − −, $p < 0.005$ (lower values in clinical positive group); NS(+), no association but higher values observed in clinically positive group; NS(−), no association but lower values observed in the clinically positive group.

with an increased frequency of HLA-DR4. Individuals who had no detectable serum antibodies to insulin showed a correlation of antibody response with an increase in the HLA-B8 and DR3 antigens (Bertrans *et al.*, 1981). Schernthauer and Mayr (1981) also demonstrated an association of HLA-DR4 with antibody to beef insulin. They also reported that the titers for insulin antibody-binding capacity were lower in HLA-DR3-positive individuals than in those individuals who were negative for this antigen. The above studies were performed on insulin-dependent diabetic patients which in effect restricted the gene pool in that there is a demonstrable increase in frequency in both HLA-DR3 and HLA-DR4 in Type I diabetic patients. In our study both Type I and Type II diabetic patients were assessed for the capability to respond to therapeutic insulins. Our results parallel those of the two previous studies in that an increase in HLA-DR3 was seen in those individuals who had no antibody response to insulin. In our study an increase in frequency of HLA-DR2 was found in those individuals who had high-affinity antibody to beef insulin. The frequency of HLA-DR4 was not different in those individuals who produced antibody and those who were antibody-negative. Our studies would, therefore, suggest that gene or genes associated with the HLA-DR2 gene are responsible for the specificity of the antibody produced against beef insulin and thus suggest a restricted immune response gene.

The results of these studies demonstrate the complexity of the immune response in humans. We have measured three parameters of the immune response: skin testing, *in vitro* lymphocyte proliferation, and antibody production. The only significant positive correlations between them was that of resistance to therapy manifested by a history of systemic reactions which were associated with antibody production. Positive skin test reactions were confined to those individuals who had a history of allergic reactions to therapeutic insulin administration. The other two measures of immune response, lymphocyte proliferation and antibody production, were not confined to the population of individuals with historical allergic reactions. Thus, the manifestations of an immune response as reflected in the skin test reactions is most probably controlled by genes other than those mapping in the *MHC*. This in fact is quite probable in that skin test reactions depend upon a cascade of reactions which result in the demonstrable skin test response.

There was no correlation observed with *in vitro* lymphocyte proliferation responses and the production of antibody to insulin. In addition, elevation in frequencies of the HLA-DR antigens were different in the populations who appeared to respond in *in vitro* lymphocyte proliferation studies and those individuals who had high titer to antibodies. The results suggested that two responses are under separate genetic control. An antibody response to the loop of the A chain of insulin is associated with *DR2*, while the proliferative response was demonstrated to be associated with *DR4*. HLA-DR3 was demonstrated to be increased in frequency in those individuals who had positive proliferative responses to both beef and pork insulin (C terminal amino acid of the B chain) and decreased in frequency in those individuals who had high-affinity antibody titers to beef insulin. We suspect that a secondary proliferative response to antigenic stimuli represents the expansion of T helper cells and that in turn would be the cooperating units in antibody production. Conversely, positive lymphocyte proliferation may represent an expansion of a suppressor cell population. One might invoke an explanation of suppressor cell expansion in the observation that the HLA-DR3 antigen was increased in frequency in those individuals who had low or no antibody response to beef insulin and a relative high frequency of this antigen in lymphocyte proliferation response to beef and pork insulin. HLA-DR3 may be associated with the suppressor gene that modifies or decreases the capability to produce antibody against the amino acid differences in the A chain in beef insulin. When insulin immunity is considered as a model, these data indicate the methodological difficulties inherent in studies of the immune response in humans as well as its relevance not only to clinical expression of disease but also to response to therapy.

REFERENCES

Amos, D. B., and Pool, P., 1976, HLA typing in: *Manual of Clinical Immunology* (E. Rose and H. Friedman, eds.), pp. 797–804, American Society of Microbiology, Washington, D.C.

Barcinski, M. A., and Rosenthal, A. S., 1977, Immune response gene control of determinant selection. 1. Intramolecular mapping of the immunogenic sites of insulin recognized by guinea pig T and B cells, *J. Exp. Med.* **145**:726–742.

Benacerraf, B., 1978, A hypothesis to relate the specificity of T lymphocytes and the activity of I region-specific Ir genes in macrophages and B lymphocytes, *J. Immunol.* **120**:1809–1812.

Benacerraf, B., and McDevitt, H. O., 1972, Histocompatibility-linked immune response genes. A new class of genes that controls the formation of specific immune responses has been identified, *Science* **175**:273–279.

Bertrans, J., Grunklee, D., 1981, HLA-DR association of humoral immunoresponsiveness to insulin in insulin-dependent (Type 1) diabetes mellitus, in: *Basic and Clinical Aspects of Immunity to Insulin* (K. Keck and P. Erb, eds.), pp. 253–261, Walter de Gruyter, Berlin.

Blundell, T., Dodson, G., Hodgkin, D., and Mercola, D., 1972, Insulin: Structure in the crystal and its reflection in chemistry and biology, *Adv. Protein Chem.* **26**:279–402.

Bunzli, H. F., Glatthaar, B., Kunz, P., Mulhaupt, E., and Humbel, R. E., 1972, Amino acid sequence of two insulins from mouse (*Mus musculus*), *Hoppe Seylers Z. Physiol. Chem.* **353**:451–485.

Corradin, G., and Chiller, J. M., 1979, Lymphocyte specificity to protein antigens. II. Fine specificity of T-cell activation with cytochrome c and derived peptides as antigenic probes. *J. Exp. Med.* **149**:436–447.

Gell, P. G. H., and Benacerraf, B., 1959, Studies on hypersensitivity. II. Delayed hypersensitivity to denatured proteins in guinea pigs, *Immunology*, **2**:64–70.

Hansen, T. H., Melvold, R. W., Arn, J. S., and Sachs, D. H., 1980, Evidence for mutation in an Ia gene, *Nature (London)* **285**:340–341.

Ishizaka, K., Kishimoto, T., Delespesse, G., and King, T. P., 1974, Immunogenic properties of modified antigen E. I. Presence of specific determinants for T cells in denatured antigen and polypeptide chains, *J. Immunol.* **113**70–77.

Kahn, R., and Rosenthal, A. S., 1979, Immunologic reactions to insulin: Insulin allergy, insulin resistance and the autoimmune insulin syndrome, *Diabetes Care* **2**:283.

Kahn, C. R., Mann, D. L., Rosenthal, A. S., Galloway, J. A., Johnson, A. H., and Mendell, N., 1982. The immune response to insulin in man. I. Interaction of HLA alloantigens and the development of the immune response, *Diabetes* **31**:16–23.

Kapp, J. A., and Strayer, D. S., 1978, H-2 linked Ir gene control of antibody response to porcine insulin. I. Development of insulin-specific antibodies in some but not all nonresponder strains injected with proinsulin, *J. Immunol.* **121**:978–982.

Kapp, J. A., Strayer, D. S., Robbins, P. F., and Perlmutter, R. M., 1979, Insulin specific murine antibodies of limited heterogeneity. I. Genetic control of spectrotypes, *J. Immunol.* **123**:109–114.

Katz, D. H., and Benacerraf, B., 1976, Genetic control of lymphocyte interactions and differentiation, in: *The Role of Products of the Histocompatibility Gene Complex in Immune Response* (Katz and Benacerraf, eds.), pp. 355–389, Academic Press, New York.

Keck, K., 1975a, Ir gene control of carrier recognition. I. Immunogenicity of bovine insulin derivatives, *Eur. J. Immunol.* **5**:801–807.

Keck, K., 1975b, Ir-gene control of immunogenicity of insulin and A-chain loop as a carrier determinant, *Nature* **254**:78–79.

Keck, K., and Erb.,P., eds., 1981, *Basic and Clinical Aspects of Immunity to Insulin,* Walter de Gruyter, Berlin.

Klein, J., Flaherty, L., VandeBerg, J. L., and Shreffler, D. C., 1978, H-2 haplotypes, genes, regions and antigens: First listing, *Immunogenetics* **6**:489–512.

Lerner, E. A., Matis, L. A., Janeway, C. A., Jr., Jones, P. P., Schwartz, R. H., and Murphy, D. B., 1980, Monoclonal antibody against an Ir gene product? *J. Exp. Med.* **152**:1085–1101.

Lin, C. C. S., Rosenthal, A. S., Passmore, H. C., and Hansen, T. H., 1981. Selective loss of antigen-specific Ir gene function in IA mutant B6.C-H2^{bm12} is an antigen presenting cell defect, *Proc. Natl. Acad. Sci. USA.* **78**:6406–6410.

Livnat, S., Klein, J., and Bach, F. H., 1973, Graft versus host reaction in strains of mice identical for H-2K and H-2D antigens, *Nature; New Biol.* **243**:42–44.

Loblay, R. H., Schroer, J., and Rosenthal, A. S., 1980, Attempts at determinant specific antibody blockade of macrophage presentation, in: *Macrophage Regulation of Immunity* (E. Unanue and A. S. Rosenthal, eds.), pp. 87–94, Academic Press, New York.

Mann, D. L., Abelson, L., Henkart, P., Honis, S., and Amos, D. B., 1975, Serologic detection of B lymphocyte antigens, in: *Histocompatibility Testing* 1975, (F. Kissmeyer-Nielsen, ed.), pp. 705–707, Aarhus, Copenhagen, Denmark.

Mann, D. L., Rosenthal, A. S., Kahn, R. C., Johnson, A. H., and Mendell, N. (1983), *In vitro* lymphocyte proliferation in diabetics to therapeutic insulin components. Evidence for genetic control by the human MHC, *J. Clin. Invest.* **72**:1130–1138.

Markussen, J., 1971, Mouse insulins—Separation and structures, *Int. J. Protein Res.* **3**:149–155.

McDevitt, H. O., 1980, Current concepts in immunology: Regulation of the immune response by the major histocompatibility system, *N. Engl. J. Med.* **303**:1514–1517.

McKenzie, I. F. C., Morgan, G. M., Sandrin, M. S., Michaelides, M. M., Melvold, R. W., and Kohn, H. I., 1979, B6.C-H.2^{bm12}, A new H-2 mutation in the I region in the mouse, *J. Exp. Med.* **150**:1323–1338.

Meo, T., David, C. S., Nabholz, M., Miggiano, U., and Shreffler, D. C., 1973, Demonstration by MLR test of a previously unsuspected intra-H-2 crossover in the BIO.HTT strain: Implications concerning location MLR determinants in the Ir region, *Transplant. Proc.* **5**:1507–1510.

Rosenthal, A. S., 1978, Determinant selection and macrophage function in genetic control of the immune response, *Immunol. Rev.* **40**:136–152.

Rosenthal, A. A., 1981, Immunological properties of insulin. Proceedings of FDA State of the Art Conference on Insulins and Growth Hormone, in: *Insulins, Growth Hormone and Recombinant DNA Technology* (J. L. Gueriguian, ed.), pp. 49–54, Raven Press, New York.

Rosenthal, A. S., and Shevach, E. M. 1973, The function of macrophages in antigen recognition by guinea pig T lymphocytes. I. Requirement for histocompatible macrophages and lymphocytes. *J. Exp. Med.* **138**:1194–1212.

Rosenwasser, L. J., Barcinski, M. A., Schwartz, R. H., and Rosenthal, A. S., 1979, Immune response gene control of determinant selection. II. Genetic control of the murine T lymphocyte proliferative response to insulin, *J. Immunol.* **123**:471–476.

Sachs, D. H., Berzofky, J. A., Pisetsky, D. S., and Schwartz, R. H., 1978, Genetic control of the immune response to staphyloccal nuclease, *Semin. Immunopathol.* **1**:51–84.

Schernthauer, G., and Mayr, W. R., 1981, Insulin antibody formation following conventional or mono component insulin treatment is influenced by genes of the HLA-DR locus, in: *Basic and Clinical Aspects of Immunity to Insulin* (K. Keck and P. Erb, eds.), pp. 263–274 Walter de Gruyter, Berlin.

Schwartz, R. H., David, C. S., Sachs, D. H., and Paul, W. E., 1976, T. lymphocyte-enriched murine peritoneal exudate cells. III. Inhibition of antigen-induced T lymphocyte proliferation with anti-Ia antisera. *J. Immunol* **117**:531–540.

Schwartz, R. H., Yano, M., Solinger, A. M., Ultee, M. E., Margoliash, E., and Paul, W. E., 1979, Gene complementation in the murine T-lymphocyte proliferative response, *J. Supramol. Struct. Suppl.* **1**:237.

Shevach, E. M., Paul, W. E., and Green, I., 1972, Histocompatibility-linked immune response gene function in guinea pigs. Specific inhibition of antigen-induced lymphocyte proliferation by alloantisera, *J.
Exp. Med.* **136**:1207–1221.

Shreffler, D. C., and David, C. S., 1974, The H-2 major histocompatibility complex and the I immune
response region: Genetic variation, function, and organization, *Adv. Immunol.* **20**:125–195.

Thomas, J. W., Schroer, J., Danho, W., Bullesbach, E., Fohles, J., and Rosenthal, A. S., 1980, Determinant selection and macrophage-mediated Ir gene function, in: *Macrophage Regulation of Immunity*, (E.
Unanue and A. S. Rosenthal, eds.), pp. 3–14, Academic Press, New York.

3

Virus and Experimental Diabetes

H. Müntefering and F. K. Jansen

I. INTRODUCTION

Special subtypes of viruses belonging to different virus families are known to be able to induce insulin-deficient diabetes or pathological glucose tolerance in experimental animals (Table 1). The development of the diabetogenic effect of viruses is dependent on the species (Table 1) and, within one species, dependent on age and sex (Friedman *et al.*, 1972), particularly on the genetic factors of the animals determining susceptibility or resistance to diabetes (Craighead and Higgins, 1974; Yoon and Notkins, 1976).

One of the important factors involved in the pathogenesis of the virus-induced diabetes is the immunological status of the host. The following discussion brings together several pieces of experimental findings in support of this hypothesis.

II. EXPERIMENTAL MODEL WITH POLYENDOCRINE DISEASE AND AUTOIMMUNITY

As a model for human type I diabetes with polyendocrine lesions produced by autoimmunreactions, Onodera *et al.* (1978, 1981) reported that reovirus type 1 produces transitory hyperglycemia in newborn mice, triggers polyendocrine disease, and induces formation of autoantibodies that react with antigens in pancreatic islets, the anterior pituitary, and gastric mucosa. One of the antibodies reacts with insulin and another with growth hormone. Using recombinant viruses the authors showed that the S1 gene segment from reovirus type 1 was required for the induction of autoantibodies to growth hormone. In addition to developing autoantibodies, many of the mice infected with reovirus type 1 developed polyendocrine disease. Twenty-five to 50% of the mice also developed a runting syndrome.

H. Müntefering • Institute of Pathology, University of Mainz, D-6500 Mainz, Federal Republic of Germany.   *F. K. Jansen* • Research Center, Klin-Midy, 34082 Montpellier Cedex, France.

Table 1. Animal Models of Virus-Induced Diabetes[a]

Virus (type)	Species affected	Pathological changes	References
		Immunopathological processes not considered as a factor of pathogenesis	
Coxsackie B (RNA)	Mice	Occasional and fine structural alterations of beta cells	Robertson, 1954
			Burch et al., 1971
			Tsui et al., 1972
			Harrison et al., 1972
			Coleman et al., 1973, 1974
Foot-and-mouth disease (RNA)	Cattle	Slight damage in both islets and acinar tissue	Barboni et al., 1962
Spontaneous (transmissible agent)	Guinea pig	Almost total absence of islets, with infiltration of round cells and some acinar and ductal necrosis	Munger and Lang, 1973
		Degranulation of beta cells, and cytoplasmatic inclusions with sparing of α and D cells	Lang and Munger, 1976
Mumps (RNA)	Monkey (in vitro)	Establishment of infection in cultured pancreatic beta cells	Prince et al., 1978
Venezuelan equine encephalomyelitis	Mice (C57KSJ db/db)	TC-83 strain: beta cell degranulation and changes in subcellular organelles, especially mitochondria	Goldberg et al., 1978
Rubella (RNA)	Rabbits	Beta cell degranulation and changes in subcellular organelles	Menser et al., 1978
		Immunological processes considered as a factor of pathogenesis	
Encephalomyocarditis, M variant (RNA)	Mice	Degranulation and coagulation necrosis with subsequent shrinking of beta cells and architectural alterations of islets	Craighead and McLane, 1968
			Müntefering et al., 1971
			Craighead and Steinke, 1971
			Müntefering, 1972
			Wellmann et al., 1972
		Degeneration and necrosis, of isolated acinar cells or acinar cells adjacent to the islets of Langerhans	Boucher and Notkins, 1973
			Hayashi et al., 1974
			Müntefering, 1972
			Wellmann et al., 1972
			Hayashi et al., 1974
			Craighead, 1975
C-type virus particles induced by multiple subdiabetogenic injections of streptozotocin (RNA)	Mice	Insulitis (mononuclear infiltration of islets)	Like and Rossini, 1976
			Rossini et al., 1977
Reovirus type 1 (RNA)	Mice	Mild beta cell damage and insulitis, with infiltration of mononuclear and plasma cells (also polyendocrine disease)	Onodera et al., 1981, 1982

[a]Modified from Rayfield and Seto (1978).

Viral antigens and inflammatory cells were found in the islets of Langerhans and in the anterior pituitary. (No quantification of the intensity of the inflammation and no identification of the inflammatory cells is presented.) The precise cause of virus-induced diabetes and the runting syndrome remains unclear.

In a recent paper, however, Onodera et al. (1982) could show that treatment with immunosuppressive agents depressed autoantibody production and prevented the development of polyendocrine disease. Thus the possibility is given that, in addition to the direct lytic effect of the virus on the cell, a virus-induced autoimmunity contributes to the pathogenesis of the disease.

Experimental results until now have not been sufficient to support this hypothesis. The question remains unanswered as to whether tissue directed autoantibodies in the reovirus-induced polyendocrine disease represent a cause or effect of the basic underlying process.

III. EXPERIMENTAL MODELS WITH IMMUNOPATHOLOGICAL REACTIONS TO THE B CELLS OF ISLETS OF LANGERHANS

A. Streptozotocin with Activated Type C Virus

Like and Rossini (1976 and Rossini et al., 1977). found that multiple subdiabetogenic injections of streptozotocin in mice produced an insulitis, progressive destruction of B cells, and subsequent hyperglycemia. Within the affected islets, they demonstrated electron microscopically type C viruses, suggesting that streptozotocin may have activated otherwise dormant murine leukemia virus in unsusceptible host. Complementary time course studies (Appel et al., 1978) suggested that type C virus induction may precede the appearance of insulitis by 2 days, and that insulitis is consistently accompanied by the presence of virus-positive islet cells.

It is proposed that the lesions in this model are the consequence of three distinct factors that interact to varying degrees to produce the final metabolic and morphologic alteration, namely (1) distinct B-cell cytotoxity, (2) viral induction within B cells and, (3) cell-mediated autoimmune reaction. Further studies are necessary to clarify the roles of streptozotocin and viruses in the pathogenesis of pancreatic insulitis.

B. EMC Virus

The most convincing data to support a viral etiology of diabetes are derived from work with the M-variant of encephalomyocarditis (EMC) virus (Craighead and McLane, 1968; Boucher and Notkins, 1973; Müntefering et al., 1971), belonging to the group of picornaviruses.

1. Insulitis

One of the striking similarities between the experimental EMC model and the human type I diabetes lies in the inflammation of the islets of Langerhans, so-called insulitis. This obligatory, but transitory phenomenon (Müntefering, 1972; Müntefering et al., 1979) is one of the most important factors suggesting autoimmunity as an explanation of the pathogenesis of diabetes. It is assumed that insulitis is a matter of an infiltration by lymphocytes, whereby the lymphocytes are taken as a sign of immunological processes (Rayfield and Seto, 1978; Jansen, 1980; Jansen *et al.*, 1979). If one further postulates that these are T lymphocytes, then the supposition of an autoimmune process is not far off (Jansen, 1980). But the histological and electron microscopic pictures of the inflammatory infiltrates of the islets of Langerhans do not support such postulates. An exact analysis, performed within short intervals during the course of the virus-induced lesions, shows a change in the intensity and composition of the infiltrates, so that the name "insulitis" covers different phenomena, possibly indicating distinct biological processes (Müntefering *et al.*, 1979).

The intensity of the inflammatory infiltration shows two peaks during the course of the infection (Fig. 1). The first sharp peak is found around the 4th day after infection, and decreases after the beginning of the 3rd week. At the end of the 4th week, the number of infiltrating cells decreases again.

While the blood glucose levels run parallel to the rise and fall in the graph of the infiltrating cells, they remain high and, in general irreversible, after the second phase. At this point, the number of B cells is greatly reduced, and the islets of Langerhans are significantly decreased in size. A rise in blood sugar can still be demonstrated, even when all inflammatory infiltration has receded (Fig. 2).

The quantitaive analysis of the inflammatory cells involved in insulitis shows that their composition during the first phase is not identical to that in the second phase.

In the 1st week one finds numerous necrotic and pyknotic cells. During this phase, the inflammatory infiltrate consists of 95% macrophages, 2% polymorphs, and

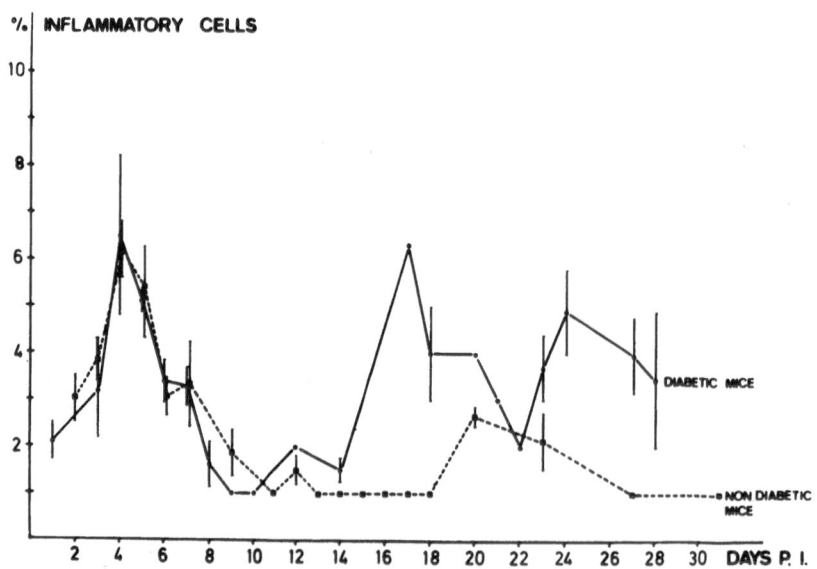

Figure 1. Inflammatory cells per 100 islets from at least 100 islets from seven or eight animals each day. Intensity of insulitis during the course of the EMC-virus lesion showing animals with (————) and without (- - - -) a manifestation of diabetes. Animals that do not develop any diabetes demonstrate insulitis only in the early phase after infection. Only diabetic animals show an infiltration of the islets after the 2nd week.

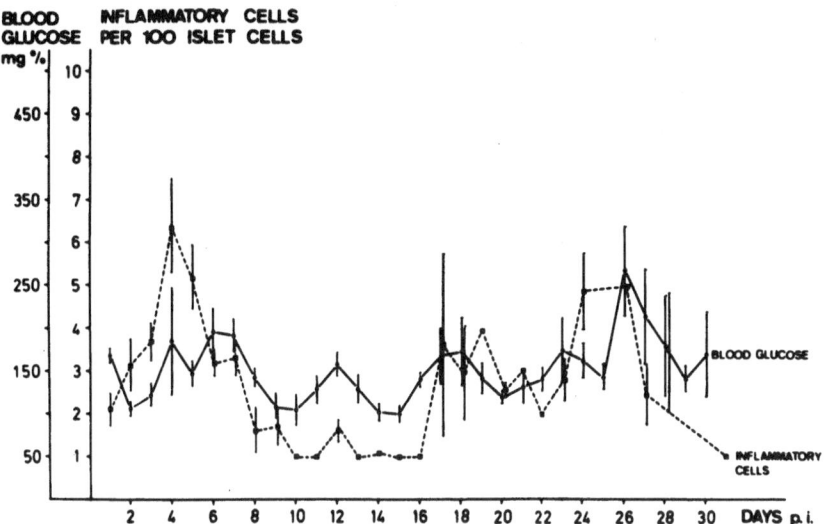

Figure 2. Relation between intensity of insulitis (- - - -) and blood glucose levels (————) during the time of the EMC virus lesion. In all infected animals blood glucose level increases and falls in relation to the density of the inflammatory infiltrates.

3% lymphocytes (Fig. 3). Between the 8th and the 22nd day, the necrosis has been amply disposed of, and so the phagocytes recede. Therefore, following this reaction, in most animals no further infiltrates can be observed.

The few infiltrates which are still to be found consist for the most part of lymphocytes and after the 25th day, 100% are lymphocytes (Fig. 4). After the 40th day at the latest, no infiltrates are found. The intensity of the infiltrates in the second phase is essentially smaller than in the first phase.

Insulitis in experiments with EMC viruses (at least in part) shows a biphasic course. The first phase is to be considered as a nonspecific reaction to the lesion caused by the virus to dispose of, not to induce, necrosis. The second phase could be regarded as a sign of a specific reaction in the context of an immunological process. But the number of immunocompetent cells involved, as a rule, is so small that this factor can only be significant when there are a great deal of preliminary lesions of the islet tissue.

2. General Immunosuppression

To study the effect of general immunosuppression on the pathogenesis of EMC-virus-induced diabetes, artificial immunodeprived animals induced by x-irradiation, chemical immunosuppression, or neonatal thymectomy, as well as naturally occurring immunodeprived athymic mice, were examined. In all these experiments the manifestation of diabetes could be inhibited.

a. Sublethal x-Irradiation. In the first approach to demonstrating virus-induced immune reactions, highly susceptible mice were artificially immunodepressed by x-irradiation or with cyclophosphamide derivative. Six days following x-irradiation

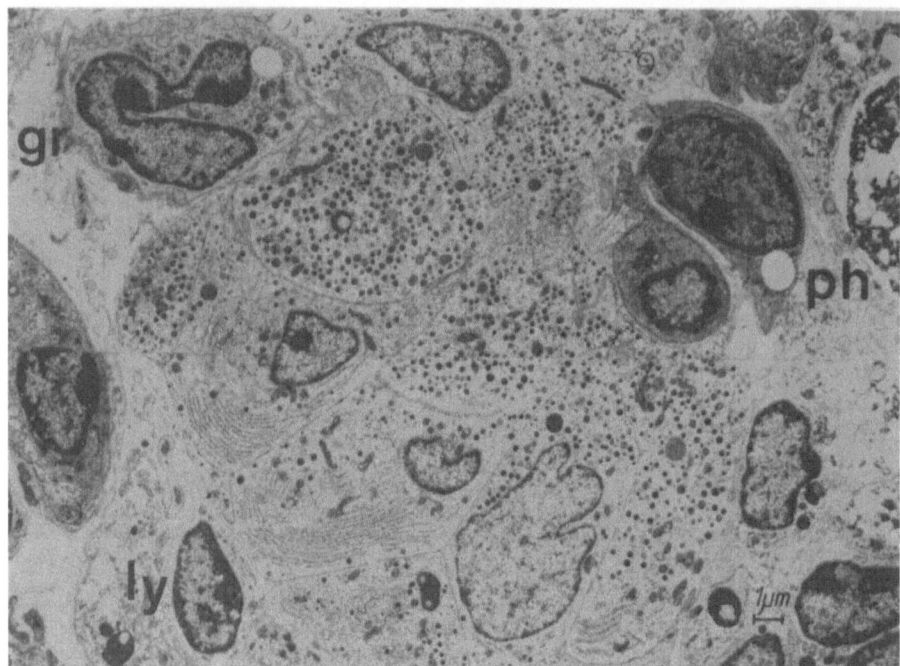

Figure 3. First phase of the EMC-virus-induced diabetes. In this early phase after virus inoculation there are inflammatory infiltrates composed mainly of phagocytes (ph) and less of granulocytes (gr) and lymphocytes (ly). Section from 12-week-old male DBA/2 mouse.

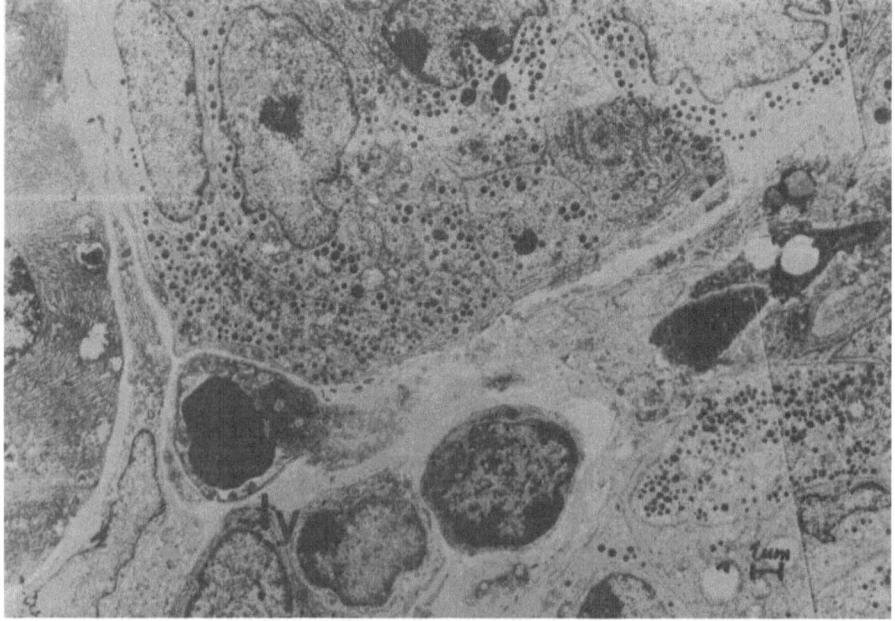

Figure 4. Late phase of the EMC-virus-induced diabetes. There are no necroses, only small inflammatory infiltrates composed exclusively of lymphocytes (ly). Section from 12-week-old male DBA/2 mouse.

with 500 R, infection with EMC virus did not lead to diabetes (Jansen *et al.*, 1977). The nonfasting mean glucose values were of the same order as those of untreated or irradiated controls, with values of about 169 ± 16 mg/100 ml. Infected, but not irradiated, positive controls showed pathological glucose levels of 286 ± 27 mg/100 ml (Fig. 5a).

This highly significant difference indicated that radiosensitive cells, probably of the immune system, are necessary for the establishment of the acute phase of virus-induced diabetes. A later phase of diabetes could not be studied, since irradiated infected mice showed a high mortality 1 week after infection.

b. Chemical Immunosuppression. With cyclophosphamide derivative, chemical immunosuppression was not able to inhibit diabetes. DBA/2 mice were infected and

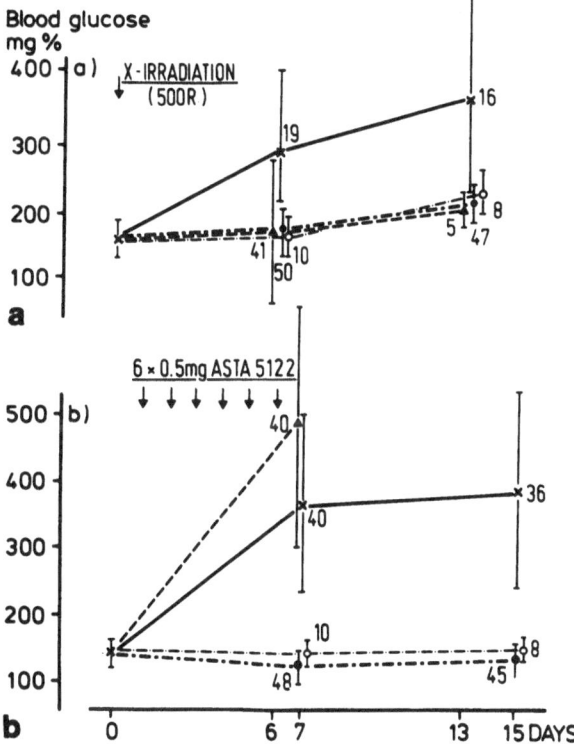

Figure 5. Virus-induced diabetes after immunosuppression. Blood glucose values are determined at weekly intervals after infection of immunosuppressed mice. (a) Immunosuppression consisted of 500-R x-irradiation a few hours before infection with EMC virus (▲ - - - ▲). A positive control group of normal mice was only infected (×———×). One negative control group received x-irradiation only (● · · · · - ●), another group was not treated at all (○ · · · · - - ○). (b) Beginning on a day of infection (▲ - - - - ▲), chemical immunosuppression was effected by six injections of 0.5 mg ASTA 5122, a cyclophosphamide derivative. A positive control group of normal mice received the virus dose only (×———×). One negative control group received the cyclophosphamide derivative only (● · · · · - ●) and another group was not treated at all (○ · · · · - ○).

treated with six daily injections of 0.5 mg ASTA 5122. No decrease in pathological glucose values could be noted on day 7 compared to untreated but infected controls (Fig. 5b).

These controversial results were explained by the fact that cyclophosphamide inhibits suppressor T lymphocytes, so that cytotoxic T lymphocytes are not inactivated during their destruction of B cells in the islets (Jansen et al., 1977).

c. Athymic Nude Mice. Nude mice, lacking the thymus and not able to effect T-cell-dependent immune reactions would be an ideal model to test the hypothesis. However, up to now no nude variants of the highly susceptible strains, in particular the DBA/2 strain, could be examined. So experiments were performed only with nude mice strains and their corresponding normal strains which are less susceptible to virus diabetes.

In a first approach Buschard et al. (1976) infected C 57B1/6 mice and their corresponding nude variants with EMC virus. The normal C57B1/6 mice, known to be relatively resistant to virus-induced diabetes, did not develop clinical diabetes. However a pathological glucose tolerance could be obtained at 30 and 60 min after the glucose load. In the corresponding nude mice, a normal glucose tolerance was maintained after infection, indicating that the immune system was necessary to obtain the pathological glucose tolerance.

In order to obtain more clear-cut findings for normal and nude mice, BALB/C nu/+ and BALB/C nu/nu mice bred by Bomholdgard were infected with different doses of virus (Jansen et al., 1979b). At an optimal virus dose, and after 7 days of viral infection, the normal BALB/C mice showed mean glucose values of about 400 mg/100 ml. The corresponding BALB/C nu/nu mice did not become diabetic at any virus dose tested, showing nonfasting mean glucose values between 100 and 120 mg/100 ml during the 2 weeks after infection.

These experiments were recently repeated using mice bred by Charles river, complemented by the additional examination of highly susceptible DBA/2 mice. This provided confirmation of the earlier results (Fig. 6a, b).

It was verified that viruses could be recovered from the pancreas of normal and nude mice. Normal mice produced high titers of neutralizing anitbodies against the virus, whereas nude mice showed low titers.

While insulitis occurred in the majority of normal mice it was almost lacking in nude mice. B cell necrosis was important in normal mice (up to 30 necroses per 100 islet cells), but it was less intense and not absent in nude mice, (maximally five necrosis per 100 islet cells) (Table 2).

The clear difference between highly diabetic mice with normal functioning immune system and normal glucose values in mice without a functioning immune system emphasizes the hypothesis of immune reactions. The explanation may be that the virus alone destroys only an insufficient number of B cells. However, if immunocytes are present in insulitis, they kill the remaining functioning B cells not containing cytocidal viruses, and diabetes manifests. Therefore only the combination of virus infection plus immune destruction may be able to eliminate a large enough number of B cells to induce diabetes. The morphological findings are, in principle, in agreement with this explanation. But the question remains unanswered as to whether necrosis or infiltrates

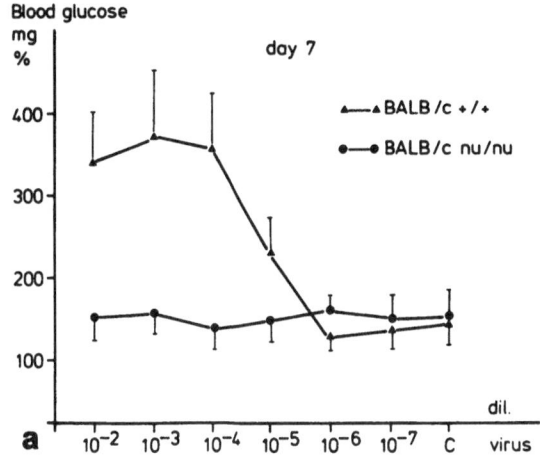

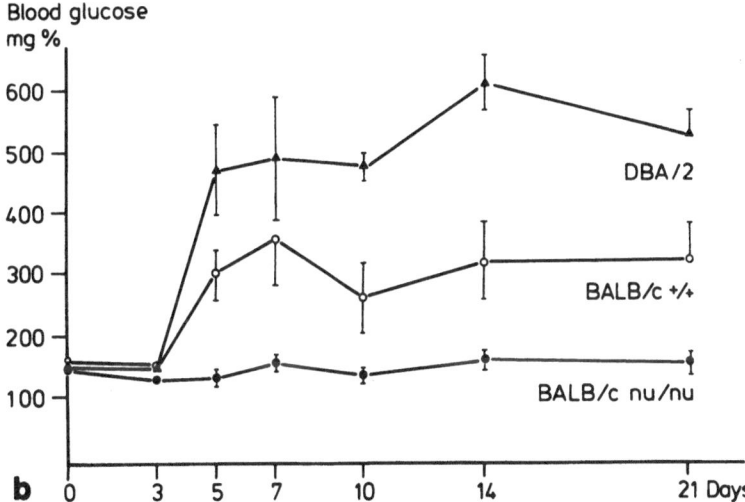

Figure 6. Different diabetogenic effect of EMC virus infection in nude and normal mice. (a) BALB/c +/+ and BALB/c nu/nu mice (bred by Charles River) were infected with different doses of virus and blood glucose concentrations determined on day 7 after infection. (b) DBA/2, BALB/c +/+, and BALB/c nu/nu mice (bred by Charles River) were infected with the optimal virus dose (10^{-3} diluted solution) and hyperglycemia tested over 21 days (solution: one heart of an EMC-virus-infected moribund mouse, homogenized and suspended in 1 ml Earl's medium).

are the leading phenomena in the virus-induced lesions. It would be, for example, also possible that the absence of diabetes in nude mice is a consequence of a change in virus kinetics.* In these animals, small numbers of islet cells are affected by virus and so the extent of necrosis will be smaller.

*Experiments in comparative virus kinetics are in progress.

Table 2.   Histologic Findings 6 Days after Infection of BALB/C nu/+ and nu/nu Mice

BALB/C mice	Insulitis				B cell necrosis				Blood/glucose (mg/100ml)	P
	N	0	+	++	0	(+)	+	++		
nu/+	26	6	13	7	0	2	19	5	296 ± 30	
nu/nu	30	21	7	2	2	28	0	0	115 ± 3	0.001

d. Neonatal Thymectomy.   (Miller, 1961; Miller and Osaba, 1967) prevents the development of T-cell-dependent cellular immunity while the function of B lymphocytes is relatively unimpaired. Thus the immunological status of neonatal thymectomized animals is similar to that of the naturally immunodeprived nude mice. The advantage of using these, as opposed to nude mice, is that a highly susceptible strain may be chosen for thymectomy. So the effects of neonatal thymectomy on hyperglycemia and insulitis after EMC infection in DBA/2 mice could be investigated (Petersen *et al.*, 1982). Male neonatal sham-operated controls and male neonatal thymectomized mice were infected by the M variant of EMC virus. Effectiveness of inoculation with EMC virus was confirmed by antibody titers in thymectomized mice and controls. Blood glucose was measured every second day. From the 4th day on male controls showed a significant increase in blood glucose, which was not observed in thymectomized mice (Fig. 7). Histological examination was performed on days 4 and 7 in two animals each of the thymectomized and control groups. Typical necroses and insulitis, identical to that well-known from untreated infected mice, were seen in sham-operated controls. Infected thymectomized mice showed no necrosis or insulitis on day 4. Only isolated necrotic cells, and only a very few or isolated mononuclear infiltrating cells within the otherwise intact islets of Langerhans on day 7 were observed.

The results show that, in DBA/2 mice, development of the typical EMC-virus-induced lesion in the islets of Langerhans with necroses and insulitis and subsequent hyperglycemia is prevented by neonatal thymectomy. Because the thymus regulates T lymphocytes, the development of diabetes after EMC virus infection must be related to events in which the thymus-dependent cell system participates.

3. Specific Activity of Sensitized T Lymphocytes

To test specific activity of sensitized lymphocytes attempts were made to *augment* a marginal diabetes by the *transfer* of well-characterized immunocompetent cells from infected animals and *to prevent* diabetes by *elimination* of specific immunocompetent cells with monoclonal antibodies in animals susceptible to the virus-induced diabetes.

a. Lymphocyte Transfer into Normal Mice.   Buchard (1978) reported a successful transfer of pathological glucose tolerance from infected C57B1/6 mice to normal mice of the same strain. Glucose levels increased in 30 min after the glucose load. In our hands transfer of overt diabetes from infected to normal mice has never been successful. Different experiments were undertaken with transfer of spleen cells from infected into normal mice, into sublethally x-irradiated mice, or into nude mice presenting no

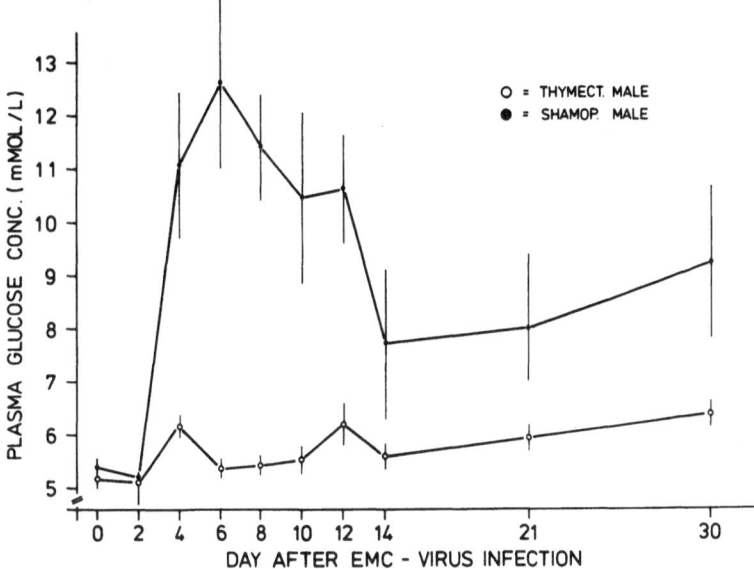

Figure 7. Blood glucose levels after EMC virus infection in thymectomized and sham operated male mice of the DBA/2 strain. Only in the sham operated group with a sufficient immune system did blood glucose levels rise in the expected manner.

suppressor lymphocytes. Even donor lymphocytes, stimulated by concanavalin A before transfer, did not induce diabetes. in one of these experiments a slight increase in nonfasting glucose level was obtained 7 days after transfer of sensitized live lymphocytes as compared to normal live or sensitized dead lymphocytes (Jansen, 1980). However, on day 10 blood glucose values decreased to normal levels and this experiment could not be reproduced.

The explanation for these results could be that lymphocytes directed only against B cells which are infected with virus will not find the corresponding antigen in noninfected B cells.

b. Lymphocyte Transfer into Suboptimally Infected Mice.   In a series of five experiments spleem lymphocytes from heavily diabetic DBA/2 mice were transferred into the peritoneum of suboptimally infected mice (Derocq *et al.,* 1982). By purifying the lymphocyte subpopulations it could be ensured that only the T cell and not the B cell subpopulation was able to enhance the appearance of diabetes. As seen in Fig. 8 total spleen lymphocytes as well as the T cell population augmented hyperglycemia while B lymphocytes or osmolyzed T lymphocytes did not.

c. Depletion of T Lymphocytes in Vivo.   Complementary to the augmentation of hyperglycemia by transfer of lymphocytes, which could be repeatedly obtained in infected recipients, the prevention of hyperglycemia could be obtained in the opposite experiment, consisting of the depletion of T cells *in vivo* by application of antibodies against the thy 1,2 marker (Derocq *et al.,* 1982). DBA/2 mice were injected with a

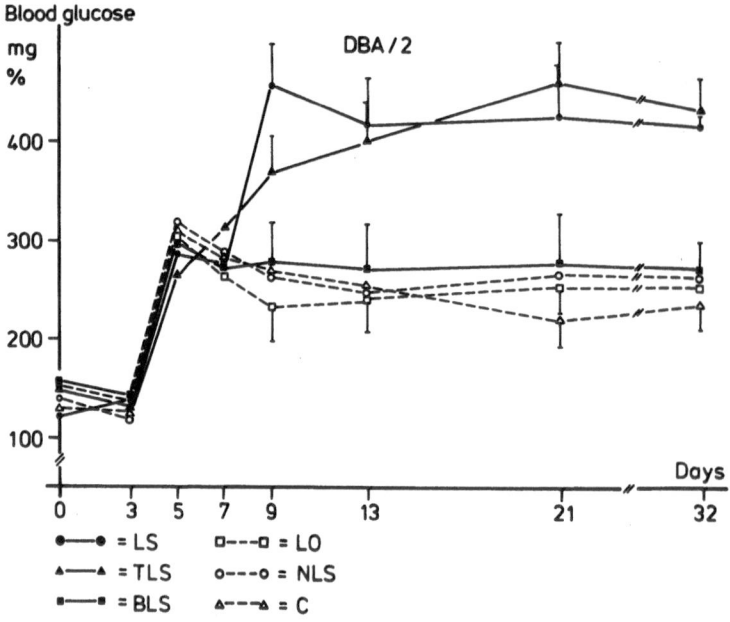

Figure 8. Transfer of sensitized lymphocytes into suboptimally infected mice. DBA/2 recipient mice (10 per group) were infected with a suboptimal virus dose (10^{-5} diluted solution) 6 days before transfer. They then received 10^8 total lymphocytes or 40×10^6 T or B lymphocytes from donor animals infected with a high virus dose 6 days before. Control groups received normal lymphocytes, salt solution, or sensitized total lymphocytes lysed by 1/10 dilution PBS.

monoclonal IgM antibody plus guinea pig complement 4 and 2 days before, as well as 3 and 5 days after, the EMC virus infection. They did not develop diabetes, while mice without treatment or with injections of complement alone showed a long-lasting diabetes with hyperglycemia of 350–400 mg/100 ml (Fig. 9).

The twofold proof of the influence of T lymphocytes on diabetes in the infected animal confirms the idea that both the virus infections and immunopathological reactions are necessary for the pathogenesis of diabetes.

IV. CRITICAL EVALUATION

The occurrence of a number of different putative autoimmune conditions in human insulin-dependent diabetics, especially the association of the disease with distinct HLA types and the occasional finding of multiple endocrinopathies in such patients, seems to be compelling evidence for an immunological component in the pathogenesis of the disease. Hypothetically this could be a cell-mediated or a humoral immune process, probably occurring as a phenomenon initiated by a sensitizing insult to the B cells of the islets of Langerhans such as might result from an infection or chemical injury. But at the present time concrete evidence supporting such a process is lacking.

Experimental studies have been undertaken to establish an environmental factor as a mechanism accounting for the initiation of the lesion on one hand, and to establish an immunologic basis for the development of an insulin-dependent diabetes on the other hand.

Because it has long been suspected that some cases of insulin-dependent diabetes might have a viral etiology, it seemed reasonable to choose models with a virus infection as the initial lesion.

Interestingly, in the model reported by Like and Rossini, which uses streptozotocin to produce an initial lesion, viruses were found unexpectedly. These type-C viruses certainly do not play any part in the disease of humans; our studies of the sera of 200 freshly diagnosed juvenile diabetics gave no indication of an infection with type-C viruses. However, in the animal experimental model, where the morphological findings in the islets bear a great resemblance to insulitis in humans with early-onset diabetes, the viruses do seem to have some significance. It is to be hoped that further experiments will succeed in clarifying whether, as we postulate, repeated applications of streptozotocin do initiate an autoimmune process, and if so, what part the viruses take in this.

The model of virus-induced diabetes with polyendocrinopathy and autoimmunity, reported by Onodera et al. (1981; 1982), as the most recent model, still leaves many

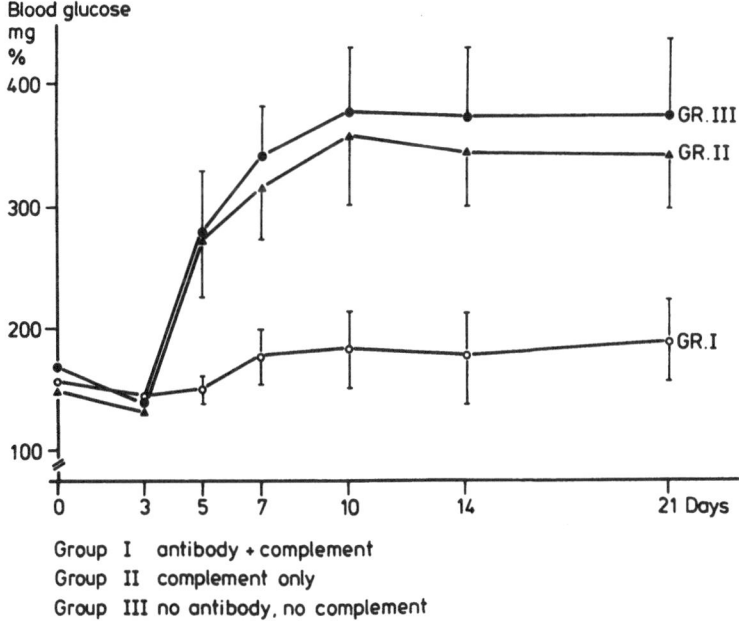

Group I   antibody + complement
Group II   complement only
Group III no antibody, no complement

Figure 9. Prevention of EMC virus diabetes by T lymphocyte depletion *in vivo*. DBA/2 mice (groups of 10 animals) were injected with 1 mg IgM anti-Thy 1,2 monoclonal mouse antibody plus 0.1 ml guinea pig complement on days -4, -2, 0, $+3$, and $+5$. One control group received the complement only, while another group was not treated with antibody or complement. All mice were infected with the 10^{-3} diluted virus solution on day 0 and hyperglycemia followed over 21 days.

questions unanswered, particularly, whether the insulitis as described until now can be taken as a sign of a cell-mediated immunity, and what part in the pathogenesis of the disease is played by the autoantibodies. The most interesting finding in this model until now is that a special gene segment (S 1) is required for the induction of autoantibodies to growth hormone and insulin. How the reovirus type 1 induces autoantibody formation, is however, still an open question. It remains to be clarified, in this respect, whether the virus, or parts of it, is involved in the immunogenic substance or whether the fabric of the cells destroyed by viruses is in itself an effective autoantigen.

In the event of the successful solution to these questions this model may serve as an experimental example for the disease of the small group of patients, who, besides having insulin-dependent diabetes, also experience a more generalized polyendocrine disorder and have autoantibodies in their sera that react with other hormone-producing cells, for example, thyroid, gastric mucosa, adrenal, and pituitary.

Most notably, the diabetes mellitus of mice in the EMC virus model demonstrates in the genetically susceptible host of juvenile-type-diabetes state. From the results of the different experiments utilizing general immunosuppression and the specific activity of sensitized lymphocytes, there is evidence that one side of the pathogenesis of the virus-induced disease is related to events in which T lymphocytes participate. This may be mediated by different mechanisms. Firstly, T-cell-mediated cytotoxicity directed against antigens of the virus and the surface of the B cells might induce autoaggressive insulitis. EMC virus, however, has no envelope structures that could enter the cytomembrane and therefore does not produce antigens on the cell surface, as do, for example, herpes simplex or lymphocytic choriomeningitis virus. So the presumed absence of viral antigens on the cell surface seems to exclude a direct T-lymphocyte-mediated cytotoxicity. This view, however, does not take into account, that B cells differ from other cells in having emiocytosis by which vesicle structures containing viral antigen become part of the cytomembrane, thus stimulating the immune response.

Secondly the protective effect of neonatal thymectomy and depletion of T lymphocytes could be due to a depression of lymphocyte–macrophage interaction, probably involving a lack of lymphokines as "migration inhibiting factor" and "macrophage arming factor." Therefore a macrophage-mediated aggression against B cells might be inhibited. The absence of macrophage accumulation in the islets of nude and neonatal thymectomized mice on the 4th day after EMC virus infection could be consistent with such a mechanism. The morphological findings in the pancreas of the immunologically intact animals, which appear during the course of the virus-induced lesion are compatible with the hypothesis of a T-cell-mediated cytotoxicity or a macrophage-mediated aggression against the B cells or parts of them. It must, however, be emphasized that the small intensity and the always transitory nature of the inflammatory infiltrates provide evidence against a classic immunological type IV reaction as a cause of the diabetes.

If there is a T-cell-mediated or a macrophage-mediated cytotoxicity involved at all then certainly it is only in the sense that only a few cells remaining after the initial damage are destroyed by them. Thus, a great deal of preliminary damage by the virus itself is necessary.

Therefore, further experiments must clarify whether the undoubted significance of the thymus-dependent immune system for the EMC virus model should not be sought instead in quite different mechanisms, such as an influence of virus kinetics or other interactions between viruses and the immune system.

Studies of the human pancreas in juvenile-type diabetes have not yet uncovered any proof of the lymphocytic infiltration well-known from other diseases that are definitely mediated by T cells.

The insulitis found in those cases with a rapid course corresponds in its intensity and cell composition to the insulitis of the EMC-model. For this reason a classic immunological type IV reaction is not to be expected in humans.

REFERENCES

Appel, M. C., Rossini, A. A., Williams, R. M., and Like, A. A., 1978, Viral studies in streptozotocin-induced pancreatic insulitis, *Diabetologia* **15**: 327–336.

Barboni, E., and Manocchio, I., 1962, Alterazionia pancreatiche in bovini con diabète mellito post-aftoso, *Arch. Vet. Ital.* **13**:477–89.

Boucher, D. W., and Notkins, A. L., 1973, Virus-induced diabetes mellitus: I. Hyperglycemia and hypoinsulinemia in mice infected with encephalomyocarditis virus, *J. Exp. Med.* **137**:1226–39.

Burch, G. E., Tsui, C. Y., Harb, J. M., and Colcolough, H. L., 1971, Pathologic findings in the pancreas of mice infected with Coxsackie B4, *Arch, Intern. Med.* **128**:40–47.

Buschard, K., 1978, Passive transfer of virus induced diabetes mellitus with spleen cells, *Acta Pathol. Microbiol. Scand. [C]* **86**:29–32.

Buschard, K., Rygaard, J., and Lund, E., 1976, The inability of a diabetogenic virus to induce diabetes mellitus in athymic (nude) mice, *Acta Pathol. Microbiol. Scand. [C]* **84**:299–303.

Coleman, T. J., Gamble, D. R., and Taylor, K. W., 1973, Diabetes in mice after Coxsackie B4 virus infection, *Br. Med. J.* **3**:25–27.

Coleman, T. J., Taylor, K. W., and Gamble, D. R., 1974, The development of diabetes following Coxsackie B virus infection in mice, *Diabetologia* **10**:755–759.

Craighead, J. E., 1975, The role of viruses in the pathogenesis of pancreatic disease and diabetes mellitus, *Prog. Med. Virol.* **19**:161–214.

Craighead, J. E., and Higgins, D. A., 1974, Genetic influences affecting the occurrence of a diabetes mellitus-like disease in mice infected with the encephalomyocarditis virus, *J. Exp. Med.* **139**:414–26.

Craighead, J. E., and McLane, M. F., 1968, Diabetes mellitus: Induction in mice by encephalomyocarditis virus, *Science* **162**:913–914.

Craighead, J. E., and Steinke, J., 1971, Diabetes mellitus-like syndrome in mice infected with encephalomyocarditis virus, *Am. J. Pathol.* **63**:119–30.

Derocq, J. M., Müntefering, H., and Jansen, F. K., 1982, Influence du système immunitaire dans le diabète viroinduit de la souris (submitted).

Friedman, S. F., Grota, L. J., and Glasgow, L. A., 1972, Differential susceptibility of male and female mice to encephalomyocarditis virus: Effects of castration, adrenalectomy, and the administration of sex hormones, *Infect. Immun.* **5**:637–644.

Goldberg, S. L., Kochicheril, N. M., Schulman, R., Walker, G. F., and Rayfield, E. J., 1978, Venezuelan encephalitis virus-induced defects in carbohydrate metabolism in genetically diabetic mice. *Diabetes* **27(Suppl. 2)**:477.

Harrison, A. K., Bauer, S. P., and Murphy, F. A., 1972, Viral pancreatitis: Ultra-structural pathological effects of Coxsackie virus B3 infection in newborn mouse pancreas, *Exp. Mol. Pathol.* **17**:206–219.

Hayashi, K., Boucher, D. W., and Notkins, A. L., 1974, Virus-induced diabetes mellitus. II. Relationship between beta cell damage and hyperglycemia in mice infected with encephalomyocarditis virus, *Am. J. Pathol.* **75**:91–102.

Jansen, F. K., 1980, The possible relationship between viral infection and autoimmunity, in: *Immunology of Diabetes* (J. Irvine, ed.), pp. 243–254, Teviot Scientific Publications, Edinburgh.

Jansen, F. K., Müntefering, H., and Schmidt, W. A. K., 1977, Virus induced diabetes and the immune system. I. Suggestion that appearance of diabetes depends on immune reactions, *Diabetologia* **13**:545–549.

Jansen, F. K., Müntefering, H., Thurneyssen, O., and Derocq, J. M., 1979a, Possible interaction between viral infection and autoimmunity, in: *Diabetes, International Congress Series No. 500, Diabetes 1979, Proceedings of the 10th Congress of the International Diabetes Federation,* Vienna, Austria, Sept. 9-14, 1979, (W. K. Waldhäusl ed.), pp. 373–378, Excerpta Medica, Amsterdam.

Jansen, F. K., Thurneyssen, O., and Müntefering, H., 1979b, Virus induced diabetes and the immune system II—Evidence for an immune pathogenesis of the acute phase of diabetes, *Biomedicine* **31**:1–2.

Lang, C. M., and Munger, B. L., 1976, Diabetes mellitus in the guinea pig, *Diabetes* **25**:434–43.

Like, A. A., and Rossini, A. A., 1976, Streptozotocin-induced pancreatic insulitis: New model of diabetes mellitus, *Science* **193**:415–17.

Menser, M. A., Forrest, J. M., Bransby, R. D., 1978, Rubella infection and diabetes mellitus, *Lancet* **1**:57–60.

Miller, J. F. A. P., 1961, Immunological function of the thymus, *Lancet* **2**:748–749.

Miller, J. F. A. P., Osoba, D., 1967, Current concepts of immunological function of the thymus, *Physiol. Rev.* **47**:437–520.

Müntefering, H., 1972, Zur Pathologie des Diabetes Mellitus der weißen Muas bei der EMC-Virusinfektion. Histologische, elektronenmikroskopische und quantitativmorphologische Befunde an den Langerhansschen Inseln, *Virchows Arch.* [Pathol. Anat.] **356**:207–234.

Müntefering, H., Schmidt, W. A. K., and Körber, W., 1971, Zur Virusgenese des Diabetes Mellitus bei der weißen Maus, *Dtsch. Med. Wochenschr.* **96**:693–697.

Müntefering, H., Schmitz, W., Jansen, F. K., and Petersen, K. G., 1979, The role of transitory insulitis in the pathogenesis of experimental virus-diabetes, *International Congress series No. 500, Diabetes 1979, Proceedings of the 10th Congress of the International Diabetes Federation,* Vienna, Austria, Sept. 9–14, 1979, (W. K. Wandäusl ed.), pp. 395–401, Excerpta Medica, Amsterdam.

Munger, B. L., and Lang, C. M., 1973, Spontaneous diabetes mellitus in guinea pigs: The acute cytopathology of the islets of Langerhans, *Lab. Invest.* **29**:285–702.

Onodera, T., Jenson, A. B., Yoon, J. W., and Notkins, A. L., 1978, Virus-induced diabetes mellitus: Reovirus infection of pancreatic β cells in mice, *Science* **201**:529–531.

Onodera, T., Toniolo, A., Ray, U. R., Jenson, A. B., Knazek, R. A., and Notkins, A. L., 1981, Virus-induced diabetes mellitus. XX. Polyendocrinopathy and autoimmunity *J. Exp. Med.* **153**:1457–1473.

Onodera, T., Ray, U. R., Melez, K. A., Suzuki, H., Toniolo, A., and Notkins, A. L., 1982, Virus-induced diabetes mellitus: Autoimmunity and polyendocrine disease prevented by immunosuppression, *Nature* **297**:66–68.

Petersen, K. G., Müntefering, H., Schmidt, W. A. K., Schlüter, K., Kasemir, H., Treiber, A., Herbst, D., and Kerp, L., 1982, Prevention of EMC virus induced diabetes of mice of neonatal thymectomy, (accepted by *Diabetologia*).

Prince, G. A., Jenson, A. B., Billups, L. C., and Notkins, A. L., 1978, Infection of human pancreatic beta cell cultures with mumps virus, *Nature* **271**:158–161.

Rayfield, E. J., and Seto, Y., 1978, Viruses and the pathogenesis of diabetes mellitus, *Diabetes* **27**:1126–1142.

Robertson, J. S., 1954, The pancreatic lesion in adult mice infected with a strain of pleurodynia virus. I. Electron microscopical observations, *Aust. J. Exp. Biol. Med. Sci.* **32**:393–409.

Rossini, A. A., Like, A. A., Chick, W. L., Appel, M. C., and Cahill, G. F., 1977, Studies of streptozotocin-induced insulitis and diabetes, *Proc. Natl. Acad. Sci. USA* **74**:2485–2489.

Tsui, C. Y., Burch, G. E., and Harb, J. M., 1972, Pancreatitis in mice infected with Coxsackie B1, *Arch. Pathol.* **93**:379–389.

Wellmann, K. F., Amsterdam, D., Brancato, P., and Volk, P. W., 1972, Fine structure of pancreatic islets of mice infected with the M variant of the encephalomyocarditis virus, *Diabetologia* **8**:349–357.

Yoon, J -W., and Notkins, A. L., 1976, Virus-induced diabetes mellitus. VI. Genetically determined host differences in the replication of encephalomyocarditis virus in pancreatic beta cells, *J. Exp. Med.* **143**:1170–1185.

4

Animal Models of Human Type I Diabetes

Ali Naji and Clyde F. Barker

I. APPLICABILITY OF ANIMAL MODELS OF DIABETES

Experimental and clinical evidence indicates that human diabetes is not a single disease, but a heterogeneous group of syndromes having hyperglycemia as the common denominator (Fajans *et al.*, 1978; Rotter and Rimoin., 1981; Nerup and Lernmark, 1981; Rizza *et al.*, 1981). The diabetic syndromes in animals are similarly complex and include a broad spectrum of pathophysiology. Since hyperglyemic states in animals may or may not parallel the human diseases, (which are themselves ill-defined), animal syndromes should not be expected to serve as exact "models" of various types of diabetes in humans. However, they can be used to simulate certain genotypic or phenotypic expressions that may have a role in human diabetes. The availability of nondiabetic animals of genetic makeup similar or identical to their diabetic counterparts constitutes an important resource for diabetes research because these nondiabetic control animals can be used for physiological comparisons as well as tissue transplantation studies.

Spontaneous diabetes in animals of various species has been known for many years to be relatively common (Cameron *et al.*, 1972; Renold *et al.*, 1974). Diabeteslike syndromes can also be induced in animals by pancreatectomy, chemical destruction of beta cells (Dulin and Soret, 1979), viral infection (Craighead, 1981), hormonal antagonism of insulin action (Volk and Wellmann, 1979), and immunologic mechanisms which inactivate insulin or destroy pancreatic islets (Toreson *et al.*, 1968). The study of animal diabetes offers several distinct advantages over the study of the disease in humans. Animals are suitable for manipulation of important etiologic factors (genetic, environmental, and immunologic) which would not be feasible in hu-

Ali Naji and Clyde F. Barker • Department of Surgery, School of Medicine, University of Pennsylvania, Philadelphia, Pennsylvania 19104

mans. The use of relatively short-lived rodents allows the study of many generations in a short period of time facilitating genetic studies involving controlled breeding which would be impossible in humans. Animal colonies permit control of environmental factors of possible etiologic significance, such as diet, drugs, toxins, and infectious agents, while ethical as well as practical considerations prevent such research in human subjects. The known and stable incidence of diabetes in some inbred animal colonies affords a powerful tool for assessment of possible preventive therapies for the disease. Provocation of human diabetes is, of course, not permissible and consequently the effectiveness and reliability of new treatments to prevent or reverse the disease must first be established in experimental animals. The short life span of rodents is also ideal for investigation of pathogenesis and complications of the disease. Since diabetes is a chronic disease in humans, defining the underlying pathology of its complications would require serial studies over many years. Therefore, relatively little information is ever obtained from any one patient. Since insulin therapy prevents early deaths pathological data are very rarely obtained in the acute phases of the human illness, when it would be of greatest interest. Study of animal models is useful for all of these reasons.

The human type I diabetes mellitus (insulin-dependent, ketosis-prone, juvenile-onset) is currently defined by an absolute deficiency of insulin and is caused by severe β cell lesions and necrosis. The major focus of this chapter will be on several recently described and extensively studied diabetic syndromes in animals which mimic human Type I diabetes. We will deal with both experimentally induced and spontaneous insulin deficiency states and with the underlying pathology of the pancreatic islets. Special emphasis will be placed on the immune system and its role in the insulitis lesion which appears to be present in the human disease as well as in several of the most pertinent animal models.

II. EXPERIMENTALLY INDUCED DIABETES

A. Chemical Agents

The use of chemical agents to induce diabetes permits detailed study of the biochemical, hormonal, and morphologic events occurring at the time of induction of a diabetic state and thereafter. The two most commonly used chemical agents producing hyperglycemia by their beta cell specific toxicity are alloxan and streptozotocin.

1. Alloxan

Alloxan is a pyrimidine with structural similarities to uric acid and glucose (Dulin and Soret, 1979). When inoculated it has a half-life in the blood stream of approximately 1 min. Alloxan can produce diabetes in several species such as rat, dog, cat, and mouse but the guinea pig and chicken are resistant to its diabetogenic action. In humans, alloxan has been administered to relieve the hypoglycemia in patients with islet cell tumors. There is evidence that it causes destruction of normal pancreatic islets while exerting no significant effect on malignant islet cell tumors. The mechanism by which alloxan induces beta cell destruction is apparently an extracellular process, which results in increasing the membrane permeability of islet cells (to which it binds instantly) culminating in inhibition of the insulin secretory mechanism (Cooperstein and Lazarow, 1964). That the action of alloxan may be at the glucose receptor site on the beta cell membrane is supported by the observation that glucose can protect against the diabetogenic effect of alloxan and that alloxan blocks glucose-stimulated insulin release (Tomita et al., 1974). Administration of alloxan results in a triphasic blood sugar response (Dulin and Soret, 1979). There is an initial mild hyperglycemia lasting 2–4 hr after injection followed by marked hypoglycemia (due to beta cell lysis) and increased plasma insulin in 12 hr and finally after 24 hr a permanent hyperglycemia with low levels of plasma insulin.

The earliest histological changes in islets of Langerhans of rats and rabbits were noted within 5 min after administration of alloxan (Dulin and Soret, 1979). These were loss of granules from beta cells associated with cytoplasmic fragmentation. Within 15 minutes there is damage to the nuclei of most beta cells. Several months after alloxan administration, islets are decreased in size with few beta cells but relatively normal alpha cells. No insulitis or circulating islet cell antibodies are observed after alloxan administration. The metabolic events of alloxan-induced diabetes are insulinopenia, increased gluconeogenesis and glycogenolysis, increased protein catabolism, and hyperlipidemia (Grodsky et al., 1982).

2. Streptozotocin

This is a 2-deoxy-2-(3 methyl-3-nitrosourea)-d-glucopyranose with antitumoral, oncogenic, and antibacterial as well as diabetogenic properties. It induces irreversible damage to beta cells within 24 hr with a triphasic blood glucose response similar to alloxan (Dulin and Soret, 1979). Therefore, the metabolic effects result from hypoinsulinemia with marked reduction of both plasma and pancreatic insulin content. It has been observed that nicotinamide inhibits the diabetogenic activity of streptozotocin and reverses its effect if given prior to its administration (Anderson et al., 1974). Thus, it is suggested that streptozotocin may act by decreasing the levels of nicotine adenine dinucleotide (NAD) within the beta cells either by decreasing its synthesis or increasing its breakdown. The nitrosourea moiety of streptozotocin can produce beta cell necrosis and diabetes as well as reduce islet NAD levels. Therefore, it is believed that this portion provides the cytotoxic effect of the compound and the 2-deoxyglucose confers specificity for the beta cells.

The earliest morphological changes after streptozotocin injection occur at 1 hr and include hypertrophy of Golgi apparatus and occasional pyknosis of nuclei of beta cells (Dulin and Soret, 1979). By 24 hr after streptozotocin injection in most species the beta cell destruction is essentially complete. In most species the alpha and D cells are not significantly affected by streptozotocin. In long-term examination the islets in streptozotocin-treated animals are small in size and contain infrequent beta cells and large numbers of alpha cells. A single large dose of streptozotocin that induces diabetes does not produce mononuclear infiltration of pancratic islets (insulitis), and an immune response to the agent when given in this manner apparently has no role in islet cell destruction.

3. Streptozotocin-Induced Insulitis

Streptozotocin is customarily administered as a single dose to induce diabetes in the experimental recipients. However, if streptozotocin is injected in multiple (five) subdiabetogenic doses (no one of which alone is diabetogenic) it produces a delayed but progressive loss of beta cells and hyperglycemia associated with intense pancreatic insulitis (Like and Rossini, 1976). The effect is both sex- and strain-dependent. Thus, when randomly bred CD-1 male mice were treated with "low" doses of streptozotocin (40 mg/kg of body weight) daily for 5 days, severe diabetes and insulitis were produced within 5–6 days after the last streptozotocin injection. In addition to insulitis, electron microscopy indicated the appearance and induction of endogenous type C viruses within pancreatic beta cells (Appel et al., 1978). In general, males are more susceptible to development of diabetes than females and the suceptibility of the males decreases upon castration (Rossini et al., 1978). In order to study the importance of genetic background and the contribution of the major histocompatibility complex (MHC) to development of insulitis and diabetes, several mouse strains of different H-2 haplotype have been studied (Rossini et al., 1977). Of eight inbred mouse strains tested, only C57BL/KSJ which are H-2^d at the MHC developed diabetes and insulitis comparable in severity to that observed in the outbred CD-1 mice. Other mice of the H-2^d haplotype were noted to have only mild insulitis with minimal elevation of blood glucose. Moreover, in recent studies by Kromann et al., (1982) the development of diabetes and insulitis did not differ in four congenic resistant lines of mice on the C57BL/10 (susceptible strain) genetic background, indicating that MHC genes are not likely to determine susceptibility to the streptozotocin-induced insulitis model of diabetes.

The development of insulitis and the appearance of type C viruses in beta cells suggest that a cell-mediated immune pathogenesis may be involved in this diabetic model. Moreover, the finding that administration of rabbit antimouse lymphocyte serum leads to effective protection of mice from streptozotocin-induced insulitis and diabetes also argues in favor of an immune etiology (Rossini et al., 1977). Therefore, it has been hypothesized that in susceptible hosts, a triad of direct beta cell cytotoxicity, virus induction within beta cells, and cell-mediated autoimmune reactions are operative to induce diabetes.

In an attempt to transfer the postulated (auto) immune diabetes, Buschard and Rygaard (1978) inoculated spleen cells from multiple-dose streptozotocin-induced diabetic donors to naive syngeneic and allogeneic recipients and reported appearance of hyperglycemia in the recipients. However, in similar studies by other investigators these findings have not been substantiated. Rossini et al., (1980), using various experimental protocols, such as parabiosis experiments and passive transfer of T lymphocytes from diabetic donors, failed to induce either hyperglycemia or insulitis.

Paik et al., (1980) studied the obligatory etiologic role of thymic function in the development of streptozotocin-induced insulitis in athymic nude (nu/nu) and euthymic heterozygous (+/nu) littermates of BALB/c mice. They reported that only the thymus competent +/nu and not the nu/nu mice developed diabetes as a result of multiple subdiabetogenic doses of streptozotocin. Restoration of the thymic immunity in nu/nu mice by thymus grafts from +/nu mice restored the susceptibility to diabetes.

The role of inbred background, sex, and thymus in susceptibility of low-dose streptozotocin-induced diabetes and insulitis in C57BL mice has also been examined by Leiter (1982). In this study the effect of neonatal thymectomy on the subsequent susceptibility of the C57BL/KsJ (susceptible strain) mice to low-dose streptozotocin-induced insulitis and diabetes was examined. Neonatal thymectomy of C57BL/KsJ mice failed to block the susceptibility of the males to induction of diabetes and insulitis. Females (both thymus-intact and thymectomized) were less susceptible than males to hyperglycemia but displayed an equally severe insulitis. Therefore, the detection of an underlying insulitis was not necessarily predictive of severe hyperglycemia. The role of the thymus, and therefore the obligatory role of T-effector-cell-mediated immunity, in susceptibility to low-dose streptozotocin-induced insulitis and diabetes was also investigated in C57B1/6J NICrOu (nu/nu) mice and their euthymic normal (+/?) littermates. The genetically athymic C57BL/6J nu/nu males and their thymus-intact +/? littermate controls were susceptible to low-dose streptozotocin-induced hyperglycemia but resistant to insulitis, the implications being that presence of severe hyperglycemia after low-dose streptozotocin treatment cannot necessarily be correleated with underlying insulitis.

In summary, to what extent the beta call damage induced by multiple subdiabetogenic doses of streptozotocin is due to direct cytotoxic action of the drug or to a cell-mediated immune process remains unclear. However, it seems clear that the diabetogenic effect of multiple low-dose streptozotocin is, at least in part, dependent on simple beta cell toxicity of the cumulative total dose given but also that some additional interaction between streptozotocin and the beta cells (which results in the insulitis) is also a prerequisite in the pathogenesis. The following transplantation experiment also provides evidence of this.

When syngeneic islets were transplanted into healthy C57BL/Ks mice prior to induction of streptozotocin insulitis, the transplanted islets suffered the same destruction by insulitis as observed in the hosts' native islets. However, when islets were transplanted 4 days after the last of five streptozotocin injections, they were not destroyed as the host islets had been but were able to ameliorate the streptozotocin-induced diabetes (Sandler and Andersson, 1981).

B. Virus-Induced Diabetes

The etiologic role of viruses in pathogenesis of human diabetes (Chapter 10) as well as virally induced diabetic syndromes in various experimental animals (Chapter 3) has been detailed in other chapters.

III. SPONTANEOUS DIABETES

Animals with spontaneous diabetes can be classified into two categories. The first group consists of animals in which the occurrence of hyperglycemia is associated with obesity, hyperphagia, hyperinsulinemia, peripheral insulin resistance, and reduced number of insulin receptors in various tissues, for example, C57BL/6J, ob/ob or C57/KsJ, db/db mice (Coleman, 1982). These animals provide genotypic and pheno-

Table 1.   Characteristics of Some Animals with Spontaneous Diabetes

Animals	Obesity	Plasma insulin	Pancreatic insulin	Insulitis	Ketosis
Yellow mouse	+	High	High	—	—
Obese mouse	+				
C57BL/6J, ob/ob		Early, high	High	—	—
C57BL/K₅J, db/db	+	Early, high; late, low	Early, high; late, low	—	—
KK mouse	+	High	High	—	—
T-KK mouse	+	High	High	—	—
Wellesley hybrid					
mouse (C₃hf×I)	+	High	High	—	—
Spiny mouse					
(Acomys cahirinus)	+	Normal to low	Very high	—	Rarely
NOD mouse	—	Low	Low	+	+ +
Chinese hamster					
(Cricetulus griseus)	—	Normal to low	Low	—	+
South African hamster					
(Mystromys alb.)	—	?	Low	—	+
BB rat	—	Very low	Very low	+	+ + +
Sand rat					
(Psammomys obesus)	+	High	Occasionally low	—	Rarely
New Zealand					
white rabbit	—	Low	?	—	—
Keeshond dog	—	Low	Low	—	+
Celebes black ape	—	Low	Low	—	—

typic expressions reminiscent of maturity onset (insulin-independent) human diabetes and as such are useful to our understanding of the nature of gene–host interaction in such disorders. However, since they seem to be models of human type II rather than type I diabetes they will not be discussed here (Chapter 5).

The second group, to which this discussion is limited, consists of nonobese animals with spontaneous hyperglycemia in association with insulin deficiency, low pancreatic insulin secretion (with attendant beta cell destruction), ketosis, and no peripheral insulin resistance. Table 1 provides an outline of some of the characteristics of animal models with spontaneous diabetes.

A. Chinese Hamster (Cricetulus Griseus)

Meier and Yerganian (1959) reported spontaneous development of diabetes in their Chinese hamster colony after four to five generations of inbreeding. Since 1963, a concerted inbreeding program has been carried out in the Upjohn Company's colony of Chinese hamsters, which were derived from Dr. Yerganian's animals (Gerritsen, 1982). A program of brother–sister mating and selection for diabetes has resulted in generation of six inbred sublines of Chinese hamsters that have an incidence of glycosuria close to 100%. In addition, two inbred nonglycosuric sublines have been derived that are virtually free of diabetes. The Chinese hamster is a nonobese model. Of particular interest have been studies of animals in the prediabetic stage, that is, individuals known to be genetically diabetic but which at the time of study are phenotypically nondiabetic. The onset of appearance of glycosuria varies from 2 weeks to 4 months of age and the onset of ketonuria usually occurs several months after the onset of glycosuria or within 6–12 months of age. There is variation in the phenotypic expression of the disease among the various diabetic sublines with respect to the time of the onset of glycosuria, ketonuria, blood glucose, and plasma insulin. In general, diabetic sublines are characterized by mild hyperglycemia (150–200 mg/dl) but hybrid lines from pure-bred parents may show severe hyperglycemia and ketosis more consistently. The pancreatic insulin levels are consistently low in all diabetic sublines as compared with nondiabetics. Conversely, pancreatic glucagon is elevated and alpha cells show ultratructural alterations of membrane systems.

Pancreatic islets of the spontaneously diabetic Chinese hamsters display several abnormalities of the beta cells. Although not a characteristic feature, very occasionally in early stages minimal lymphocytic infiltration has been reported in islets of diabetic Chinese hamsters soon after the onset of the disease (Boquist, 1979). However, at the onset of overt symptoms of the disease, the most notable changes in the islets are the degranulation of beta cells and hydropic changes such as cytoplasmic vacuolation and deposition of glycogen masses (Like, 1979).

The diabetic syndrome is considered to be the result of a polygenic inheritance with at least four genes involved. Experimental breeding data indicate the requirement of a minimum of two homozygous recessive genes for development of diabetes. Whether the inbred diabetic lines are of similar diabetic genotype is not known, and there is a high probability that modifier background genes may vary in members of different sublines (Gerritsen, 1982).

The pathogenesis of diabetes in Chinese hamsters appears to be related to an increased demand for insulin. Soon after birth there is a compensatory response on the part of beta cells by an increase in their number and size. However, this response of beta cells to the continuous demand for insulin is not sufficient and functional exhaustion occurs followed by gradual decrease in the beta cell mass (Gerritsen, 1982).

There is dramatic correlation between the nutrition and caloric restriction on the prevention or retardation of onset of hyperglycemia and ketonuria in prediabetic Chinese hamsters (perhaps by reducing insulin demand). Therefore, this model is particularly useful in study of the effect of nutrition in nonobese diabetes.

Diabetes in the Chinese hamster is a progressively severe condition and several late-onset morphologic changes in the kidney, nerve, blood vessels, eyes, brain, and genitourinary systems have been reported. In kidney, a thickening of glomerular capillary basement membrane and increase in mesangial matrix have been observed (Soret et al., 1973). The aorta of the diabetic Chinese hamster has been reported to show mild preatheroscleroticlike changes (Soret et al., 1976). In metahypophyseal diabetic Chinese hamsters treated with cortisol and growth hormone, retinal arteriolar and capillary aneurysms develop after 4–6 months of hyperglcyemia. However, no microaneurysms have been observed in spontaneously diabetic Chinese hamsters (Soret et al., 1973). In peripheral nerves, segmental demyelination and axonal degeneration and reduced conduction velocity of nerves have been reported and the severity of these changes appears to be related to duration and severity of diabetes (Gerritsen, 1982).

B. South African Hamsters (Mystromys Alb.)

Another insulinopenic nonobese diabetic animal model is the South African hamster or white-tailed rat. The genetics are unknown in this species and their diabetes is characterized by mild hyperglycemia and occasional ketonuria (Stuhlman, 1979).

C. Nonobese Diabetic Mouse

In 1980, Makino *et al.* reported the development of polyuria and glycosuria in a subline of CTS mice, a line of JCL-ICR mice maintained in Japan. Two sublines have been produced, one diabetic and one normal and not diabetes-prone. In the diabetes-prone line the onset of diabetes is abrupt and usually occurs at 60 days of age with a higher percentage of females afflicted than the males. Severe manifestations of the disease such as polyuria, glycosuria, ketonuria, and weight loss can be controlled only by regular injections of exogenous insulin. Morphologically, the pancreas displays lymphocytic infiltration of the islets of Langerhans (insulitis) with reduction in the number and the size of the islets in chronically diabetic mice. Although the genetic components involved in this form of insulinopenic diabetes are not defined, genetic susceptibility of certain members of the strain is assumed to play a role in the development of the overt diabetes. Because of the preponderance of females afflicted, the effect of sex hormones has been studied. Castration of males causes an increase in the incidence of severe diabetes to that normally found in females. In contrast, castration of females prevents the development of diabetes (Makino *et al.*, 1981).

Since an autoimmune factor has been suspected in the pathogenesis of this disease, assessment of immunologic functions has been carried out (Toyota *et al.*, 1982). Natural killer cell activity was found to be reduced in nonobese diabetic (NOD) mice but the number of antibody-producing spleen cells, and therefore antibody production against sheep red blood cells, was increased in NOD mouse. Furthermore, the number of T cells identified with thy 1.2 antigen was diminished. In addition, autoantibody to islets has been reported to be detectable in NOD mouse at 14 days of age. Lymphocytic infiltration in other endocrine organs as well as the islets of the diabetic NOD mice has been observed. Recently Yamada *et al.*, (1982) have reported that administration of large doses of nicotinamide ameliorated the diabetes of NOD mice with restoration of normal glucose tolerance while also improving the insulitis lesion.

Although several features of the syndrome are similar to the diabetes observed in the better-studied BB rat model, further studies are needed to characterize the pathophysiology and possible causative factors.

D. Guinea Pig

Lang *et al.* (1977) have reported development of diabetes in approximately 50% of a specific colony of guinea pigs. This diabetes usually occurs at 5 months of age and is characterized by decreased pancreatic insulin and islet degeneration. The diabetes is apparently due to an unknown endemic viral infection since other guinea pigs placed in this colony develop diabetes after several weeks. The transient nature of diabetes in guinea pigs is reminiscent of the syndrome of encephalomyocarditis-virus-infected mice (Craighead, 1981).

E. New Zealand White Rabbit

Spontaneous development of insulin-dependent diabetes in a closed inbred colony of nonobese New Zealand white rabbits has been described by Roth *et al.* (1980). The affected members show various degrees of hyperglycemia or glucose intolerance. The pancreatic islets show β cells to be hypergranulated with normal α and D cells, suggesting a defect in insulin secretion.

F. Canine Models

Historically, dogs with induced diabetes (β cell toxin or pancreatectomy) have played important roles in diabetes research. It was in this species that von Mering and Minkowski recognized the role of the pancreas in diabetes and, of course, the pioneering works of Banting and Best on the effect of the insulin-containing pancreatic extracts was done in pancreatectomized diabetic dogs.

A familial early-onset diabetes mellitus was recently described in golden retrievers by Williams *et al.* (1980). The genetics are not clear, but the animals are nonobese, become diabetic between 2 and 5 months of age, and are insulin-deficient. Another genetically determined (autosomal recessive condition) diabetes has been identified in a line of nonobese keeshond dogs (Engerman and Kramer, 1982). The pancreatic islets are hypoplastic and pancreatic insulin and glucagon are reduced.

G. Nonhuman Primates

Several nonhuman primate species with spontaneous diabetes have been reported (Howard, 1982). Among them the spontaneous diabetes that occurs in black celebes apes (*Macaca nigra*) has been well characterized. Overtly diabetic monkeys are nonobese, hyperglycemic, and have impaired responses to glucose tolerance tests. At least 50% have mild to moderate diabetes and 10% are overtly diabetic and require insulin therapy. The hormonal changes occur concurrently with morphological alterations in islet structure (islet amyloid). With progressive deterioration of secretory cells and amyloid deposition clinical diabetes eventually develops. The size of these colonies is small: the animals are not available for general scientific community and are being studied only at few institutions.

H. BB Rat

The spontaneously diabetic BB rat was discovered serendipitously in 1974 at the BioBreeding Laboratories, (thus BB) Ltd., Ottawa, Canada (Chappel and Chappel, 1975). This rat syndrome has many similarities to human type I diabetes and is generally considered the closest animal model to the human condition (Marliss *et al.*, 1982; Seemayer *et al.*, 1980). The syndrome appeared in a commercial outbred but closed colony of Wistar-derived albino rats. The characteristics of the diabetic syndrome were first reported by Nakhooda *et al.* (1977, 1978, 1979). Genetically susceptible rats develop an abrupt onset of glycosuria and hyperglycemia between 60 and 140 days of age (60 days being the approximate time of sexual maturation in this species). Both male and female rats are nonobese and develop diabetes with equal frequency.

The affected animals demonstrate a spectrum of clinical severity with respect to hyperglycemia, hypoinsulinemia, and hyperketonemia (Nakhooda *et al.*, 1978). The severely ketotic (6–13 mM) rats show rapid loss of weight and dehydration over 1–6 days after detection of the disease. The moderately ketotic (1–5 mM) rats show gradual decline in weight over 15 days and in stable diabetic rats (ketonemia less than 1 mM), there is stabilization of weight, polyuria, and glycosuria for a longer period of time. Diabetic rats always require daily injections of insulin to promote or maintain stable weight and to prevent dehydration, emaciation, ketoacidosis, coma, and death. In all groups the circulating levels of plasma immunoreactive insulin (IRI) and pancreatic IRI content are diminished. The plasma immunoreactive glucagon (IRG) levels are significantly elevated in both severely and moderately ketotic rats but are within the normal range in stable insulin treated diabetic rats. The pancreatic IRG content is reduced to two-thirds normal in the moderately ketotic and stable diabetic rats and to one-third normal in the severely ketotic animals. The plasma-free fatty acid levels and branched chain animo acids are elevated in relation to the clinical severity of the syndrome.

Tannenbaum *et al.* (1981a) studied the dynamic time course profiles of plasma growth hormone (GH), IRI, and glucose at various times before and after the onset of diabetes. In the prediabetic state (preglycosuric) normal patterns of GH secretion, basal plasma IRI, and glucose levels were noted in all rats. After the onset of diabetes there was marked hyperglycemia and hypoinsulinemia but no significant effect on the GH rhythm in the early phase of the disease. As the disease progressed the GH secretory episodes were markedly suppressed, probably via reduced synthesis by the pituitary gland.

Although Nakhooda (1978) reported decreased pancreatic glucagon contents, Patel *et al.* (1980) found no significant changes in the pancreatic glucagon content in control vs. diabetic BB rats, although portal venous and inferior vena cava glucagon levels were increased. Tannebaum *et al.* (1981b) also found no significant alteration of pancreatic glucagon concentrations in the early and stable groups of diabetic BB rats. However, the unstable group had significantly lower levels of glucagon as compared to nondiabetic control littermates. Thus, the paradoxical hyperglucagonemia could originate either from the hyperactive residual cells in the islets or from nonpancreatic sources.

Boden *et al.* (1980, 1982) have studied the effect of spontaneous diabetes in BB rats on hormone release in response to amino acids and to amino acids plus glucose from isolated perfused pancreas (P) or pancreas/stomach/duodenum/spleen (PSDS) preparations. Spontaneous diabetes virtually abolished the total integrated insulin output from the PSDS by 97%, a fact consistent with major pancreatic beta cell loss as well as a major reduction of pancreatic and circulating plasma IRI. The combined IRG output from the PSDS, representing essentially all major IRG-releasing tissues, was reduced by 50% compared to nondiabetic controls (indicating that alpha cell function was compromised) while somatostatin output did not change. Integrated pancreatic glucagon output fell by 91% while integrated somatostatin output more than doubled. Intestinal glucagon and somatostatin contribution was estimated by comparing hormone release from the PSDS with that from the P preparations. In nondiabetic BB rats, the pancreas was the only source for the release of glucagon and insulin; and the intestinal tract secreted more somatostatin than the pancreas. In diabetic BB rats, pancreatic glucagon and insulin release was markedly reduced while glucagon secretion from the intestinal tract increased and somatostatin decreased.

In untreated diabetic BB rats the concentration of immunoreactive somatostatin (IRS) in portal vein (PV) and inferior vena cava (IVC) was elevated (Patel *et al.*, 1980). Insulin treatment restored both values to normal. The pancreatic IRS content in both untreated and treated diabetic BB rats was reduced by 60% (Tannenbaum *et al.*, 1981b; Patel *et al.*, 1980). Seemayer *et al.* (1982b) studied the effect of diabetes on pancreatic alpha, beta, and D cells. The loss of beta cells was evident at all stages of the disease. However, the number of alpha and D cells appeared normal in stable BB diabetics though reduced in unstable diabetics. Therefore, the morphological changes in the pancreas correlated with the extractable pancreatic hormone contents.

The morphological hallmark of recent-onset-insulin-dependent diabetes is lymphocytic infiltration of pancreatic islets associated with beta cell destruction (Gepts and LeCompte, 1981). The islet cell alterations in the BB rat strikingly resemble those found in human diabetics. Morphologically, the pancreatic islets at the onset of the disease display a pronounced insulitis (Fig. 1) with the predominant cell types being lymphocytes, macrophages, and few eosinophils (Nakhooda *et al.*, 1977; Naji *et al.*, 1979a; Seemayer *et al.*, 1982b). This is associated with marked beta cell degranulation and necrosis without a consistent change in alpha and D cells. As the disease prog-

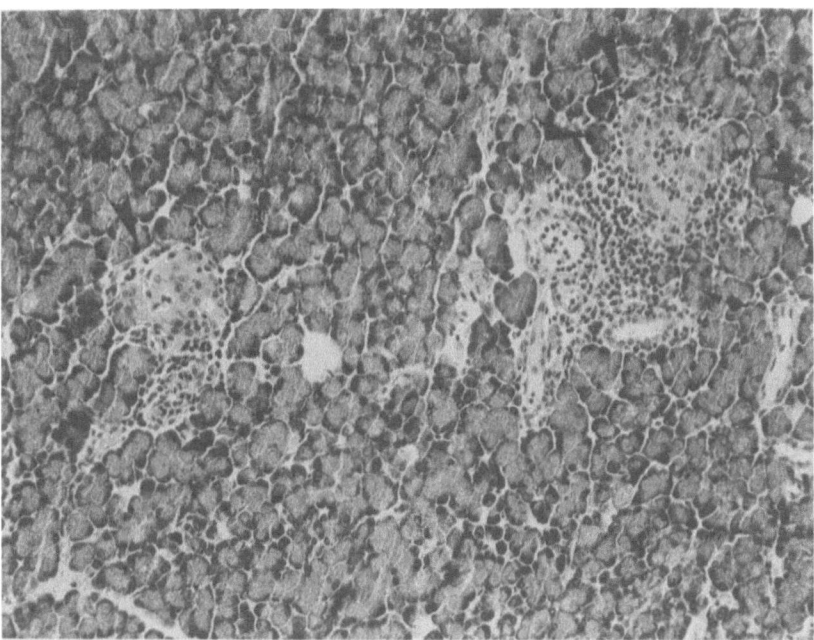

Figure 1. Pancreatic islets from a BB rat 4 days after the onset of hyperglycemia. Note the severe mononuclear infiltration throughout and around the periphery of the islet (extending into adjacent exocrine and parenchyma) (hematoxylin and eosin, 160X).

resses, there is virtual destruction of the beta cells in the pancreatic islets followed by a decreasing intensity of cellular infiltration. The end-stage disease islet is composed virtually only of glucagon, somatostatin, and pancreatic-polypeptide-synthesizing islet cells. The fate of the alpha and D cells in the course of progressive beta cell failure is less clear. In the unstable diabetics both alpha and D cells appear to be decreased (Seemayer et al., 1982b). Therefore, the suggestion has been made that although the beta cell appears to be the principle target of injury, the alpha and D cell may also be involved to a lesser extent in the same cellular damage that destroys the beta cells. Alternatively the integrity of these non-beta cells may depend upon a minimal local concentration of insulin, the loss of which eventually leads to their demise. In addition to pronounced insulitis in diabetic BB rats variable degrees of insulitis and beta cell damage have been documented in young (65-day-old) normoglycemic BB rats, suggesting that the destructive process in the islets is initiated well in advance of the onset of the clinical hyperglycemia (Seemayer et al., 1982b; Like et al., 1982b).

Therefore, the spectrum of events with respect to islet morphology and clinical presentation of diabetes in BB rats could be summarized as follows: The genetically susceptible rats may remain completely normal, may progress suddenly to insulin-dependent diabetes (without a preceding recognizable period of glucose intolerance), or may become frankly hyperglycemic only after a preceding period of impaired glucose tolerance (Marliss et al., 1982).

Individual BB rats with persistent impaired glucose tolerance (but normal fasting plasma glucose) may remain as such but the majority progress to overt insulin-dependent diabetes. Impaired glucose tolerance has been reported to be present in 10–25% of littermates of diabetic rats, the frequency varying with the genetic origin of the litter being studied (Marliss et al., 1982; Like et al., 1982b). A consistent impaired glucose tolerance is almost invariably associated with insulitis. Spontaneous remission from overt diabetes appears to occur very infrequently (5 in more than 1000 diabetic rats) (Rossini, personal communication, 1982).

The exact mode of inheritance of diabetes in BB rats remains to be defined. Genetic background is an important factor in susceptibility to diabetes as evidenced by the incidence of diabetes among sibs from various mating protocols. The observed frequency of diabetes varies from 20% (if one parent is diabetic) to 50% (when both parents are phenotypically diabetic). Butler et al. (1983) reasoned that phenotypically diabetic animals would be homozygous for the diabetic gene. In their studies, the offspring of diabetic matings were mated in diallelic crosses in which phenotypically diabetic and phenotypically normal rats were mated sequentially with diabetic and normal siblings (Like et al., 1982b). It was found that diabetics were produced with equal frequency by all the mating combinations regardless of the phenotypic characteristics of the mating pair. Hence, matings between diabetic females and their phenotypically diabetic or phenotypically nondiabetic male siblings, respectively, produced 48% and 41% frequency of diabetics in offsprings. Moreover, when normal females were mated with their diabetic or normal male siblings, the frequency of diabetes in their offspring was 51% and 42% respectively. Interpretation of the available genetic analyses suggests that diabetes is polygenic and is transmitted as an autosomal recessive gene but that the phenotypic expression of the diabetic genes occurs in only 50% of the genotypically diabetic animals (i.e., 50% penetrance).

In humans there is well-known genetic predisposition to the development of insulin-dependent diabetes mellitus (IDDM). Susceptibility genes are linked to certain cell surface determinants encoded by genes located in the MHC (HLA-DR3/DR4) (Nerup et al., 1980; Cudworth et al., 1980). Therefore it is germane to carry out immunogenetic analysis of BB rats to find whether the susceptibility (or resistance) is linked to the MHC or the RT1 locus. The MHC of BB rats, tested by serotyping and mixed lymphocyte reactions were found by Naji et al. (1979a, 1981b) to be RT1^u. F$_1$ populations produced by mating diabetic BB and normal inbred rat strains never produced any diabetic animals (Naji et al., 1981b; Colle et al., 1981). When F$_1$ hybrids were backcrossed to diabetic BB, all diabetic backcross progeny were homozygous for RT1^u (Naji et al., 1981b). Moreover, when F$_2$ hybrids were produced by intercrossing F$_1$ hybrids all the affected animals were homozygous RT1 u/u, suggesting that, as in the human case, the susceptibility is associated with gene products of the MHC (Colle et al., 1981). More recently, Colle et al. (1982) noted the appearance of diabetes in a few rats which had only one u haplotype, suggesting that homozygosity for $RT1^u$ is not obligatory.

Several etiologic possibilities have been examined. The role of viruses in initiation of the islet damage and diabetes has been extensively studied in several laboratories. In no instance has a virus been implicated (Naji et al., 1981b). However, since the identity of the suspected diabetogenic virus is unknown (as well as its culture requirements), such negative studies remain inconclusive. The etiologic role of some environmental pathogens is further reduced by the occurrence of diabetes in cesarean-derived gnobiotic rats (Rossini et al., 1979). Common viral, bacterial, and parasitic pathogens were excluded by negative cultures, stains, and serologic assay. However, the possibilities of transplacentally transferred or unidentified viruses cannot be excluded.

The possibility that a perturbed immune system is responsible for type 1 human IDDM has been suggested by the increased association of this disease with certain autoimmune endocrinopathies, presence of islet cell antibody, as well as the characteristic mononuclear infiltration of pancreatic islets (Irvine, 1980). The BB rat is the first animal model to be extensively studied to investigate role of the immune system in pathogenesis of a diabetes. Several findings suggest that an altered humoral or cell-mediated immunity may be importantly involved in the pathogenesis of spontaneous diabetes in BB rats. The insulitis lesion which is highly reminiscent of lesions found in early human type I diabetics remains one of the strongest pieces of evidence. Naji et al. (1981b) reported that BB rats of diabetic sublines were generally less robust and more susceptible to environmental pathogens than other inbred rats or sublines of BB rats known to lack susceptibility to diabetes. Furthermore, a high incidence of malignant lymphoma (a tumor unusual in rats) was also found among members of a diabetic subline (Kalant and Seemayer, 1979; Naji et al., 1981b; Seemayer et al., 1982a). These findings raised the possibility that members of the diabetes-prone BB lines experience an immunological debilitation which increased their susceptibility to infections, tumors, and also to diabetes. A systematic analysis of lymphoid organs of members of diabetic subline was done and compared to those of other rats and rats of a nondiabetes-prone BB subline (Naji et al., 1981b). It was found that both overtly diabetic and normoglycemic members of the diabetic subline experienced marked lymphocytopenia that was evident in all lymphoid compartments such as lymph nodes, spleen, and thoracic duct lymph. Moreover, histological examination of lymph nodes and spleens of diabetic BB rats also indicated a marked paucity of small lymphocytes in T-cell-dependent anatomical zones.

In addition to impaired protective immunity, Naji *et al.* (1981b) found that members of the diabetes-prone subline displayed feeble transplantation immunity to skin allografts, as compared to members of the non-diabetes-prone BB subline. The above findings were highly suggestive of immunological deficiency, especially of T cells, both in overtly diabetic BB rats and their normoglycemic littermates. The presence of lymphocytopenia has been confirmed in other BB colonies (Poussier *et al.*, 1981; Jackson *et al.*, 1981; Elder and Maclaren, 1982a). It is present in young weaning BB rats during the time when no detectable metabolic disorder is noted (Bellgrau *et al.*, 1982). It has been reported that lymphocytopenia is consistently associated with insulitis (whether or not the host becomes overtly hyperglycemic) and therefore may be used as a marker for susceptibility to the syndrome (Poussier *et al.*, 1982).

Serologic and immunofluorescent studies of lymphocyte populations of BB rats have indicated that a major loss of T (rather than B) lymphocytes accounts for the observed lymphocytopenia (Naji *et al.*, 1981b, 1982a; Jackson *et al.*, 1981; Bellgrau *et al.*, 1982; Poussier *et al.*, 1982; Elder and Maclaren, 1982a). Jackson *et al.* (1981) analyzed the T-cell subsets using immunofluorescent microscopy and reported that reduction in the T helper subset (reactive with monoclonal antibody W3/25) is the major cause of T lymphocytopenia. However, in recent studies Naji *et al.* (1983b) systematically analyzed the composition of lymphocytes of BB rats of diabetic and non-diabetes-prone BB sublines using monoclonal antibodies specific for all currently defined rat T-cell subsets (Mason *et al.*, 1980) with the aid of the fluorescence-activated cell sorter. Like Jackson *et al.* (1981), they found that T helper cells were reduced. However, there was a much more striking reduction in the suppressor/cytotoxic T-cell subset (not examined by Jackson *et al.*) as identified by the monoclonal antibody OX8 (Table 2).

Additional evidence of immune etiology of BB diabetes is provided by the influence of immunosuppression or neonatal thymectomy on the disease. Like *et al.* (1979) noted that administration of rabbit antirat lymphocyte serum (ALS) to newly diagnosed overtly diabetic rats reversed the hyperglycemia in 36% and prevented the development of diabetes in normoglycemic diabetes-prone littermates. A similar beneficial effect of ALS was also noted by Naji *et al.* (1979a, b) who also found that discontinuation of ALS resulted in recurrence of hyperglycemia in ALS-cured rats (Naji *et al.*, 1981a).

Like *et al.* (1982c) have also obtained evidence that a thymus-dependent, cell-mediated autoimmune destruction of pancreatic beta cells is responsible for the pathogenesis of diabetes in BB rats by subjecting BB rats to neonatal thymectomy within 24 hr of birth. Total thymectomy reduced the frequency of spontaneous diabetes in BB rats from 27 to 3%. Incomplete thymectomy was less effective but also reduced the incidence of diabetes.

Additional evidence of the immune etiology of diabetes in BB rats was provided by the islet and bone marrow transplantation studies, which also suggest a possible

Table 2. Analysis of Surface Marker Composition of Lymphocytes
of BB Rats[a]

BB Rat	Tissue	Percentage of marker-positive cells			
		W3/13+	W3/25+	OX8+	OX6+
BBND	LN	71 ± 1.2	51 ± 2.1	20 ± 1.6	21 ± 2.3
	TDL	87 ± 3.5	65 ± 4	23 ± 2.1	12 ± 1.5
BBDP	LN	46 ± 3.5	37 ± 3.6	9 ± 0.5	55 ± 5.9
	TDL	57 ± 2.3	46 ± 4	11 ± 1.8	36 ± 2
BBDP tol. WF	LN	68 ± 3.2	49 ± 1.1	21 ± 2.4	24 ± 3.1
	TDL	91 ± 4.5	64 ± 2.3	30 ± 2.1	11 ± 3.4

[a]Cells were labeled with mouse monoclonal antibodies (W3/13, pan-T; W3/25, T-helper; OX8, T-suppressor/cytotoxic; OX6, B-cells) and analyzed by fluorescent-activated cell sorter. Numbers indicate the mean % of positive cells ± SEM. BBND = Normal BB control; BBDP = diabetes-prone BB (normoglycemic or diabetic); tol. BBDP = bone-marrow-inoculated BBDP; LN = lymph node; TDL = thoracic duct lymphocytes.

therapeutic or preventive maneuver. Naji *et al.* (1981a) noted that transplanted allogeneic BB islets from nondiabetic donors to *nonimmunosuppressed* BB recipients were rapidly destroyed. Rejection by the nonimmunosuppressed outbred BB rats was a possible cause of the transplant islet failure despite the use of closely histocompatible donors (identical with the recipient at the MHC but differing at other loci). Therefore, islet transplantation was carried out in BB rats that had been rendered immunologically tolerant to the prospective islet donor strain (Naji *et al*, 1981b, c). Tolerance induction was accomplished by inoculation of the prospective recipients with bone marrow from normal Wistar Furth (WF) donors during the first 24 hr of life (Billingham and Silvers, 1971). Tolerance was confirmed by permanent acceptance of donor (WF) skin allografts by these hosts. In adulthood only a few of these tolerant BB rats developed spontaneous diabetes and received transplanted islets from WF donors. The transplanted islet cells failed to sustain normoglycemia for more than 1–11 days prior to recurrent diabetes. In tolerant hosts the transplant islet failure could not be attributed to rejection. In all cases of recurrent diabetes, a histological picture of insulitis was found in the transplanted islets. This experiment provided conclusive evidence that the original disease process was responsible for the destruction of transplanted islets.

A serendipitous finding in BB rats rendered immunologically tolerant to WF cells was even more important. The incidence of diabetes was noted to be unexpectedly low in BB rats that had received bone marrow from normal allogeneic donors compared to untreated BB rats (Naji *et al.*, 1981b, c; 1982b). This was corroborated when half of each additional litter of highly diabetes susceptible BB rats was randomly selected and rendered tolerant by inoculation with WF bone marrow, while the remaining pups were left untreated as controls (Table 3). The incidence of diabetes in bone-marrow-inoculated animals was 8% as compared to 41% in their noninoculated littermates. The inoculated members also fared significantly better in other ways than their untreated

Table 3. Prospective Study of Incidence of Diabetes[a]

Group	Number of rats	Diabetics	Percentage
Marrow inoculated	61	5	8[b]
Noninoculated littermates	61	25	41

[a]Fourteen litters of BB rats were studied: half of each litter was inoculated with WF bone marrow at birth.
[b]Significantly different from noninoculated (control) value at $p < 0.001$.

littermates. They were more vigorous and had a much reduced vulnerability to patho-genic microorganisms. Evidence was also obtained that the neonatal marrow treatment improved the immunodeficiency of BB rats and corrected the T-cell microenvironmental defects that were present in noninoculated littermates (Naji *et al.*, 1982b; 1983c). While, in accordance with previous findings, the noninoculated BB rats were lymphocytopenic, their bone-marrow inoculated littermates had higher total lymphocyte contents in various lymphoid organs. Also several T-cell functions were restored towards normal in marrow inoculated rats, such as *in vitro* alloreactivity of their cells in mixed lymphocyte cultures and humoral response of their lymphocytes to thymus-dependent antigens (functional assays that were always depressed in noninoculated BB rats) (Bellgrau *et al.*, 1982; Naji *et al.*, 1983a). Furthermore the composition and ratio of T lymphocytes and their subsets were normalized. Whereas, as previously noted the unmodified BB rats had reduced markers of T helper (W3/25[+]) cells and an even more pronounced reduction of T cytotoxic/suppressor (OX8[+]) cells, the proportions of these cells were restored to normal in their marrow-inoculated littermates (Naji *et al.*, 1983b, c).

Passive transfer of the disease with putatively immune lymphoid cells would be the *sine qua non* for demonstration of its autoimmune nature. In this regard, Naji *et al.* (1981b) inoculated large numbers of thoracic duct lymphocytes from acutely diabetic BB rats into sublethally irradiated nondiabetic BB recipients. Pancreatic biopsy speci-mens taken 6 days after cell transfer were normal in all recipients, but after 16 days mild to moderate insulitis was found to be present in 20% of the recipients. However, in none of the animals was hyperglycemia noted. A similar outcome was reported by Nakhooda *et al.* (1981). Following their intraperitoneal inoculation with blood or spleen cells from newly detected BB diabetics, 37% of athymic nude mice displayed varying degrees of insulitis but none were hyperglycemic. Results of such cell transfer protocols should be interpreted with caution since BB rats are not as yet isogenic and transfer of lymphocytes could lead to varying degrees of graft-versus-host disease. Pancreatic islets of mice during active graft-versus-host disease have been shown by Kolb *et al.*(1981) to display insulitis.

The presence of islet cell antibodies in human insulin-dependent diabetics, partic-ularly during early stages after diagnosis, has been well documented (Cudworth *et al.*, 1980). Therefore, such autoantibodies were sought in the BB rat. Several laboratories have failed to demonstrate islet cell cytoplasmic antibodies by immunofluorescence on frozen sections of the rat pancreas (Naji *et al.*, 1981b; Dryberg *et al.*, 1982; Elder *et al.*, 1982b; Like *et al.*, 1982a), in contrast to the presence of such circulating antibodies in more than 60% of human diabetics. Islet cell surface antibodies have also been investigated by a protein-A radioligand assay (Dryberg *et al.*, 1982) using dispersed beta cells of non-BB Wistar rats as targets. These workers found cell surface antibodies in 85% of diabetic BB rats 3–11 days after diagnosis, a result which provides further analogy of the diabetes of BB rats to that of insulin-dependent human diabetics.

Because of the increased frequency of autoantibodies to a variety of tissue and cell constituents (e.g., thyroid, gastric mucosa) in human IDDM, such autoantibodies were also sought in BB rats (Neufeld *et al.*, 1980). Elder *et al.*, (1982b), in longitudinal studies of circulating autoantibodies in sera of BB rats, found no adrenocortical or thyroid microsomal autoantibodies but autoantibodies reactive to gastric parietal cells, smooth muscle, and thyroid colloidal antigens were identified in high frequencies in the BB rats. Furthermore, it was found that the time of the first appearance of parietal cell antibodies correlated with the onset of the diabetes in BB rats, suggesting that BB rats may have an underlying autoimmune diathesis. Like *et al.*, (1982a) have also found anti-smooth-muscle and antithyroid colloid antibodies with great frequency in diabetic as well as in normoglycemic offsprings of diabetic rats. Such antibodies were rarely found in nondiabetic lines of BB rats, suggesting that they may be useful markers for the diabetic gene(s).

Several investigators have studied BB rats for the development of complications such as neuropathy, angiopathy, and retinopathy. The earliest neuropathic change is a decrease in motor nerve conduction velocity to 80% of control after 3 weeks of diabetes (Sima, 1980; Sima and Hay, 1981; Mendell *et al.*, 1980). After 4 months a further decrease in conduction velocity is associated with the first structural change, abnormal accumulation of glycogens in distal axons. After more prolonged diabetes degenerative changes are noted within myelinated and unmyelinated nerve fibers.

Like *et al.*, (1980) have demonstrated deposits of IgG, IgM, and complement within the mesangial region of the glomeruli of diabetic BB rats. These changes resemble those observed in kidneys of streptozotocin-induced diabetic rats (Mauer *et al.*, 1972).

In addition to their interest to diabetologists, BB rats may represent a model of multiple autoimmune endocrinopathy. In view of the well-recognized association of human IDDM with other autoimmune endocrinopathies (e.g., Hashimoto's thyroiditis) diabetic BB rats were studied to determine the frequency of lympocytic thyroiditis. Sternthal *et al.*, (1981) have reported that the incidence of lymphocytic thyroiditis was strikingly increased (59%) in diabetic rats compared with their nondiabetic cohorts (11%). Lymphocytic thyroiditis was not associated with abnormal thyroid function test results.

From the exponentially increasing literature on BB rat, a number of speculations can now be drawn as to the etiology and pathogenesis of the diabetic syndrome. Genetic factors are obviously crucial in predisposition to the disease. The nature of additional etiological factors which seem likely to be involved is less clear. Since BB rats are genetically heterogeneous it is tempting to speculate that a mutation in immune response genes coupled with some environmental agent (e.g., viruses that either directly injure the beta cells or indirectly invite an aberrant immune response to it) might be likely candidates. Therefore, as in the case of humans, in BB rats, an interaction between a genetically susceptible host and a yet-to-be-identified environmental triggering agent is a likely prerequisite for the expression of the disease. Immunogenetic analysis of the MHC of BB rats and its linkage to disease suscepibility should yield valuable information.

Islet transplantation experiments in BB rats have proved especially interesting, both as possible treatments and as probes of the etiology of the disease. The rapid recurrence of diabetes in tolerant islet recipients incapable of rejection has a counterpart in the failure of many human renal isografts transplanted to victims of another autoimmune disease, glomerulonephritis, and perhaps argues against successful islet transplantation in human diabetics (Glassock et al.,1968).

That BB rats experience an immunoregulatory disorder is now firmly established. Whether the immunodeficiency and propensity for diabetes are causally related remains to be resolved. However, the finding that inoculation of highly susceptible diabetes-prone BB rats with bone marrow from normal donors strikingly reduces the incidence of diabetes further stresses the importance of the immune etiology in the diabetes of BB rats. Moreover, the finding that bone marrow inoculation reverses both the immunodeficiency and their T-cell subset abnormalities provides persuasive evidence that a normal T-cell repertoire is intricately involved in conferring protection against the disease. It seems likely that much of this information may have relevance to human diabetes. If so, some type of immunologic manipulation may eventually be useful in humans known to be genetically predisposed to the disease.

REFERENCES

Anderson, T., Schein, P. S., McMenamin, M. G., and Cooney, D. A., 1974, Streptozotocin diabetes, correlation with extent of depression of pancreatic islet NAD, J. Clin. Invest. 54:672–677.

Appel, M. C., Rossini, A. A., Williams, R. M., and Like, A. A., 1978, Viral studies in streptozotocin-induced pancreatic insulitis, Diabetologia 15:327–336.

Bellgrau, D., Naji, A., Silvers, W. K., Markmann, J. F., and Barker, C. F., 1982, Spontaneous diabetes in BB rats: Evidence for a T cell dependent immune response defect, Diabetologia 23:359–364.

Billingham, R., and Silvers, W. K., 1971, Immunological tolerance, in: The Immunobiology of Transplantation (R. Billingham and W. K. Silvers, eds.), pp. 132–148, Prentice Hall, Englewood Cliffs, New Jersey.

Boden, G., Barker, C., Naji, A., and Matchinsky, F., 1980, Reduced A cell and increased D cell responsiveness in spontaneously diabetic BB/W rats with absolute insulin deficiency, Diabetes 29:41 (abstract).

Boden, G., Naji, A., Barker, C. F., June, V., and Matschinsky, F. M., 1983, Effect of spontaneous diabetes on hormone release in BB/Phi rats. Comparison between the isolated perfused pancreas/stomach/duodenum/spleen and the isolated perfused pancreas, Endocrinology 112:1777–1781.

Boquist, L., 1979, Histochemistry and electron microscopy of islets, in The Diabetic Pancreas (B. W. Volk and K. F. Wellman, eds.), pp. 129–169, Plenum Press, New York.

Buschard, K., and Rygaard, J., 1978, T-lymphocytes transfer streptozotocin induced diabetes mellitus in mice, Acta. Pathol. Microbiol. Scand. [C.] 86:277–282.

Butler, L., Guberski, D. C., and Like, A. A., 1983, Genetic analysis of the BB/W diabetic rat, Can. J. Genet. Cytol. 25: 7–15.

Cameron, D., Renold, A. E., Stauffacher, N., 1972, Spontaneous hyperglycemia and obesity in laboratory rodents, in: Handbook of Physiology (R. O. Greep, E. B. Astwood, and D. F. Steiner, eds.), Vol. 7, pp. 611–625, American Physiology Society, Washington.

Chappel, C. I., and Chappel, W. R., 1975, Spontaneous insulin-deficient diabetes in the Wistar rats, *Proc. Can. Fed. Biol. Sci.* **18**:97.

Coleman, D. L., 1982, Diabetes–obesity syndromes in mice, *Diabetes* **31**(Suppl. 7):1–6.

Colle, E., Guttmann, R. D., and Seemayer, T., 1981, Spontaneous diabetes mellitus syndrome in the rat. 1. Association with the major histocompatibility complex, *J. Exp. Med.* **154**:1237–1242.

Colle, E., Guttmann, R. D., Michel, F., Seemayer, T. A., and Belmonte, M. M., 1982, Genetics of T lymphopenia in the syndrome of spontaneous diabetes mellitus in the rat, *Diabetes* **31**(Suppl. 2):46 (abstract) 184.

Cooperstein, S. J., and Lazarow, A., 1964, Distribution of alloxan-C^{14} in islet and other tissues of the toadfish (*opsanus tau*), *Am. J. Physiol.* **207**:423–430.

Craighead, J. E., 1981, Viral diabetes in man and experimental animals, *Am. J. Med.* **70**:127–134.

Cudworth, A. G., Bottazzo, G. F., and Doniach, D., 1980, Genetic and immuological factors in Type I diabetes, in: *Immunology of Diabetes* (W. J. Irvine, ed.), pp. 67–99, Teviot Scientific Publications, Edinburgh, United Kingdom.

Dulin, W. E., and Soret, M. G., 1979, Chemically and Hormonally induced diabetes, in: *The Diabetic Pancreas* (B. W. Volk and K. F. Wellman, eds.), pp. 425–465, Plenum Press, New York.

Dryberg, T., Nakhooda, A. F., Baekkeskow, S., Lernmark, A., Poussier, P., and Marliss, E. B., 1982, Islet cell surface antibodies and lymphocyte antibodies in the spontaneously diabetic 'BB' Wistar rat, *Diabetes* **31**:278–281.

Elder, M., and Maclaren, N., 1982, Immunoincompetence in the BB rat, *Diabetes* **31**(Suppl. 2):48 (abstract) 189.

Elder, M., Maclaren, N., Riley, W., and McConnel, T., 1982, Gastric parietal cell and other autoantibodies in the BB rat, *Diabetes* **31**:313–318.

Engerman, R. L., and Kramer, J. W., 1982, Dogs with induced or spontaneous diabetes as models for the study of human diabetes mellitus, *Diabetes* **31**(Suppl. 1):26–29.

Fajans, S. S., Cloutier, M. C., and Crowther, R. L., 1978, Clinical and etiologic heterogeneity of idiopathic diabetes mellitus, *Diabetes* **27**:1112–1125.

Gepts, W., and LeCompte, P. M., 1981, The pancreatic islets in diabetes, *Am. J. Med.* **70**:105–115.

Gerritsen, G. C., 1982, The Chinese hamster as a model for the study of diabetes mellitus, *Diabetes* **31**(Suppl. 1):14–23.

Glassock, R. J., Feldman, D., Reynolds, E. S., Dammin, J., and Merrill, J. P., 1968, Human renal isografts, a clinical and pathologic analysis, *Medicine* **47**:411.

Grodsky, G. M., Anderson, C. E., Coleman, D. L., Craighead, J. E., Gerritsen, G. C., Hansen, C. T., Herberg, L., Howard, C. F., Lernmark, A., Matschinsky, F. M., Rayfield, E., Riley, W. J., and Rossini, A. A., 1982, Metabolic and underlying causes of diabetes mellitus, *Diabetes* **31**(Suppl. 7):45–53.

Howard, C. F., 1982, Nonhuman primates as models for the study of human diabetes mellitus, *Diabetes* **31**(Suppl. 7):37–42.

Irvine, W. J., 1980, Immunological aspects of diabetes mellitus: A review (including the salient points of the NDDG report on the classification of diabetes), in: *Immunology of Diabetes* (W. J. Irvine, ed.), pp. 1–53, Teviot Scientific Publications, Edinburgh, United Kingdom.

Jackson, R., Rassi, N., Crump, T., Haynes, B., and Eisenbarth, G. S., 1981, The BB diabetic rat: Profound T-cell lymphocytopenia, *Diabetes* **30**:887–889.

Kalant, N., and Seemayer, T., 1979, Malignant lymphoma in spontaneously diabetic rats, *N. Engl. J. Med.* **300**:737 (letter).

Kolb, H., Freytag, G., Kiesel, U., and Kolb-Bachogen, V., 1981, Cellular immune reactions against pancreatic islets as a consequence of graft versus host disease, *Clin. Exp. Immunol.* **43**:121–127.

Kromann, H., Christy, M., Egeberg, J., Lernmark, A., and Nerup, J., 1982, Absence of H-2 genetic influence on streptozotocin-induced diabetes in mice, *Diabetologia* **23**:114–118.

Lang, C. M., Munger, B. L., and Rapp, F., 1977, The guinea pig as an animal model of diabetes mellitus, *Lab. Anim. Sci.* **27**:789–805.

Leiter, E., 1982, Multiple low-dose streptozotocin-induced hyperglycemia and insulitis in C57BL mice: Influence of inbred background, sex and thymus, *Proc. Natl. Acad. Sci. USA* **79**:630–634.

Like, A. A., 1979, Spontaneous diabetes in animals, in: *The Diabetic Pancreas* (B. W. Volk and K. F. Wellman, eds.), pp. 381–423, Plenum Press, New York.

Like, A. A., and Rossini, A. A., 1976, Streptozotocin-induced pancreatic insulitis: New model of diabetes, *Science* **293:**415–418.

Like, A. A., Rossini, A. A., Guberski, D. L., Appel, M. C., and Williams, R. M., 1979, Spontaneous diabetes mellitus: Reversal and prevention in the BB/W rat with antiserum to rat lymphocytes, *Science* **206:**2421–2423.

Like, A. A., Appel, M. C., and Ericson, S., 1980, Renal glomerular studies in bio breeding/worchester (BB/W) diabetic rats, *Diabetes* **129***(Suppl. 2):*80 (abstract) 314.

Like, A. A., Appel, M. C., and Rossini, A. A., 1982a, Autoantibodies in the BB/W rat, *Diabetes* **31:**816–820.

Like, A. A., Butler, L., Williams, R. M., Appel, M. C., Weringer, E. J., and Rossini, A. A., 1982b, Spontaneous autoimmune diabetes mellitus in the BB rat, *Diabetes* **31**(Suppl. 1):7–13.

Like, A. A., Kislauskis, E., Williams, R. M., and Rossini, A. A., 1982c, Neonatal thymectomy prevents spontaneous diabetes mellitus in the BB/W rat, *Science* **216:**644–656.

Makino, S., Kunimoto, K., Muraoka, Y., Mizushima, Y., Katagari, K., and Tochino, Y., 1980, Breeding of non-obese, diabetic strain of mice, *Exp. Animal* **29:**1–13.

Makino, S., Kunimoto, K., Muraoka, Y., and Katagiri, K., 1981, Effect of castration on the appearance of diabetes in the NOD mouse, *Exp. Animal* **30:**137–140.

Marliss, E. B., Nakhooda, A. F., Poussier, P., and Sima, A. A. F., 1982, The diabetic syndrome of the BB Wistar rat: Possible relevance to Type I (Insulin-dependent) diabetes in man, *Diabetologia* **22**():225–232.

Mason, D. W., Brideau, R. J., McMaster, W. R., Webb, M., White, R. A. H., and Williams, A. F., 1980, Monoclonal antibodies that define T-lymphocyte subsets in the rat, in: *Monoclonal Antibodies, Hybridomas: A New Dimension in Biological Analyses* (R. H. Kennett, T. J. McKearn, and K. B. Bechtol, eds.), pp. 251–273, Plenum Press, New York.

Mauer, A. M., Michael, A. F., Fish, A. J., and Brown, D. M., 1972, Spontaneous immunoglobulin and complement deposition in glomeruli of diabetic rats, *Lab. Invest.* **27:**488–494.

Meier, H., and Yerganian, G. A., 1959, Spontaneous hereditary diabetes mellitus in Chinese hamster (*Cricetulus griseus*). 1. Pathologic findings, *Proc. Soc. Exp. Biol. Med.* **100:**810–815.

Mendell, J. R., Sohenk, Z., and Warmolts, J. R., 1980, Peripheral nerve abnormalities in the spontaneously diabetic "BB" wistar rat, *Neurology* **30:**434 (abstract).

Naji, A., Silvers, W. K., Plotkin, S. A., Dafoe, D., and Barker, C. F., 1979a, Successful islet transplantation in spontaneous diabetes, *Surgery* **60:**218–226.

Naji, A., Silvers, W. K., and Barker, C. F., 1979b, Treatment of diabetes in BB rats with immunosuppression and islet transplantation, *Diabetes* **28**(Suppl. 2):383 (abstract) 153.

Naji, A., Silvers, W. K., and Barker, C. F., 1981a, Islet transplantation in spontaneously diabetic rats, *Transplant. Proc.* **13:**826–828.

Naji, A., Silvers, W. K., Bellgrau, D., Anderson, A., Plotkin, S., and Barker, C. F., 1981b, Prevention of diabetes in rats by bone marrow transplantation, *Ann. Surg.* **194:**328–338.

Naji, A., Silvers, W. K., Bellgrau, D., and Barker, C. F., 1981c, Spontaneous diabetes in rats: Destruction of islets is prevented by immunological tolerance, *Science* **213:**1390–1392.

Naji, A., Silvers, W. K., Bellgrau, D., and Barker, C. F., 1982a, Restoration of T cell dependent immune response defect in BB rats, *Diabetes* **31**(Suppl. 2):47 (abstract) 188.

Naji, A., Bellgrau, D., Anderson, A., Silvers, W. K., and Barker, C. F., 1982b, Transplantation of islets and bone marrow cells to animals with immune insulitis, *Diabetes* **31** (Suppl. 4):84–89.

Naji, A., Silvers, W. K., Kimura, H., Bellgrau, D., Anderson, A. O., and Barker, C. F., 1983a, Correction of the peripheral T-cell functional and microenvironmental defects in BB rats by bone marrow transplantation, *Transplant. Proc.* **15:**1424–1426.

Naji, A., Silvers, W. K., Kimura, H., Bellgrau, D., Markmann, J. F., and Barker, C. F., 1983b, Spontaneous diabetes mellitus in rats. Analytical and functional studies of the T cells of untreated and immunologically tolerant diabetes prone rats, *J. Immunol.* **130:**2168–2172.

Naji, A., Silvers, W. K., Kimura, H., Bellgrau, D., Anderson, A. O., and Barker, C. F., 1983c, Influence of islet and bone marrow transplantation on the diabetes and immunodeficiency of BB rats, *Metabolism* **32**(Suppl. 1):62–68.

Nakhooda, A. F., Like, A. A., Chappel, C. I., Murray, F. T., and Marliss, E. B., 1977, The spontaneously diabetic Wistar rat, Metabolic and morphologic studies, *Diabetes* **26**:100–112.

Nakhooda, A. F., Like, A. A., Chappel, C. I., Wei, C. N., and Marliss, E. B., 1978, The spontaneously diabetic Wistar rat. Studies prior to and during development of overt syndrome, *Diabetologia* **14**:199–207.

Nakhooda, A. F., Like, A. A., and Marliss, E. B., 1979, Diabetes mellitus in the 'BB' Wistar rat, in: *Spontaneous Animal Models of Human Disease* (E. J. Andrews, B. C. Ward, and N. H. Altman, eds.), pp. 131–135, Academic Press, New York.

Nakhooda, A. F., Sima, A. A. F., Poussier, P., and Marliss, E. B., 1981, Passive transfer of insulitis from the 'BB' rat to the nude mouse, *Endocrinology* **109**:2264–2266.

Nerup, J., and Lernmark, A., 1981, Autoimmunity in insulin-dependent diabetes mellitus, *Am. J. Med.* **70**:135–141.

Nerup, J. Christy, M., Kromann, H., Andersen, O. O., Platz, P., Ryder, L. P., Thomsen, M., and Svejgaard, A., 1980, Genetic susceptibility and resistance to insulin-dependent diabetes mellitus (IDDM), in: *Immunology of Diabetes* (W. J. Irvine, ed.), pp. 55–66, Teviot Scientific Publications, Edinburgh, United Kingdom.

Neufeld, M., Maclaren, N., Riley, W., Lozotte, D., McLaughlin, J., Silverstein, J., and Rosenbloom, A., 1980, Islet cell and other organ-specific antibodies in U.S. caucasians and blacks with insulin-dependent diabetes mellitus, *Diabetes* **29**:589–592.

Paik, S., Fleischer, N., and Shin, S., 1980, Insulin-dependent diabetes mellitus induced by subdiabetogenic doses of streptozotocin: Obligatory role of cell-mediated autoimmune process, *Proc. Natl. Acad. Sci. USA* **77**:6129–6133.

Patel, Y. C., Wheatley, T., Mallaise-Lagae, F., and Orci, L., 1980, Elevated portal and peripheral blood concentration of immunoreactive somatostatin in spontaneously diabetic (BBL) Wistar rats. Suppression with insulin, *Diabetes* **29**:757–761.

Poussier, P., Nakhooda, A. F., Sima, A. A. F., and Marliss, E. B., 1981, Lymphopenia in the spontaneously diabetic 'BB' rat, *Diabetologia* **21**:317 (abstract).

Poussier, P., Nakhooda, A. F., Falk, J. A., Lee, C., and Marliss, E. B., 1982, Lymphopenia and abnormal lymphocyte subsets in the 'BB' rat: Relationship to the diabetic syndrome, *Endocrinology* **110**:1825–1827.

Renold, A. E., Chang, A. Y., and Muller, W. A., 1974, Third Brook Lodge Workshop on spontaneous diabetes in laboratory animals, *Diabetologia* **10**:491–701.

Rizza, R. A., Mandarino, L. J., and Gerich, J. E., 1981, Mechanisms of insulin resistance in man. Assessment using the insulin dose-response curve in conjunction with insulin-receptor binding, *Am. J. Med.* **70**:168–176.

Rossini, A. A., Like, A. A., Chick, W. L., Appel, M. C., and Cahill, G. F., 1977, Studies of streptozocin-induced insulitis and diabetes, *Proc. Natl. Acad. Sci.* **74**:2485–2489.

Rossini, A. A., Williams, R. M., Appel, M. C., and Like, A. A., 1978, Sex differences in the multiple-dose streptozotocin model of diabetes, *Endocrinology* **103**:1518–1520.

Rossini, A. A., Williams, R. M., Mourdes, J. P., Appel, M. C., and Like, A. A., 1979, Spontaneous diabetes in the gnotobiotic BB/W rat, *Diabetes* **23**:1031–1032.

Rossini, A. A., Williams, R. M., Appel, M. C., and Like, A. A., 1980, Animal models of type I diabetes, in: *Immunology of Diabetes* (W. J. Irvine, ed.), pp. 275–290, Teviot Publications, Edinburgh, United Kingdom.

Roth, S. I., Conaway, H. H., Sanders, L. L., Casali, R. E., and Boyd, A. E., 1980, Spontaneous diabetes mellitus in the New Zealand white rabbit, *Lab. Invest.* **42**:571–579.

Rotter, J. I., and Rimoin, D. L., 1981, The genetics of the glucose intolerance disorders, *Am. J. Med.* **70**:116–126.

Sandler, S., and Andersson, A., 1981, Islet implantation into diabetic mice with pancreatic insulitis, *Acta. Pathol. Microbiol. Scand. [A.]* **89**:107:12.

Seemayer, T. A., Oligny, L., Tannenbaum, G. S., Goldman, H., and Colle, E., 1980, Animal model: Spontaneous diabetes mellitus in the BB Wistar rat, *Am. J. Pathol.* **101**:485–488.

Seemayer, T. A., Schurch, W., and Kalant, N ., 1982a, B Cell lymphoproliferation in spontaneously diabetic 'BB' wistar rats, *Diabetologia* **23**:261–265.

Seemayer, T., Tannenbaum, G., Goldman, H., and Colle, E., 1982b, Dynamic time course studies of the spontaneously diabetic BB wistar rat, III. Light-microscopic and ultrastructural observations of pancreatic islets of Langerhans, *Am. J. Pathol.* **106**:237–249.

Sima, A. A. F., 1980, Peripheral neuropathy in the spontaneously diabetic BB-Wistar rat. An ultrastructural study, *Acta. Neuropathol.* **51**:223–227.

Sima, A. A. F., and Hay, K., 1981, Functional aspects and pathogenic considerations of the neuropathy in the spontaneously diabetic 'BB' wistar rat, *Neuropathol. Appl. Neurobiol.* **7**:341–350.

Soret, M. G., Dulin, W. E., and Gerritsen, G. C., 1973, Microangiopathy in animals with spontaneous diabetes, in: *Early Diabetes, Advances in Metabolic Disorders* (R. Camerini-Davalos, and H. S. Cole, eds.), pp. 291–98, Academic Press, New York.

Soret, M. G., Peterson, T., and Block, E. M., 1976, Electron microscopy of the aorta in young and adult Chinese hamsters, *Artery* **2**:109–128.

Sternthal, E., Like, A. A., Sarantis, K., and Brauerman, L. E., 1981, Lymphocytic thyroiditis and diabetes in the BB/W rat: A new model of autoimmune endocrinopathy, *Diabetes* **30**:1058–1061.

Stuhlman, R. A., 1979, Animal model: Spontaneous diabetes mellitus in Mystromys albicaudatus, *Am. J. Pathol.* **94**:685–688.

Tannenbaum, G. S., Colle, E., Gurd, W., and Wanamaker, L., 1981a, Dynamic time-course studies of the spontaneously diabetic BB wistar rat. I. Longitudinal profiles of plasma growth hormone, insulin and glucose, *Endocrinology* **109**:1872–1879.

Tannenbaum, G. S., Colle, E., Wanamaker, L., Gurd, W., Goldman, H., and Seemayer, T. A., 1981b, Dynamic time-course studies of the spontaneously diabetic BB wistar rat. II. Insulin, glucagon, and somatostatin-reactive cells in the pancreas, *Endocrinology* **109**:1880–1887.

Tomita, T., Lacy, P. E., Matschinsky, F. M., and McDaniel, M. L., 1974, Effect of alloxan on insulin secretion in isolated rat islets perifused in vitro, *Diabetes* **23**:517–524.

Toreson, W. E., Lee, J. C., and Grodsky, G. H., 1968, the histopathology of immune diabetes in the rabbit, *Am. J. Pathol.* **52**:1099–1015.

Toyota, T., Kataoka, S., Fujiya, H., Sato, J., and Goto, Y., 1982, Immunological analysis of NOD mice as a model of insulin-dependent diabetes mellitus, *Diabetes* **31**(Suppl. 2):20 (abstract) 77.

Volk, B. W., and Wellman, K. F., 1979, Hormonal diabetes, in: *The Diabetic Pancreas* (B. W. Volk and K. F. Wellman, eds.), pp. 271–290, Plenum Press, New York.

Williams, M., Gregory, R., Schall, W., Rovner, D., and Padgett, G., 1980, Diabetes mellitus in a colony of golden retrievers, *Fed. Proc.* **39**:637 (abstract).

Yamada, K., Nonaka, K., Hanafusa, T., Miyazaki, A., Toyoshima, H., and Tarui, S., 1982, Preventive and therapeutic effects of large-dose nicotinamide injections on diabetes associated with insulitis, An observation in non-obese diabetic (NOD) mice, *Diabetes* **31**:749–753.

5

Immune Function in Obese, Diabetic, Hyperinsulinemic C57BL/KsJ-db+/db+ and C57BL/6J-ob/ob Mice

Barry S. Handwerger, Gabriel Fernandes, and David M. Brown

I. THE C57BL/KsJ-db+/db+ MOUSE

A. Introduction

The mutant C57BL/KsJ-db+/db+ (db/db) mouse was first described by Hummel and co-workers of the Jackson Laboratory (Hummel *et al.*, 1966). The mutant diabetes *(db)* gene is inherited as an autosomal recessive with full penetrance. In the homozygous state, the *db* gene is associated with a metabolic disturbance closely resembling adult-oneset, insulin-independent diabetes mellitus. The diabetic syndrome in db/db mice is characterized by obesity, hyperphagia, polydypsia, polyuria, and marked hyperglycemia (Hummel *et al.*, 1966; Coleman and Hummel, 1967, 1969; Herberg and Coleman, 1977; Coleman 1978, 1982). Adult db/db mice weigh up to 70 g, while age- and sex-matched littermates only weight up to 30 g. On an *ad libitum* diet, the

Barry S. Handwerger • Rheumatology Research Unit, Departments of Medicine and Immunology, Mayo Clinic and Mayo Medical School, Rochester, Minnesota 55905.   *Gabriel Fernandes* • Division of Clinical Immunology and Arthritis, Department of Medicine, University of Texas, San Antonio, San Antonio, Texas 78284.   *David M. Brown* • Departments of Pediatrics and Laboratory Medicine and Pathology, University of Minnesota School of Medicine, Minneapolis, Minnesota 55455.

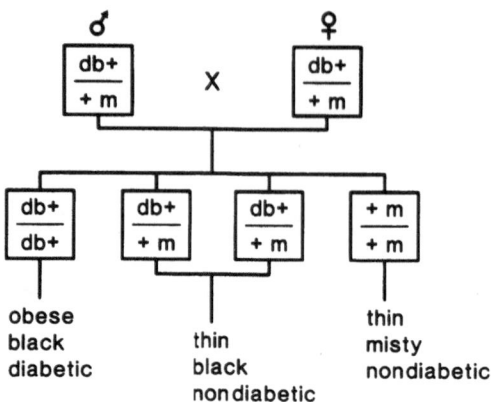

Figure 1. Breeding of db/db mice.

average daily food intake of mice is approximately twice normal. Blood sugars run between 350 and 650 mg/dl (normal 100–200 mg/dl). During the first 4–6 months of age plasma insulin concentrations are markedly elevated in the range of 300–600 μU/ml. After approximately 6 months of age, plasma insulin concentrations fall to within the normal range of 10–100 μU/ml. Early in the course of the disease, during the period of hyperinsulinemia, the islets of Langerhans are characterized by β cell hypertrophy and hyperplasia with β cell degranulation (Like and Chick 1970). The mice are insulin-resistant and have a decrease in the number of insulin receptors on insulin-sensitive target tissues (Kahn *et al.,* 1973, Chang *et al.,* 1975, Raizada *et al.,* 1980). Later in the disease, concomitant with the drop in plasma insulin concentration, progressive atrophy of islet cells occurs (Like and Chick, 1970).

Because homozygous db/db mice are sterile, heterozygous carriers are used for breeding. The diabetes (*db*) gene is in close linkage with the misty (*m*) color coat gene (both are located on chromosome 4, linkage group VIII). As demonstrated in Figure 1, when the misty gene is maintained in repulsion on the opposite chromosome to the *db* gene, mating of heterozygous carriers results in the production of mice of three distinct genotypes (Chick and Like, 1970): obese, black, diabetic mice homozygous for the *db* locus (db+/db+ or db/db); lean, black, phenotypically nondiabetic mice heterozygous for both *db* and *m* (db+/+m or db/m); and (C) lean, misty, nondiabetic mice homozygous for *m* but lacking the *db* gene (+m/+m or m/m).

B. Alterations in Immunological Function

During the past several years, increasing evidence has documented the existence of marked alterations in immunological function in *db/db* mice.

1. In Vivo Immunological Function in db/db Mice

a. Cellularity of Lymphoid Organs. Db/db mice have a significant decrease in spleen and thymus weight and diminished ^{125}I-iododeoxyuridine uptake by the thymus gland (Fernandes *et al.*, 1978). The number of nucleated cells in the spleens of 3–6-month-old db/db mice (72 ± 4 million nucleated cells/spleen) is significantly lower than that in their nondiabetic littermates (116 ± 5 million nucleated cells/spleen). Paski and co-workers (1981) have documented that the spleens of db/db mice have fewer germinal centers and less cells in the white pulp and that the thymic cortex is thinner and the thymic medulla less dense than in their nondiabetic littermates. The number and percentage of T cells and complement-receptor-bearing lymphocytes in the spleens of db/db are significantly reduced (Pasko *et al.*, 1981). Lymph node cells in the db/db mouse are markedly underdeveloped and difficult to find. The number of macrophages recovered from the peritoneal cavity of db/db mice 4–5 days after intraperitoneal inoculation of light mineral oil is significantly depressed compared to the recovery of macrophages from their nondiabetic littermates. The mean recovery of peritoneal macrophages was 5.05×10^6 per db/m mouse compared to 0.23×10^6 per db/db mouse (Pasko *et al.*, 1981). This difference, however, may have been due in part to incomplete recovery of macrophages from the peritoneal cavity of db/db mice due to their tremendous intraperitoneal adiposity. Kazura *et al.*, (1979) have reported that the total number of cells recovered from the peritoneal cavity of db/db mice 48 hr after intraperitoneal injection of 10% proteose peptone is normal.

Db/db mice have a normal hemoglobin, hematocrit, and peripheral blood red blood cell count, reticulocyte count, white blood cell count, and platelet count (Table 1) (Roodman *et al.*, 1982). Bone marrow CFU-E (erythroid-colony-forming units) and BFU-E (erythroid-burst-forming units) are similar in db/db, db/m, and m/m mice. In contrast, bone marrow CFU-GM (granulocyte–macrophage-colony-forming units) are significantly higher in db/db mice than in db/m mice. Interestingly, the number of CFU-GM in db/m bone marrow, in turn, is about twice that in the bone marrow of m/m mice (Table 2) (Roodman *et al.*, 1982). These data suggest that the db mutation may affect the number of CFU-GM in a gene dose-dependent fashion. It is possible that genes controlling CFU-GM differentiation and/or proliferation from precursor cells may be linked to the *db* locus.

b. Skin Graft Survival.   Db/db mice have a significantly diminished capacity to reject allogeneic skin grafts. In our studies (Fernandes *et al.*, 1978), db/db (H-2^d) mice rejected *H-2* nonidentical allogeneic full-thickness C57BL/6 (H-2^b) skin grafts in 13.5

Table 1.   *Hematologic Parameters in m/m, db/m, and db/db Mice*

	Mice		
Variable	m/m	db/m	db/db
Hemoglobin (g/dl)	13.6 ± 0.5	12.7 ± 0.5	13.5 ± 0.5[a]
Red blood cell count ($\times 10^6$)	6.69 ± 0.26	6.84 ± 0.13	7.47 ± 0.26
Hematocrit (%)	32.5 ± 1.2	31.0 ± 0.8	34.4 ± 1.3
Reticulocytes (%)	1.1 ± 0.2	1.1 ± 0.1	1.4 ± 0.2
White blood cell count ($\times 10^3$)	5.6 ± 0.6	6.5 ± 0.9	7.6 ± 0.8
Platelets ($\times 10^3$)	925 ± 43	810 ± 35	889 ± 31

[a]Results are presented as the mean ± SEM of five independent determinations and are per μl of blood.

*Table 2.   Hematopoietic Progenitors in Bone Marrow Samples from m/m,
db/m, and db/db Mice*

	m/m	db/m	db/db
Erythroid colony-forming unit	227 ± 27[a]	332 ± 83	251 ± 50
Erythroid burst-forming unit	14 ± 1	20 ± 2	19 ± 2
Granulocyte–macrophage colony-forming unit	49 ± 5	83 ± 3	127 ± 5

[a]Results are presented as the mean ± SEM of at least three independent experiments.

± 1.1 days (mean ± SEM), while nondiabetic db/m and C57BL/Ks controls rejected similar grafts in 7.8 ± 0.2 days and 8.0 ± 0.4 days, respectively. Mandel (1978; Mandel and Mahmond, 1979) has reported that db/db reject H-2-identical allogeneic BALB/c skin grafts in 17.8 ± 1.2 days compared to 9.7 ± 0.3 days for control nondiabetic littermates. Second-set grafts survived 10.1 ± 0.5 days in db/db mice and 6.0 ± 0.3 days in control mice.

c. *In Vivo Generation of Cytotoxic T Cells following Allogeneic Stimulation.* Db/db mice have a significantly diminished ability to generate a splenic cytotoxic T cell response following intraperitoneal immunization with allogeneic EL4 (H-2^b) lymphoma cells (Fernandes *et al.*, 1978). Cytotoxic cell activity was examined on days 10–20 following *in vivo* immunization. The cytotoxic cell response of db/db mice was defective throughout that time course. Table 3 illustrates the cytotoxic cell responses of spleen cells from db/db and db/m mice on day 10 following *in vivo* immunization with 5 × 10^6 EL4 cells. A similar defect in the cytotoxic cell response of spleen cells from db/db mice was also apparent after *in vivo* immunization with 1 × 10^6 and 10 × 10^6 of EL4 cells.

*Table 3.   Cell-Mediated Cytotoxicity of Spleen Cells from db/db and
db/m Mice Immunized in Vivo with EL4 Cells (5 × 10^6)*

Experiment	Mice	(No.)	% Cytotoxicity (mean ± SEM) Day 10[a]		
			100:1[b]	50:1	25:1
1	db/db	(4)	4 ± 1	2 ± 1	1 ± 1
	db/m	(4)	66 ± 4	59 ± 7	44 ± 7
2	db/db	(4)	7 ± 2	3 ± 1	2 ± 1
	db/m	(4)	73 ± 2	61 ± 5	42 ± 3
3	db/db	(3)	7 ± 2	5 ± 1	3 ± 0
	db/m	(3)	78 ± 2	70 ± 1	58 ± 2
4	db/db	(6)	11 ± 1	8 ± 1	5 ± 1
	db/m	(3)	77 ± 3	73 ± 5	59 ± 7

[a]Db/db and db/m mice (3–5 months old) were immunized intraperitoneally with 5 × 10^6 allogeneic EL4 (H-2^b) lymphoma cells. Ten days later their spleens were removed and their cytotoxic activity against EL4 target cells determined in a 4-hr microtiter ^{51}Cr-release assay system.
[b]Effector-to-target-cell ratio.

Table 4. Cytotoxicity of Cells Infiltrating Alloantigen-Containing Sponges in db/db and db/m Mice[a]

Days after sponge implantation	Mice	(No.)	% Cytotoxicity (mean ± SEM)				Lymphocytes recovered per sponge × 10^6
			32:1	16:1	8:1	4:1	
10	db/db	(5)	—	0	0	0	0.2
	db/m	(3)	—	9 ± 1	6 ± 1	—	1.7
14	db/db	(5)	0	1 ± 1	1 ± 1	—	0.2
	db/m	(3)	65 ± 2	64 ± 1	59 ± 1	—	1.4
22	db/db	(5)	42 ± 1	58 ± 1	58 ± 1	40 ± 1	0.7
	db/m	(6)	23 ± 1	22 ± 1	16 ± 1	8 ± 1	0.5

[a]Sponges coated with peritoneal exudate cells from C57BL/6 (H-2[b]) mice were implanted subcutaneously into db/db and db/m mice. On days 10, 14, and 22 following implantation, the sponges were removed, the nonadherent cells obtained, and their cytotoxicity activity against EL4 (H-2[b]) target cells determined in a 4-hr microtiter ^{51}Cr-release assay system. The total and differential cell counts were also determined for each cell population.

To explore further the nature of the cytotoxic T cell defect in db/db mice, we have examined the cytotoxicity in db/db and db/m mice of cells infiltrating alloantigen-containing sponge matrix allografts (Hoffman *et al.*, unpublished data, 1983). The sponge matrix allograft model used in these studies was adopted from the procedure of Roberts and Hayry (1976). Sponges containing C57BL/6 (H-2[b]) alloantigens were implanted subcutaneously into 3- to 6-month-old db/db and db/m mice. At varying time points thereafter, the sponges were removed, the nonadherent cells obtained, and their cytotoxicity against EL4 (*H-2[b]*) target cells determined in a 4-hr microtiter ^{51}Cr-release assay system. Table 4 demonstrates that db/db mice were able to mount a cytotoxic cell response in the sponge allograft. The peak cytotoxic response of db/db mice, however, was delayed, and, in terms of total lytic activity, of less magnitude than the peak response in db/m mice. On day 22, the day of maximal response for db/db mice, the total number of lymphocytes recovered per sponge was only $0.7 × 10^6$ compared to $1.4 × 10^6$ db/m lymphocytes recovered per sponge on day 14, the day of peak db/m response. As a result, the total lytic activity of lymphocytes infiltratign the sponge grafts at the time of peak response in db/db mice was significantly less than in the db/m mice. These data, which demonstrate that db/db mice have a diminished and kinetically delayed cytotoxic cell response at the implantation site of an alloantigen-containing sponge graft, are consistent with the observed prolongation of skin allograft rejection times in db/db mice (Fernandes *et al.*, 1978; Mandel and Mahmond, 1978; Mandel 1979).

d. In Vivo Plaque-Forming Cell (PFC) Responses. We have previously reported that 2- to 6-month-old db/db mice have a significantly enhanced (1.4–3.0 fold) splenic direct IgM PFC response on day 4 after primary intraperitoneal immunization with sheep red blood cells (SRBC), a T-dependent antigen (Fernandes *et al.*, 1978). Db/db mice also have enhanced splenic indirect IgG PFC responses on day 7 following primary (Table 5) and day 4 following secondary (Table 6) *in vivo* immunization with SRBC. In addition, db/db mice have enhanced splenic primary direct IgM PFC responses fol-

Table 5.   Indirect (IgG) PFC Response following Primary in Vivo Immunization with SRBC: db/db, db/m, and m/m Mice

Experiment	Mice	(No.)	PFC (day 7)[a]	
			Per 10^6 spleen cells	Per spleen
1	db/db	(3)	$1,977 \pm 35$[b]	$165,000 \pm 10,800$
	db/m	(3)	616 ± 79	$78,800 \pm 7,400$
	m/m	(4)	665 ± 114	$73,700 \pm 14,775$
2	db/db	(3)	$1,985 \pm 642$	$188,200 \pm 77,400$
	db/m	(3)	940 ± 67	$69,500 \pm 24,300$
	m/m	(3)	856 ± 67	$73,100 \pm 7,910$
3	db/db	(3)	967 ± 171	$95,700 \pm 17,900$
	db/m	(3)	309 ± 12	$34,800 \pm 3,100$
	m/m	(3)	348 ± 77	$40,400 \pm 8,100$

[a]Mice (3–6 months of age) were immunized intraperitoneally with 10×10^8 SRBC and 7 days later the indirect IgG PFC response of their spleen cells was determined in a modified Jerne plaque assay.
[b]Mean $\pm$ SEM.

Table 6.   Indirect (IgG) PFC Response following Secondary in Vivo Immunization with SRBC

Experiment	Mice	(No.)	PFC (mean $\pm$ SEM)[a]	
			Per 10^6 spleen cells	Per spleen
1	db/db	(3)	815 ± 67	$53,000 \pm 4,700$
	db/m	(4)	359 ± 32	$32,300 \pm 6,200$
2	db/db	(4)	$1,148 \pm 113$	$93,800 \pm 9,300$
	db/m	(4)	490 ± 56	$52,800 \pm 6,000$

[a]Mice (4–5 months of age) were immunized intraperitoneally with 10×10^8 SRBC on day 0 and boosted with 5×10^8 SRBC given on day 30. The indirect IgG PFC response of their spleen cells was determined 4 days after the secondary immunization in a modified Jerne plaque assay.

Table 7.   Direct (IgG) PFC Response following Primary in Vivo Immunization with Pneumococcal Polysaccharide S III

Experiment	Mice	(No.)	PFC (day 5)[a]	
			Per 10^6 spleen cells	Per spleen
1	db/db	(4)	59 ± 5[b]	4642 ± 697
	db/m	(4)	31 ± 2	2600 ± 369
2	db/db	(4)	87 ± 3	6195 ± 483
	db/m	(4)	36 ± 1	4810 ± 350
3	db/db	(4)	70 ± 1	6680 ± 1400
	db/m	(4)	34 ± 1	3560 ± 217

[a]Mice (age 4–5 months) were immunized intraperitoneally with 0.5 μg pneumococcal polysaccharide SIII and 5 days later the direct IgM PFC response of their spleen cells determined in a modified Jerne plaque assay using SIII-coated sheep erythrocytes as indicator cells.
[b]Mean $\pm$ SEM.

lowing *in vivo* immunization with the T-independent antigen, pneumococcal polysac-charide SIII (Table 7) (Torseth *et al.*, 1983).

e. Delayed-Type Hypersensitivity Responses.   Mahmoud, Mandel, and co-workers (Mahmoud *et al.*, 1976, Mandel and Mahmoud 1978; Mandel, 1979) have demon-strated that Schistosoma-immunized db/db mice have markedly diminished delayed-type hypersensitivity responses (as measured by delayed foot-pad swelling) following *in vivo* challenge with Schistosoma antigens. The net increase in foot-pad swelling 24 hr after injection of antigen in immunized db/db mice was only 0.09 ± 0.01 mm com-pared to 0.38 ± 0.09 mm in nondiabetic db/m controls. Pasko *et al.*, (1981) have reported that bacille Calmette-Guérin (BCG)-immunized db/db mice have a marked defect in delayed-type hypersensitivity responses to purified protein derivative (PPD), manifested by only an 11% increase in foot-pad swelling after antigenic challenge com-pared to a 98% increase in swelling in control db/m mice.

f. In Vivo Induction of Suppressor Cells.   Rich and Rich (1975) demonstrated that suppressor T cells can be induced *in vivo* by intravenous injection of concanavalin A. We have examined the *in vivo* induction of suppressor cells in 3–6 month-old db/db and db/m mice injected intravenously with concanavalin A (200 μg per mouse). The model system used to assess suppressor cell activity was the ability of spleen cells from con-A-treated and control mice to inhibit the generation of cytotoxic cells in an *in vitro* mixed lymphocyte culture of db/m (H-2^d) responder cells and C57BL/6 (H-2^b) stimu-lator cells. As demonstrated in Figure 2, spleen cells from con-A-treated db/db and

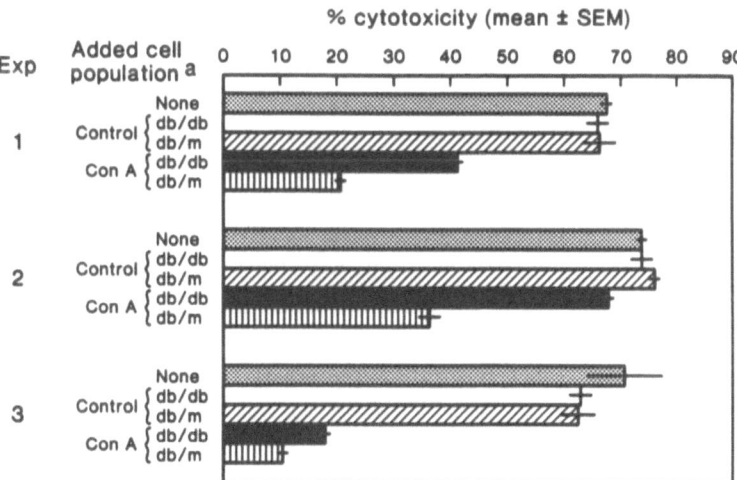

Figure 2.   Suppression of the *in vitro* generation of cytotoxic cells by suppressor cells induced *in vivo* with concanavalin A. Spleen cells (2 × 10^6) from db/m mice were cultured for 5 days in allogeneic mixed lym-phocyte culture with C57BL/6 (H-2^b) spleen cells as stimulators. At the initiation of culture no additional cells or 2 × 10^6 spleen cells were added from db/db or db/m mice which had been injected intravenously 24 hr previously with either 200 μg/mouse con A (dissolved in phosphate-buffered saline) or phosphate-buffered saline alone (control mice). On day 5, the cells were harvested and tested for cytotoxic activity against EL4 (H-2^b) target cells in a 4-hr microtiter ^{31}Cr-release assay system.

db/m mice were both able to suppress the *in vitro* generation of alloantigen-stimulated cytotoxic cells. The degree of suppression induced by spleen cells from con-A-treated db/db mice, however, was significantly less than that induced by spleen cells from con-A-treated db/m mice, suggesting that suppressor cell induction *in vivo* is impaired in db/db mice. The comparative ability of db/db and db/m spleen cells to respond to suppressor signals from con-A-induced suppressor cells was also evaluated. Db/db responder cells in mixed lymphocyte culture were inhibited to the same degree as db/m responder cells by *in vivo* con-A-activated db/db or db/m suppressor cells. These data suggest that the *in vitro* response of db/db spleen cells to immunoregulatory signals from con-A-activated suppressor cells is normal.

g. Tolerance Induction in Vivo.   The induction of immunological tolerance following *in vivo* administration of toleragen in normal in 2- to 4-month-old db/db mice (Azar *et al.*, 1983). As illustrated in Table 8, 20 days following tolerization with 0.1 mg or 1 mg. of deaggregated human gammaglobulin (HGG), db/db and db/m mice exhibit equivalent degrees of tolerance, as measured in an immune elimination assay.

h. Fc-Receptor-Mediated Clearance of ^{125}I-Labeled Heat-Aggregated Human IgG.   The clearance of heat-aggregated human IgG from the blood of nonimmune hosts is macrophage-dependent and related to the binding of the IgG to Fc receptors on liver macrophages (Kupffer cells) and, to a lesser extent, splenic macrophages. Keane *et al.* (1983) have demonstrated that the rate of clearance of ^{125}I-labeled heat-aggregated human IgG from blood is significantly diminished in nonimmune db/db mice compared to normal db/m mice. Following intravenous injection, the half-life of ^{125}I-labeled heat-aggregated human IgG in the blood of db/db mice was 39.1 $\pm$ 4.8 min compared to 18.6 $\pm$ 2.3 min for db/m mice. These data suggest the presence in db/db mice of a defect in *in vivo* Fc-receptor-mediated macrophage function.

i. Immune Complex Deposition in Kidney.   Db/db mice have more IgG, IgM, and C3 deposited in their glomeruli than their nondiabetic littermates (Meade *et al.*, 1981). The pattern of glomerular staining with fluoresceinated antisera to immunoglobulins or

Table 8.   *In Vivo Induction of Tolerance to Human Gamma Globulin*[a]

Tolerization dose (mg)	Mice	(No.)	%^{131}I-Ag remaining at 24 hr
1.0	db/db	(15)	71 $\pm$ 3
	db/db	(21)	62 $\pm$ 2
0.1	db/db	(16)	64 $\pm$ 4
	db/m	(20)	66 $\pm$ 4

[a]Db/db and db/m mice (2–4 months of age) were tolerized by intraperitoneal injection of 0.1 mg or 1.0 mg of deaggregated HGG on day 0. On day 14, the mice were immunized with 0.1 mg of aggregated HGG. On day 20 the mice were injected intraperitoneally with ^{131}I-HGG and the percent radioactivity remaining after 24 hr determined. In control (naive) db/db and db/m mice, 88 $\pm$ 8% and 80 $\pm$ 12%, respectively, of the injected antigen was present at 24 hr; in immune db/db and db/m mice, 14 $\pm$ 1% and 14 $\pm$ 3%, respectively, was detected at 24 hr.

C3 was irregular and granular with deposits predominantly seen within the mesangium with occasional deposition within the juxtamesangial portions of the capillary loops. In fixed sections stained with haemotoxylin and eosin, mesangial thickening secondary to an increase in mesangial matrix with proliferation and clustering of mesangial cells was observed. Limited insulin deposits were present in the kidneys of 8 out of 15 db/db mice and immunoglobulin eluted from kidney of db/db mice had a significant increase in insulin-binding capacity compared to immunoglobulin from control kidneys.

j. Immunity to Infectious Agents

i. Staphylococcal and β-Hemolytic Streptococcal Infections. Db/db mice injected intraperitoneally with either coagulase-positive *Staphylococcus aureus* or β-hemolytic streptococci (Lancefield, Group A) do not contain the infection as well as their nondiabetic littermate controls and consequently have a significantly higher mortality (Mandel, 1979). The mean 50% survival time of staphylococcus-infected db/db mice was 4 days compared to 10 days for db/m mice; streptococcus-infected db/db mice survived 5 days compared to 19 days for db/m mice.

ii. Schistosoma mansoni Infections. Mahoud and co-workers (Mahmoud *et al.*, 1976, Mandel and Mahmoud, 1978, Mandel, 1979) have demonstrated that db/db mice have a significant reduction in the areas of granulomatous inflammation around *Schistosoma mansoni* eggs injected via the tail vein into the pulmonary microvasculature. In db/db mice, the mean granuloma area was 10.8×10^3 μm², compared to 35.4×10^3 μm² in nondiabetic controls. Hepatic granulomas were also smaller in *S.-mansoni*-infected db/db mice.

The granulomas that occur in *S.-mansoni*-infected db/db mice contained a decreased number of eosinophils, which normally constitute approximately 50% of the host's granulomatous response (Mahmoud *et al.*, 1976). Granuloma formation to *S. mansoni* eggs is a T-cell-dependent phenomenon (Warren 1976). As outlined above, T-cell-mediated immunity to *S.-mansoni* egg antigens, as determined by delayed-type hypersensitivity reactions, is markedly impaired in Schistosoma-sensitized db/db mice (Mahmoud *et al.*, 1976, Mandel and Mahmoud, 1978, Mandel, 1979). Kazura *et al.*, (1979) have reported that db/db mice and db/m mice infected subcutaneously with the cercariae of *S. mansoni* have similar numbers of total cells and eosinophils in peritoneal exudates 48 hr after stimulation with 10% proteose peptone. The peritoneal exudate cells of db/db mice, however, displayed a significantly diminished eosinophil migration in response to soluble *S. mansoni* egg antigen (SEA). Migration was measured in the direct eosinophil stimulation promoter (ESP) assay described by Colley (1973). At 25 μg/ml SEA, for example, eosinophils from db/db had mean value of $-24.6 \pm 6.1\%$ enhanced migration vs. $114.9 \pm 4.5\%$ for nondiabetic db/m controls (Kazura *et al.*, 1979). The defect in eosinophil migration appeared to be secondary to a defect in the ability of db/db spleen cells to produce or secrete the lymphokine ESP.

iii. Candida albicans Infections. Db/db mice injected intravenously with 1.5×10^4 *Candida albicans* organisms develop a progressive infection, while their nondiabetic db/m littermates are resistant (Pasko *et al.*, 1981). Intravenous injection of 4×10^4 *C. albicans* into db/db mice resulted in death within 14 days and recovery of approximately 10^8 yeast organisms per db/db kidney. Db/m mice were alive at 14 days and only 10^5 yeast were recovered per kidney (0.1% of the number recovered per db/db kidney) (Pasko *et al.*, 1981). Peritoneal macrophages from db/db mice were deficient in their *in vitro* ability to phagocytose *C. albicans*. The percentage of phagocytic macrophages and number of yeast phagocytosed per macrophage were decreased in db/db mice.

iv. Group B Coxsackievirus Infections.   The diabetic (*db*) gene influences the susceptibility of C57BL/Ks mice to infection with coxsackie B4 virus (Webb *et al.*, 1976). Heterozygous, nondiabetic db/m mice were more susceptible to coxsackie B4 virus infection than the parental background strain (C57BL/Ks) and developed more severe pathologic changes and manifested a higher mortality. Db/db mice were more susceptible than either db/m or C57BL/Ks mice to coxsackie B4 infection and showed much more extensive and severe pancreatic involvement and greater mortality.

k. In Vivo Transfer Experiments.   The alterations in *in vivo* immunological function in db/db mice appear to be a consequence of the abnormal metabolic millieu present in the diabetic mice (Fernandes *et al.*, 1978). This conclusion is supported by the observation that spleen cells from db/db mice transferred into 900-R irradiated db/m mice are able in that nondiabetic environment to generate a normal cytotoxic cell response following *in vivo* allogeneic stimulation (Table 9) (Handwerger *et al.*, 1979). In contrast, when studied 10–14 days after reconstitution, 900-R irradiated db/m mice reconstituted with spleen cells from db/db mice have enhanced direct PFC responses following primary *in vivo* immunization with SRBC (Table 10) an enhancement similar to that seen in intact db/db mice. These data suggest that the enhanced PFC responsiveness of db/db mice may be due to a more profound alteration in splenic lymphoid cell function, which might require a longer period of time in a normal metabolic environment before normal immunological activity can be restored. To evaluate this possibility, the PFC responsiveness of db/db spleen cells in irradiated db/m hosts was evalu-

Table 9.   *In Vivo Cytotoxic Cell Response of Spleen Cells from 900-R Irradiated db/m Mice Reconstituted with db/db or db/m Spleen Cells*

Experiment	Donor strain	(No. of mice)	% Cytotoxicity (mean ± SEM)		
			$100:1^a$	$50:1$	$25:1$
1	db/db	(5)	24 ± 3	23 ± 3	16 ± 2
	db/m	(5)	20 ± 7	18 ± 7	12 ± 5
2	db/db	(5)	22 ± 3	18 ± 2	11 ± 2
	db/m	(3)	19 ± 5	17 ± 5	10 ± 2

[a]Db/m mice were irradiated with 900-R and reconstituted with 45×10^6 spleen cells from db/db or db/m mice. Seven days later the mice were immunized intraperitoneally with allogeneic EL4 (H-2^b) lymphoma cells. The cytotoxic response of their spleen cells was determined 10 days after immunization in a 4 hr microtiter ^{51}Cr-release assay system using EL4 target cells.

Table 10.   In Vivo PFC Response of 900-R Irradiated db/m Mice Reconstituted with db/db or db/m Spleen Cells

Experiment	Donor strain	(No. of mice)	Direct PFC/spleen (mean ± SEM)[a]
1	db/db	(4)	17,345 ± 1,313
	db/m	(5)	5,548 ± 929
2	db/db	(5)	22,087 ± 3,319
	db/m	(5)	9,951 ± 1,175

[a]Db/m mice (3–5 months of age) were irradiated with 900-R and reconstituted with 45×10^6 spleen cells from db/db or db/m mice. Eight days later the mice were immunized intraperitoneally with 10×10^8 SRBC and the direct PFC response of their spleen cells determined in a modified Jerne plaque technique (4 days after immunization).

Table 11.   In Vitro Responses of Thymectomized, 900-R Irradiated db/m Mice Reconstituted with db/db, db/m, and m/m Spleen Cells

Donor strain	(No. of mice)	Direct PFC/spleen (mean ± SEM)[a]
db/db	(3)	17,424 ± 3,182
db/m	(4)	8,240 ± 1,920
m/m	(4)	7,472 ± 1,175

[a]Db/m mice were thymectomized at 2 months of age. Ten days later the mice were irradiated with 900-R and reconstituted with 45×10^6 spleen cells from db/db/, db/m, or m/m mice. Thirty-five days after reconstitution, the mice were immunized intraperitoneally with 10×10^8 SRBC, and 4 days after immunization, the direct PFC response of their spleen cells was determined.

ated 5 weeks following spleen cell transfer. Because host thymic function begins to return about 3 weeks after irradiation, the db/m hosts were thymectomized prior to 900-R whole-body irradiation. As illustrated in Table 11, thymectomized, irradiated db/m mice reconstituted with db/db spleen cells still demonstrated an enhanced direct PFC response following primary *in vivo* immunization with SRBC. The enhanced PFC response of db/db spleen cells therefore appears to be due to an alteration in a subpopulation of spleen cells whose function requires the presence of an intact thymus gland.

2. In Vitro Immunological Function of db/db Lymphoid Cells

a. Mixed Lymphocyte Culture, in Vitro PFC, and in Vitro Cytotoxic T Cell Responses.   In contrast to the marked alterations in *in vivo* immunological function in db/db mice, spleen cells from young (2–6 month-old) db/db mice demonstrate only minimal or no alteration in their blastogenic responses to alloantigenic stimulation in mixed lymphocyte culture with C57BL/6 (H-2^b) or CBA/H (H-2^k) stimulator cells, direct IgM PFC responses following *in vitro* stimulation with SRBC, or cytotoxic T cell responses following *in vitro* sensitization with C57BL/6 alloantigens (Fernandes *et al.*, 1978).

Table 12.   Mitogenic Responses of Spleen Cells from db/db and db/m Mice[a]

Experiment	Mice	(No.)	PHA	Con A	LPS	No added mitogen
1	db/db	(3)	54,347 ± 790[b]	61,458 ± 6,745	77,338 ± 3,983	7,947 ± 1,037
	db/m	(4)	51,078 ± 4,213	92,102 ± 3,593	72,430 ± 10,083	12,581 ± 2,221
2	db/db	(3)	129,434 ± 10,091	97,667 ± 7,401	27,872 ± 225	12,114 ± 2,112
	db/m	(4)	130,883 ± 15,926	80,131 ± 8,975	42,963 ± 2,574	16,091 ± 2,759
3	db/db	(4)	29,590 ± 5,714	50,649 ± 5,198	7,489 ± 1,503	2,510 ± 566
	db/m	(4)	23,230 ± 978	49,347 ± 2,447	11,341 ± 1,586	1,169 ± 266

[a]Spleen cells (5 × 10^5 cells per well) from 3–6-month-old db/db and db/m mice were cultured for 68 hr in the presence or absence of varying concentrations of mitogen. During the final 16 hr of culture 0.5μCi of [^{3}H]thymidine was added per well.
[b]The data represent the mean ± SEM of the maximal responses of each individual mouse.

b. Mitogenic Responses to PHA, ConA, and LPS.   Mandel and Mahmoud (1978) and Pasko *et al.* (1981) have reported that spleen cells from db/db mice are markedly defective in their blastogeneic response to phytohemagglutinin (PHA) and concanavalin A (Con A). In contrast, we have found no consistent defect in the blastogenic responsiveness of db/db spleen cells to mitogenic stimulation with PHA, Con A, or LPS (lipopolysaccharide) when cultured in media containing either 2% fetal calf serum (Fernandes *et al.*, 1978) or 5% fetal calf serum (Table 12). In six experiments, the maximal blastogenic response of spleen cells from db/db mice to stimulation with PHA, Con A, and LPS was 127 ± 18%, 116 ± 20%, and 128 ± 31%, respectively, of the maximal response of db/m spleen cells.

c. Effector Cell Function in Antibody-Dependent Cell-Mediated Cytotoxicity (ADCC).   The ADCC effector cell activity of spleen cells from db/db mice has been examined in a 3 hr microtiter ^{51}Cr-release cytotoxcity assay system using chicken red blood cells (CRBC) as targets and rabbit anti-CRBC antibodies. In this ADCC system, macrophages are the major effector cell (Handwerger and Koren, 1976, Tada *et. al.*, 1980). As illustrated in Table 13, spleen cells from db/db mice on a per cell basis had

Table 13.   Effector Cell Activity of Spleen Cells in
Antibody-Dependent, Cell-Mediated Cytotoxicity

Experiment	Mice	(No.)	% Cytotoxicity (mean ± SEM)[a]		
			100:1[b]	50:1	25:1
1	db/db	(4)	41 ± 2	29 ± 1	14 ± 1
	db/m	(4)	23 ± 2	14 ± 1	6 ± 1
2	db/db	(4)	72 ± 4	65 ± 3	43 ± 4
	db/m	(4)	53 ± 4	34 ± 3	16 ± 2
3	db/db	(3)	31 ± 5	17 ± 5	9 ± 5
	db/m	(4)	21 ± 4	10 ± 2	8 ± 1
4	db/db	(3)	32 ± 3	21 ± 2	13 ± 1
	db/m	(4)	17 ± 1	10 ± 1	4 ± 1

[a]Spleen cells were removed from 3–4-month-old db/db and db/m mice and their cytolytic activity determined against antibody-coated chicken erythrocytes in a 3-hr microtiter ^{51}Cr-release assay system.
[b]Effector-to-target-cell ratio.

Table 14. Uninduced Splenic Natural Killer Cell Activity

Mice	(No.)	Target cell	% Cytotoxicity (mean ± SEM)[a]		
			200:1[b]	100:1	50:1
db/db	(8)	RL♂ 1	7 ± 1	4 ± 1	2 ± 1
db/m	(8)	RL♂ 1	10 ± 1	7 ± 1	3 ± 1
db/db	(16)	YAC	3 ± 1	2 ± 1	1 ± 1
db/m	(16)	YAC-1	22 ± 2	18 ± 1	9 ± 3

[a]Spleen cells were prepared from 3–4-month-old db/db and db/m mice and the cytotoxic activity against the natural-killer-cell-sensitive target cells RL♂ 1 and YAC-1 determined in a 3-hr microtiter ^{51}Cr-release assay system.
[b]Effector-to-target-cell ratio.

Table 15. In Vivo Induction of Natural Killer Cell Activity by Poly I·C

Mice	(No.)	In vivo poly I·C	% Cytotoxicity (mean ± SEM)[a]		
			200:1[b]	100:1	50:1
db/db	(12)	−	4 ± 1	3 ± 1	1 ± 1
		+	25 ± 2	21 ± 2	12 ± 2
db/m	(12)	−	20 ± 2	17 ± 1	9 ± 1
		+	41 ± 2	33 ± 1	21 ± 2

[a]Db/db and db/m mice (3–4 months of age) were injected intraperitoneally with 100 μg poly I·C in 0.1 ml phosphate-buffered saline (PBS). Control mice were injected with PBS alone. Twenty-four hours later, spleen cells were removed and their cytotoxic activity against NK-sensitive YAC-1 target cells determined in a 3-hr microtiter ^{51}Cr-release assay system.

normal to enhanced ADCC effector cell activity when compared nondiabetic db/m controls *et al.*, 1982).

d. Uninduced and Poly I·C-Induced Natural Killer (NK) Cell Activity.
Spleen cells from db/db mice and db/m mice, 3–4 months of age, have low but relatively comparable natural killer cytotoxicity cell activity against NK-sensitive RL♂ 1 target cells (Table 14) (Handwerger *et al.*, 1982). In contrast, NK-sensitive YAC-1 cells are killed well by db/m spleen cells, but very poorly by spleen cells from db/db mice (Table 14). Poly I·C (polyinosinic-polycytidylic acid) is a known inducer (enhancer) of NK cell activity (Djeu *et al.*, 1978). When db/db and db/m mice were treated *in vivo* with poly I·C, 24 hr later splenic NK cell activity against YAC-1 targets was markedly enhanced in both groups of mice (Table 15). Nevertheless, the NK effector activity of spleen cells from poly-I·C-treated db/db mice was still diminished compared to the activity of spleen cells from poly-I·C-treated db/m mice.

II. THE C57BL/6J-ob/ob MOUSE

A. Introduction

The obese (ob) mutation was first observed at the Jackson Laboratories in the noninbred V strain of mice (Ingalls *et al.*, 1950). Subsequently, the *ob* gene was transferred into the C57BL/6J and C57BL/KsJ strains by a series of cross-intercross matings. On the C57BL/6 background, homozygosity at the *ob* locus is characterized by obesity, hyperphasia, transient hyperglycemia, mild glucose intolerance, markedly elevated plasma insulin concentrations, insulin resistance, a decreased number of insulin receptors on insulin-sensitive tissues, and persistent hypertrophy and hyperplasia of pancreatic beta cells (Bray and York 1971; Herberg and Coleman 1977; Coleman 1978, 1982). On the C57BL/KsJ background, the syndrome associated with homozygosity at the *ob* locus is very similar to that seen in C57BL/KsJ db+/db+ mice with persistent and marked hyperglycemia and transient hyperinsulinemia. Ob/ob mice are infertile; as a result, known heterozygotes (ob/+ mice) must be used to propagate the strain.

B. Alterations in Immunological Function

Several laboratories have investigated immunological competence in C57BL/6J–ob/ob mice and have demonstrated the existence of abnormalities analogous to those present in C57BL/KsJ–db+/db+ mice (Sheena and Meade 1978; Nichols *et al.*, 1978; Meade *et al.*, 1979).

1. In Vivo Immunological Function

a. Cellularity of Lymphoid Organs.   Spleens of C57BL/6J–ob/ob mice are significantly smaller in weight and contain fewer nucleated cells than the spleens of their lean (+/ob or +/+) littermates (Meade *et al.*, 1979). The mean ± SEM spleen weight of ob/ob mice is 76 ± 7 mg compared to 95 ± 4 mg for ob/+ or +/+ mice. The spleens of ob/ob mice contain a mean of 72×10^6 nucleated cells/spleen compared to 111×10^6 nucleated cells/spleens for their lean littermates. The percentage of T cells, as defined by lysis with anti-Thy 1.2 antibodies plus complement, in the spleens of ob/ob mice is normal (Meade *et al.*, 1979).

b. Skin Graft Survival.   The median survival time of male tail skin grafts from C57BL/6J mice on female C57BL/6J–ob/ob mice is longer than on their lean female littermates for both first and second set skin grafts (Sheena and Meade, 1978).

c. In Vivo Generation of Cytotoxic Cells following Allogeneic Stimulation. Meade and co-workers (1979) have demonstrated that C57BL/6J–ob/ob (H-2^b) mice have a significant defect in the ability to generate a splenic cytoxic T cells response following intraperitoneal injection of 3×10^7 allogeneic P815 (H-2^d) mastocytoma cells.

d. Delayed-Type Hypersensitivity Responses.   Ob/ob mice have a significantly depressed delayed-type hypersensitivity response as measured by ear swelling following contact sensitization and ear lobe challenge with picryl chloride. Twenty-four hours after antigenic challenge, the mean ± SEM increase in ear thickness of ob/ob mice was 0.103 ± 0.008 mm compared to 0.185 ± 0.014 mm in lean littermate controls (Sheena and Meade, 1978).

e. Graft-versus-Host Reactions. Spleen cells from ob/ob, ob/+ and +/+ mice do not differ significantly in their ability to cause a graft-versus-host reaction, as measured in a spleen weight assay in B6D2F$_1$ mice (Sheena and Meade, 1978).

2. In Vitro Immunological Function

In contrast to the abnormalities in *in vivo* immunological function, lymphoid cells from ob/ob mice appear to function relatively normally *in vitro*. Spleen cells from C57BL/ 6J–ob/ob mice undergo a normal blastogenic response to stimulation with the T cell mitogen, concanavalin A, and the B cell mitogen, lipopolysaccharide (Nichols *et al.*, 1978). The peak blastogenic response of spleen cells of C57BL/6J–ob/ob mice to alloantigenic stimulation in mixed lymphocyte culture with DBA/2 stimulator cells is mildly but not statistically depressed (Nichols *et al.*, 1978). Spleen cells from C57BL/ 6–ob/ob J mice have no impairment in their ability to generate a cytotoxic T cell response following *in vitro* stimulation with either allogeneic DBA/2 cells (Meade *et al.*, 1979) or TNP-modified syngeneic spleen cells (Nichols *et al.*, 1978).

III. SUMMARY AND CONCLUSIONS

Obese, hyperinsulinemic, diabetic C57BL/KsJ–db+/db+ mice have a marked alteration in *in vivo* immunological function characterized by: (1) the decrease in the size and an alteration in the morphology of spleen and thymus; (2) an increased bone marrow CFU-GM; (3) a significantly diminished capacity to reject allogeneic skin grafts; (4) a markedly diminished ability to generate a splenic cytotoxic T cell response following intraperitoneal immunization with allogeneic tumor cells; (5) a delayed and reduced cytotoxic cell response at the local site of a sponge allograft; (6) significantly enhanced primary direct IgM and indirect IgG PFC responses and increased secondary indirect IgG PFC responses following intraperitoneal immunization with SRBC, a T-dependent antigen; (7) signficantly enahanced primary direct IgM PFC responses following intraperitoneal immunization with pneumococcal polysaccharide SIII, a T-independent antigen; (8) markedly diminished delayed-type hypersensitivity responses to Schistosoma antigens and PPD; (9) decreased induction of suppressor cell activity following *in vivo* administration of concanavalin A; (10) delayed Fc receptor-mediated clearance of ^{125}I-labeled heat-aggregated human IgG; (11) increased IgG, IgM and C3 deposition in renal glomeruli; (12) diminished resistance to infection with staphylococci, β-hemolytic streptococci, *Candida albicans,* and group B coxsackie-virus; and (13) decreased immunological reactivity to *Candida albicans* and *Schistosoma mansoni.* In marked contrast, except for natural killer cell function, *in vitro* immunological activity of db/db spleen cells is essentially normal. These data strongly suggest that the abnormalities in *in vivo* immunological function in db/db mice are secondary to the altered *in vivo* metabolic state and not to an intrinsic defect in db/db lymphoid cells. This conclusion is supported by the observation that db/db spleen cells are able to generate normal cytotoxic cell responses following *in vivo* transfer into irradiated db/m hosts.

Obese hyperinsulinemic C57BL/6–ob/ob also have abnormalities in *in vivo* immunological function characterized by: (1) a decrease in spleen cell size; (2) a decreased ability to reject skin grafts across minor histocompatibility (H-Y) differences; (3) a signiciantly diminished ability to generate a splenic cytotoxic T cell response following intraperitoneal immunization with allogeneic tumor cells; and (4) a diminished delayed hypersensitivity response following contact sensitization with picryl chloride. Like db/db mice, lymphoid cells from ob/ob mice appear to function relatively normally *in vitro*. Spleen cells from ob/ob mice have normal blastogenic response to mitogenic stimulation and alloantigenic stimulation and no impairment in their ability to generate the cytotoxic T cell response following *in vivo* stimulation with either allogeneic spleen cells or TNP-modified syngeneic spleen cells. This discrepancy between *in vivo* and *in vitro* immunological function of ob/ob lymphoid cells highly suggests that the *in vivo* abnormalities in immunological function are a direct consequence of the abnormal metabolic environment present in ob/ob mice. The nature of the alteration in *in vivo* environment in db/db and ob/ob mice responsible for the alteration in *in vivo* immunological function is unknown but may be related to hyperinsulinemia, down regulation of the number of insulin receptors on thymocytes (Goldfine *et al.*, 1972), activated T lymphocytes (Helderman and Strom, 1978) or macrophages (Schwartz *et al.*, 1975), alterations in the concentration of corticosteroids or other hormones, a change in the composition of serum or membrane lipids, or abnormalities in other as yet undefined metabolic parameters.

Levine *et al.* (1981), for example, have recently reported that zinc levels in epididymal fat, femur, and pooled sera of db/db mice were significantly lower than in nondiabetic control (m/m) mice. Zinc deficiency in other systems has been associated with defective cell-mediated immunity (Fernandes *et al.*, 1979; Chandra and Au, 1980). During the next several years the definition of the exact interrelationship of *in vivo* immunological function and metabolic milieu in db/db/ and ob/ob mice should be an exciting and productive area of investigation.

ACKNOWLEDGMENTS.   The authors thank Martha Bennington, Barbara Goodspeed, Terri Riehm, Arlymae Rand, Margo Stich, and James Peterson for excellent technical assistance and Shirley Behnken for assistance in preparing the manuscript. These investigations were supported by U.S. Public Health Service research grants AM25879, AM 31802, CA 21672, CA 021084, AG 03417, the Juvenile Diabetes Foundation, the American Diabetes Association, and the American Diabetes Association (Minnesota Chapter). Dr. Handwerger was a recipient of a Veterans Administration Clinical Investigatorship.

REFERENCES

Azar, M., Brown, D. M. and Handwerger, B.S., 1983, unpublished observations.
Bray, G. A., and York, D. A., 1971, Genetically transmitted obesity in rodents, *Physiol. Rev.* **51**:598–646.
Chandra, R. K., and Au, B., 1980, Single nutrient deficiency and cell-mediated immune responses. I. Zinc, *Am. J. Clin. Nutr.* **33**:736–738.

Chang, K-J, Huang, D., and Cuatrecasas, P., 1975, The defect in insulin receptors in obese, hyperinsulinemic mice: A probable accompaniment of more generalized alterations in membrane glycoproteins, *Biochem. Biophys. Res. Commun.* **64**:566–573.

Chic, W. L., and Like A. A., 1970, Studies in the diabetic mutant mouse: IV. DBM, a modified diabetic mutant produced by outcrossing the original strain. *Diabetologia* **6**:252–256.

Coleman, D. L., 1978, Obesity and diabetes: Two mutant genes causing diabetes–obesity syndromes in mice, *Diabetologia* **14**:141-148.

Coleman, D. L., 1982, Diabetes–obesity syndromes in mice, *Diabetes* **31**:1–6.

Coleman, D. L., and Hummel K. P., 1967, Studies of the mutation, diabetes, in the mouse, *Diabetologia* **3**:238-248.

Coleman, D. L., and Hummel, K. P., 1969, The mutation diabetes, in the mouse, in: *Diabetes Proceedings of the Sixth Congress of the International Diabetes Foundation* (J. Ostman and R. D. G. Milner, eds), pp.813–820, Excerpta Medica Foundation, Amsterdam.

Colley, D. G., 1973, Eosinophils and immune mechanisms. I. Eosinophil stimulation promoter (ESP): A lymphokine induced by specific antigen or phytohemagglutinin, *J. Immunol.* **110**:1419–1423.

Djeu, J. Y., Heinbaugh, J. A. Holden, H. T., and Herberman, R. B., 1978, Augmentation of mouse natural killer cell activity by interferon and interferon inducers, *J. Immunol.* **122**:175–181.

Fernandes, G., Handwerger, B. S. Yunis, E. J., and Brown, D. M., 1978, Immune response in the mutant diabetic C57BL/Ks-db+ mouse: Discrepancies between in vitro and in vivo immunological assays, *J. Clin. Invest.* **61**:243–250.

Fernandes, G., Nair, M., Onoe, K. Tanaka, T., Floyd, R. and Good, R. A., 1979, Impairment of cell-mediated immunity functions by dietary zinc deficiency in mice, *Proc. Natl. Acad. Sci. USA* **76**:457–461.

Goldfine, I. D., Gardner, J. D., and Neville, D. M., Jr., 1972, Insulin action in isolated rat thymocytes: I. Binding of ^{125}I-insulin and stimulation of a-aminoisobutyric acid transport, *J. Biol. Chem.* **247**:6919–6926.

Handwerger, B. S., Fernandes, G., and Brown, D. M., 1979, Immune response in diabetic mice: Influence of in vivo metabolic environment, *Diabetes* **28**:398.

Handwerger, B. S., and Koren, K. S., 1976, The nature of the effector cell in antibody-dependent, cell-mediated cytolysis (ADCC): The cytolytic activity of murine tumor cells and peritoneal macrophages, *Clin. Immunol. Immunopathol.* **5**:272–281.

Handwerger, B. S., Toseth, J., Riehm, T., Fernandes, G., and Brown, D. M. 1982, Immunologic function in obese, diabetic C57BL/Ks-db+/db+ mice and streptozotocin-induced murine diabetes: Further characterization of the defects in plaque-forming cell (PFC) and cytotoxic cell responses, *Diabetes* **31(Suppl. 2)**: 20A.

Helderman, J. H., and Strom, T. B., 1978, Specific insulin binding sites on T and B lymphocytes as a marker of cell activation, *Nature* **274**:62–63.

Herberg, L., and Coleman, D. L., 1977, Laboratory animals exhibiting obesity and diabetes syndromes, *Metabolism* **26**:59–99.

Hoffman, R. A., Simmonds, R. L., Brown, D. M. and Handwerger, B. S., 1983, unpublished observations.

Hummel, K. P., Dickie, M. M., and Coleman, D. L., 1966, Diabetes, a new mutation in the mouse, *Science* **153**:1127–1128.

Ingalls, A. M., Dickie, M. M., Snell, G. D., 1950, Obese, a new mutation in the house mouse, *J. Hered.* **41**:317–318, 1950.

Kahn, C. R., Soll, A., Neville, D. M., Jr., and Roth, J., 1973, Severe deficiency in insulin receptors: A common denominator in the insulin resistance of obesity, *Clin. Res.* **21:+628.**

Kazura, J. W., Gandola, C., Rodman, H. R., and Mahmoud, A. A. F., 1979, Deficient production of the lymphokine eosinophil stimulation promoter in chemically induced and mutant diabetes mellitus in mice, *J. Immunol.* **123**:2114–2117.

Keane, W. F., Brown, D. M. and Handwerger, B. S., 1983, unpublished observations.

Levine, A. S., Morley, J. R., McClain, J. E., Handwerger, B. S., and Brown, D.M., 1981, Zinc status in diabetic mice, *Clin. Res.* **29**:703A.

Like, A. A., and Chick, W. L., 1970, Studies in the diabetic mutant mouse. I. Light microscopy and radioautography of pancreatic islets, *Diabetologia* **6**:207–215.

Mahmoud, A. A., Rodman, H. M., Mandel, M. A., and Warren, K. S.., 1976, Induced and spontaneous diabetes mellitus and suppression of cell-mediated immunologic responses. Granuloma formation delayed dermal reactivity and allograft rejection, *J. Clin. Invest.* **57**:362–367.

Mandel, M. A., 1979, Immune competence and diabetes mellitus. II. Experimental mouse studies, *J. Surg. Res.* **26**:199–205.

Mandel, M. A., and Mahmoud, A. A. F., 1978, Impairment of cell-mediated immunity in mutant diabetic mice (db/db), *J. Immunol.* **120**:1375–1377.

Meade, C. J., Brandon, D. R., Smith, W., Simmonds, R. G., Harris, S., and Sowter, C. 1981, The relationship between hyperglycaemia and renal immune complex deposition in mice with inherited diabetes, *Clin. Exp. Immunol.* **43**:109–120.

Meade, C. J., Sheena, J., and Martin, J., 1979, Effects of the obese (ob/ob) genotype on spleen cell immune function, *Int. Arch. Allergy Appl. Immunol.* **58**:121–127.

Nichols, W. K., Spellman, J. B., and Daynes, R. A., 1978, Immune responses of diabetic animals: Comparison of genetically obese and streptozotocin-diabetic mice, *Diabetologia* **14**:343–349.

Pasko, K. L., Salvin, S. B., and Winkelstein, A., 1981, Mechanisms in the *in vivo* release of lymphokines. V. Responses of alloxan-treated and genetically diabetic mice, *Cell. Immunol.* **62**:205–209.

Raizada, M. H., Tan, G., Deo, R., and Fellows, R. E., 1980, Cells cultured from the diabetic (db/db) mouse have a permanent decrease in insulin receptors, *Endocrinology* **107**:1652–1655.

Rich, R. R., and Rich, S. S., 1975, Biological expressions of lymphocyte activation IV. Concanavalin A-activated suppressor cells in mouse mixed lymphocyte reactions. *J. Immunol.* **114:1112–1115.**

Roberts, P. J., and Hayry, P., 1976, Spone matrix allografts: A model for analysis of killer cells infiltrating mouse allografts, *Transplantation* **21**: 437–445.

Roodman, G. D., Asconsao J. L., Kenyon, P. D., Zanjami, E. D. Brown, D. M., and Handwerger, B. S., 1982, unpublished observations.

Schwartz, R. H. Bianco, A. R., Handwerger, B. S., and Kahn, C. R., 1975, A demonstration that monocytes, rather than lymphocytes, are the insulin binding cells in human periperal blood mononuclear leukocyte preparations. Application for studies of insulin resistance in man. *Proc. Natl. Acad. Sci. USA* **72:474–478.**

Sheena, J., and Meade, C. J., 1978, Mice bearing the ob/ob mutation have impaired immunity, *Int. Arch. Allergy Appl. Immunol.* **57**:263–268.

Tada, M., Honuma, S., Abo, T., and Kumagai, K., 1980, Murine antibody-dependent cell-mediated cytotoxicity: Failure to detect effector cells equivalent to human K cells, *J. Immunol.* **124**:1929–1936.

Torseth J., Brown, D. M., and Handwerger, B. A., 1983, unpublished observations.

Warren, K. S., 1976, Schistosomiasis: A multiplicity of immunopathology, *J. Invest. Dermatol.* **67**:464–469.

Webb, S. R., Loria, R. M., Madge, G. E., and Kibrick, S., 1976, Susceptibility of mice to group B coxsackie virus is influenced by the diabetic gene, *J. Exp. Med.* **143**:1239–1248.

6

The Influence of Sex Hormones on Immunological Processes in the Induction of Diabetes

Young Tai Kim and Charles E. Moody, Jr.

I. INTRODUCTION

Although diabetes mellitus in humans and experimental animals has been studied for many years, the basic mechanisms underlying the induction of diabetes are still not clear. Recent studies, including our own results, suggest that immune mechanisms may play important roles in the induction and pathogenesis of diabetes mellitus. The evidence supporting the idea of an immune mechanism for induction of diabetes includes the following observations: (1) the occurrence of lymphocyte infiltration of pancreatic islets in acute juvenile-onset- (Type I) diabetes (Gepts, 1965, 1972), (2) the occurrence of autoantibodies to islet cells in Type 1 (Bottazzo *et al.*, 1974; MacCuish *et al.*, 1974a,b), (3) the finding that diabetes mellitus could not be induced in athymic nude mice by diabetogenic M-strain encephalomyocarditis virus (EMC virus) (Buschard and Rygaard, 1976), or diabetogenic chemicals (Buschard and Rygaard, 1978; Paik *et al.*, 1980), and (4) the finding that diabetes mellitus could be transferred to normal mice by the passive transfer of spleen cells from diabetic mice induced by streptozotocin (SZ) (Buschard and Rygaard, 1978; Kiesel *et al.*, 1980).

The diabetogeneic property of streptozotocin, a methylnitrosourea derivative of 2-deoxyglocose produced by *Streptomyces achromogenes,* was first reported in 1963 (Rakieter *et al.,* 1963). It is generally accepted that the induction of diabetes by streptozotocin results from the destruction of beta cells. Morphological changes in the beta cells of streptozotocin-treated mice have been extensively demonstrated

Young Tai Kim and Charles E. Moody, Jr. • Divisions of Allergy and Immunology, and Geriatrics and Gerontology, Department of Medicine, Cornell University Medical College, New York, New York 10021.

(Patterson *et al.*, 1970; Findlay *et al.*, 1973). However, it is possible that damage to beta cells by streptozotocin may also activate an autoimmune response which then leads to the further destruction of beta cells. When mice are injected with a single dose of 200 mg streptozotocin/kg body weight, hyperglycemia appears within a few hours. It is therefore unlikely that hyperglycemia induced by such an injection of streptozotocin is mediated by immunological mechanisms. Direct physical destruction of beta cells by streptozotocin is undoubtedly the primary mechanism for the induction of diabetes under these circumstances. However, when mice are injected with 40 mg streptozotocin/kg body weight for 5 consecutive days, hyperglycemia appears slowly. Five to seven days after the last injection of streptozotocin the animals become hyperglycemic and lymphocyte infiltration of the pancreatic islet can be observed. Thus, immunological mechanisms may play a role in induction of diabetes by multiple injections of low doses of streptozotocin. It is interesting to note that diabetes induced by streptozotocin in experimental animal shows a pathogenesis similar to that observed in insulin-dependent diabetes in humans.

The diabetogenic action of streptozotocin is strongly influenced by the gender of the animal; males are in general significantly more susceptible than females (Paik *et al.*, 1980, Rossini *et al.*, 1978). In studies in our laboratory utilizing mice of the C57BL/6J strain, 100% of the males given the multiple low-dosage injections of SZ developed severe and permanent insulin-dependent hyperglycemia, but less than 15% of the females treated identically became hyperglycemic (Kim, 1983). Predominance in male susceptibility has also been reported in the development of experimental diabetes in mice after infection by a diabetogenic virus (Boucher *et al.*, 1975; Morrow *et al.*, 1980) and in rats treated with alloxan (Goodman and Hazelwood, 1974), or after a nearly total pancreatomy (Houssay, 1951; Rodriguez, 1965). Recent epidemiologic data suggest that the incidence of type I diabetes in postpubescent children may also be higher in boys than in girls (West, 1978). It seems possible, therefore, that hormonal influences may play a role in the susceptibility to insulin-dependent diabetes, both in humans and in experimental animals. An understanding of the sex dependency in streptozotocin-induced diabetes might therefore provide an insight into the pathogenesis of insulin-dependent diabetes in general.

In contrast to diabetes, most forms of human autoimmune diseases occur more frequently in the female. Autoimmune-prone strains of mice also show a striking female predominance. Nevertheless, both the induction of diabetes and the occurrence of autoimmunity are influenced by sex difference. It is widely recognized that in most species studied, females show stronger humoral immune response than male (Butterworth *et al.*, 1967; Terres *et al.*, 1968; Batchelor, 1968) Thus, in these autoimmune diseases caused by humoral autoantibodies, females tend to be predominant. Recent reports have suggested that estrogen tends to suppress graft-versus-host reaction and delayed hypersensitivity (Kalland and Forsberg, 1977; Luster *et al.*, 1979) and natural killer cell activity (Seaman *et al.*, 1978; 1979) and thus may protect females from cell-mediated autoimmune diseases. Therefore, autoimmune diseases caused by cellular immunity tend to affect males more often than females. In addition, cytotoxic cell activity generated by virus infection in females is lower than that of males (Wong *et al.*, 1977).

For many years, an explanation for female predominance in autoimmunity was not apparent. However, it is now clear that sex hormones significantly modulate the expression of autoimmunity (Kalland, 1980; Eidinger and Garrett, 1972). It is also clear that sex hormones influence the induction of diabetes by multiple injections of low-dosage streptozotocin or by injecting of M-strains of EMC virus. Furthermore, insulin-independent diabetes in humans and diabetes induced in experimental animals by multiple injection of low-dosage streptozotocin appears to be mediated by immunological processes. In this chapter we will discuss whether the influence of sex hormones on the induction of diabetes by streptozotocin is mediated through immunological mechanisms.

II. SEX HORMONES AND IMMUNE RESPONSE

For many years, an explanation for the female predominance of autoimmunity was not apparent. In humans, systemic lupus erthyematosus (SLE) occurs approximately 10 times more frequently in females than in males and the ratio of chronic thyroiditis in males and females is stated to be 1:4 (Okayasu et al., 1981). This female bias seems to occur only after puberty, because a ratio of approximately 1:1 is found in prepubertal onset of thyroid autoantibodies in asymptomatic children. Several lines of evidence have suggested that sex hormones are important modulators of the immune response. For example, females have fewer infections, higher baseline IgM levels, and better humoral responses to antigens (Cohn, 1979). The capacity of enhanced antibody response in females is manifested both in secondary and primary immune responses (Butterworth et al., 1967; Terres et al., 1968). The enhanced immunological capability, as perhaps might have been predicted, has been associated with numerous additional observations and consequences. For example, it is apparently easier to produce immunological tolerance in the male than in the female (Dresser, 1962). Females are more susceptible to autoimmune disease produced by circulating antibody (Steinberg et al., 1971; Helyer and Howie, 1963) as well as by immune complexes (Halstead, 1969).

Occurrence of antinuclear antibodies is one of the characteristics of SLE, both in humans and mice. These antibodies are heterogeneous and react with single-stranded (ss) and double-stranded (ds) DNA and RNA as well as with DNA–RNA hybrids (Talal and Gallo, 1972). Antibodies to ds DNA occur almost exclusively in SLE, and are associated with disease activity and immune-complex nephritis. Antibodies to ss DNA and RNA occur in other rheumatic diseases as well. In NZB/NZW F_1 mice, a severe lupuslike disorder develops first in females. Prepubertal castration of male mice results in a female pattern of disease characterized by earlier formation of high-titer antibodies to nucleic acids, more severe immune complex glomerulonephritis, and increased mortality. Prepubertal castration of female mice does not significantly alter survival. However, prepubertal castration of females combined with androgen administration results in less autoantibody formation and nephritis and prolonged survival. There is evidence that the presence of the thymus is required for these effects to occur. When castration or treatment with androgen is delayed until an age when disease is

already established, there is again less immune-complex nephritis and prolonged survival. Under these circumstances, however, there is no fall in autoantibody level. In
these older mice, the male hormone may by acting through mechanisms involving
complement or the handling of immune complexes. The antiestrogenic drug nafoxidine
is also therapeutic in female NZB/NZW F_1 mice, resulting in less autoantibody formation and prolonged survival (Duvic et al., 1978).

Female mice of many normal strains generally show enhanced immunological reactivity in comparison with males (Butterworth et al., 1976; Terres et al., 1968). A
greater response of females is observed to a variety of antigens, both thymic-dependent
and thymic-independent. Castration of males can augment immune reactivity, making
it comparable to the female response. The thymus is required for these effects. Their
results may be explained by sex hormones acting on T-lymphocyte subpopulations,
possibly influencing the equilibrium between helper and suppressor cells. Experiments
with autoimmune prone MLR/lpr strain of mice showed that androgen treatment led to
reduced anti-DNA antibodies and prolonged survival without significant reduction in
lymphadenopathy (Steinberg et al., 1980).

Since the immune response is fundamentally dependent on the physiological state
of the lymphoid tissue, it is evident that natural, pathological, or experimental conditions perturbing the lymphoid system will be reflected in changes of immune expression. Calzolari first noted in 1898 that the thymus glands of rabbits castrated before
sexual maturity were larger than those of uncastrated controls. In spite of the formidable volume of work on thymic involution and atrophy inducible by the injection of sex
hormones or gonadotrophic substances, and of the enhancement of these responses by
castration, it is still not possible to predict the effect of sex hormones on the immune
response. Thymic involution during pregnancy has been studied for a long time in
various mammalian species, especially in humans and mice (Persike, 1940; Pepper,
1961). These previous reports were based mainly on histological and morphological
observation showing that the initial involution of the thymus is apparently linked to a
reduction of the thymic cortex. Recently, Phuc and his associates (1981) reported the
characterization of the thymocyte subpopulation in pregnant mice. They found that
cortical thymocytes were greatly reduced in number, whereas medullary thymocytes
appeared unchanged in pregnant mice.

We have studied the influence of sex hormones on the lymphoid tissue in mice
using silastic tube implants containing either androgen or estrogen (Kim et al., 1983).
The influence of implants containing sex hormones on the weight of the thymus and the
number of cells recovered from the thymus and spleen was determined as shown in
Table 1. The weight of the thymus from male mice with estrogen implants was only
one-fourth that of thymus from mice with sham implants. The weight of the thymus
from the female mice with androgen implants was two-thirds that from female mice
with sham implants. Similarly, the number of thymocytes prepared from the thymus
obtained from the male mice with estrogen implants was only one-fifth that from controls. While the number of thymocytes from female mice with androgen implants was
more than half the number from controls. Thus, implants containing estrogen lead to a
greater depletion of thymocytes than do implants containing androgens. However, the
number of spleen cells from the male mice implanted with estrogen was about the same

Table 1. Influence of Sex Hormones on Thymus[a]

Strain/sex	Implants	Weight of thymus (mg)	Number of thymocytes ($\times 10^6$)	Number of spleen cells ($\times 10^6$)
C57BL/6J male	Sham	39	74	84
	Estrogen	10	15	82
C57BL/6J female	Sham	26	68	78
	Androgen	18	38	79

[a]A silastic tube containing 5 mg of estrogen or androgen was implanted subcutaneously in male and female mice respectively. Sham animals received empty silastic tube. Three weeks after implant thymus and spleen were taken out from individual animals and measured wet weight and single cell suspensions were prepared.

as that from the control mice. Therefore, the estrogen or androgen implanted in the either male or female mice, respectively, influences the development of thymus but do not influence the number of spleen cells.

Thus, the influence of sex hormone on immune response may be mediated through the modulation in the growth and function of lymphoid organs. It has been reported that administration of high doses of estrogen is thymolytic and produces a depression of cell-mediated immunity (Money et al., 1952, Luz et al., 1969, Bimes et al., 1975, Shiff et al., 1975, Greenman et al., 1977). Also, high doses of estrogen inhibit antibody production, whereas low doses enhance antibody production and the number of antibody-producing cells in spleens of mice (Kenny et al., 1976). The effects of estrogen on antibody production have been postulated to be directly on the immunocompetent cells, since the presence of estrogen during in vitro induction of antibody-producing cells increased the response. In addition, the phagocytic activity of the reticuloendothelial system is stimulated by exogeneous estrogen(Steven and Snook, 1975). Kalland (1980) demonstrated that treatment of neonatal female mice with estrogen resulted in a decreased number of antibody-producing cells in spleens of adult animals. This depression was due to the reduced helper T-cell activity from estrogen-treated animals which was a reflection of a reduced proportion of Lyt 1 cells. No difference in suppressor activity of primed Lyt 2,3 cells was found.

Ablin and his associates (1974) reported that the phytohemagglutinin (PHA) response of human lymphocyte in vitro was suppressed by the presence of estrogen. Seaman and his co-workers (1978,1979) demonstrated the effect of estrogen on natural killer cells in mice. Natural killer cell activity in mice is most prominent in the spleen and the peripheral blood and appears in the spleen when the mouse is about 20 days old. It then rises rapidly, but declines after 3–4 months. Administration of estrogen to mice causes a substantial reduction in natural killer cell activity in the spleens of either sex. Administration of androgen did not reduce natural killer cell activity. The effects of estrogen were not dependent on the thymus, since estrogen reduced natural killers in mice that had been neonatally thymectomized.

Sex-related difference in the generation of cytotoxic T lymphocytes in the spleen of adult mice infected with Coxsacksie B3 virus (Wong et al., 1977) has been reported. Male mice exhibited a stronger response and significant levels of cytotoxicity were evident by day 3 after injection. Virus-specific cytotoxicity in male mice peaked on

Table 2. Influence of Sex Hormones on Generation of Cellular-Mediated Cytotoxicity[a]

Strain/sex	Implant	Allo[b] MLR (cpm)	Cells recovered after MLR[c]	TLU[d]	Incidence of diabetes by SZ
C57BL/6J male	Sham	72,065	7.2	90.4	15/15
	Estrogen	47,745	1.7	19.2	0/15
C57BL/6J female	Sham	54,536	6.0	41.4	1/10
	Androgen	83,276	10.6	84.1	8/15

[a]Silastic tube containing 5 mg of estrogen or androgen was placed subcutaneously in male and female mice. Sham mice received empty silastic tube. Three weeks after implantation, spleen cells were prepared from individual mice.
[b]Allogeneic mixed lymphocyte cultures were set up with 4×10^5 spleen cells of respective C57BL/6J mice as responder and irradiated 4×10^5 spleen cells of BALB/c mice as stimulator.
[c]Cells were recovered after 4 days of allogeneic mixed culture with whole spleen cells of individual C57BL/6J and appropriate number of irradiated spleen cells of BALB/c mice.
[d](TLU) Total lytic units.

day 7 after infection. In marked contrast, little or no target cell lysis was detected in females on day 7 after injection.

Our recent data also suggest that sex hormones influence generation of cytotoxic cells (Kim et al., 1983). Spleen cells from C57BL/6J with empty or hormone-containing implants were used as responder cells in an allogeneic mixed lymphocyte reaction (MLR). The mixed lymphoycte cultures (MLC) were incubated for 4 days. Eight hours before the end of incubation 1 μCi [^{3}H]thymidine ([^{3}H]-Tdr) was added to the mixed lymphocyte cultures as shown in Table 2. Spleen cells from male mice with estrogen implants incorporated less [^{3}H]-Tdr than did spleen cells from control male mice in cultures with irradiated BALB/c spleen cells. In contrast, the spleen cells from female mice with androgen implants incorporated more [^{3}H]-Tdr in MLC than did control female mice. [^{3}H]-Tdr incorporation by spleen cells from male mice given estrogen implants approximated that of female controls and female mice given androgen implants approximated male control. The number of viable cells recovered 4 days after MLC was comparable in male and female control mice. The number of cells recovered after MLC was increased in female mice receiving androgen and markedly decreased in male mice receiving estrogen.

Finally, total cytotoxic lytic units generated during the MLR were measured in the four groups of mice studied. The total lytic units (TLU) was twice as high in the MLR of control male than in control female mice. Estrogen treatment markedly depressed the number of TLU while androgen increased the number of TLU (Table 3). Furthermore, neonatal exposure of female mice to estrogen has been reported to diminish delayed hypersensitivity and graft versus host reaction (Kalland and Forsberg, 1977; Luster et al., 1979).

III. SEX HORMONES AND DIABETES

Insulitis and diabetes mellitus have been induced experimentally in mice by injecting the M-strain of EMC virus or by injecting multiple low dosages of streptozotocin (40 mg/kg). Suspectibility of mice to EMC virus depends on both genetic background and gender (Craighead and McLane, 1968; Craighead and Steinke, 1971; Boucher and Notkins, 1973; Like and Rossini, 1976). Genetic variation in susceptibility to multiple low-dosage SZ injection in experimental animals has also been shown (Paik *et al.*, 1980; Rossini *et al.*, 1978). Using inbred strain of mice, the susceptibility to multiple low-dose SZ injection for induction of diabetes has been reported by several investigators. Rossini and his associates showed that major histocompatibility complex (*H-2*) genes are not the sole determinants of the severity of hypoglycemia and insulitis in the streptozotocin model (Rossini *et al.*, 1977a). Kromann and his associates (1979) also showed that *H-2* genes influence the diabetogenic effect of EMC virus. However, they suggested that the glucose intolerance following heterologous and homologous immunization with pancreatic antigens appeared to be under *H-2* influence.

As shown in Table 3, our studies showed striking differences in the susceptibility of various inbred strains of mice to the induction of diabetes by multiple injections of low dosages of streptozotocin. We have found that streptozotocin induced hyperglycemia in male mice of some strains but not of other strains (Kim, 1983). It should be noted that certain strains of mice were resistant not only to multiple injections of low-dosage streptozotocin, but also to the single high dose of streptozotocin (200 mg/kg body weight). Single (200 mg/kg body weight) or multiple (40 mg/kg body weight) injections of streptozotocin induced hyperglycemia in CD-1, C57BL/6J, and BALB/c mice from two separate colonies (obtained from Dr. M. Bosma, The Institute for Cancer Research and Dr. S. Shin, Einstein Medical College). In contrast, neither single nor multiple injections of streptozotocin induced hyperglycemia in AKR/J and BALB/c mice (obtained from Jackson Laboratories). In LAF$_1$ mice a single injection of streptozotocin (200 mg/kg body weight) induced diabetes while multiple injections of low dosage failed to induce hyperglycemia. It is of interest to note that BALB/c mice obtained from different colonies differed in their susceptibility to streptozotocin; 12 mice of each line have been studied. All BALB/c mice from Dr. Bosma and the Einstein Medical College colonies developed hyperglycemia following multiple injec-

Table 3. Strain Differences in the Induction of Hyperglycemia by Streptozotocin

Strain	Glucose concentration (mg/dl) ± SD[a]	
	1 × 200 mg/kg SZ[b]	5 × 40 mg/kg SZ[c]
AKR/J	—	177 ± 34 (0/5)
C57BL/6J	525 ± 138 (5/5)	379 ± 121 (15/15)
LAF$_1$	569 ± 209 (4/5)	176 ± 17 (0/11)
CD-1	556 ± 18 (5/5)	397 ± 200 (5/6)
BALB/c (Jackson Lab.)	212 ± 124 (2/5)	215 ± 48 (1/5)
BALB/c AnNIcr (Dr. Bosma)	488 ± 122 (6/6)	318 ± 83 (6/6)
BALB/c (Dr. Shin)	510 ± 62 (14/14)	475 ± 210 (14/15)

[a]Glucose concentration was measured with the serum samples obtained from each animal 14 days after the final injection of streptozotocin.
[b]Each mouse received a single injection of 200 mg streptozotocin/kg body weight.
[c]Each mouse received five injections daily with 40 mg streptozotocin/kg body weight.
[d]Number of animals hyperglycemic after streptozotocin (>200 mg/dl) per total number of animals used.

tions of the low dose of steptozotocin. In contrast, only 2 out of 12 BALB/c mice from Jackson Labs developed hyperglycemia after similar treatment.

Sex difference in development of diabetes in humans has been reported by many investigators. Even though more elderly women develop diabetes mellitus than men, there is less agreement about the incidence according to sex in earlier life. Fitzgerald and his associates (1961) have examined the effect of sex and parity on incidence of diabetes in a large number of patients and conclude that the incidence of diabetes before the age of 40 is actually higher in men than in women. Recent epidemiologic data suggest that the incidence of insulin-dependent diabetes in postpubescent children may also be higher in boys than in girls (West, 1978).

In 95% depancreatized animals, removal of the ovaries increases the incidence and severity of diabetes, which indicates that the ovarian hormones may be protective (Houssay, 1951). In ovarectomized, pancreatectomized rats, estrogen decreases the incidence and severity of diabetes (Lewis *et al.*, 1950). Diabetes has also been shown to be attenuated in animals with estrogen treatment (Sloan and Oliver, 1975; Beck, 1969).

More recently, Morrow and his associates (1980) reported that a diabeticlike disease was induced in male DBA/2 mice by injection of the M-strain of EMC virus, whereas, female mice of this strain sustained systemic infection, but rarely exhibit hyperglycemia. Similarly, Paik and his associates (1980) showed that 100% of the BALB/c male mice given multiple low-dosage injections of SZ developed severe and permanent insulin-dependent hyperglycemia, but less than 15% of the BALB/c female mice treated identically developed the syndrome. As shown in Table 4, our recent data showed similar results with C57BL/6J mice (Kim *et al.*, 1983). The male and female C57BL/6J mice were injected with 40 mg streptozotocin/kg body weight daily for 5 consecutive days. There was a marked difference in the susceptibility of male and female mice to the induction of hyperglycemia by multiple injections of low-dose streptozotocin. The multiple injections of low-dosage streptozotocin induce hyperglycemia in all of 15 C57BL/6 male mice but in none of 10 C57BL/6 female mice. A single injection of a high dosage of streptozotocin (200 mg/kg body weight)

Table 4. Sex Difference in the Induction of Hyperglycemia by Streptozotocin

Strain	Sex	Glucose concentration (mg/dl) $\pm$ SD[a]	
		1×200 mg/kg SZ[b]	5×40 mg/kg SZ[c]
BALB/c (Dr. Shin)	Male	—	475 ± 210 (10/10)[d]
BALB/c (Dr. Shin)	Female	—	210 ± 26 (1/10)
C57BL/6J	Male	525 ± 138 (10/10)	379 ± 121 (15/15)
C57BL/6J	Female	237 ± 138 (10/10)	150 ± 18 (0/10)

[a]Glucose concentration was measured with the serum samples obtained from each animal 14 days after the final injection of streptozotocin.
[b]Each mouse received a single injection of 200 mg streptozotocin/kg body weight.
[c]Each mouse received five injections daily with 40 mg streptozotocin/kg body weight.
[d]Number of animals hyperglycermic after streptozotocin (>200 mg/dl) per total number of animals used.

Table 5. Influence of Sex Hormones in the Induction of Hyperglycemia in C57BL/6 Mice by Multiple Injections of Streptozotocin[a]

Sex	Implant	Glucose concentration (mg/dl) + SD[b]
Male	β-Estradiol	177 ± 34 (0/10)[c]
	Sham	383 ± 81 (15/15)
Female	5α-Androstan-17β-OL-3-one	285 ± 62 (8/15)
	Sham	195 ± 40 (1/10)

[a]Silastic tubes containing 5 mg of estrogen or androgen were placed subcutaneously in male and female mice. Sham mice received empty tubes. Three weeks after implant, each mouse was injected with 40 mg/kg streptozotocin for 5 consecutive days.
[b]Glucose concentration was measured with the serum samples obtained from each animal 14 days after the final injection of streptozotocin.
[c]Number of animals hyperglycemic per total number of animals used.

induced hyperglycemia in all 10 male but in only 3 out of 10 female mice. A similar finding was found in BALB/c mice (obtained from Dr. S. Shin) in which multiple doses of SZ induced hyperglycemia in all 10 male mice but only in 1 of 10 female mice (Table 5). To determine if the difference in suspectibility to hyperglycemia induced by streptozotocin was due to sex hormones, male or female C57BL/6 mice were treated with female or male hormones, respectively, prior to injection of streptozotocin. Plastic tubes containing 5 mg β-estradiol (estrogen), were implanted subcutaneously in male mice and plastic tubes containing 5 mg of 5α-androstan-17β-OL-3-one (androgen) were implanted subcutaneously in female mice. Control male and female mice were implanted with empty plastic tubes. Three weeks after implantation of sex hormones, the concentration of estrogen and androgen in plasma was measured by radioimmunoassay. Male mice implanted with plastic tubes containing estrogen had 0.78 ng estrogen/ml plasma. Male mice with empty implants had less than 0.10 ng androgen/ml plasma. Female mice with empty implants had 0.42 ng estrogen/ml plasma and less than 0.10 ng androgen/ml plasma. Thus, male mice implanted with plastic tubes containing estrogen had higher plasma estrogen levels than control female mice. Female mice implanted with the plastic tube containing androgen had 0.85 ng androgen per ml plasma. Thus, female mice implanted with androgen had a higher concentration of androgen in plasma than did control male mice. The high concentrations of estrogen in male mice implanted with estrogen and of androgen in female mice implanted with androgen continued for 6 months after implantation of hormone-containing tubes.

Four weeks after implantation, all mice were given multiple injections of low-dosage streptozotocin. As shown in Table 5, all male mice that received empty plastic implants developed hyperglycemia as expected. In contrast, none of the male mice given implants containing 5 mg estrogen developed hyperglycemia. Only 1 of 15 female mice given empty plastic implants developed hyperglycemia while 8 of 15 female mice that received implants containing 5 mg androgen developed hyperglycemia. These results suggest that sex hormones influence the induction of hyperglycemia by repeated low doses of streptozotocin. Thus, it appears that estrogen inhibits, and androgen facilitates, the induction of hyperglycemia by repeated low doses of streptozotocin. How these sex hormones influence the induction of hyperglycemia is not clear, but the known influence of these hormones on immune function suggests that they may be operating through an immunological pathway influencing the induction of hyperglycemia by streptozotocin.

IV. DISCUSSION AND CONCLUSION

It has been demonstrated that immunological mechanisms may play an important role in induction of diabetes in both humans and experimental animals. The observation of lymphocyte infiltration in pancreatic islets of acute Type 1 diabetic patients and of diabetic mice treated with multiple injections of low-dose streptozotocin suggests that an immune mechanism may be involved in induction of diabetes. Additional support for this hypothesis was obtained from the experiments in which T-lymphocyte-depleted mice and athymic nude were shown to be resistant to the induction of diabetes by multiple injections of low-dose streptozotocin (Table 6 and Figure 1). Furthermore, diabetes can be transferred into normal mice after injection of spleen cells from mice which are rendered diabetic by multiple injections of low-dose streptozotocin.

Since streptozotocin is a cytotoxic substance for insulin-producing beta cells of pancreatic islets, a single injection of high-dose streptozotocin induces a rapid onset of hyperglycemia presumably due to the physical destruction of beta cells. In contrast,

Table 6.   Correlation between the Induction of Diabetes by Five Daily Doses of SZ and the Response to SRBC by Thymectomized, Lethally Irradiated Mice Reconstituted with Spleen Cells or T-Cell-Depleted Bone Marrow

Thymectomized, irradiated recipient reconstituted with	Glucose concentration 10 days[a] after 5 × 40 mg/kg SZ	Anti-SRBC[b] PFC/spleen
Anti-thy-1.2-treated bone marrow[c]	181	270
	185	1,200
	198	360
	200	1,110
	257	1,860
	268	8,340
	302	4,170
	547	13,080
Normal spleen cells[d]	245	15,180
	325	7,800
	416	18,000
	532	27,360
	540	31,900

[a]Irradiated mice were reconstituted with bone marrow cells treated with anti-thy 1.2 antibody and complement. The mice received five injections daily of 40 mg streptozotocin/kg body weight.
[b]Irradiated mice were reconstituted with normal spleen cells, and received five injections daily of 40 mg streptozotocin/kg body weight.
[c]Glucose concentration was measured with serum samples obtained 10 days after the final injection of streptozotocin.
[d]All experimental mice were immunized with SRBC intravenously 10 days after the final injection of streptozotocin. Spleen cells suspensions were prepared and then anti-SRBC PFC was determined by the method described by Dresser (1962).

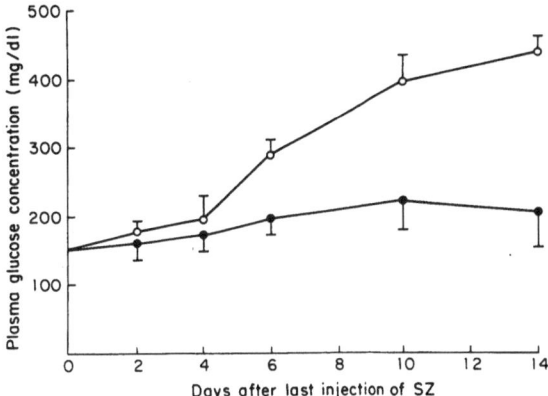

Figure 1. Requirement for T lymphocytes for the induction of diabetes by repeated low doses of SZ. C57BL/6J mice were thymectomized followed by lethal irradiation and reconstitution with anti-Thy 1.2 plus complement-treated bone marrow (●). Controls were not thymectomized and were reconstituted with spleen cells after lethal irradiation (○). All mice were given five daily injections of 40 mg SZ/kg body weight starting 4 weeks after cell transfer. Average blood glucose levels (±SD) for 19 T-cell-depleted and 10 control mice are presented.

when mice are injected with multiple low doses of streptozotocin, hyperglycemia appears slowly after a latent period of 5 or 6 days which is preceded by lymphocyte infiltration in pancreatic islets. These results strongly suggest that autoimmune processes take place in the induction of diabetes by this protocol. A likely mechanism would be the generation of cytotoxic T cells directed against streptozotocin-modified beta cells. These cytotoxic cells may directly damage the beta cells, thereby inducing insulin-dependent diabetes. The cytotoxic cells generated by streptozotocin-modified beta cells would recognize preferentially the SZ modified beta cells as target cells. This hypothesis is supported by our experimental data in Figure 2 on the transfer of diabetes into normal mice by spleen cells from diabetic mice. Also, our findings that diabetes could not be induced in T-cell-depleted animals support this hypothesis.

The requirement of T lymphocytes for induction of diabetes through injection of diabetogenic agents could also be interpreted as necessary for the production of autoantibodies to SZ modified beta cells. Immunologically mediated destruction of beta cells after injection of diabetogenic agents could be accomplished by either generation of cytotoxic cells or production of autoantibodies. Both cases would require the presence of T lymphocytes. Presently, we favor the hypothesis that induction of diabetes by diabetogenic agents is due to the generation of cytotoxic cells, because our preliminary experimental data suggest that no autoantibodies against beta cells are found in the serum sample from diabetic mice induced by multiple injections of low-dose streptozotocin.

For many years, an explanation for the female predominance of autoimmunity was not clear. However, it is now apparent that sex hormones significantly modulate the expression of autoimmunity. It is a curious finding that induction of diabetes by diabetogenic agents is predominant in males, since most other autoimmune diseases

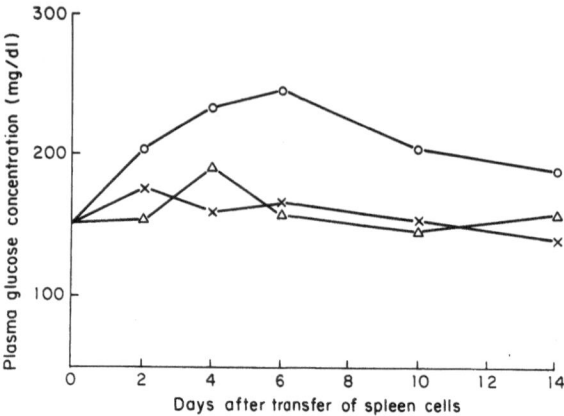

Figure 2. Transfer of diabetes from mice treated with five daily injections of 40 mg SZ/kg body weight to normal syngeneic mice by spleen cells. C57BL/6 mice were sacrificed 12 days after completing a 5-day course of SZ injections and their spleen cells were transferred into normal syngeneic mice or into mice that had received one injection of 40 mg SZ/kg body weight 5 days before cell transfer. Blood glucose levels were assayed periodically and average values for groups of eight mice are presented. (×) Normal spleen cells donors and recipients treated with one injection of 40 mg SZ/kg body weight. (△) SZ-treated donors (five doses) and normal recipients. (○) SZ-treated donors (five doses) and recipients treated with one injection of 40 mg SZ/kg body weight.

are predominant in females. It has been demonstrated that female sex hormones augment humoral immune responses, which may be due to the fact that they influence suppressor-T-cell activity. On the other hand, it has been demonstrated that estrogen tends to suppress the phytohemagglutinin response of lymphocytes, delayed hypersensitivity reaction, and graft versus host reaction. These results suggest that female sex hormones are suppressing cell-mediated immunity. Therefore, we propose the hypothesis that autoimmune disorders caused by humoral autoantibodies may be predominant in females, whereas autoimmune disorders caused by cellular immunity may be predominant in males. In fact, our experimental results show that generation of cytotoxic cells in allogeneic mixed lymphocyte cultures *in vitro* from estrogen-treated mice is much less than that from the androgen-treated animals. Thus, the influences of sex hormones on induction of diabetes by multiple injections of low dose streptozotocin are mediated by immunological mechanisms. It is our hypothesis that induction of diabetes in experimental animals by streptozotocin may be due to generation of cytotoxic cells against SZ-modified beta cells of pancreatic islets through autoimmune processes and that sex hormones may influence the generation of these cytotoxic cells.

ACKNOWLEDGMENTS. This research was supported by U.S. Public Health Service Grants AM28263 and AG 00842 and by the New York American Diabetes Association. The authors are grateful to Drs. S. Shin, Einstein Medical College, New York, and M. Bosma, The Institute for Cancer Research, Philadelphia, for making available to us mice from their colonies, and to Drs. G. W. Siskind and M. E. Weksler for their encouragement and advice.

REFERENCES

Ablin, R. J., Bruns, G. R., Guinin, P., and Bush, I. M., 1974, The effect of oestrogen on the incorporation of 3H-thymidine by PHA-stimulated human peripheral blood lymphocytes, *J. Immunol.* 113:705–707.

Batchelor, J. R., 1968, Hormonal control of antibody formation, in: *Regulation of the Antibody Response.* (B. Cinader, ed.), p. 276–282. Charles C. Thomas, Springfield, Ill.

Beck, P., 1969, Progestin enhancement of the plasma insulin response to glucose in rhesus monkeys, *Diabetes* 18:146–152.

Bimes, C. P., Graeve, P., Guilhem A., and Amiel, S., 1975, La cytologie thymique sous l'action des hormones genitales chez la coboye, *R. Soc. Biol. (Paris)* 169:233.

Bottazzo, G. F., Florin-Christensen, A., and Donaich, D., 1974, Islet-cell antibodies in diabetes mellitus with autoimmune polyendocrine deficiencies, *Lancet* 2:1279–1283.

Boucher, D. W., and Notkins, A. L., 1973, Virus-induced diabetes mellitus. I. Hyperglycemia hypoinsulinemia in mice infected with encephalomyocarditis virus, *J. Exp. Med.* 137:1226–1239.

Boucher, D. W., Hayashi, K., Rosenthal, J., and Notkins, A. L., 1975, Virus-induced diabetes mellitus. III. Influence of the sex and strain of the host, *J. Infect. Dis.* 131:462–466.

Buschard, K., Rygaard, J., 1978, Is the diabetogenic effect of streptozotocin in part thymus-dependent?, *Acta Pathol. Microbiol. Scand.* [C] 86:23–27.

Buschard, K., Rygaard, J., and Lund, E., 1976, The inability of a diabetogenic virus to induce diabetes mellitus in athymic (nude) mice, *Acta Pathol. Microbiol. Scand.* [C] 84:299–303.

Buschard, K., Madsbad, S., and Rygaard, J., 1978, Passive transfer of diabetes mellitus from man to mouse, *Lancet* 908–910.

Butterworth, M., McClellanen, B., and Allansmith, M., 1967, Influence of sex on immunoglobulin level, *Nature* 214:1224–1225.

Calzolari, A., 1898, Rechérches experimentales sur un rapport probable entre la fonction du thymus et celle des testicules, *Arch. Ital. Biol.* 30:71–77.

Cohn, D. A., 1979, High sensitivity to androgen as a contributing factor in sex difference in the immune response, *Arthritis Rheum.* 22:1218–1223.

Craighead, J. E., and McLane, M. F., 1968, Diabetes mellitus: Induction in mice by encepholomyocarditis virus, *Science* 162:913–914.

Craighead, J. E., and Steinke, J., 1971, Diabetes mellitus-like syndrome in mice infected with encephalomyocarditis virus, *Am. J. Pathol.* 63:119–134.

Dresser, D. W., 1962, Specific inhibition of antibody production. I. Protein overloading paralysis, *Immunology* 5:161–168.

Duvic, M., Steinberg, A. D., and Klassen, L. W., 1978, Effect of the anti-estrogen, nafoxidine on NZB/W autoimmune disease, *Arthritis Rheum.* 21:414–417.

Eidinger, D., and Garrett, T. J., 1972, Studies of the regulatory effects of the sex hormones on antibody formation and stem cell differentiation, *J. Exp. Med.* 136:1098–1116.

Findlay, J. A., Rookledge, K. A., Beloff-Chain, A., and Lever, J., 1973, A combined biochemical and histological study of the islets of Langerhans in the genetically obese hyperglycemic mouse and the lean mouse including observations on the effect of streptozotocin treatment, *J. Endocrinol.* 56:571–583.

Fitzgerald, M. G., Mallines, J. M., O'Sullivan, D. J., and Wall, M., 1961, The effect of sex and parity on the incidence of diabetes mellitus. *Q. J. Med.* 117:57–70.

Gepts, W., 1965, Pathologic anatomy of the pancreas in juvenile diabetes mellitus, *Diabetes* 14:619–633.

Gepts, W., 1972, Pathology of islet tissue in human diabetes, in: *Handbood of Physiology,* sect. VII, vol. 1 (D. F. Steiner, and N. Freinkel, eds.), pp. 289–363, American Physiology Society Washington.

Goodman, M. N., and Hazelwood, R. L., 1974, Short-term effects of oestradiol benzoate in normal hypophysectomized and alloxan-diabetic male rats. *J. Endocrinol.* 62:439–449.

Greenman, D. L., Dooley, L. K., Breeden, C. R., and Gass, G. H., 1977, Strain differences in the response of the mouse to diethylstilbestrol, *J. Toxicol. Environ. Health* 3:589–597.

Halstead, S. B., 1969, Observations related to pathogenesis to dengue hemorhagic fever. VI. Hypothesis and discussion, *J. Biol. Med.* 42:350.

Hammer, J. A., 1926, Die Menschen Thymusdrüse in Gesundheit and Krankheit. Das Normale Organismus, *Z. Mikrosk. Anat. Forsch.* (Suppl. 6):1.

Helyer, B. J., and Howie, J. B., 1963, Spontaneous autoimmune disease in NZB/BL mice, *Br. Med. J.* **2**:505–510.

Kalland, T., 1980, Alterations of antibody response in female mice after neonatal exposure to diethylstilbestrol, *J. Immunol.* **124**:194–198.

Kalland, T., and Forsberg, J. G., 1977, Delayed hypersensitivity to oxagolone in neonatally estrogenized mice, *Cancer Lett.* **4**:141–146.

Kenny, J. F., Pangburn, P. C., and Trial, G., 1976, Effect of estradiol on immune competence *in vivo* and *in vitro* studies, *Infect. Immun.* **13**:448–456.

Kiesel, U., Freytag, G., Biener, J., and Kolb, H., 1980, Transfer of experimental autoimmune insulitis by spleen cells in mice, *Diabetologia* **19**:516–520.

Kim, Y. T., 1983, Immunological studies on induction of diabetes in experimental animals. I. Cellular basis of induction of diabetes by streptozotocin, *Diabetes,* in press.

Kim, Y. T., Michaelis, M. A., Tomonari, K. H., and Weksler, M. E., 1983, Immunological studies on induction of diabetes in experimental animals. II. Effects of sex hormones on induction of diabetes by streptozotocin, *Diabetes,* in press.

Kromann, H., Lernmark, A., Vestergaard, B. F., and Nerup, J., 1979, The influence of the major histocompatibility complex (H-2) on experimental diabetes in mice, *Diabetologia* **16**:107–114.

Lewis, J. T., Foglia, V. G., and Rodrigues, R. R., 1950, The effects of steroids on the incidence of diabetes in rats after subtotal pancreatectomy, *Endocrinology* **46**:111–121.

Like, A. A., and Rossini, A. A., 1976, Streptozotocin-induced pancreatic insulitis: New model of diabetes mellitus, *Science* **193**:415–417.

Luster, M. I., Faith, R. E., McLachlan, J. A., and Clark, G. C., 1979, Effect of *in vitro* exposure to diethylstilbesterol on the immune response in mice, *Toxicol. Appl. Pharmacol.* **47**:279–285.

Luz, N. P., Marques, M., Ayub, A. C., and Correa, P. R., 1969, Effects of estradiol upon the thymus and lymphoid organs of immature female rats, *Am. J. Obstet. Gynecol.* **105**:525–528.

MacCuish, A. C., Barnes, E. W., Irvine, W. J., and Duncan, L. J. P., 1974a, Antibodies to pancreatic islet-cells in insulin-dependent diabetics with coexistent autoimmune disease, *Lancet* **2**:1529–1531.

MacCuish, A. C., Jordan, J., Campbell, C. J., Duncan, L. J. P., and Irvine, W. J. 1974b, Cell-mediated immunity to human pancreas in diabetes mellitus, *Diabetes* **23**:693–697.

Money, W. L., Fager, J., and Rawson, W., 1952, The comparative effects of various steroids on lymphoid tissue of the rat, *Cancer Res.* **12**:206.

Morrow, P. L., Freedman, A., and Craighead, J. E., 1980, Testosterone effect on experimental diabetes mellitus in encephalomyocarditis (EMC) virus infected mice, *Diabetologica* **18**:247–249.

Okayasu, I., Kong, Y. M., and Rose, N. R., 1981, Effect of castration and sex hormones on experimental autoimmune thyroiditis, *Clin. Immunol. Immunopathol.* **20**:240–245.

Paik, S. G., Fleischer, M., and Shin, S., 1980, Insulin-dependent diabetes mellitus induced by subdiabetogenic doses of streptozotocin: Obligatory role of cell-mediated autoimmune process, *Proc. Natl. Acad. Sci. USA* **77**:6129–6133.

Patterson, B., Hellerstrom, C., and Gunnarsson, R., 1970, Structure and metabolism of the pancreatic islets in streptozotocin treated guinea pigs, *Horm. Metab. Res.* **2**:313–317.

Pepper, F. J., 1961, The effect of age, pregnancy, and lactation on the thymus gland and lymph nodes of the mouse, *J. Endocrinol.* **22**:335–348.

Persike, E. D., 1940, Involution of thymus during pregnancy in young mice, *Proc. Soc. Exp. Biol.* **45**:315–317.

Phuc, L. H., Papiernik, M., Berrik, S., and Duval, D., 1981, Thymus involution in pregnant mice. I. Characterization of the remaining thymocyte subpopulation. *Clin. Exp. Immunol.* **44**:247–252.

Rakieter, N., Rakieter, M. C., and Nadkarni, M. W., 1963, Studies on the diabetogenic action of streptozotocin (NSC-37917). *Cancer Chemother. Res.* **29**:91–98.

Rodriguez, R. R., 1965, Influence of osetrogens and androgens on the production and prevention of diabetes, in: *On the Nature and Treatment of Diabetes* (G. A., Wrenshell, and B. S., Liebel, eds.), pp. 288–307. Excerpta Medical Foundations, Amsterdam.

Rossini, A. A., Appel, M. C., Wiliam, R. M., and Like, A. A., 1977a, Genetic influence of streptozotocin-induced insulitis and hyperglycemia. *Diabetes* **26**:916–920.

Rossini, A. A., Like, A. A., Chick, W. L., Appel, M. C., and Cahil, G. F., 1977b, Studies of streptozotocin induced insulitis and diabetes. *Proc. Natl. Acad. Sci. USA* **74**:2485–2489.

Rossini, A. A., Williams, R. M., Appel, M. C., and Like, A. A., 1978, Sex differences in the multiple-dose streptozotocin model of diabetes, *Endocrinology* **103**:1518–1520.

Seaman, W. E., Blackman, M. A., Gindhart, T. D., Roubinian, J. R., Loeb, J. M., and Talal, N., 1978, B-estradiol reduces natural killer cells in mice, *J. Immunol.* **121**:2193–2198.

Seaman, W. R., Merigan, T. C., and Talal, N., 1979, Natural killing in estrogen-treated mice responds poorly to poly I-C despite normal stimulation of circulating interferon, *J. Immunol.* **123**:2903–2905.

Shiff, R. I., Mercier, D., and Buckley, R. H., 1975, Inability of lactational hormones to account for the inhibitory effects of pregnancy plasmas on lymphocyte responses *in vitro*, *Cell. Immunol.* **20**:69–80.

Sloan, J. M., and Oliver, I. M. 1975. Progestogen-induced diabetes in the dog, *Diabetes* **24**:337–344.

Steinberg, A. D., Pincus, T., and Talal, N., 1971, The pathogenesis of autoimmunity in new zealand mice. III. Factors influencing the formation of anti-nucleic acid antibodies, *Immunology* **20**:523–531.

Steinberg, A. D., Roths, J. B., Murphy, E. D., Steinberg, R. T., and Raveche, E. S., 1980, Effect of thymectomy or androgen administration upon the autoimmune disease of MRL/Mp-1pr/1pr mice, *J. Immunol.* **125**:871–873.

Steven, W. M., and Snook, T., 1975, The stimulatory effects of diethylstilbestrol and diethylstilbestrol diphosphate on the reticuloendothelial cells of the rat spleen, *Am. J. Anat.* **144**:339–360.

Talal, N., and Gallo, R. C., 1972, Antibodies to a DNA:RNA hybrid measured by cellulose ester filter immune assay, *Nature* **240**:240–241.

Terres, G., Morrison, S. L., and Habicht, G. S., 1968, Quantitative difference in the immune response between male and female mice, *Proc. Soc. Exp. Biol. Med.* **127**:664–667.

West, K. M., 1978, *Epidemiology of Diabetes and its Vascular Lesion*, Elsevier, Amsterdam.

Wong, C. Y., Woodruff, J. J., and Woodruff, J. F., 1977, Generation of cytotoxic T lymphocytes during coxsackie virus B-3 infection. III. Role of sex, *J. Immunol.* **119**:591–597.

7

Transplantation of Pancreas and Islets

David E. R. Sutherland, Patricia L. Chinn, and Charles E. Morrow

I. RATIONALE AND STATEMENT OF THE PROBLEMS

Total endocrine replacement therapy for insulin-dependent diabetes mellitus is possible by transplantation of either immediately vascularized pancreatic allografts or the islets of Langerhans as free grafts. The rationale for these treatments rests on the hypothesis that the microangiopathic and other lesions associated with diabetes mellitus are secondary to disordered metabolism. Presumably, perfect control of carbohydrate metabolism would prevent the development or halt the progression of the lesions affecting the eye, kidney, nervous, and other systems. Although the point is controversial, clinical and experimental observations support this hypothesis (see reviews by Brownlee and Cahill, 1979; Tchobroutsky, 1978; Mauer *et al.*, 1981).

Nondiabetic individuals maintain plasma glucose concentrations within an extraordinarily narrow range. In diabetic individuals, exogenous insulin, administered by standard techniques, cannot reliably prevent wide excursions of plasma glucose levels (Molnar *et al.*, 1972). Systems designed to administer insulin continuously may be able to do so, but they will probably never be as efficient as functioning beta cells (Ungar, 1982).

The first attempts at clinical pancreas transplantation showed that immediately vascularized pancreatic grafts were unequivocally able to normalize plasma glucose levels and obviate the need for exogenous insulin, but technical complications were frequent and the success rate was low (see review by Sutherland, 1981b). For that reason, a surge of interest developed in experimental transplantation of free grafts of islet

David E. R. Sutherland, Patricia L. Chinn, and Charles E. Morrow • Department of Surgery, University of Minnesota Health Sciences Center, Minneapolis, Minnesota 55455.

tissue (Sutherland, 1981a). Transplanted islets can reverse diabetes in a variety of animal models, but isolation of islets in large numbers is difficult, free grafts of allogeneic islets are extremely vulnerable to rejection effector mechanisms, and clinical attempts at islet allotransplantation, almost without exception, have not been successful (Sutherland, 1982). However, there are no inherent biological reasons why these problems cannot be solved, as pointed out by Barker *et al*. (1982a) in a recent commentary. Much progress has been made in the past few years, both in islet procurement and in reduction of graft immunogenicity, using methods that have not yet been applied clinically. Concomitantly, the results of clinical pancreas transplantation have improved with the development of safe techniques for handling exocrine secretions and advances in immunosuppression (Sutherland, 1983).

Experiments on various aspects of pancreas and islet transplantation in animals are summarized separately here. These investigations define the problems and form the basis for future application of pancreas and islet transplantation to the treatment of human diabetes.

II. EXPERIMENTAL TRANSPLANTATION

Allograft rejection is ultimately the limiting factor in the application of pancreas transplantation to the treatment of diabetes, but the technical aspects of pancreas transplantation have to be solved first. Provision for drainage of exocrine enzymes is the major technical consideration.

Pancreatic grafts can be either (1) pancreaticoduodenal; (2) whole organ; or (3) segmental (tail, or body and tail of the pancreas). The technical variations of pancreas transplantation can also be divided into those that establish exocrine drainage into the bowel or another viscus, and those that do not (duct ligated, ductal system obliterated, duct left open).

The difficulties with pancreas transplantation are apparent from the variety of techniques employed. There are further difficulties with interpretation of the results of experimental pancreas transplantation because of limitations imposed by the models used (whether they are autografts or allografts, immunosuppressed or nonimmunosuppressed, diabetic or not diabetic).

Most experiments with pancreas transplantation have been done in large outbred animals, usually dogs. If the method of transplantation is to be evaluated without the influence of immunological factors, an autograft model must be used, imposing further technical difficulties, such as preserving blood supply to other vital organs during pancreatectomy. Allograft models are technically easier to use, since the donor can be sacrificed, but allograft rejection makes assessment of the technique employed more difficult. Immunosuppression is unquestionably able to delay graft rejection in a large animal model, but has not always been employed. Thus allograft rejection may result in graft failure before technical problems become manifest; conversely, technical problems may result in graft failure even though a satisfactory immunosuppressive regimen is employed.

A. Pancreas with Exocrine Drainage Established

1. Pancreaticoduodenal and Whole-Organ Grafts

The earliest attempts at transplantation of the canine pancreas (reviewed by Lillehei *et al.*, 1970) utilized the duodenum as a conduit to the skin for exocrine secretions. Largiader *et al.* (1967) first successfully transplanted an entire pancreaticoduodenal allograft and established exocrine drainage to the bowel of recipient dogs. Uchida *et al.* (1971) modified this technique for use in an autograft model.

The technique of pancreaticoduodenal grafting in large animals has been used by Ruiz *et al.* (1972), Choudhury (1973), and Toledo-Pereyra *et al.* (1975) in dogs, and by Bitter-Suermann *et al.* (1979) and van Hoorn *et al.* (1978) in pigs. Vascular torsion and thrombosis, duodenal anastomotic leaks of activated exocrine enzymes, hemorrhage, and fistula formation have consistently frustrated these efforts (De Jode and Howard, 1967). Heterotopic pancreaticoduodenal transplantation can ameliorate diabetes in rats (Lee *et al.*, 1972; Orloff *et al.*, 1975), but the operative mortality is high, particularly if combined with *en bloc* transplantation of other organs (Maki *et al.*, 1977).

Acquino *et al.* (1973), in both autograft and allograft experiments, obviated some of these problems by transplanting the entire pancreas without the duodenum except for the papilla of Vater, and Nozawa *et al.* (1974) developed a similar technique for use in rats. Bewick (1976) has used this method with only a 7.7% morbidity and mortality rate from technical complications in canine recipients of whole-pancreas allografts, but the procedure is technically demanding and has been largely superceded by the segmental technique.

2. Segmental Pancreatic Grafts

Segmental pancreas transplantation is simpler than pancreaticoduodenal transplantation and avoids some of the problems related to the grafted duodenum. Gleidman *et al.* (1973) transplanted the tail (left limb) of the pancreas in dogs and anastomosed the pancreatic duct to the recipient ureter. The pancreatic exocrine enzymes are inactive and injury to the urinary tract does not occur. Although this technique has been applied clinically, Toledo-Pereyra *et al.* (1975), Dickerman *et al.* (1975), and Baumgartner *et al.* (1981) were unable to achieve satisfactory duct-to-ureter anastomoses in dogs. Cook *et al.* (1983) directly anastomosed the graft pancreatic duct to the bladder of ducts, and demonstrated patency at > 60 days in immunosuppressed recipients.

Several investigators (Toledo-Pereyra *et al.* 1975; Bitter-Suermann *et al.*, 1979; Rausis *et al.*, 1970; Piegari *et al.*, 1981) established exocrine drainage of segmental pancreatic grafts by anastomosing the pancreas to recipient bowel. Anastomotic leaks with enzyme activation and local necrosis occurred with high frequency. Dickerman *et al.* (1975) minimized, but did not completely avoid, these complications by a staged procedure in which a Roux-en-Y jejunal loop was first placed in the retroperitoneal iliac fossa; later, the pancreas graft was anastomosed to the loop.

B. Segmental Pancreas Transplantation without Provision for Exocrine Drainage

1. Duct-Ligated Pancreatic Grafts

Transplantation of the tail of the pancreas followed by ductal obliteration or no further manuevers, although less physiological, is technically easier than those described above and can be applied to large-animal auto- or allograft models as well as to the rat. The anatomical considerations in dogs (van Schilfgaarde *et al.*, 1983) and rats (Squifflet *et al.*, 1983a) have been well described. Pancreas transplantation in inbred rats, with immunological factors controlled, has been used with increasing frequency in recent years. Nolan *et al.* (1982) have described a simplified method in which a cuff of donor aorta is interposed over a tube in the recipient. In large animals some investigators have attempted to prevent vascular thrombosis (the pancreas is a low-blood-flow organ) by performing an arteriovenous (A-V) fistula of the graft, splenic vessels (Collin, 1978; Calne *et al.*, 1980; DuToit *et al.*, 1981; van Schilfgaarde, 1983), although some investigators (Florack *et al.*, 1982b; Kyriakides *et al.*, 1981b) have found the incidence of thrombosis to be very low without this maneuver. In baboons the creation of an A-V fistula results in hemorrhagic pancreatitis (DuToit *et al.*, 1983).

Exocrine tissue atrophy occurs but endocrine tissue, theoretically, remains intact after duct ligation. However, several investigators (Rausis *et al.*, 1970; Toledo-Pereyra and Castellanos, 1979) have described acute and chronic inflammatory reactions in the pancreas which may involve the islets and result in impaired function (Bewick *et al.*, 1983). Various attempts to decrease pancreatic exocrine function following duct ligation have been made. These include direct irradiation of the pancreas (Merkel *et al.*, 1968; Terisigni *et al.*, 1980), intraductal injection of radioisotopes in dogs (Faure *et al.*, 1980) or rats (Devonec *et al.*, 1980), and administration of steroids (Kyriakides *et al.*, 1976) or of drugs that inhibit pancreatic exocrine enzyme synthesis or secretion (Castellanos *et al.*, 1975). These maneuvers may not be necessary. Verschoor *et al.* (1975) found that 1 year after duct ligation in dogs, fasting plasma glucose levels were unchanged. Although glucose tolerance test k values were 75% and insulin levels were 60% of normal, no further deterioration occurred over a 3-year period, constituting adequate function for transplantation purposes.

In rats, duct-ligated pancreatic isografts undergo acute inflammatory reactions followed by progressive fibrosis. Orloff *et al.* (1975) could not detect any differences in the islet function of ligated and nonligated pancreatic grafts tested up to 2 years after transplantation, although others have (Fairbrothers *et al.*, 1980a, b; Nolan *et al.*, 1980, 1982; Satake *et al.*, 1983) and some have not (Brynger *et al.*, 1980) detected mild deterioration in function in the long term (> 6 months) by glucose tolerance testing and serum insulin assays that correlated with the histological changes.

Duct ligation does not completely prevent fluid leakages from the pancreas, and this can give rise to local problems (Kyriakides *et al.*, 1976). However, Kyriakides *et al.* (1979b) found that duct-ligated pancreatic allografts transplanted to the peritoneal cavity of totally pancreatectomized pigs did not result in local complications. These observations suggested that if contamination is avoided, by not opening the donor or recipient bowel, the peritoneal cavity can tolerate leakage of fluid from the pancreatic graft.

2. Duct-Obliterated Pancreatic Grafts

Various liquid synthetic or semisynthetic polymers have been injected into the pancreatic ducts of dogs to obliterate the ductal system totally, including neoprene (Dubernard *et al.*, 1978), prolamine (Land *et al.*, 1980; Wayand *et al.*, 1980), cyanoacrylate (Papachristou and Fortner, 1979), polyisoprene (McMaster *et al.*, 1980a), and silicone rubber (Germain *et al.*, 1979; Weiser *et al.*, 1980; White *et al.*, 1981a,b). These polymers liberate chemicals that damage exocrine cells and harden almost immediately after injection, forming a solid cast within the major duct and its radicals, suppressing exocrine function, and eliminating or reducing secretions. All remain permanently, except prolamine which is absorbable (Gebhardt and Stolte, 1978), and all result in inflammatory reactions and ultimate fibrosis of the gland. Nevertheless, good long-term endocrine function has been demonstrated in canine autografts injected with neoprene (Dubernard *et al.*, 1979), prolamine (DuToit *et al.*, 1982c), or cyanoacrylate (Papachristou and Fortner, 1980) and blood flow is not disturbed (Gooszen *et al.*, 1983). Histological examination of duct-obliterated animal pancreases has shown variable results. Blanc-Brunat *et al.* (1983) described severe fibrosis that involved the islets in some pancreases, while other pancreases were atrophic with normal-appearing islets.

Serial observations by Baumgartner *et al.* (1980d, 1981) of dogs with neoprene-injected pancreatic autografts showed that most remain normoglycemic and that glucose tolerance was only slightly impaired, although histological examination at 1 year showed persistent inflammation and distortion of islets. Piegari *et al.* (1981) also observed good function in neoprene-injected canine pancreas autografts, with well-preserved islets within a fibrotic gland at 6 months, similar to the findings of Nolan *et al.* (1982) in latex-injected rat pancreatic isografts and White *et al.* (1981a,b) with silicone-rubber-injected dog pancreases. There are no long-term observations on duct-injected pancreas allografts, but Kyriakides *et al.* (1979a) and Abri *et al.* (1982) found neoprene to be associated with more complications and less satisfactory function than with duct-open or prolamine injection, while McMaster *et al.* (1980b) observed nearly normal function of polyisoprene-injected canine pancreas allografts prior to rejection. The long-term effect of the pancreatic fibrosis induced by polymer injection remains to be determined but, at least in dogs, loss of endocrine function does not occur from this problem alone.

3. Intraperitoneal Transplantation of Segmental Pancreatic Grafts without Duct Ligation

Pancreatic enzymes do not necessarily have a deleterious effect on the peritoneum. Kyriakides *et al.* (1979a,b), Sutherland *et al.* (1979b), and Agnes *et al.*, (1980), in pancreatic allograft experiments in pigs and dogs, found that free intraperitoneal drainage of exocrine secretions from immediately vascularized, segmental pancreatic grafts with unligated ducts was well tolerated without any harmful effect to the host. The peritoneal cavity of animals can usually absorb pancreatic secretions since the pancreatic proenzymes are not activated when the intestine is not violated and the proenzymes are not exposed to enterokinase. The serum amylase concentration is initially increased after transplantation of a graft with an open duct, but the duct gradually closes and levels return to normal within a week (Sutherland et al., 1980a). In long-term grafts, exocrine tissue disappears and islets coalesce; the fibrosis that occurs is less in dogs immunosuppressed with azathioprine and prednisone than in those who do not require immunosuppression to maintain long-term graft function, attributable to the antiinflammatory effect of steroid (Kyriakides et al., 1981b). Early and late examinations of in situ pancreatic segments (Bewick et al., 1983) or of pancreases transplanted with the duct left open have shown less inflammation and fibrosis than if the duct was ligated immediately (Toledo-Pereyra and Castellanos, 1979; Satake et al., in press) or injected with synthetic polymers (Baumgartner et al., 1980d, 1981; Piegari et al., 1981; Abri et al., 1982). Intraperitoneal transplantation of segmental pancreatic grafts with open ducts is now used as a standard technique for pancreas transplant experiments in dogs (DuToit et al., 1981; Florack et al., 1982a; Severyn et al., 1982), baboons (DuToit et al., 1983), and rats (Satake et al., 1979; Squifflet, 1982a).

C. Metabolic Efficiency of Pancreatic Transplantation

Successful transplantation of immediately vascularized pancreatic grafts to animals made diabetic either by drugs or by pancreatectomy uniformly restores plasma glucose to normal if more than 20% of the normal pancreatic mass is transplanted (Toledo-Pereyra et al., 1979a).

Blood glucose and insulin levels during glucose, tolbutamide, or arginine tolerance tests have been reported as low, normal, or elevated (Sutherland, 1981a; Berlastky et al., 1982; Brekke et al., 1980a; Dutoit et al., 1982c; Florack et al., 1982a,c; Liquori et al., 1979; Meister et al., 1981; Satake et al., in press). The factors responsible for the different results are difficult to sort out because of the variations in the models studied: whole or segmental grafts, autografts or allografts, immunosuppressed or not immunosuppressed.

Autograft experiments in totally pancreatectomized recipients give the most useful information, of which the most relevant to humans may be experiments with heterotopic transplantation of open duct grafts in baboons by DuToit et al. (in press). In these experiments k values were reduced at 6 weeks after transplantation compared to normal animals, but the recipients were euglycemic. Restoration of normoglycemia by pancreas transplantation has effects on other metabolic aberrations, such as the increased somatostatin release from the pancreas (Kadowaki et al., 1980), increased gastric somatostatin (Chiba et al., 1981), plasma lipids (Brekke et al., 1980b), and hyperglucagonemia (Brekke et al., 1982) in rats with beta-cell-toxin-induced diabetes. Rats have shown reversal of the abnormalities, although hyperglucogenemia may recur. Satake et al. (1983) have also observed improvement in the exocrine function of the native pancreas in rats with diabetes ameliorated by whole-pancreas isotransplantation.

Most pancreas transplants have been done with venous drainage of the pancreatic graft into the iliac vein or vena cava of the recipient, which tends to elevate systemic insulin levels over what they would be otherwise since the liver—the major site of insulin degradation—is initially bypassed. In some experiments metabolic profiles were improved by portal as opposed to systemic drainage of the pancreas graft venous effluent (Sells *et al.*, 1972; Piegari *et al.*, 1980), while in others an advantage in terms of glucose metabolism could not be established (Ruiz *et al.*, 1972; Baumgartner *et al.*, 1980a; Bewick *et al.*, 1981b; Collin *et al.*, 1983; Martin *et al.*, 1980a,b) although serum insulin levels were generally lower. Baumgartner *et al.* (1980a) found that reduction in islet mass was an important factor in alteration of glucose tolerance after pancreatectomy and segmental pancreas transplantation. The other data from partial pancreatectomy experiments in rats or dogs would support this contention (Merrell *et al.*, 1982; Weir and Bonner-Weir, 1982). Because of the reduction in islet mass by segmental pancreas transplantation in pancreatectomized recipients, insulin levels are lower than normal even with systemic drainage (Florack *et al.*, 1982a,c), but higher than in dogs with simple partial pancreatectomy.

Bewick *et al.* (1981a,b) and Florack *et al.* (1982c) have shown that the elevation in plasma insulin after heterotopic transplantation, of the entire pancreas relative to normal and to segmental grafts to partially pancreatectomized recipients, is due to a combination of systemic venous drainage and pancreatic denervation. In physiological preparations, transposition of the portal venous drainage into the systemic circulation alone or denervation of the pancreas alone had little effect on systemic insulin or glucose levels. Only the combination of the two duplicated the findings after heterotopic pancreas transplantation. With heterotopic segmental pancreas transplantation, local venous effluent insulin concentration is higher than in the portal vein of partially pancreatectomized dogs, suggesting that the pancreas secretes more insulin to compensate for lack of initial passage to the liver. As long as this compensation is maintained glucose levels are normal and therefore k values depend only on islet mass.

Comparison of endocrine function of heterotopic segmental pancreas transplants and intrasplenic islet transplants in dogs has shown the latter to be less efficient, but probably because of greater islet mass in the former (G. Florack, D. E. R. Sutherland, S. Ward, C. E. Morrow, and J. S. Najarian, unpublished observations). In rats, intrahepatic islet transplants are as efficient metabolically as heterotopic microsegmental grafts with the same islet mass, although neither provides the normal metabolism seen with standard heterotopic segmental pancreas grafts (Squifflet *et al.*, 1982a).

D. Immunological Aspects of Pancreatic Allotransplantation

Pancreatic allografts will be rejected like any other organ (Sutherland, 1981a; Savas *et al.*, 1981; van Hoorn *et al.*, 1978; McMaster *et al.*, 1980b; Bewick *et al.*, 1981c). Pancreas-specific alloantigens exist (Metzgar, 1980), but a role in allograft rejection has not been defined. The functional criteria used to define rejection differ for various organs and make it appear that the pancreas is more or less susceptible to rejection than another organ (Lillehei *et al.*, 1970). Severyn *et al.* (1982) found that serum creatinine elevation precedes glucose elevation in beagle recipients of simultaneous kidney and pancreas allografts and that antirejection treatment is effective only if initiated prior to occurrence of hyperglycemia. Similarly, in rats, pancreas allografts are rejected more readily than heterotopic heart allografts when recurrence of hyperglycemia and cessation of heart beat are the criteria of rejection (Klempnauer *et al.*, 1982a; Squifflet *et al.*, 1982b). However, in experiments with *en bloc* allotransplantation of the pancreas, duodenum, liver, spleen, and kidney in rats, histological evidence of rejection was seen in all organs either simultaneously or within a few days of each other (Maki *et al.*, 1977).

Pancreas allografts will survive indefinitely in rats in whom tolerance is induced by injection of donor-strain bone marrow in the neonatal period (Perloff *et al.*, 1980), but adult immunological enhancement protocols that prolong the survival of heart or renal allografts are ineffective (Perloff *et al.*, 1981). In certain rat strain combinations (Wag-Agus), spleen allografts are not rejected and will protect a simultaneously placed pancreas allograft from rejection (Bitter-Suermann and Save-Soderburg, 1978; Shah *et al.*, 1980), but in others (ACI-Lewis) simultaneous pancreas and spleen allografts are both rejected (Squifflet *et al.*, 1983b). There is also a differential effect of major histocompatibility complex (MHC) subregions on pancreas allograft rejection in the rate, with AB or ABC disparate grafts being rapidly rejected, while rejection is delayed for B-region-only differences and some C-region-only disparate grafts survive indefinitely (Klempnauer *et al.*, 1983).

Canine pancreatic allografts are rejected within a few days in nonimmunosuppressed animals (Sutherland, 1981a). Various combinations of azathioprine, corticosteroids, and antilymphocyte serum have prolonged the mean graft functional survival or recipient survival times to several weeks in immunosuppressed mongrel dogs (Sutherland, 1981a; Bewick *et al.*, 1981c; Kyriakides *et al.*, 1979a; Verschoor *et al.*, 1975) and indefinitely in DLA-matched beagles (Severyn *et al.*, 1982).

Kyriakides *et al.* (1981c) found that the duration of pancreas graft survival in beagles correlated most strongly with the recipients reactivity in mixed lymphocyte culture (MLC) to the donor. In MLC-reactive recipients immunosuppressed with azathioprine and prednisone, graft survival ranged from 25 to 260 days. MLC nonreactive nonimmunosuppressed beagles had graft survival range from 9 to 55 days. Severyn *et al.* (1982) showed that donor-specific cell-mediated lymphocytotoxicity developed shortly before onset of hyperglycemia in pancreas allograft recipients, but that this was a relatively late finding since serum creatinine elevation preceded glucose elevation in renal allograft recipients. An interesting aspect of experiments by Kyriakides *et al.* (1981b) was the finding that pancreatic allografts from DLA-identical donors who had previously given a kidney to donors treated by whole-body irradiation and autologous bone marrow transplantation survived indefinitely.

In the initial experiments with cyclosporine, rejection of pancreatic allografts in rats (Rynasiewicz *et al.*, 1980a; Garvey *et al.*, 1980b; Morris *et al.*, 1980) and dogs (McMaster *et al.*, 1980b) was delayed, but not prevented indefinitely. Subsequent experiments in rats using various dosages and routes of administration have shown that cyclosporine by itself is not as effective in preventing rejection of pancreas allografts as of other organs, particularly the heart (Klempnauer *et al.*, 1982a; Rynasiewicz *et al.*, 1982). For that reason Squifflet *et al.* (1982b) used cyclosporine in combination with azathioprine but were unable to find doses that would prevent rejection of ACI pancreases in Lewis recipients without toxic effects, even though such combinations were effective in other allograft models. Low-dose cyclosporine and prednisone are very effective in preventing rejection of rat heart allografts (Rynasiewicz et al., 1982; Squifflet et al., 1983a), but have not yet been tested in the rat pancreas allograft model. More recent experiments have shown that cyclosporine can prevent rejection of pancreas allografts in dogs if the oral dosage is raised to a level (40 mg/kg per day) to compensate for the decreased absorption from exocrine deficiency in recipients made diabetic by total pancreatectomy (DuToit et al., 1982c). DuToit et al. (1982c) had five of eight dogs who were normoglycemic and survived greater than 100 days on this regimen; reduction of the dosage to 5 mg/kg per day resulted in rejection episodes that were reversed by steroid administration and by an increase in cyclosporine A dosage in three of four dogs. Kyriakides et al. (1981a) used parenteral cyclosporine (25 mg/kg per day) in combination with oral prednisone to prevent pancreas allograft rejection indefinitely in four of seven dogs with strong reactivity in MLC to their donor. In addition, Kyriakides et al. (1982) found that cyclosporine could prevent pancreas allograft rejection even when given after serum creatinine elevation occurred in canine recipients of combined pancreas and renal allografts.

Total lymphoid irradiation has been used to prevent rejection of pancreas allografts in rats by Rynasiewicz et al. (1980b) and is very effective when combined with cyclosporine (Rynasiewicz et al., 1982). More recently Hardy et al., (1982) have used a technique of selective lymphoid irradiation using 109-palladium hematoporphyrin which selectively homes to the lymphatic tissue and distal bone marrow, in combination with ALG, to delay or prevent rejection of WF pancreas allografts in diabetic recipients. Those that did not reject accepted subsequent heart allografts from the same donor strain.

In the absence of a renal allograft from the same donor, in which case an elevation of creatinine will occur from rejection of that organ and will precede glucose elevation from pancreas rejection (Severyn et al., 1982), the diagnosis of rejection is usually made when hyperglycemia recurs. Serum amylase measurements are usually not helpful (Dickerman et al., 1975), although with duct open segmental pancreatic allografts, the serum amylase is high initially and may be seen to decline precipitously and simultaneously with hyperglycemia if rejection recurs early (Kyriakides et al., 1979a).

Bewick et al. (1981c) found that the insulin reserve of pancreatic allografts in dogs fell 2–3 days before overt rejection. Paradoxically, a temporary rise in serum insulin levels preceded a rise in fasting blood sugar levels. However, insulin levels then declined as hyperglycemia recurred. In contrast, Kyriakides et al. (1981b) found that changes in glucose clearance during glucose tolerance tests, or in tolerance tests, or in serum insulin response did not precede rejection, and that the occurrence of hyperglycemia was rapid and unpredictable. They were however, able to demonstrate changes in cell-mediated lymphocytotoxicity against the donors before overt rejection, but not in time to initiate treatment to reverse rejection (Kyriakides et al., 1981b). Currently, except in the situation where a simultaneously placed renal allograft in an anephric recipient allows serum creatinine to be used to monitor rejection activity on the part of the recipient, there is not a reliable method for early diagnosis of pancreas allograft rejection.

Histological examinations of rejecting pancreatic allografts have usually been performed late (Lillehei et al.,1970; Ruiz et al., 1972; Bewick, 1976), and have shown edema, interstitial hemorrhage, and round-cell infiltration. In serial studies, Umeyama et al.(1980) found that the histological lesions are less severe in the islets than in the exocrine pancreas early in the process, an observation consistent with functional studies.

An important question is whether there is a difference in susceptibility to rejection between intact, immediately vascularized pancreatic allografts and free grafts of allogeneic islets. In nonimmunosuppressed animals, the interval between transplantation and recurrence of hyperglycemia has been longer with pancreas than with islet allografts (Hardy et al., 1982; Perloff et al., 1980; Sutherland et al., 1980b; Zammit et al., 1979). However, the free quantity of islets engrafted in these early studies was less than that contained in the pancreas grafts, and it was uncertain whether the physiological manifestation of rejection occurred earlier with islet allografts simply because their beta cell mass and functional reserve was less than that of pancreas grafts, or for immunological reasons. Squifflet et al. (1983b) answered this question definitively in rats by transplanting immediately vascularized microsegmental grafts whose beta cell mass was less than that engrafted by intraportal injection of islets (determined in parallel syngeneic transplant recipients), from the same donor strain (ACI) in nonimmunosuppressed diabetic Lewis recipients. The mean time to rejection was 9.8 days with microsegmental and 4.5 days with islet allografts. There is only a small influence of the beta cell mass engrafted on the rejection times of pancreas or islet allografts, since standard segmental grafts, with an insulin content more than double that of the micrografts were not rejected until 11.1 days (Squifflet et al., 1983b). It is clear, then, that immediately vascularized pancreas grafts are less vulnerable to rejection effector mechanisms than free islet grafts. In accordance with these results, Reckard et al. (1981) showed that rats with long-term enhanced renal allografts would accept immediately vascularized pancreas grafts but not islet grafts from the same donor strain without rejection. Similarly, Morris et al. (1980) found that immunosuppressive regimens are also more effective at preventing rejection of pancreas than of islet grafts if the histocompatibility barriers are similar. On the other hand, Hardy et al. (1982) found that palladium-110–hematoporphyrin plus antilymphocyte globulin prolonged islet allograft survival to > 60 days in 8 of 10 Lewis recipients of Wistar Furth islets and only 3 of 7 recipients of Wistar Furth pancreas allografts. Again, however, it is more difficult to prevent rejection of pancreas allografts than of heart allografts by generalized immunosuppression in the rat model (Rynasiewicz et al., 1982; Hardy et al., 1982).

In spite of the difficulties inherent in pancreas allotransplantation, there is room for optimism. The long-term function of pancreas allografts in mongrel dogs receiving cyclosporine observed by DuToit et al. (1982c) indicates that clinical pancreas transplantation with generalized immunosuppression is feasible, although ultimately, if it is to have a major impact on the treatment of diabetes, specific measures to prevent rejection that do not require generalized immunosuppression must be developed and made applicable to humans.

E. Preservation of the Intact Pancreas

For cadaveric organ transplantation to be logistically feasible on a large scale, preservation is essential (Idezuki *et al.*, 1968a, b). The current status of the two basic techniques used for kidney preservation—cold storage in intracellular salt solutions and hypothermic pulsatile perfusion with plasmalike solutions—has been recently reviewed by Toledo-Pereyra (1981) and their application to the pancreas by Sutherland *et al.* (1983b). Attempts at pancreas freezing, although unsuccessful, have also been reviewed (Toledo-Pereyra *et al.*, 1982a).

Cold storage is the simplest technique for pancreas preservation and the electrolyte solutions designed for kidney preservation have been used for 24-hour preservation of the pancreas by several investigators in experiments in dogs (Baumgartner *et al.*, 1980c; Brynger *et al.*, 1975; DuToit *et al.*, 1982a; Florack *et al.*, 1982b; Toledo-Pereyra *et al.*, 1979c; Westbroek *et al.*, 1974) and rats (Klempnauer *et al.*, 1982b; Nolan *et al.*, 1983). Most, but not all, pancreas grafts function after storage for this time, although DuToit *et al.* (1982a), who used citrate solution, found evidence for impaired function at 1 month. On the other hand, in rats, Nolan *et al.* (1983) found Collins' solution to be better than either citrate solution or Sachs' solution. Most of the investigators have found that the results are best if the cold storage solution is hyperosmolar; otherwise, considerable edema results during storage which is exacerbated after revascularization. Toledo-Pereyra *et al.* (1979b) were able to preserve the pancreas for 48 hr by addition of Collins' to the solution. Florack *et al.* (1982b) also had a relatively high success rate in preserving pancreas at 48 hr using a hyperosmolar silica-gel-filtered plasma.

DeGruyl *et al.* (1973, 1977), using the Belzer machine, and Brynger *et al.* (1975), using the Gambro machine, were able to preserve segmental pancreas grafts for 24 hr by pulsatile perfusion and had success rates similar to those achieved by cold storage in electrolyte solutions. Toledo-Peyrera *et al.* (1979c) were able to use the Mox 100 machine for 24 hr preservation of whole pancreas grafts, but Baumgartner *et al.* (1980b) experienced difficulty with perfusion of segmental grafts on the Mox 100 machine. These machines are designed to perfuse kidneys at a high flow rate, but the pancreas is a low-flow organ and machine perfusion results in excessive pressure within the system. Baumgartner *et al.* (1980d) modified the Mox 100 machine by leaving one port open, converting it into a low-pressure system. Florack *et al.* (1983b) used this modification for successful preservation up to 24 hr, but in comparative experiments, machine perfusion was not successful for 48 hr while cold storage and hyperosmolar silica gel plasma were (Florack *et al.*, 1983a). It thus appears that cold storage is superior to pulsatile perfusion for pancreas preservation.

In vitro tests to predict viability of pancreas grafts after transplantation have not shown a very good correlation with the *in vivo* function (Pegg *et al.*, 1982). Other questions relevant to pancreas transplantation and preservation include the tolerance of the gland to warm ischemia. In rats, warm ischemia up to 90 min followed by immediate transplantation is associated with good function (Schulak *et al.*, 1981, 1983) and 1 hr of ischemia combined with 4 hr in cold storage in Collins' solution has been successful in rats (Nolan *et al.*, 1983). In dogs, satisfactory pancreas graft functioned after one-half hour of warm ischemia (Westbroek et al., 1974; Florack et al., in press).

If the methods used for preservation of animal pancreases are applicable to humans, it should be possible to perform the logistical maneuvers of histocompatibility matching and preparation of the recipient for transplantation after removal of the graft from a donor. It should also be noted that the above experiments on pancreas preservation in dogs were performed in the allograft models by all investigators except Baumgartner et al. (1980b,c,d) and Florack et al. (1982b; 1983a,b); the latter used autograft models, so immunological factors did not influence interpretation of the results. The rat experiments were carried out in syngeneic models.

III. EXPERIMENTAL TRANSPLANTATION OF FREE GRAFTS OF ISLET TISSUE

The earliest attempts at transplantation of free pancreatic fragments (reviewed by Brooks and Gifford, 1959, and Hegre and Lazarow, 1977) either did not reverse diabetes, or were performed in nondiabetic animals and the results were evaluated by morphological or in vivo techniques. For more than a decade, amelioration of diabetes in experimental animals has been possible by transplantation of free grafts including (1) islets specifically isolated from the adult pancreas; (2) dispersed adult pancreatic tissue, either prepared from donors previously depleted of exocrine enzymes or transplanted to sites tolerating the introduction of exocrine enzymes; (3) intact or dispersed exocrine-poor, islet-rich fetal or neonatal pancreas; and (4) insulinoma fragments.

The bulk of the experimental work has been done in rodents. Inbred strains allow the effect of transplantation to be evaluated independently of immunological factors. In addition, one of the major problems of islet transplantation (obtaining sufficient islets for an effective transplant) is easily bypassed by using multiple isologous donors for a single recipient. On the other hand, the problems for clinical application have to be solved in large animal models, and experiments in these models deserve to be emphasized.

Most investigations have been performed in rodents with diabetes induced by either alloxan or streptozotocin (Sutherland, 1981a) but pancreatectomy has been used (Helmke et al., 1975; Lorenz et al., 1975; Champault et al., 1978; Reece-Smith et al., 1983), and some experiments have been done in animals with viral-induced or naturally occurring diabetes (reviewed by Barker et al., 1982b). In large animals, diabetes has been induced either by total pancreatectomy (Markowitz, 1959), an absolutely reliable model for both autograft and allograft experiments, but complicated by exocrine deficiency; or by streptozotocin and alloxan with or without partial pancreatectomy (Scharp et al., 1975; Lorenz et al., 1979a,b,c), a less reliable model of diabetes and one that makes autotransplant experiments difficult (Noel et al., 1982). This is an important drawback because the lack of inbred strains may dictate the use of allogenic donors in situations where immunological and metabolic consequences of the transplant are not easily distinguished.

The experiments on islet transplantation are reviewed according to the source and technique of tissue preparation, the metabolic effects, and the immunological aspects in the allogenic situation. The results often differ according to the animal model used.

A. Source and Preparation

1. Isolation from Adult Pancreases

The basic technique used for isolation of islets from adult rat pancreases is a composite of innovations introduced by various investigators. The exocrine tissue is disrupted by retrograde perfusion of the pancreatic duct (Lacy et al., 1972). The pancreas is then minced and the exocrine and endocrine tissue are dissociated by collagenase digestion (Moskalewski, 1965) The islets can be hand-picked or they can be separated from physically more dense pancreatic component by centifugation on a discontinuous density gradient of Percoll (Buitrago et al., 1977; Brundstedt, 1980), and Ficoll (Lindall et al., 1969), either dialyzed (Scharp et al., 1973) or adjusted to isotonicity with hypaque (Tze et al., 1976b). Some contamination with lymphatic or other tissue is inevitable, but a clean preparation can be obtained by handpicking Ficoll-separated rat islets suspended in phenol red solution under a dissecting microscope with a reflected green light (Finke et al., 1979). The islets appear pink, while lymph nodes are green. Between 150 and 500 islets can be isolated from an adult rat pancreas by the collagenase technique. Approximately 5–10% islets are obtained according to estimates of the number of islets in a rat pancreas (Hess and Root, 1938).

The same method has been applied to mouse pancreas (Panijayanond et al., 1973) except that the pancreas is distended by direct injection prior to mincing and collagenase digestion, with yields of approximately 50 islets per pancreas (Faustman et al., 1983). Alternatively, mechanical mincing is not done before serial collagenase digestion and liberations of islets from the smaller mouse pancreas (Steffes et al., 1981), and close to 200 islets per pancreas can be isolated (Parr et al., 1982; Morrow et al., 1983).

Although the islets can be used for functional studies in vitro (Lacy et al., 1972), there are no quantitative data on the percentage of islets viable at the end of the isolation procedure. In general, several donors are required to obtain sufficient islets for successful transplantation to a single recipient (Sutherland, 1981a).

Various modifications in the basic technique of islet isolation in rodents have been tried in attempts to improve yield and viability. The largest number of islets are obtained from rats weighing 451–500 g (Tze and Tai, 1982a). Scharp et al. (1975) used a filtration chamber to remove islets from the digestion mixture as they were liberated. A larger number of small islets is obtained, but the final islet mass isolated was only slightly increased (Shibata et al., 1976). Trypsin, hyaluronidase, and other proteolytic enzymes have been added to the digestion mixture (Henriksson et al., 1977b). The yield of islets can be increased by pretreating rat (Vrbova et al., 1979; Theodorou et al., 1980b) or mouse (Parr et al., 1982) donors with pilocarpine to reduce exocrine enzyme content, and islet viability may be enhanced by donor pretreatment with steroids and glucagon (Toledo-Pereyra *et al.*, 1980b,c). Single-cell preparations from rat islets will reaggregate into pseudoislets during culture, and will consist of 98% endocrine cells with almost no endothelial ductal or passenger leukocyte cells (Tze and Tai, 1982b), a finding that can be exploited to determine the importance of the various cell types in initiating an immune response to allogenic islets.

The standard collagenase digestion–Ficoll gradient separation technique is less satisfactory for isolation of islets from large-animal pancreases (Scharp *et al.*, 1980), but it has been used in dogs (Lorenz *et al.*, 1979a), pigs (Sutherland *et al.*, 1974), and monkeys (Scharp *et al.*, 1975) and humans (Najarian *et al.*, 1975). In general, application to large animals has been difficult because such pancreases are more fibrous, identification of islets by gross morphology is unreliable, the yield is low, there is variability between pancreases, and lots of collagenase differ in activity and content of various (and perhaps essential) impurities (Mehigan *et al.*, 1981) resulting in underdigestion and decreased liberation of islets, or overdigestion with destruction of islets (Sutherland, 1981a). Special instruments can help with mechanical mincing (Matas *et al.*, 1976c; Gray *et al.*, 1979; Gordon *et al.*, 1981) of large-animal pancreases, including those from rodents (MacDonald, 1980).

New approaches to islet purification are being tried (Scharp *et al.*, 1981). Downing *et al.* (1980) found that disruption of the acinar tissue by venous, rather than ductal, distention resulted in a higher yield of islets from the canine pancreas. Merrel *et al.* (1979) reported that isolated single-cell suspension of the pancreas would selectively reaggregate in gyrotational culture, but these islet preparations were not tested by transplantation. Tze and Tai (1982b), however, have shown that pseudoislets prepared from rat pancreas will ameliorate diabetes after syngeneic transplantation.

Lacy *et al.* (1982b) have used a technique for isolation of islets from beef or pig pancreas in which pancreatic fragments are placed on Velcro strips. During digestion islets are liberated while residual pancreatic fibrous tissue is retained on the Velcro. The islets appear viable on *in vitro* testing and have temporarily ameliorated diabetes by xenotransplantation to mice, but the technique has not been adapted for large-scale isolation and transplantation for auto- or allotransplantation. Horaguchi and Merrell (1981) and Noel *et al.* (1982) have used methods in which the initial maneuver is to perfuse the duct of canine pancreases with collagenase solution at 37°C prior to mincing for the collagenase digestion in the cold followed by screen filtration (Horaguchi and Merrell, 1981) or culture overnight followed by Ficoll separation (Noel *et al.*, 1982). They estimated islet yields of 57% (Horaguchi and Merrell, 1981) and 30% (Noel *et al.*, 1982) based on tissue insulin measurements. Both groups and Warnock *et al.* (1983) have autotransplanted the islets in a small number of animals with moderate success. Long *et al.* (1983) have automated the method of Horaguchi *et al.* (1982) by using an islet autoisolation chamber, and have been able to obtain enough islets from one pancreas to induce euglycemia and normal results of glucose tolerance tests in pancreatectomized recipients after autotransplantation. Some variations of these new techniques would seem to be appropriate for ultimate application to human pancreases, but it must be emphasized that the latter are much more fibrous. New methods, such as use of fluorescence-labeled monoclonal antibodies directed against the cells, for automatic isolation in a cell sorter, are also being explored (Rabinovitch *et al.*, 1982b), but such methods have so far been used for *in vitro* studies only.

A unique method for preparing adult islets isolated by the standard collagenase technique for transplantation in rats has been used by Reece-Smith *et al.* (1981). The islets are placed under the kidney capsule of a diabetic or nondiabetic (Reece-Smith *et al.*, 1983) syngeneic animal for 1–2 weeks prior to secondary transplantation as a composite, now immediately vacularized, kidney islet graft to a diabetic recipient. This latter method is similar to that employed by Mullen *et al.* (1977a,b) for transplantation of fetal pancreas grafts and probably does not have clinical applicability, but is quite useful for various immunological studies of islet allografts. For experiments designed to prolong the survival of the composite islet–kidney allograft, the results are best if the intermediate host has streptozotocin-induced diabetes, as opposed to a normal or pancreatectomized diabetic host. Thus the administration of streptozotocin has some influence on immunogenicity of the composite graft derived from the intermediate host (Reece-Smith *et al.*, 1983).

2. Dispersion of Adult Pancreatic Tissue without Specific Islet Isolation

Although purified islets may be desirable for immunological reasons (Lafferty *et al.*, 1983), it is not necessary to isolate adult islets for transplantation. However, simple mincing of otherwise unaltered pancreas does not result in a preparation suitable for free grafting. Since islet isolation is relatively easy from rodent and difficult from large-animal pancreases, most investigators have focused on the latter for preparation of dispersed pancreatic islet tissue for transplantation, but such preparations are also useful in rodent experiments. For example, Kramp *et al.* (1975) simply mince pancreatic tissue of adult donor mice 6–8 weeks after induction of exocrine atrophy by pancreatic duct ligation. This preparation is suitable for transplantation as a free graft of islet tissue to diabetic mice (Kramp *et al.*, 1976).

Payne *et al.* (1979) induced exocrine atrophy in adult rats by a few weeks of chronic oral administration of DL-ethionine, a methionine analogue that is selectively toxic to the exocrine pancreas. Tissue insulin content and islet architecture are preserved, and tissue can be prepared for transplantation by retrograde injection of the pancreatic duct followed by simple mincing collagenase digestion. Mendez-Picon and McGeorge (1983) have also used this technique to prepare islet tissue for transplantation in rats used to induce exocrine atrophy in dogs before islet preparation by Cobb *et al.* (1982), but the preparations have not been tested by transplantation.

Maneuvers to reduce exocrine tissue prior to donor pancreatectomy and tissue dispersal may not be necessary in all species. Champault *et al.* (1978) and Hinshaw *et al.* (1981) have had moderate success in rabbits with a purely mechanical technique. Most investigators, however, have relied on collagenase digestion for tissue dispersal. Mirkovitch and Campiche (1976, 1977) first showed totally pancreatectomized dogs became normoglycemic after autotransplantation to the spleen or portal vein of pancreatic tissue dispersed by mincing and collagenase digestion alone. Kretschmer *et al.* (1977a) used a mechanical tissue chopper (Matas *et al.*, 1976c), as did Gordon *et al.*

(1981) and Gray *et al.* (1979), and defined the conditions that give the optimal balance between the degree of tissue dispersal, depletion of exocrine enzyme content, and islet recovery after collagenase digestion (Kretschmer *et al.*, 1977b). Mehigan *et al.* (1980b) found that prior duct ligation gave a less satisfactory preparation. Elimination of the steps required for purification shortens the islet prepartion time, increases the recovery, and reduces the need for multiple donors. This technique of tissue preparation has been extended to pigs (Kiviluoto *et al.*, 1982) and nonhuman primates (Mieny and Smit, 1978; Nash *et al.*, 1981), but even in dogs certain factors such as collagenase lot (Mehigan *et al.*, 1981) and the method of gland distention before mincing (Hanson *et al.*, 1981) are critical to success.

The contaminating exocrine tissue does not seem to be a problem and even though some may engraft (Kretschmer *et al.*, 1977b), acinar cell function could not be demonstrated (Hadji-Georgopoulos *et al.*, 1982). Measurements of insulin and amylase tissue content indicated greater destruction of exocrine than of cell tissue during preparation, but in general maximum islet yield ranges from 40 to 60% (Ward *et al.*, 1983). Thus yields by the techniques that are not designed for purification are not much greater than those described by other investigators (Noel *et al.*, 1982; Horaguchi *et al.*, 1981; Long *et al.*, 1983; Warnock *et al.*, 1983), who are attempting to purify the islets. However, these latter techniques do not result in absolutely pure islets.

3. Neonatal Pancreas

Neonatal rodent pancreas has a low exocrine enzyme content and a large proportion of islet tissue relative to other pancreatic components (Leonard *et al.*, 1974; Matas *et al.*, 1976a, 1977b). Although only 4% by weight of an adult pancreas, neonatal rat pancreas possesses 11% of the adult islet mass (Matas *et al.*, 1976a). These properties permit neonatal rat (Leonard *et al.*, 1973) or mouse (Matas *et al.*, 1977b) pancreas to be minced, dispersed by collagenase digestion, and transplanted intraperitoneally or intravenously without specific islet isolation. Although > 70% of islet tissue is lost during the usual dispersal process (Matas *et al.*, 1976a) and although shorter digestion period is less destructive (Matas *et al.*, 1976b), minimally digested tissue from a few donors is not as effective as transplantation of more extensively digested tissue from multiple donors, even though the insulin content of the transplanted tissue may be similar. Thus, a balance exists between the final islet mass obtained and the optimal dispersion needed for the tissue to take as a free graft.

Neonatal rat islets may be partially purified from dispersed pancreas by a period of tissue culture (Axen and Pi-Sunyer, 1981). Hegre *et al.* (in press) have also developed a nonenzymatic method to isolate islets by culture in 5%–95% CO_2 of minced neonatal pancreases in which fibroblast migration is induced by polystyrene to leave behind islets which are further purified by subculture. Gyrotational culture has been used to form pseudoislets from neonatal pig pancreas dispersed with collagenase and trypsin (Britt *et al.*, 1981); although the latter were not tested by transplantation. Yasunami *et al.* (1982b) modified this technique by dispersion of islet cells with dispase followed by reaggregation during tissue culture before xenotransplantation to ameliorate hyperglycemia transiently in diabetic mice. New techniques to isolate islets from cultured neonatal rat pancreas, such as identification by specific staining with monoclonal antibodies, are also being attempted (Kortz *et al.*, 1982).

Intact neonatal pancreases have been transplanted as free grafts under the renal capsule in mice (DaFoe *et al.*, 1980) and rats (Korec *et al.*, 1977; Strubbe and van Wachem, 1982; Woo and Pi-Sunyer, 1982) and intrasplenically in rats (Banks *et al.*, 1982). The interval between transplantation of neonatal pancreatic islet tissue and reversal of diabetes is relatively long unless very large numbers of donors are used, which presents some problems for allogeneic experiments.

4. Fetal Pancreas

Fetal pancreas has the same favorable rationale of high islet volume and low exocrine enzyme content (Brown *et al.*, 1978), even though the total beta cell mass of one pancreas is small. Fetal rat (Brown *et al.*, 1976; McEvoy *et al.*, 1978) or fetal mouse (Mandel and Higginbotham, 1979) pancreas can be transplanted as an intact, whole-organ graft usually obtained at between 17 and 18 days of gestation. If no further maneuvers are done, at least four fetal pancreases must be transplanted if diabetes in the recipient is to be completely ameliorated. Mullen *et al.* (1977a) found that one fetal pancreas was sufficient if placed under the kidney capsule of nondiabetic hosts and allowed to grow for 3 weeks before transplantation *en bloc* with the kidney as a composite vacularized graft. Growth of the fetal pancreas can also take place in tissue culture (Mandel *et al.*, 1981b) with an increase in insulin content (Hoffman *et al.*, 1982) and acinar degeneration (Mandel *et al.*, 1982a), but the culture conditions are important (Collier *et al.*, 1981) with high glucose concentration being detrimental (Collier *et al.*, 1982). Under optimal conditions, the insulin content will increase fivefold and even one-half of a pancreas will be sufficient for transplantation if a long interval is acceptable to ameliorate diabetes (Mandel *et al.*, 1983).

Hegre *et al.* (1976a) have dispersed multiple fetal rat pancreases by the same collagenase digestion technique that they used for neonatal pancreas. They found that less fetal than neonatal tissue was required for successful transplantation. Fetal pancreatic fragments have also been transplanted after mechanical disaggregation alone (Feldman *et al.*, 1980; Usadel *et al.*, 1974), but semipurified or proislets may be obtained by mincing and collagenase digestion without (Hegre *et al.*, 1981, in press) or with (Hellerstrom *et al.*, 1979) a 4-day period culture before handpicking for transplantation (Simeonovic and Lafferty, 1981).

There is a long latent period between transplantation of fetal pancreatic islets and reversal of diabetes (Brown *et al.*, 1978; Hegre *et al.*, 1979; Mandel *et al.*, 1982a), reflecting the need for growth and maturation of the endocrine component of fetal pancreas (Hegre, 1976a). Although the delay may not be a problem for experiments in the syngeneic situation, it can make allograft experiments difficult to interpret.

5. Use of Insulinoma Tissue for Transplantation

Chick *et al.* (1977b) first described a radiation-induced insulinoma in the NEDH strain of rats that could be propagated by serial subcutaneous transplantation of tumor fragments. Most experiments with this tumor have been performed in nondiabetic animals to study insulin secretion (Sopwith *et al.*, 1981), but it has also been used for subcutaneous transplantation into diabetic hamsters (Reintgen *et al.*, 1980a) and into allogeneic rats to study the immunological consequences (Reintgen *et al.*, 1980b). Islet adenomas with slow (biphasic) or fast insulin release can also be induced in rats by streptozotocin–nicotinomide injection, and such tumors can be simply minced into 1-mm fragments and tranplanted under the kidney capsule with variable amelioration of diabetes (Dixit *et al.*, 1982). The occurrence of hypoglycemia in the recipients is a drawback to the use of insulinomas in transplant experiments. The NEDH insulinomas almost always produced hyperglycemia; however, some streptozotocin–nicotinomide-induced beta cell tumors appear to respond partially to insulin secretory regulatory mechanisms.

B. Results in Rodents

1. Isolated Adult Islets

Younoszai *et al.* (1970) first transplanted isolated adult islets in outbred rats but the diabetes was only temporarily ameliorated because rejection occurred. Ballinger and Lacy (1972) observed partial amelioration of diabetes by transplantation of 400–600 isologous islets to the peritoneal cavity of rats. They were the first to demonstrate sustained function of transplanted islets. In 1973 Reckard *et al.* in rats and Panijayanond *et al.* (1973) in mice were able to normalize plasma glucose levels completely by transplantation of a larger number of islets to the peritoneal cavity (see review by Sutherland, 1981a).

A major contribution was the demonstration by Kemp *et al.* (1973a) that the same number of islets that were only partially effective when transplanted intraperitoneally completely cured diabetes when embolized to the liver via the portal vein. Presumably more islets engrafted because a blood supply was immediately available, or there was physiological advantage to this site because of the secretion of insulin into the portal system. Since this discovery many groups have successfully applied intraportal injections of islets for long-term reversal of experimental diabetes in rodents (see review by Sutherland, 1981a).

The number of islets required for successful transplantation depends on several factors besides the site, including the integrity of the islets isolated by various investigators or the severity of the preexisting diabetic state (Koncz *et al.*, 1976; Mennini *et al.*, 1978). As few as 240 islets (Henriksson *et al.*, 1977a; Henriksson, 1978a,b) or as many as 2100 islets may be required (Rumpf *et al.*, 1977) to restore normoglycemia in rats. The latent period between transplantation and amelioration of diabetes is shortened (Vialettes *et al.*, 1979a) and glucose tolerance improved if larger numbers of islets are injected. In general, if more than 1000 islets are injected, normoglycemia usually occurs within a day or two of transplantation (Scharp *et al.*, 1982; Wojcikowski and Arendarczyk, 1982). Islets from young adult donors seem to function better than islets from older donors (Selawry *et al.*, 1978).

Therefore, if adequate numbers of isologous islets are transplanted, the metabolic abnormalities in diabetic rats are reversed: Plasma glucose levels return to normal, circulating insulin levels become nearly normal or elevated, glucose tolerance test curves are improved or normalized, glycosuria is abolished, weight gain is restored, polyuria, polydipsia, and polyphagia are alleviated (see review by Sutherland, 1981a). Elevated pancreatic glucagon (Pipeleers-Marichal et al., 1976), plasma lipid (Vialettes et al., 1979c), and articular cartilage enzyme (Silberberg et al., 1977), or decreased liver guanylate cyclase (Vesely et al., 1979; Mangnall et al., 1977) and serum gastrin (Fabri et al., 1983) levels and depressed exocrine function of the recipients native pancreas (Satake et al., in press), as well as defects in neutrophil function (Payne et al., 1983b) and alterations in immune function (Handwerger et al., in press) disappear. Subtle pertubations in glucose tolerance (Louis-Sylvestre, 1978)—such as delayed insulin release after oral glucose administration (Trimble et al., 1980b)—may be attributed to the ectopic location of the islets (Pipeleers et al., 1978), lack of sympathetic or parasympathetic innervation (Berthoud et al., 1980; Trimble et al., 1981), disruption of the enteroinsular axis (Siegel et al., 1980a,b) or less-than-normal islet mass (Scharp et al., 1982). The latter may be particularly important, since if enough islets are transplanted even responses under stress are normal (Woo and Xavier-PiSunger, 1982).

Transplanted islets lodge within the hepatic portal venules immediately after intraportal transplantation (Pipeleers-Marichal et al., 1976) but are eventually found in interstitial tissue in direct apposition to hepatocyte (Franklin et al., 1979). Neovascularization occurs rapidly (Griffith et al., 1977) and both insulin- and glucagon-containing cells can be demonstrated in the liver by immunofluorescent techniques (Lorenz et al., 1975).

Quantitative studies suggest that at least one-half of the islets that are embolized into the portal vein survive in the liver (Pipeleers-Marichal et al., 1976). Between 50 and 90% of the insulin content of the originally transplanted tissue has been recovered in the liver of rats completely ameliorated of diabetes (Rabinovitch et al., 1976; Vialettes et al., 1978a; Trimble et al., 1980a). Ziegler et al. (1975) caused reversion to the diabetic state by partial hepatectomy in rats bearing islets selectively infused into the right branch of the portal vein, suggesting that the majority, if not all, of the islets were confined to the liver.

The effect of embolization of islets to the portal vein on liver function in rats is minimal (Amamoo et al., 1975). Oakes et al. (1978) found that serum liver enyzme levels increased acutely, but the levels returned to baseline by 3 days and remained normal in long-term follow-up after intraportal islet transplantation.

Isolated islets have been transplanted to other sites with variable results. In rodents intrasplenic injection is nearly as efficient as intraportal injection (Feldman et al., 1977; Finch et al., 1977c; Reckard et al., 1978; Franklin et al., 1979), although some islets may escape into the liver (Feldman et al., 1977). Embolization of islets to the lung via a systemic vein (Slijepcevic et al., 1975) and direct injection into the liver (Eloy et al., 1977) only partially ameliorated diabetes. Diabetes has not or has rarely or only partially been reversed after subcutaneous, intramuscular, intratesticular, intrapancreatic, or intrasalivary gland implantation of isolated adult rodent islets (Georgakais, 1979), although histological survival has been observed in some instances (see review by Sutherland, 1981a). Some of these sites may still be appropriate, since large quantities of neonatal islet tissue have been successfully transplanted subcutaneously or intramuscularly with amelioration of diabetes (Pi-Sunyer et al., 1979; Axen and Pi-Sunyer, 1981). Even isolated adult islets can be transplanted to a closed space, since rat-to-mouse intratesticular xenografts have reversed diabetes (Bobzien et al., 1983) as have pancreatic fragments transplanted to the gastric submucosa of rabbits (Champault et al., 1978). The cleared mammary fat pad has also been used for transplantation of isolated adult mouse islets, primarily for histological studies, but also with partial amelioration of diabetes (Outzen and Leiter, 1981).

The best alternative site to intraportal transplantation, however, appears to be kidney capsule (Reece-Smith et al., 1981a), since amelioration of diabetes can occur with even fewer islets than needed for intraportal injection (Lacy et al., 1981a,b). Reece-Smith et al. (1981a) found that transplantation of 1000–1200 islets under the kidney capsule of diabetic rats ameliorated diabetes but intravenous glucose tolerance test k values were 1.7%, as opposed to 2.4% in normal animals. Experiments testing transplantation of larger numbers of islets, similar to those of Scharp et al. (1982), who were able completely to correct metabolic abnormalities by intraportal transplantation of > 2000 islets in rats, need to be done using the renal subcapsular site. Reece-Smith et al. (1982b) demonstrated the k values can be increased by performing a renal portal shunt after transplantation under the kidney capsule. Reece-Smith et al. (1981c) also transplanted islets placed under the kidney capsule of syngeneic rats as a secondary immediately vascularized composite graft with reversal of diabetes in the secondary recipients. Vascularization of the islets under the kidney capsule occurs very rapidly, within 48 hr (Reece-Smith et al., 1981d). Islet transplant experiments in diabetic mice also appear to indicate that the renal capsule is superior to the intrasplenic or portal vein route for amelioration of diabetes (Lacy et al., 1981b; Faustman et al., 1982b).

2. Dispersed Adult Pancreas without Islet Purification

Kramp et al. (1975) were the first to produce long-term amelioration of experimental diabetes by transplantation of adult pancreatic fragments without specific islet isolation. Fragments from three to four duct-ligated hemipancreases were transplanted subcutaneously to syngeneic mildly diabetic mice. Most recipients became normoglycemic over 3–14 weeks, although glucose tolerance test results were abnormal. Measurement of tissue insulin content showed that approximately 15% of the transplanted islets survived (Kramp et al., 1976). In a series of experiments Kramp and Burr (1981) studied the relationship between carbohydrate tolerance and hormone content of the transplanted pancreas, and were not able to achieve normal results of glucose tolerance tests, perhaps because the final islet mass (by tissue insulin content) was <22% of normal.

Payne et al. obtained better results by intraportal transplantation of unpurified islet tissue prepared by collagenase digestion of pancreases harvested from donor rats in whom exocrine atrophy had been induced by prior administration of DL-ethionine (DLE). Diabetes was ameliorated in almost all of the rats who received tissue prepared from a single or a half and in two-thirds of the rats who received tissue prepared from one-third or one-fourth of a pancreas. The interval between transplantation and normoglycemia was shortest in rats that received the largest amount of tissue. Glucose tolerance test results in successfully transplanted animals were the same as for normal animals. This method has been used for a variety of islet isograft (Morrow *et al.*, 1982; Payne *et al.*, 1982) and allograft (Rynasiewicz *et al.*, 1982; Squifflet *et al.*, 1982b; Mendez-Picon and McGeorge, 1983) experiments in rats.

Pancreatic islet tissue from DLE-treated donors (one donor per recipient) has also been transplanted to the spleen of diabetic rats (Sutherland *et al.*, 1979a). Normoglycemia occurred less rapidly after intrasplenic than intraportal transplantation, but the results of glucose tolerance tests were similar and normal when tested at 8 weeks. Splenectomy resulted in recurrence of diabetes.

Measurements of tissue insulin content (Sutherland *et al.*, 1980b) have shown that approximately 40% of the original islet mass was recovered after adequate dispersal of DLE-treated donor pancreas by collagenase digestion. Several weeks after intraportal transplantation, between 50 and 70% of the original insulin content of the transplanted tissue could be detected in the liver of recipient rats (Squifflet *et al.*, 1983b). If adequate quantities of islet tissue are engrafted intraperitoneally, glucose tolerance is nearly normal and equal to or better than that achieved with heterotopic pancreas transplantation (Squifflet *et al.*, 1982a). This technique is efficient for laboratory investigations, since intraportal injection of islet tissue prepared from two DLE-treated donors can rapidly restore normoglycemia in diabetic rats, as required for allograft experiments (Rynasiewicz *et al.*, 1982).

3. Neonatal Pancreas

Almost all of the studies with transplantation of neonatal pancreatic tissue have been with rodent donors. Leonard *et al.* (1973) were the first to ameliorate diabetes by intraperitoneal transplantation of multiple neonatal pancreases dispersed by collagenase digestion without specific islet isolation. Subsequent studies by several investigators have shown that the diabetic state in rats and mice can be reversed by intraperitoneal, intraportal, intrasplenic, or intravenous transplantation of dispersed neonatal pancreas (see review by Sutherland, 1981a). The portal vein route appears to be best (Mennini *et al.*, 1978), but even the intramuscular route can ameliorate diabetes and restore nearly normal metabolism if more than 30 donors are used (Axen and Pi-Sunyer, 1981). There are no reports on transplantation of dispersed neonatal islet tissue to under the kidney capsule, the most efficient site for transplantation of adult islets and intact free grafts of neonatal and fetal pancreases (see previous and subsequent sections). Comparative studies of tissue preparation and sites, such as those done earlier by Pi-Sunyer *et al.* (1979) need to be repeated.

The amount of dispersed neonatal pancreatic tissue required to reverse the diabetic state, as well as the latent period between transplantation and the reversal of diabetes, depends upon the quantity of tissue transplanted and the site of transplantation, and can range from a few days to weeks. If a sufficient quantity of dispersed neonatal pancreas is transplanted, permanent normoglycemia occurs, glycosuria is abolished, weight gain is restored, and glucose tolerance test result curves in rats receiving intraportal or intravenous transplants are almost always, and after intraperitoneal transplantation usually but not always, normal. Plasma insulin levels have been low, normal, or elevated in the fasting or nonfasting state or during glucose tolerance testing (see review by Sutherland, 1981a). These differences may be related to the quantity of islet tissue transplanted, or variations in the distribution of islet implants and whether their result- ant venous drainage is systemic or portal. Most likely, the most critical issue is islet mass since Woo and Xavier-PiSunyer (1982) found that rats ameliorated of diabetes by intraportal transplantation of dispersed neonatal pancreas as well as with intact pan- creas to the renal subcapsule had normal metabolic responses even when stressed with epinephrine and cortisone. There was no evidence of an exaggerated denervated re- sponse as seen in studies by Trimble *et al.* (1981) with transplantation of relatively small numbers of adult islets.

Immunohistochemical studies after intraperitoneal (Hegre *et al.*, 1976a), intraportal (Grotting *et al.*, 1978), or intravenous (Matas *et al.*, 1977a) transplantation of dispersed neonatal pancreas have shown insulin-, glucagon-, and somatostatin and pancreatic polypeptide-containing cells in the implants or target organs. Islets of nor- mal architecture as well as of one cell type can be identified. Mitotic figures are some- times present (Leonard *et al.*, 1973). Acinar elements largely disappear, and serial studies of the liver after intraportal transplantation have shown that islet cells become endothelized and gradually move into the hepatic lobules from the portal spaces (Grotting *et al.*, 1978).

The quantitative aspects of transplantation of dispersed neonatal pancreases to di- abetic rats have been studied in detail by Matas *et al.* (1976a, b, 1977a). The interval between transplantation and occurrence of normoglycemia was clearly related to islet mass transplanted. Once normoglycemia was achieved, however, there were no ob- servable differences in the rats receiving larger or smaller amounts of tissue; plasma glucose and insulin levels and the results of glucose tolerance tests were similar. The beta cell mass of one neonatal pancreas after collagenase digestion is 6% of the normal adult beta cell mass (Matas *et al.*, 1976a), suggesting that proliferation of neonatal islets is required for amelioration of diabetes when small quantities of tissue are trans- planted. Even when adequate quantities of dispersed neonatal pancreas are trans- planted, the interval between transplantation and occurrence of normoglycemia is longer than when equivalent quantities of isolated adult islets are transplanted (Mennini *et al.*, 1978). Vialettes *et al.* (1978a) transplanted adult islets or dispersed neonatal pancreas with the same tissue insulin content to the portal vein of diabetic rats; the decline of plasma glucose was more rapid with adult islets even though the beta cell mass that ultimately survived in the liver was higher from neonatal than from adult donors (70% vs. 50%, according to tissue insulin content).

Dispersed neonatal pig pancreatic tissue that has been allowed to form pseudoislets has been transplanted intraportally as xenografts with temporary ameliora- tion of diabetes in mice (Yasunami *et al.*, 1982). Transplantation of dispersed neonatal pancreatic tissue in large animals has not yet been reported.

Intact neonatal pancreases can be transplanted as free grafts (Korec *et al.*, 1977). DaFoe *et al.* (1980) reversed diabetes in mice by implantation of four to nine neonatal pancreases under the renal capsule. Strubbe (1982) has done likewise in the rats to study insulin secretion in relation to various glucose loads. Banks *et al.* (1982) performed histological studies in rats following partial amelioration of diabetes by intrasplenic transplantation of intact neonatal pancreases. They demonstrated preservation of endocrine cells but degeneration of acinar cells with adjacent adipose tissue proliferation.

4. Fetal Pancreas

Fetal islets have the capacity to grow and differentiate after transplantation (Brown *et al.*, 1981; Mandel *et al.*, 1982a), and the latent period between transplantation and reversal of hyperglycemia is usually several weeks (Brown *et al.*, 1978; Hegre *et al.*, 1976b).

Most investigators have transplanted fetal islets as intact free pancreas grafts, but there are a few reports on transplantation of mechanically dissociated fetal pancreas (Usadel *et al.*, 1974) or intraportally (Feldman *et al.*, 1980), or of collagenase-dispersed tissue transplanted intraperitoneally (Hegre *et al.*, 1976a, 1979). The latter is more efficient than similarly prepared neonatal tissue on a weight basis, but a long interval to cure was still required.

Transplantation of at least four intact fetal pancreases to under the kidney capsule (Brown *et al.*, 1976) and two to the spleen (Spence *et al.*, 1979) consistently ameliorates diabetes within 2–3 weeks in rats temporarily treated with insulin, and restores circulating insulin levels and glucose tolerance test results to nearly normal. Modulating the severity of the diabetic state by temporary administration of insulin enhances engraftment and allows even one fetal pancreas to ameliorate diabetes (Brown *et al.*, 1981). This makes unnecessary the maneuver of Mullen *et al.* (1977b) in which one fetal pancreas was sufficient to ameliorate diabetes if it was placed in the kidney capsule of syngeneic normal hosts and allowed to mature for 3 weeks before *en bloc* transplantation of the kidney and intact pancreas to the recipient. Even without these maneuvers, three fetal pancreases are sufficient if a renal vein portal caval shunt is performed after grafting to under the renal capsule. The studies by Brown *et al.* (1979) support the concept that there is a physiological benefit from diversion of secreted insulin into the hepatic portal circulation. Mandel *et al.* (1983a) reversed hyperglycemia after transplantation of one cultured fetal pancreas to the kidney of sygeneic diabetic mice. Tissue culture (Mandel *et al.*, 1980) provided a period of growth that continued after transplantation in mice treated with insulin (Hoffman *et al.*, 1981).

McEvoy *et al.* (1978), McEvoy and Hegre (1978, 1979), and Hegre *et al.* (1979) have also performed detailed quantitative studies of transplantation of intact fetal rat pancreases. The beta cell mass of implants increased eightfold after transplantation and 1 week of insulin treatment. Further 2–3 weeks of insulin treatment had variable outcome after transplantation. These paradoxical results suggest that control of extreme hyperglycemia may be beneficial during the period needed for neovascularization, growth, and differentiation, but that an endocrine deficiency state is also important for establishment of graft function. According to studies by Weisman *et al.* (1980), however, a period of normoglycemia, although not essential, is optimal for development of insulin-release capabilities in transplanted fetal rat pancreases. These observations may relate to those of Louis-Sylvestre (1978) on the absence of cephalic-phase insulin release from transplanted fetal pancreases. The abnormalities are probably not physiologically important since rats cured of diabetes by transplantation of one fetal pancreas are euglycemic even when subjected to stress, for example, a normal pregnancy (Brown et al., 1982). The main drawback to the use of fetal pancreases is the long latent period between transplantation and reversal of diabetes, complicating the interpretations of allograft experiments.

5. Insulinoma Tissue

Although transplantation of NEDM insulinoma tissue can reverse diabetes in rats, hypoglycemia also occurs (Chick et al., 1977b; Reintgen et al., 1980). However, Dixit et al. (1982) have reversed diabetes in syngeneic rats with transplantation of nicotinamide–streptozotocin-induced islet adenoma fragments and observed only mild hypoglycemia after engraftment. The NEDM insulinoma (Reintgen et al., 1980a,b), but not the chemically induced islet adenomas, has been used for allograft and xenograft experiments.

C. Results in Large Animals

1. Isolated Islets

There are only a few reports on transplantation of isolated adult islets in large animals. The problems of islet yield are formidable. If multiple donors are used, allogeneic islets may be rejected before function of a technically successful transplant is established. If rejection is avoided by using an autotransplant model, the number of islets may be too few to have a significant effect on the diabetic state. A minimal effect on diabetes was observed in the earliest experiments on islet transplantation in large animals (see review by Sutherland, 1981a), except for those of Lorenz et al. (1979a,b,c) in which a relatively mild diabetes induced by 80% pancreatectomy and streptozotocin injection in partially inbred german sheperd dogs was ameliorated by intraportal transplantation of minimally histoincompatible allogeneic islets. Because of the uncertainty over the reliability of the model, these results are difficult to interpret, as are similar experiments by Araki et al. (1979) in a totally pancreatectomized model.

More recently, the methods of Noel et al. (1982) and Horaguchi et al. (1981), designed to isolate a large number of viable islets from the canine pancreas by initial ductal perfusion of collagenase, have been used for transplantation, in a small number of animals. Noel et al. (1982) used the 80% pancreatectomy and streptozotocin technique which is not an entirely reliable model of diabetes, but observed return to normoglycemia in two of three dogs receiving the islets intrasplenically. However, no subsequent splenectomy or residual pancreatectomy was done to determine whether the reversal was due to the transplanted islets or the residual pancreas (Matas et al., 1977e). Horaguchi et al. (1981) used a total pancreatectomy model, and found that three of five dogs receiving islets into the liver and two of two receiving islets into the spleen became normoglycemic after autotransplantation. Warnock et al. (1983) and Long et al. (1982) obtained excellent results using modified versions of the Horaguchi *et al.* (1981) technique for intrasplenic islet autotransplantation to totally pancreatectomized dogs, all of whom had normal results of glucose tolerance tests 1 month after transplant.

2. Dispersed Adult Pancreas without Islet Purification

The problem of yield of purified islets in large animals is gradually being solved (see Sections III.A.1 and III.C.1) but islet purification is not absolutely necessary. In 1976, Mirkovitch and Campiche *et al.* ameliorated diabetes in totally pancreatectomized dogs by intrasplenic autotransplantation of dispersed pancreatic tissue prepared from the left limb (pancreatic tail) by collagenase digestion alone.

Kretschmer *et al.* (1977b) dispersed the entire pancreas and found that dogs receiving transplants of tissue digested with collagenase for 20 min had the best outcome. However, metabolic studies in recipient dogs were not completely normal. The animals had fasting normoglycemia, but k values during glucose tolerance tests were only half those of normal controls and peripheral vein insulin levels were very low (Kretschmer *et al.*, 1977a). The results of splenectomy and histological examination were similar to those of Mirkovitch and Campiche (1976). The efficiency of engraftment is low. In studies by Ward *et al.* (1983) on transplantation of dispersed pancreatic tissue prepared only from the right and left limbs of totally pancreatectomized dogs, an average of 13% of the insulin content of the tissue transplanted was recovered in the spleen at 3 weeks. The metabolic effect correlated with the insulin content of the spleen. Because of attrition of tissue during preparation, the splenic insulin content averaged < 10% of that of a normal canine pancreas, but 80% of animals with a splenic insulin content of > 6% that of the normal pancreas were normoglycemic.

Several investigators have used the model of intrasplenic transplantation of dispersed pancreatic tissue in dogs to study a variety of problems, including preservation (Sutherland *et al.*, 1977; Schulak *et al.*, 1978), systemic vs. portal venous drainage (Schulak *et al.*, 1979), the effect of endogenous pancreatic tryptic activity on the islet preparation (Traverso *et al.*, 1978), and the metabolic responses after transplantation (Gray *et al.*, 1979; Kolb *et al.*, 1977; Hadji-Georgopoulos *et al.*, 1982). In the experiments of Hadji-Georgopoulos *et al.* (1982), portal vein insulin levels were lower than normal in pancreatectomized transplanted dogs, but the response was biphasic; no exocrine function was demonstrated. Mehigan *et al.* (1980b) found that the success rate was lower with transplantation of tissue prepared from dogs with chronic pancreatitis induced by duct ligation even though the insulin reserve of the pancreas before dispersion was nearly normal. Mehigan *et al.* (1981) have also documented the inherent variability of success or failure in this model based on critical factors in techniques and collagenase lots.

Mirkovitch *et al.* (1979a) found that if completion of the pancreatectomy was delayed to more than 3 weeks after intrasplenic transplantation of dispersed tissue prepared from the left limb, the animals became diabetic. This outcome suggests that an endocrine deficiency state is important for engraftment. The results are interesting because of their similarity to the paradoxical results on the effect of insulin treatment after islet transplantation in rats (McEvoy *et al.*, 1978).

Diabetes has also been ameliorated by infusion of collagenase-dispersed pancreatic tissue into the portal vein of pancreatectomized dogs (Kolb *et al.*, 1977; Kretschmer *et al.*, 1978; Matas *et al.*, 1977e; Mehigan *et al.*, 1980b). Serum liver enzyme levels are transiently elevated. Dogs are particularly susceptible to the development of portal hypertension. Kretschmer *et al.* (1978) found transplantation by this route not to be as effective as transplantation to the spleen. Mehigan *et al.* (1980a) described disseminated intravascular coagulation and portal hypertension after intraportal transplantation. This syndrome was secondary to tissue thromboplastin in the preparation and could be prevented by prophylactic administration of heparin and aprotinin. Intraportal embolization to the liver can also occur during intrasplenic transplantation of dispersed pancreatic tissue. DuToit *et al.* (1980) found that this occurrence gave rise to portal hypertension and hemodynamic disturbances in puppies.

Diabetes has also been obviated in three of four baboons (Mieny *et al.*, 1978) and in six of eight baboons (Nash *et al.*, 1981) after total pancreatectomy by infusion of colleagenase-dispersed autologous pancreatic tissue into the portal vein. Nash *et al.* (1981) also performed allograft experiments in baboons using this technique, but with poor results.

In summary, experiments in large animals show that pancreatic tissue dispersed by mincing and collagenase digestion alone can ameliorate severe diabetes after autotransplantation to the spleen or portal vein. Elimination of the steps for purification allows sufficient islet tissue to be obtained from one donor for an effective transplant, but similar results are now being obtained with semipurified islet tissue (Long *et al.*, 1983). Further experiments are needed to show whether the purification process provides mechanical, metabolic, or immunological advantages.

D. Islet Transplantation in Natural Models of Diabetes

Most islet transplant experiments have been in animals with diabetes induced by either beta cell toxins or total pancreatectomy. The syndrome produced—insulinopenic hyperglycemia—resembles juvenile-onset insulin-dependent diabetes mellitus, but it is an artificial counterpart. In addition, pancreatectomy causes metabolic and nutritional changes that complicate the animal studies. For these reasons animals with spontaneous diabetes are useful for evaluation, although not all of the models are akin to human diabetes (Barker *et al.*, 1982b).

Two inbred strains—the C57BL/6J (ob/ob) and the C57BL/KsJ (db/db) mice—are characterized by hyperinsulinemia, hyperphagia, hyperglycemia, islet hyperplasia early in life, and, particularly in db/db mice, insulin resistance (Coleman, 1978). (C3HF X I) F_1 male hybrids (Dafoe *et al.*, 1982) also exhibit this syndrome. These animals are models for human Type 2 diabetes.

Strautz (1970) reported that islet transplantation partially reversed the syndrome in ob/ob mice and suggested that the islets supplied a missing satiety factor. Barker *et al.* (1977) obtained slightly different results. They found that transplantation of histocompatible normal islets resulted in reduction of plasma glucose for only 2–3 weeks; hyperglycemia and progressive weight gain then recurred, suggesting that the transplanted islets either became involved in the pathological process or eventually failed to function for nonimmunological reasons. Andersson *et al.* (1981) did not even observe a temporary effect of intrasplenic transplantation of histocompatible islets from congeneic lean normal mice on plasma glucose levels in ob/ob mice, even though islets from lean mice or old ob/ob islets would cure drug-induced diabetes in lean mice. Similarly, Barker *et al.* (1977) showed no effect on diabetes in db/db mice after transplantation of histocompatible normal islets, even though the transplants were done at an age when plasma insulin concentrations were falling from endogenous islet exhaustion. However, they also found that transplantation of islets derived from db/db mice completely reversed the diabetic state in congeneic mice with streptozotocin-induced diabetes. DaFoe *et al.* (1983) also found that parental-strain neonatal pancreas transplanted to (C3HexI) F_1 diabetic male mice would not ameliorate diabetes in C3H mice with streptozotocin-induced diabetes treated with antilymphocyte serum (ALS) after transplantation to prevent rejection. This observation seems to provide definitive proof that whatever the defect in db/db or ob/ob mice, it does not reside in their islets.

New Zealand obese (NZO) mice have only mild elevations of basal blood glucose levels; but they are hyperinsulinemic and glucose tolerance test results are abnormal. Gates *et al.* (1972) reported that transplantation of islets enclosed within millipore filter chambers corrected the abnormalities, although Swenne *et al.* (1979) could not reproduce these results. Barker *et al.* (1977) found that after transplantation of rat islets to immunosuppressed NZO mice, glucose tolerance test results returned to normal. Normal islets may produce a factor that decreases insulin resistance and alleviates the syndrome (Gates *et al.*, 1974).

Although the results of the experiments in the obese hyperinsulinemic mice models indicate that transplantation may not be appropriate treatment for all forms of diabetes, the syndromes in these mice bear little resemblance to juvenile-onset insulin-dependent diabetes in humans. Other animal models of naturally occurring diabetes are more appropriate for comparison to the human situation (Barker *et al.*, 1982b).

Viruses have been implicated in the etiology of some cases of human diabetes (Rayfield and Seto, 1978). Howard *et al.* (1979) reversed the diabetic state that follows infection with encephalomyocarditis virus (EMCV) in SWR/J mice by intrasplenic transplantation of islet tissue from uninfected isologous donors. Following transplantation, reexposure to the virus was not followed by recurrence of diabetes. This finding is not surprising, since the mice would be expected to be resistant to secondary infection; however, SWR/J mice that previously had been cured of streptozotocin-induced diabetes by islet transplantation to the spleen also did not become diabetic after primary exposure to the virus. Normal littermates infected at the same time became diabetic. This finding is surprising and suggest that either intrasplenic islets are not susceptible to infection or that streptozotocin induces changes in the mice that make them resistant to the virus.

Naji *et al.* (1979b) reversed EMCV-induced severe diabetes in DBA mice by transplantation of syngeneic fetal pancreas to under the kidney capsule. Removal of the graft 30 days later was followed by recurrence of the diabetes. DaFoe *et al.* (1980, 1981) performed islet transplantation in F1 hybrids of mice strains either susceptible or resistant to viral-induced diabetes in mice with susceptibility or resistance dependent upon their sex. The hybrids had intermediate susceptibility. Transplantation of islets from one or the other parental strain to hybrids or from donors of the opposite sex ameliorated streptozotocin-induced diabetes. Subsequent infections with virus resulted in diabetes with the same frequency as normal hybrids or as in the recipient's sex. Together, these experiments show that (1) islet transplantation can reverse virus induced diabetes, (2) latent virus or recurrent virus does not damage the transplanted islets, and (3) host factors are more important than intrinsic pancreatic factors in determining susceptibility to virus-induced diabetes (Barker et al., 1982a,b).

One other animal model with spontaneous diabetes has been used for islet transplantation: the "BB" Wistar rat (see review by Marliss et al., 1982). A variable percentage of rats in this outbred line develop isletitis, and rapidly become hypoinsulinemic, severely hyperglycemic, and ketosis-prone (Barket et al., 1982b). The animals also have an immune deficiency syndrome (Bellgran et al., 1982; Naji et al., 1982), which can be corrected by allogeneic bone marrow transplantation (Naji et al., 1983) to induce tolerance (Naji et al., 1981d) and such treatment also usually prevents the development of diabetes (Naji et al., 1981c).

Autoimmunity is probably involved in the pathogenesis of diabetes in BB rats, since administration of antilymphocyte serum soon (but not late) after the onset will restore normoglycemia (Nagi et al., 1979b). Naji et al. (1981b) restored normoglycemia by intraportal transplantation of allogeneic islets from normal histocompatible donors to immunosuppressed "BB" recipients. If the recipients are not immunosuppressed, diabetes will recur even before rejection of the allogeneic islets. A few BB rats who do develop diabetes after induction of tolerance to WF rats by neonatal bone marrow injection will have recurrence of diabetes from insulinitis in transplanted WF islets, even though they cannot reject the islets. The BB rat is currently the most useful animal for studying the effect of islet transplantation in a natural model of diabetes as well as for research into the etiology of diabetes (Barker et al., 1982b).

Spontaneous diabetes has occasionally been observed in mice (Prowse et al., 1982a). Prowse et al. (1982b) were able to cure one such CBA mouse by transplantation of cultured Balb/C islets without the use of immunosuppression. This animal might differ considerably from the BB rat, and might possibly be even more representative of human diabetes. The other natural models of diabetes—hyperglycemia associated with obesity and islet hyperplasia—are more akin to maturity-onset diabetes. Not even all of these animals become hyperglycemic, such as the 129/JDB 3J/DB3J mouse which has hyperplastic islets that are extremely sensitive to streptozotocin. However, transplantation can ameliorate diabetes in syngeneic or allogeneic mice (Outzen and Leiter, 1981).

Although not a natural model, isologous islets can reverse drug-induced diabetes in mice accompanied by cell-mediated insulitis in the absence of immunosuppression (Andersson, 1979; Sandler and Andersson, 1981). Autoimmune phenomena associated with diabetes will not necessarily persist to affect transplanted islets adversely (Sandler and Andersson, 1981).

In summary, islet transplantation can reverse diabetes in natural models characterized by beta cell destruction and insulin deficiency. These results strongly argue that transplantation in humans with juvenile-onset diabetes will be similarly effective if technical and immunological problems can be overcome.

E. Immunological Aspects of Islet Allo- and Xenotransplantation

Multiple factors make it difficult to interpret and compare the results of the islet allograft experiments reported by various investigators (Barker *et al.,* 1982a). These factors include (1) heterogeneous combinations of donor-recipient pairs; (2) variability in the donor source, the site of transplantation, and the number of islets transplanted or engrafted; (3) variations in the potency of biological immunosuppressants, such as antilymphocyte serum and enhancing antibodies; (4) the effect of immunosuppressive agents, such as corticosteroids, on the severity of diabetes; and (5) the lack of uniformity in the definition of rejection. At least 2 consecutive days of normoglycemia should be a minimum criterion for successful islet engraftment (Matas *et al.,* 1978a). Since a fall in blood glucose on the first day of transplantation may be due to release of insulin from damaged islets, experiments reporting allograft survival data of 1–2 days' duration should be viewed with caution, particularly if there are no isologous controls. Rejection may have occurred before the islets were physiologically effective, since in many isograft models there is a latent period of days to weeks before sustained normoglycemia occurs. Ideally, in allograft experiments a large number of islets should be transplanted to an appropriate site so that normoglycemia is established definitely before rejection occurs. Many but not all islet allograft experiments have met this criterion.

As the technical aspects of transplantation have improved, islet allograft experiments have become more sophisticated and in rodent models it is even possible to prevent rejection of full histoincompatibility islets without systemic immunosuppression. The mechanisms involved are not necessarily unique to islets, but methods to prevent rejection of other types of organ allografts have not always been effective for islets. Conversely some of the methods that had been developed to prevent rejection of islet allografts have not been tested in other models so their general applicability is not known. The most recent experiments must be interpreted in the light of modern immunological concepts: These include the knowledge that dendritic cells (see review by Steinman, 1981) may be the most important for the immunogenicity of foreign tissues; the hypothesis on the origin and mechanism of the allograft reaction in which two signals, one provided by histocompatibility antigens and the other by specific response of T cells, are necessary to initiate an allogeneic response (see reviews by Lafferty, 1980; Lafferty and Woolnough, 1977; Lafferty *et al.,* 1983); and the genetic control of transplant rejection via immune response genes (Butcher and Howard, 1982). The specific application of some of these concepts to islet transplantation has been succinctly stated by Prowse *et al.* (1982a).

It is generally believed that surface determinants encoded by Class I genes of the MHC (murine H-2 K/D, human HLA-A, B, C) are expressed on virtually all nucleated cells (Klein, 1975) and molecular products of Class II genes (mouse H-2 I, human HLA D/DR) are expressed only in B lymphocytes, macrophages (Cowing *et al.,* 1978), Langerhans cells in the skin, dendritic cells, and certain populations of suppressor T lymphocytes (Hammerling *et al.,* 1979). Since certain tissues, for example, the cornea (Streilein *et al.* 1979), do not express Ia antigens at all, the presence or absence of H-2 antigens in pancreatic islets is of great importance, especially in view of the apparent extreme sensitivity of islets to rejection, a phenomenon which may be separate from their immunogenicity (Mandel *et al.*, 1982). The results of experiments designed to study this problem are summarized in the following section.

1. Islet Antigenicity and Susceptibility to Rejection

Although Parr (1979), using an immunoferratin labeling technique, was not able to detect H-2 antigens on mouse islet beta cells, it is now apparent from cytotoxicity and absorption experiments and from studies using other labeling techniques that Class I antigens are present on islets (Faustman *et al.*, 1980; Baekkeskov *et al.*, 1981), although their density may be low (Parr *et al.*, 1982). Class II antigens, however, cannot be detected on beta cells (Parr *et al.*, 1980b; Faustman *et al.*, 1980; Baekkeskov *et al.*, 1981) but are present in passenger leukocytes and endothelial cells (Rabinovitch, 1982a) and the rare dendritic cells (Hart and Fabres, 1981) in rat islets. Class II antigens have also been demonstrated in dendritic cells in adult (Alejandro *et al.*, 1982b; Natali *et al.*, 1981a,b; Shienvold *et al.*, 1982; and Daar *et al.*, 1983) and fetal (Danilovs *et al.*, 1982) pancreatic islet tissue or periislet tissue by immunoperoxidase or immunofluorescent techniques that may be more sensitive than the absorptive, microcytotoxicity, or immunoprecipitation techniques. Mouse pancreatic endothelial cells do not express Class II antigens (Parr *et al.*, 1980b, 1982). Hart and Fabres (1981) were not able to detect Class II antigens on rat endothelium, but Class II antigens have been detected on endothelial mouse cells of rats and humans (Alejandro *et al.*, 1982b) and such cells may be immunogenic (Hirschberg *et al.*, 1980; Ashida *et al.*, 1981). Islets can initiate immune response *in vitro* (Alejandro *et al.*, 1982a; Miller *et al.*, 1981; Rabinovitch *et al.*, 1981). Although islet specific antigens may be responsible, the stimulation could also be from contaminating passenger leukocytes or dendritic cells, the latter being more potent stimulators than other lymphoid tissue (Steinman, 1981).

There may be pure islets, in which dendritic cells are fortuitously absent or passenger leukocytes have been eliminated, which are not immunogenic either because of the absence of Class II antigens, or because the cells (which happen to express Class II antigens) necessary to provide one of the signals for initiation of the immune response are absent (Lafferty *et al.*, 1983). However, the islets would remain susceptible to rejection if the immune response were initiated because of Class I antigens, which are expressed on the beta cells that could serve as targets unless the donors and recipients are identical for these antigens (Morrow *et al.*, 1983). In reviewing the experiments on islet allotransplantation, it must be kept in mind that the islet preparations used by the various invest gators differ considerably in purity and possible leukocyte contamination, and such differences may influence the results obtained and disparities observed.

Adult islets as ordinarily isolated are definitely immunogenic. Ziegler *et al.* (1974) showed that Fischer rats injected with handpicked Lewis islets rejected Lewis skin grafts in an accelerated fashion. Reemstma *et al.* (1981) demonstrated that Lewis recipients of WF islets developed cytotoxic antibodies (unless they were treated with antilymphocyte globulin) and after rejection of islets would reject WF hearts in a hyperacute fashion whether or not cytotoxic antibodies were detectable. These experiments do not indicate what component of the islets or contaminating tissue are immunogenic. Lacy *et al.* (1979a) and Bowen *et al.* (1980) first provided evidence that rat islets depleted of putatively passenger leukocytes by culture or treatment with lympholytic agents are not or are weakly immunogenic. Rat beta cells are definitely susceptible to immune destruction once the afferent arc of the immune response is activated by injection of the appropriate allogeneic cells (Lacy *et al.*, 1979b; Zitron *et al.*, 1981a). T cells are most potent in this regard whereas peritoneal exudate cells (PECs) and B lymphocytes are unable to induce rejection of established islet (Zitron *et al.*, 1981b). Bowen *et al.* (1981) also found that PECs had a variable effect, since only three of six CBA mice bearing cultured Balb/C islets greater than > 100 days rejected the islets after injection with Balb/C PECs. In those that did reject the effect was specific since previous injection of foreign antigen alone was not able to induce rejection. The mechanisms for unresponsiveness in some mice are unclear. It may be time-dependent since injection of Balb/C spleen cells at 30 days after transplantation of cultured islets to CBA mice induced rejection, unless irradiated spleen cells had been administered previously, in which case a specific unresponsiveness to the donor strain appeared to be induced (Prowse *et al.*, 1982a).

The immunogenicity and vulnerability of neoplastic islet tissue to immune effector mechanisms is uncertain. Hamster insulinoma following subcutaneous transplantation to nonimmunosuppressed outbred Syrian hamsters was apparently not rejected but ameliorated streptozotocin-induced diabetes (Reintgen *et al.*, 1980a). However, a rat insulinoma has been shown to express histocompatibility antigens and seemed to be rejected after transplantation to allogeneic recipients (Reintgen *et al.*, 1980b). Fetal (Bowen *et al.*, 1980; Hegre *et al.*, 1976b; Mullen and Shintaku, 1980) and neonatal islets (Leonard *et al.*, 1973; Vialettes *et al.*, 1978b) are definitely antigenic and rejected just as rapidly as adult islets. Well-established fetal allografts under the renal capsule may be more resistant to immune destruction (Brown *et al.*, 1979) than intraportal allogeneic islets (Perloff *et al.*, 1981a), since the latter ceased while the former continued to fucntion after passive administration of donor-specific antiserum in nonimmunosuppressed recipients. Fresh fetal pancreatic islet allografts are almost always rejected before they have matured sufficiently to reverse diabetes (Garvey *et al.*, 1979b). Simeonovic and Lafferty (1982) have some histological evidence that isolated fetal mouse proislets, which are derived after only 4 days of culture of collagenase-dispersed fetal pancreas, are not very immunogenic in comparison to intact fetal pancreas (Prowse *et al.*, 1982a).

The importance of histocompatibility factors and passenger leukocytes is also apparent. Faustman *et al.* (1981) demonstrated that isolated rat islet allografts treated with donor-specific anti-Ia serum and complement prior to transplantation across a major histocompatibility barrier (*H-2 K* + *I* + *D*-disparate) in mice were not rejected. Elimination of Ia-positive contaminating passenger leukocyte or dendritic cells (which also express Class I antigens) presumably rendered the islets nonimmunogenic.

However, Morrow *et al.* (1983b) found that the simple absence of *I* region (Class II) antigenic disparities does not result in prolonged survival of islet allografts. Mice of the B10 background that are disparate at the *H-2 K* and *D* loci (Class I only) with donors of allogeneic islets reject the islets even though they are identical for *I* region (Class II) antigens. The protocol of Morrow *et al.* (1983a) did not eliminate dendritic or passenger cells from the islets, but Class II antigen disparities were eliminated genetically. Even though the donor islets were histocompatible for Class II antigens with the recipient, they were able to present Class I antigens in an immunogenic fashion. According to the two-signal hypothesis of Lafferty *et al.* (1977, 1981, 1982) these results mean that the recognition of a foreign Ia epitope itself is not essential to activate an allogeneic immune response, but only those that also express Class II antigens (whether the latter are disparate or not with the recipient) are immunostimulatory. Thus, unmodified islets are immunogenic as long as Class I (*H-2 K* or *D*) disparities between the donor and recipient exist; while if *Ia* cells are eliminated or if only Class II (*H-2 I* regions) antigenic disparities exist between the donor and recipients, the islets are not immunogenic. This theory is also consistent with the hypothesis of Silvers *et al.* (1982), in other allograft systems, that grafts can provoke a strong immune response only if the donor macrophages are included.

The isolated effects of *H-2, K, D,* and *I* region histocompatibility differences on rejection and survival of allogeneic islets transplanted under the kidney capsule of diabetic mice were studied by Morrow *et al.* (1983b). The percentage of islet allografts functioning at < 70 days in mice disparate at the *I* locus only, *D* locus only, or *K* locus only were 92%, 89%, and 27%, respectively. For mice disparate at *K* + *D*(*I* region identical) only 29% of the grafts functioned > 79 days, a rejection rate similar to that of mice disparate at the entire *H-2* complex (*K* + *I* + *D*), where only 20% had allografts functioning at 70 days. The immune response genes as well as the specific allelic differences could influence the results (Butcher and Howard, 1982), but the results clearly indicate that the Class II antigen disparities do not have to be present to initiate islet allograft rejection, and that Class I antigen disparities alone are sufficient. Faustman *et al.* (1980) selectively eliminated passenger leukocyte- or antigen-presenting dendritic cells, because such cells express Class II antigens and were susceptible to lysis upon exposure to anti-Ia serum and complement. Since beta cells do not express the Class II antigens, they survive this treatment and by themselves are nonimmunogenic. Other protocols to eliminate passenger leukocytes have this rational basis for their effectiveness. There are no reports of fresh purified islet allograft experiments, similar to those performed by Morrow *et al.* (1983a) in mice, in congeneic rats differing at various histocompatibility loci of the MHC, although some studies along these lines have been done by Klempnauer *et al.* (1983) using a pancreas allograft model.

The vulnerability of adult islets to immune destruction by both humoral and cellular mechanisms was first demonstrated in a series of experiments by Naji *et al.* (1975, 1979a). They transplanted islets and skin across a major histocompatibility barrier to diabetic rats who had been made tolerant at birth to donor strain antigens by intravenous injection of bone marrow from donor recipient strain hybrids. The rats stayed normoglycemic with no further treatment, confirming the tolerant state. However, when lymphocytes obtained from normal or sensitized recipient strain rats were injected, hyperglycemia occurred within 3–8 days and the skin grafts were also rejected. Similarly, daily injection of antiserum directed against donor antigens resulted in hyperglycemia within 1–7 days in islet allograft recipients, although skin grafts were rejected much more slowly and parathyroid grafts were not rejected at all (Naji and Barker, 1978). Damage to islets occurred even when immunological tolerance was not broken, since it was possible to restore normoglycemia by retransplantation after the effect of antiserum had dissipated (Naji et al., 1979a). Similar experiments have been done in other models, but the results have not been uniform. Tolerant mice previously ameliorated of diabetes by islets transplanted across an extremely weak histocompatibility barrier (Frangipane et al., 1977a) or an H-Y barrier (Naji et al., 1981a) did not revert to the diabetic state after administration of normal recipient-strain lymphocytes or donor-specific antiserum. However, immunosuppressed mice ameliorated of diabetes by transplantation of rat islet xenografts became hyperglycemic within 24 hr of administration of donor-specific alloantiserum (Frangipane et al., 1977b), showing that islets can be damaged very rapidly by humoral mechanisms.

The vulnerability of islets to rejection by passively administered antibody may depend, however, on factors other than the strength of the histocompatibility barrier. Agostino et al. (1982) found that established CBA islet allografts (conditioned by cultured prior to transplantation to Balb/C mice) continued to function after injection of the recipients with donor-specific antibody and complement > 100 days after transplantation. They hypothesized that the grafts were invulnerable to rejection because of neovascularization with host endothelium. However, they did not test the effect of antibody administration early after transplantation and the proposed mechanism should also have protected the islets in the experiments of Naji et al. (1979a). It is clear that established islets contain antigenic targets for rejection, since in the same model as that used by Agostino et al. (1982), Bowen et al. (1981) found that administration of donor strain PECs induced rejection of established islet allografts in half of the recipients, even though previously adminstered alloantibody had no effect. In those animals that do not reject after injection of donor strain cells, an active suppressor mechanism may be operative (Zitron et al., 1981a), but the type of cell that is injected is also important (Zitron et al., 1981b). Bowen et al. (1981) did not test the effect of injection of splenic T cells in their models. In the experiments of Zitron et al. (1981b), Lewis rats bearing long-term WF islet allografts by lieu of 7-day culture before and recipient ALS administration at the time of transplantation rejected the islets when challenged with WF spleen T cells or PECs. They also did so just as vigorously when challenged with third-party (Buffalo) splenic T cells, but with a lower incidence and less vigorously after injection of Buffalo PECs. They suggest that PECs caused rejection by a haplotype-specific mechanism while T cells induced rejection by non-haplotype-dependent mechanisms. However, cross-reactivity of histocompatibility antigens expressed on Buffalo and WFT cells could also explain their results. In either case, the mechanisms responsible for islet allograft rejection are gradually being dissected.

The importance of the type of secondary allogeneic stimulus used in attempts to induce rejection of established islet allografts, as well as the immune response status of the recipient, is also demonstrated by the experiments of Steffes et al. (1981) in which 40% of allogeneic islets transplanted between the A.TL and A.TH strains (identical for H-2 K+D antigens, but different for I-region-encoded antigens as well as Qa and minor loci) were not rejected over 13 weeks. Skin grafts from the donor strains were rejected in the recipients with functioning islet allografts, but none of the A.TL and 50% of the A.TH recipients became hyerglycemic after skin graft rejection, while donor spleen cells induced rejection in A.TH but not in A.TL recipients.

In a different model, Faustman *et al.* (1981) found that fully histoincompatible mouse islets treated with donor-specific anti-Ia antisera (to deplete the islets of passenger leukocytes) were not rejected for > 200 days, but donor spleen cells administered at that time would induce rejection, showing that the islets retained their vulnerability to rejection. Small numbers of spleen cells, however, could not induce rejection unless anti-I-J serum was also administered (putatively directed against suppressor cells), suggesting an active mechanism allows the long-term survival of such grafts (Faustman *et al.*, 1982a). Alternatively, the anti-Ia-J sera could lower the threshold for initiation of an immune response to injection of allogeneic spleen cells independent of the presence or absence of allogeneic islets. The fact that high dose of spleen cells could induce rejection (Faustman *et al.*, 1980) shows that the mice were not tolerant to the donor strain, suggesting that the anti-Ia-treated islets survived simply because they were nonimmunogenic when transplanted.

Further experiments on induction of rejection of established islet allografts have been performed by Morrow *et al.* (1983). A small proportion (11–32%) of islet allograft donors disparate for K only, $K+D$, or $K+I+D$ loci and a somewhat larger proportion (65–88%) disparate for D or D+I (60%) antigens with the recipients are not rejected. However, when the recipients with long-term functioning allografts (> 100 days) were injected intravenously with 10^6 donor strain spleen cells the islets were promptly rejected in most (80–86%) of the animals (Morrow *et al.*, 1983). On the other hand, islets are infrequently rejected when transplanted across I region disparities only (93% functioning > 100 days), and rejection could not be induced at this time by placement of donor strain skin grafts (which were rejected) or injection of donor strain splenocytes. Since skin grafts were rejected, the islet recipient mice were obviously not unresponsive to the donor strain; presumably, β cells cannot serve as targets because they do not express the disparate antigens (I region or Class II), while skin cells do express these antigens, and therefore are susceptible to rejection effector mechanisms. In the other donor–recipient strain combinations, who differed for Class I antigens and in whom primary rejection after islet transplantation alone did not occur, the islets may have been of low immunogenicity, but once donor-strain splenocytes were injected an allogeneic response was initiated. The islet allografts in these mice were susceptible to rejection because the β cells expressed the disparate antigens (Class I) which could then serve as targets for rejection. Scott *et al.* (1982) observed that islets from A.TH mice transplanted into the spleen of A.TL mice were rejected at a mean of 21 days in unsensitized animals and at 8 days if the recipients had previously received skin grafts from the donor strain. These studies show that islets can be rejected even when there are not H-2 K or D antigenic differences, but these mice also differ at the *Qa* and *Tla* regions as well as at minor loci which might be expressed on β cells and serve as targets. Thus, skin grafts are able to sensitize recipients to reject fresh islet allografts, (Scott *et al.*, 1982) and are able to stimulate rejection of established islet allografts in the situation where non-*I* disparities exist (Steffes *et al.*, 1981). They cannot induce rejection of well-established islet allografts in the situation where there are *I* region (Class II) disparities only (Morrow *et al.*, 1983).

In rats, even Class I disparities may not always lead to rejection with a secondary stimulus in recipients with well-established islet allografts. Selawry *et al.* (1981) observed rejection of donor strain skin grafts with maintenance of normoglycemia in islet allograft recipients who received donor-specific blood transfusion before and a single dose of ALS at the time of islet transplantation. However, the dependence of the skin-grafted rats on the islet allografts for maintenance of normoglycemia was not conclusively demonstrated in these experiments since islet grafts were not removed and the rats were not observed for recurrence of hyperglycemia.

The most recent islet allograft experiments in mice, taken together with the previously cited studies on the expression of histocompatibility antigens on the various cells within islets (also reviewed by Lafferty *et al.*, 1983), suggest that islets are not very immunogenic and that their immunogenicity depends on dendritic cells or contaminating passenger leukocytes. These cells, unlike beta or other parenchymal cells which express Class I antigens only, possess both Class I and Class II antigens, and unless these cells are eliminated the islets are immunogenic. The beta cells can serve as targets for the immune response generated as long as the donor–recipient combinations are disparate for Class I or other alloantigen expressed on beta cells. If the animals are identical for Class I and other related antigen, but disparate for Class II antigen (tested only in the experiments of Morrow *et al.*, 1983), beta cells are not rejected even though other tissues or organs which, unlike beta cells, express Class II antigens and can serve as targets, are rejected. These new findings and interpretations must be kept in mind when reviewing the results of the earlier islet allograft experiments in fully histocompatable rodents, which showed that islets are extremely sensitive to rejection effector mechanisms.

If immunosuppression is not used, and precautions are not made to isolate very pure islets, fresh islet allografts can be rejected very rapidly (Reckard *et al.*, 1973; Nash *et al.*, 1977). This is particularly apparent if small numbers of islets are transplanted across strong histocompatibility barriers, and if comparison is made to other organ allografts using different or less sensitive endpoints to define rejection (Barker *et al.*, 1980). The rejection time, however, depends on several factors, including the number of islets transplanted, the site of transplantation, the histocompatibility barrier, and the donor–recipient strain combinations. For example, Naji *et al.* (1981a) found that H-Y incompatibile B6 male islets grafted intraperitoneally were rejected within 3–7 days by B6 female mice, a strain in which male skin grafts are rejected between 15 and 29 days. On the other hand, C3H females respond poorly to the H-Y antigens and did not reject C3H male islets (Naji, 1981a).

In most experiments, the day of rejection has been defined in terms of graft function. The physiological manifestations of rejection depend in part on the functional reserve of the transplanted tissue. If the number of islets engrafted is just sufficient to ameliorate diabetes, the destruction of only a few islets will result in the return to the hyperglycemic state. Finch and Morris (1977a) were able to improve the functional survival of islet allografts in rats by increasing the number of islets transplanted from

600–800 to 1500–3000. On the other hand, Squifflet *et al.* (1983) found that islet mass made only a small difference in the time to recurrence of hyperglycemia after pancreas or islet transplantation across a minor histocompatibility barrier in nonimmunosuppressed hosts.

In regard to the site of transplantation, Barker *et al.* (1975) and Ziegler *et al.* (1975) found that the median functional survival of the same number of islets transplanted across a weak histocompatibility barrier was three times longer after intraportal than intraperitoneal transplantation. Although Barker *et al.* (1975) broached the possibility that the liver is an immunologically privileged site, the differences may just as well have been a reflection of the number of islets that initially survived transplantation to the respective sites, since transplantation to a vascularized bed is more efficient in the isologous situation (Pi-Sunyer *et al.*, 1979). This contention is supported by the observation of Slijepcevic *et al.* (1975) who showed that allogeneic islets embolized to the lung by intravenous injection also functioned longer than islets transplanted to the peritoneal cavity, and these results were comparable to those obtained by intraportal injection. The difference that transplant site can make is also apparent from studies of Naji *et al.* (1981a) on H-Y incompatibility. In their study Lewis male islets transplanted to unsensitized female recipients functioned > 100 days in 5 of 6 recipients of intraportal and in only 4 of 11 recipients of intraperitoneal islets (in sensitized hosts). One of seven intraportal male-to-female isografts functioned for the long term, similar to the outcome with skin grafts, but in contrast to the permanent functional survival of most male-to-female parathyroid isografts.

The functional survival of allogeneic islets transplanted across major histocompatibility barriers to the spleen or portal vein of diabetic rats has been compared. Reckard *et al.* (1978) found the mean functional survival time was 4.4 days after intrasplenic and 4.8 days after intraportal transplantation. Finch *et al.* (1977) reported rejection times of 5.4 and 4.8 days for intrasplenic versus intraportal islets, and immunosuppression with antilymphocyte serum equally prolonged grafts transplanted to either site. On the other hand, Janney *et al.* (1982b) found that fresh rat islet xenografts survived an average of only 5.1 days in the spleen, while the survival time was 8.7 days in the portal vein, and manipulations to prolong islet xenograft survival were more effective when the portal vein rather than the spleen was used for transplantation (Lacey *et al.*, 1982b). Allogeneic islets have also been transplanted to the spleen (Zammit *et al.*, 1979; Sutherland *et al.*, 1979a; Kretschmer *et al.*, 1979; Mirkovitch *et al.* 1979b) or portal vein (Kolb *et al.*, 1979) of totally pancreatectomized dogs. Comparative experiments by the same investigators have not been done, but in nonimmunosuppressed dogs, normoglycemia is not achieved or rejection occurs in a few days at either site (Mirkovitch *et al.*, 1979b; Kolb *et al.*, 1979). In immunosuppressed dogs rejection of intrasplenic islets has either been delayed (Zammit *et al.*, 1979; Kretschmer *et al.*, 1979) or prevented in one-third of the recipients (Sutherland *et al.*, 1979). The results of intrasplenic transplantation in the various models is interesting because the spleen is an immunological organ and rejection might be expected to occur earlier at this site than in the portal vein, which is not always the case.

The kidney capsule may be a better site than even the portal vein for transplantation of isolated adult islets in rodents. Reece-Smith *et al.* (1981a) found that Lewis rat islets transplanted to nonimmunosuppressed DA recipients functioned for a mean of 4.0 days after intraportal and for 8.4 days after renal subcapsular allotransplantation. The renal capsule has also proven to be a good site for xenotransplantation of rat islets to diabetic mice, with a mean survival time of fresh islets in immunosuppressed recipients of 11.2 days as opposed to 8.8 days for the portal vein and 5.1 days for the spleen (Bobzien *et al.*, 1983). On the other hand, the testicle might be even superior to the kidney as a transplant site, since Bobzien *et al.* (1983) found that 3 of 12 grafts function for > 60 days at this site (mean of > 30.8 days). This was one of the first convincing demonstrations that the testicle may be an immunologically semiprivileged site. Prolonged survival of islet allografts without immunosuppression has also been observed in the cleared mammary fat pad of mice (Outzen and Leiter, 1981).

The results of the experiments comparing the rejection time of islets and other organs have been variable when transplantation has been across a minor histocompatibility barrier (see review by Sutherland *et al.*, 1981a). Functional survival may be shorter for islets (Reckard *et al.*, 1973, 1979; Perloff *et al.*, 1980; Beyer *et al.*, 1981; Naji *et al.*, 1979a, 1981a). However, in at least three experiments intraportal (Ziegler *et al.*, 1974; Trimble *et al.*, 1979) or intraperitoneal (Frangipane *et al.*, 1977b) islet allografts were rejected less rapidly (Ziegler *et al.*, 1974; Frangipane, 1977b) or less frequently (Trimble, 1979) than skin allografts from the same donor strain in rats (Ziegler, 1974; Trimble, 1979) and mice (Frangipane, 1977b). On the other hand, Lewis male islets are rejected in some unsensitized and most sensitized female recipients while parathyroid grafts are not.

Experiments using minor H-Y histocompatibility barriers can provide useful clues to the mechanisms of the allogeneic response. Silvers *et al.* (1982), on the basis of the results of skin and parathyroid allograft experiments in such systems, have hypothesized that reduction of passenger leukocyte load has much less of an effect on survival time of grafts across a minor barrier. Also, minor histocompatibility or organ-specific alloantigens may be less likely to evoke a response in allografts depleted of passenger leukocytes if the transplants are to MHC-incompatible hosts. This is because if transplanted to MHC-compatible recipients, the hosts could provide antigen-processing cells (dendritic or macrophage cells) that could present the minor antigen to the recipients' immune system, activating the rejection process. Such a hypothesis is based on the concept of MHC restrictions in transplantation immunity.

When transplantation has been across a major barrier, islets always seem to be rejected earlier than skin (Reckard *et al.*, 1973, 1979; Nash *et al.*, 1977), heart (Rynasiewicz *et al.*, 1982; Perloff *et al.*, 1980; Nash *et al.*, 1977) or kidney allografts (Nash *et al.*, 1977) (Table 2). In addition, immunosuppressive regimens that prolong the survival of skin, kidney, or heart allografts have also been less affected in promoting the survival of islet allografts (Squifflet *et al.*, 1982b; Rynasiewicz, 1982; Reckard *et al.*, 1973, 1981; Nash *et al.*, 1977).

Islets transplanted as a free graft are also more susceptible to immune destruction than islets transplanted as part of an immediately vascularized intact pancreatic graft (Sutherland *et al.*, 1980b; Perloff *et al.*, 1980; Reckard *et al.*, 1980; Zammit *et al.*, 1979; Squifflet *et al.*, 1983b).

It is theoretically possible that the difference in the interval between allotransplantation and recurrence of hyperglycemia for islet versus pancreas grafts is

Table 1. Functional Survival (Mean Days) of Intraportal Islet Allografts Relative to Other Organ Allografts in Nonimmunosuppressed Rats

Donor: Recipient: Barrier:	AsxAg As Major	WF Lewis Major	BN Lewis Major	ACI Lewis Major	DA Lewis Major	DA ACI Minor	Fisher Lewis Minor	Lewis W=Lewis Minor	Lewis Fisher Minor	Fisher Lewis Minor	Fisher Lewis Minor
Tissue											
Islets[a]	3.2	4.3	3.5	3.6	3.3	22.0	2.1	> 77[b]	4.4	5.2	4.5
Pancreas[a]	—	9.5	7.6	6.8	8.3	—	—	—	16.5	12.1	9.8–11.1
Skin	8.2	—	—	—	—	11.4	13.2	11.5	—	—	—
Heart	7.9	—	7.5	6.5	—	—	—	—	> 40	—	—
Kidney	8.8	—	—	—	—	—	—	—	—	—	—
References	Nash et al. (1977)	Hardy et al. (1982)	Perloff et al. (1980)	Rynasiewicz et al. (1982)	Garvey et al. (1980)	Griffith et al. (1977)	Beyer et al. (1981)	Trimble et al. (1979)	Perloff et al. (1980)	Sutherland et al. (1980b)	Squifflet et al. (1983)

[a] Criteria for rejection different for each tissue except pancreas and islets.
[b] 4/12 recipients did not reject islets; the other 8 never became normoglycemic.

due to quantitative nonimmunological factors related to the final islet mass engrafted. Sutherland *et al*. (1980b) initially tried to compensate for this problem by transplanting the same islet mass in both types of grafts; while the insulin content of the islet and standard segmental pancreas grafts was equivalent in isologous controls, the final islet mass engrafted in the liver (according to tissue insulin content) was only 50–70% of the original islet mass transplanted, so the question was not satisfactorily answered. Squifflet *et al*. (1983b) compensated for this problem by transplanting microsegmental immediately vascularized pancreas grafts. In parallel syngeneic experiments, the final insulin content of the microsegmental grafts was less than that recovered in the liver 3 weeks after islet transplantation. However, in the recipients of allogeneic grafts prepared in fashions identical to the isologous grafts, the islet allografts were rejected, or hyperglycemia recurred, twice as rapidly for the islet allograft as for the microsegmental pancreas allograft recipients. These findings are consistent with the observations of Reckard *et al*. (1981) that pancreas but not islet allograft survival was prolonged following transplantation to adult recipients bearing immunologically enhanced heart or kidney allografts. Thus, it seems clear that free grafts of islets are more vulnerable to rejection than pancreas grafts.

The rapid rejection of unmodified, semipure allogeneic islets in nonimmunosuppressed hosts appears to be atypical when defined in terms of graft function. Histological studies of other organ allografts, however, have clearly shown that the rejection process is well underway before functional deterioration is grossly evident. It may be that in dissociated state islets are more vulnerable and functional deterioration occurs more rapidly. Histological studies after transplantation of adult islets to various sites have been performed by several investigators (Bowen *et al*., 1980; Prowse *et al*., 1982a; Andersson, 1982). Leonare *et al*. (1973, 1974) found degranulated beta cells surrounded by lymphocytes in peritoneal implants at the time recipients of neonatal islets became hyperglycemic. Kretschmer *et al*. (1979) observed progressive cellular infiltration and degeneration of adult allogeneic islet tissue in the spleen of totally pancreatectomized dogs. Andersson (1982) made similar observations in mice, provided the islets had been cultured. Franklin *et al*. (1979) and Slater *et al*. (1976) found that by 2 days intraportal islets were surrounded, and by 4 days infiltrated, by mononuclear cells. Beta cells were intact, but functional deterioration was evident by 4 days. By 7 days there was focal disintegration of islets and β cells were degranulated. By 2 weeks islets were hard to recognize, although there were focal collections of mononuclear cells. The findings were similar in the spleen (Franklin *et al*., 1979). Both organs remained morphologically normal (Slater *et al*., 1976; Franklin *et al*., 1979).

Outzen and Lieter (1981) have described the appearance of mouse islet allografts placed in the cleared mammary fat pad, which may be a semiprivilege site, because long-term function was demonstrated even without immunosuppression at 8 weeks. Many granulated beta cells were present in intact islets but in some a continuing rejection process was apparent as evidenced by variable degrees of mononuclear cell infiltration and fibrotic tissue interspersed between the islet cell and lymphoid elements. A very interesting histological study was performed by Marner *et al*. (in press) in which it was observed that isografted islets in either the A.TL or A.TH strains demonstrated increased proportions of glucagon-positive α cells, while in nonrejecting and successfully functioning allografted islets between these strains which differ only for the *I*, *Qa*, and *Tla* regions on MHC loci, few or no cells were present. H-2-encoded antigens may therefore influence islet cellular composition while leaving function relatively ineffective. However, a loss of alpha cells was not observed in similar experiments by Morrow *et al.* (1983).

Histological studies have been performed by Millard *et al.* (1983) on composite islet renal allograft in cyclosporine-A-treated rats. In long-term surviving allografts there was minimal evidence of rejection; the transplanted islet tissue was made up almost entirely of beta cells; only a few α cells and very rare δ and pancreatic polypeptid-positive cells were present.

The histological appearance of fetal islet allografts in diabetic (Hegre *et al.*, 1976b; Mullen and Shintaku, 1980; Garvey *et al.*, 1980a; Millard *et al.*, 1980) and nondiabetic (Simeonovic *et al.*, 1980) recipients has also been described. There is variability depending on the histocompatibility barrier, but cellular infiltration is seen as early as 3 days (Garvey *et al.*, 1980a) and beta cell deterioration and loss of insulin progresses rapidly (Mullen and Shintaku, 1980).

There is only one published study (Janney *et al.*, 1982a) in which an attempt has been made to characterize the lymphocytes that infiltrate histoincompatible islet grafts. This study was performed in the rat-to-mouse xenograft model of fresh or cultured megaislets to nonimmunosuppressed or animals immunosuppressed withALS (Lacy *et al.*, 1982a). They found that 90% of the cells were T lymphocytes, with a predominance of Ly-2 cells in the fresh islet allografts, but in the animals receiving cultured islets and ALS, the percentage of T lymphocytes and the Ly-2 population was decreased relative to Ly-1 cells. By day 70, even though there was no functional evidence of rejection, the proportion of Ly-2 cells had returned to the levels detected in the infiltrates of actively rejecting grafts in nonimmunosuppressed recipients. Janney *et al.* (1982a) speculated that the Ly-2 cells that appeared early in fresh allografts in nonimmunosuppressed animals were cytotoxic T cells, while those that appeared late in the animals that did not reject the grafts were suppressor cells. The experiments to test this hypothesis have not yet been reported.

In summary, no fundamental differences have been detected in the immune processes leading to rejection of islets and other tissue. Highly purified islets may, however, not be very immunogenic. On the other hand, islets are exquisitively sensitive to rejection effector mechanisms, at least if they differ for Class I histocompatibility antigens with the recipient (Morrow *et al.*, 1983). For example, protocols that enhance other organ allografts may actually curtail the survival of islet allografts (Perloff *et al.*, 1980; Reckard *et al.*, 1981). These results emphasize the problems that must be overcome for diabetes to be successfully treated by transplantation of free grafts of allogeneic islets.

Several approaches have been used in attempts to prevent rejection of islet allografts, some of which are remarkably effective. These include (1) immunosuppression by drugs or antilymphocyte preparations; (2) induction of specific tolerance or enhancement; (3) minimization of histocompatibility differences; (4) reduction of islet immunogenicity by tissue culture or islet or donor pretreatment with agents designated to eliminate passenger leukocytes or dendritic cells; and (5) use of immunoisolation devices or mechanical barriers to prevent contact of islets with host lymphocytes or antibodies.

2. Prevention of Rejection by Generalized Immunosuppression

A variety of drugs and immunosuppressive protocols has been tested in the various islet transplant models (see Table 2 for an update of experiments since review by Sutherland, 1981a). Experiments testing a single agent are instructive, but their failure to prolong islet allograft survival significantly does not necessarily mean they are ineffective, since combinations of drugs are usually used clinically.

The drugs currently used for clinical immunosuppression have had variable effects. Marquet and Heystack (1975) extended the funtional survival of islet allografts in two of five rats by administration of azathioprine, while P. R. F. Bell et al. (1980) and Morris et al. (1980) found azathioprine to be ineffective.

Rynasiewicz et al. (1982) and Squifflet et al. (1982b) found that azathioprine alone extended the median functional survival times of islet allografts transplanted across a minor histocompatibility barrier from 5.5 days without to 7 and 8 days, respectively, for azathioprine doses of 15 and 30 mg/kg per day. However, when azathioprine was combined with a low dosage of cyclosporine A there was a synergistic effect. In two of six animals receiving cyclosporine A 1.25 mg/kg per day plus azathioprine 15 mg/kg per day, islet allografts functioned > 100 days. When azathioprine 15 mg or 30 mg (1 kg per day) was combined with cyclosporine 2.5 mg/kg per day, the median islet allograft survival times were 71 and 49 days, but most of the animals died with functioning grafts.

Finch and Morris (1977a) prevented rejection indefinitely in two of six rats receiving greater than 1500 islets by daily administration of cyclophosphamide; only a minimal effect was observed in rats receiving 600–800 islets (Morris et al., 1980). Vialettes et al. (1978b) found that a single dose and P. R. F. Bell et al. (1980) that five doses of cyclophosphamide minimally prolonged (Vialettes et al., 1978b) or did not prolong (P. R. F. Bell et al., 1980) the survival of neonatal (Vialettes et al., 1978b) or adult rat islets (P. R. F. Bell et al., 1980) transplanted across weak (Vialettes et al., 1978b) or strong (P. R. F. Bell et al., 1980) histocompatibility barriers.

Corticosteroids are the backbone of most clinical immunosuppressive regimens, but are potentially diabetogenic. Steffes et al. (1974) found that low-dose prednisone did not have an adverse effect on the function of islet isografts in rats, but Nelken et al. (1977), P. R. F. Bell et al. (1980), Morris et al. (1980), and Rynasiewicz et al. (1982) could not prevent, and Schulak et al. (1977) could not reverse, islet allograft rejection in rats with steroids alone (Nelkens, 1978; Schulak et al., 1977; Morris et al., 1980) or in combination with azathioprine (P. R. F. Bell et al., 1980) or cyclosporin A (Rynasiewicz et al., 1982). Furthermore, Kretschmer et al. (1979) found that pancreatectomized dogs treated with azathioprine and prednisone after islet autotransplantation took longer to achieve normoglycemia and had lower k values than nonimmunosuppressed recipients. Nevertheless, one-third of canine allograft recipients treated by this regimen became normoglycemic; in the others it was difficult to distinguish the contribution of rejection or the diabetogenic action of prednisone to

graft failure (Sutherland *et al.*, 1977). Zammit *et al.* (1979) reported a slight prolongation of intrasplenic islet allograft survival in dogs treated with azathioprine and
prednisone, but Kolb *et al.* (1979) observed almost no effect with a similar regimen
after intraportal islet transplantation in dogs.

Antilymphocyte serum (ALS), or one of its derivatives, has been the most effective agent in delaying rejection of islet allografts. If islets are transplanted across a
minor histocompatibility barrier in rats (Reckard *et al.*, 1973; Nelkens *et al.*, 1977;
Griffith *et al.*, 1977; Lacy *et al.*, 1979a; Beyer and Friedman, 1979) or mice (Frangipane *et al.*, 1977a), only a few doses of ALS can prolong their survival. Lacy *et al.*
(1979a) found that even a single dose of ALS greatly prolonged the survival of
handpicked Fischer islets in Lewis rats, although their criterion for rejection (glycosuria at -1 SD below pretransplant level) was less stringent than the criterion used by
other investigators: recurrence of hyperglycemia. Gray *et al.* (1974) prevented rejection for more than 1 year in Lewis recipients of Fischer islets by chronic administration
of ALS. Beyer *et al.* (1981) were able to prolong the functional survival of islets indefinitely in some rats of this strain combination by administration of ALS whenever
plasma glucose elevated to greater than 200 mg/dl. Indeed, in their experiments ALS
was more effective in preventing rejection of islet than skin allografts.

In earlier experiments when only small numbers of islets were transplanted, a beneficial effect of ALS could not be demonstrated (Reckard *et al.*, 1973) in rats or was
minimal (Panijayanond and Monaco, 1974) in mice with intraperitoneal transplantation
of strongly histocompatible islets. In more recent experiments, ALS has uniformly prolonged the survival of intraportal islet allografts transplanted across a major
histocompatibility barrier in rats (Marquet and Heystek, 1975; Lacy *et al.*, 1979a,b,c;
Beyer, 1979; Finch and Morris, 1977b; Morris *et al.*, 1980; Reemtsma *et al.*, 1981;
Schulak *et al.*, 1980; Hardy *et al.*, 1982), indefinitely if they are transplanted as a
kidney–islet composite allograft in the strains used by Reece-Smith *et al.* (1983).

The effect of ALS has been enhanced by combining the treatment with other modalities. Lacy *et al.* (1979a) found that pretreating donors of handpicked rat islets with
irradiation and silica (to reduce passenger leukocytes) more than doubled the graft survival time seen with ALS alone after transplantation across a major histocompatibility
barrier. Islets cultured at 24°C for 1 week were not rejected in ALS-treated animals
(Lacy *et al.*, 1979c). Reemtsma *et al.* (1981) nearly doubled the graft survival time
over that seen with ALG alone by adding selective lymphatic irradiation with intravenous   palladium-109–hematoporphyrin to recipients of strongly histocompatible rat islets. Hardy *et al.* (1982) modified this protocol to achieve 80% long-term allograft
survival (> 60 days) in recipient rats. Schulak *et al.* (1980) found donor pretreatment
with irradiation of a synergistic effect with recipient ALS treatment, each modality
alone resulting in mean allograft survival times of 7.0 and 18.2 days and, when used
together, of 45.6 days.

In other experiments ALS was part of a protocol intended to induce donor-specific
immunological responsiveness, although none of the investigators showed that this was
actually the case. Panijayanond *et al.* (1974) extended the survival of islet allografts in
mice to 9 weeks by combining ALS with administration of donor strain bone marrow.
Nelken *et al.* (1977) prolonged the survival of allogeneic rat islets transplanted across a

major barrier more than threefold over that seen with ALS alone by injection of *B. pertussis* culture fluid and donor strain liver extract. Vialettes *et al.* (1978b) found that an antilymphocyte globulin regimen ineffective by itself was able to prolong the survival of neonatal rat islets transplanted across a weak histocompatibility barrier when combined with administration of donor-specific soluble antigen. On the other hand, Finch and Morris (1977b) were not able to show a synergistic effect of ALS and enhancing antiserum in diabetic rat islet allograft recipients. Mullen (1980) found that a combination of donor antigen, procarbazine, and ALS increased by more than four times the survival of fetal pancreatic islet allografts transplanted across a major histocompatibility barrier, which resulted in indefinite survival of fetal grafts transplanted across a minor barrier (Mullen and Shintaju, 1982b). Finally, Selawry *et al.* (1981) in rats (major histocompatibility barrier) and Jolley *et al.* (1982) in outbred rabbits combined pretransplant transfusions of the recipients of donor strain blood with posttransplant ALS administration and found that the combined therapy was associated with long-term amelioration of diabetes in more than half of the islet allograft recipients.

Administration of ALS has also been combined with prednisone (Scharp *et al.*, 1975) or azathioprine (Scharp *et al.*, 1975; Lorenz *et al.*, 1976c) in large-animal islet allograft models in attempt to mimic clinical protocols. Scharp *et al.* (1975) improved the diabetic status of monkeys after islet transplantation, but the experiments were short-term. Lorenz *et al.* (1979b,c) found that the duration of normoglycemia was extended from 4 months in nonimmunosuppressed recipients to greater than 1 year in dogs treated with ALG and azathioprine after transplantation of islets from closely matched donors. Although the results of the experiments with ALS are encouraging for clinical application, other drugs will be needed for long-term maintenance.

Fractionated total lymphoid irradiation (TLI) protocols, modified after those devised by Slavin *et al.* (1977) for use in other experimental systems, have also been tested in rat allograft models. Rynasiewicz *et al.* (1980, 1982) found that a short course of pretransplant TLI alone (200 rad for five doses) in rats tripled the survival time of islets transplanted across a weak histocompatibility barrier. Mendez-Picon and McGeorge (1983) obtained similar results; pretransplant administration of 200 rad per day to diabetic rats (800–1200 rad total) resulted in mean islet allograft survival times of 15–22 days, as compared to graft survival times of only 5 days with no treatment. They also found that donor-specific blood transfusions abrogated the effect of TLI. Britt *et al.* (1982) used high-dose (200 rad × 17 doses) TLI to rats prior to the induction of diabetes and islet allotransplantation. Three rats who also received donor strain bone marrow after completion of TLI (a protocol found to induce tolerance by Slavin *et al.*, 1977) experienced permanent amelioration of diabetes after transplantation of donor strain islets with no further immunosuppression. Only one of three rats treated with TLI alone experienced permanent amelioration of diabetes following islet allotransplantation. Mullen and Shintaku (1982a) administered various doses of fractionated (200 rad/ fraction) TLI (1000–3000 total rad) and varying doses of bone marrow ranging from 1 to 3×10^8 cells to recipients before fetal pancreas islet allotransplantation to the renal subcapsule across both major and minor histocompatible barriers to rats made diabetic before administration of TLI. The mortality from TLI was 9%. TLI alone (2400 rad) was used only in the minor barrier (F344 to Lewis) and prolonged the islet allograft survival from >10 day in untreated to between 28 and 41 days in treated recipients. In this donor–recipient strain combination a TLI dose of 100 rad combined with administration of 10^8 donor strain bone marrow cells was sufficient to induce chimerism and permanent acceptance (>70 days) of fetal pancreas allografts. However in the major histocompatibility barrier 3000 rad and 3×10^8 bone marrow cells were required for chimerism and permanent graft acceptance to be achieved (Mullen et al., 1983). Nakajima et al. (1982), in a hamster-to-diabetic-rat portal vein islet xenograft model, administered fractionated (200 rad) TLI during the week before transplantation in total doses ranging from 400 to 1600 rad. The high dose was associated with death of the animal within 1 week of transplantation, but in the other groups mean graft survival times were 3.1, 9.7, and 30.3 days in recipients treated with 400, 800, and 1200 rad TLI, respectively. TLI by itself can prolong graft survival, but not indefinitely, and thus it ultimately must be employed in combination with pharmacological immunosuppression (Rynasiewicz et al., 1982), or with donor bone marrow administration in attempts to induce specific immunological tolerance. The morbidity of TLI administration in diabetic animals makes it difficult to administer the dosage required to induce tolerance by bone marrow administration. However, low-dose TLI is effective and should probably be tested with other agents in the islet allograft model since such combinations in therapy has been found to be highly effective in the heart allograft model (Rynasiewicz et al., 1982).

Chemical immunosuppression has the greatest potential for clinical application as generalized immunosuppressive treatment. However, except for cyclosporine, new agents have not been very effective, at least in the dosages given and the models used. Lum et al. (1979, 1980) found that erythro-9-(2-hydroxy-3-nonyl) adenosine, an adenosine deaminase inhibitor, could prolong the survival of neonatal mouse (but not neonatal rat) islet allografts across a weak histocompatibility barrier. In rats another inhibitor, 2-deoxycoformycin, had a slight effect when combined with adeninine arabinoside (Lum et al., 1980). These agents may not have received a fair test, since fresh neonatal islet tissue is difficult to use in an allograft model because of the latent period between transplantation and amelioration of diabetes. These agents should probably be investigated in an adult islet allograft model. Nash and Bell (1979) evaluated two macrophage-suppressing agents. They found that silica, but not carageenan, prolonged the survival of allogeneic rat islets in nearly half of the recipients. This treatment was more effective than other chemical immunosuppressants (P. R. F. Bell et al., 1980).

The drug with the greatest potential for clinical application, cyclosporine A, has been tested in both rat and dog islet allograft models. Garvey et al. (1980b) found that high doses of orally administered cyclosporine (40 mg/kg per day × 14 days) were needed to prolong the survival of a small proportion of intrasplenic adult rat islets or renal subcapsular fetal pancreases transplanted across a major histocompatibility barrier (DA to Lewis). The animals either died of infection with functioning grafts or rejected after the drug was stopped (Morris et al., 1980). P. R. F. Bell et al. (1980) reported that intraportal rat islet allografts were rejected subsequent to, but not during, a 7-day course of oral cyclosporine A (20 mg/kg per day). Rynasiewicz et al. (1980)

found continuous oral administration of cyclosporine A (10–20 mg/kg per day) very effective at preventing the rejection of intraportal rat islet allografts transplanted across a weak histocompatibility barrier (Fisher to Lewis), but infections occurred at high dosages. Vialettes *et al.* (1979b) increased the survival of rat islet allografts transplanted intraportally across a strong histocompatibility barrier (Wistar to Lewis) by administration of oral cyclosporine A (50 mg/kg) for 2 weeks. Reece-Smith *et al.* (1981b) used the kidney capsule for transplantation of adult isolated islets across a major histocompatibility barrier (DA to Lewis) in rats given a 14-day course of oral cyclosporine A and observed no effect on islet allograft survival in doses of 5 and 10 mg/kg per day. However, four of six animals in the 20 ml/kg per day group and eight of eight in the 40 mg/kg per day maintained functioning grafts during the period of cyclosporine administration with median survival times of 18.5 to 24.5 days, respectively; however, three animals in the high-dose group died with functioning grafts.

The experiments of Reece *et al.* (1981b) were performed in a donor–recipient strain combination in which a short course of cyclosporine A results in indefinite survival of renal or other immediately vascularized allografts (Homan *et al.*, 1980; Reece-Smith *et al.*, 1981c; Fabri, 1982) a phenomenon not seen in other donor–recipient strain combinations (Rynasiewicz *et al.*, 1982). Accordingly, Reece-Smith *et al.* (1981c) transplanted kidney islet composite allografts (in which islets had been placed under the kidney capsule of the renal donor 2 weeks previously) to diabetic recipients, and found that cyclosporine A 5 mg/kg per day for 14 days (a regimen that is effective in promoting indefinitely survival of renal allografts but that usually does not prevent rejection of islet allografts alone) was followed by indefinite amelioration of diabetes. In subsequent experiments Reece-Smith *et al.* (1981a) determined that 48 hr of residence of islets under the kidney capsule of the intermediate renal donor was sufficient time for the islets to become vascularized and to be transplanted as a composite graft without rejection in cyclosporine A-treated recipients. It was essential that the intermediate host be diabetic from streptozoticin administration and not be a normal or a pancreatectomized diabetic intermediate host if only 5 mg/kg for 14 days was given to the ultimate recipient of renal islet composite allografts. The intermediate host could be a nondiabetic normal animal if 10 mg/kg were given to the ultimate recipient (Reece-Smith *et al.*, 1983). Islets transplanted at the time of a renal allograft were rejected even though the animals were given 5 mg/kg per day of cyclosporine A (Reece-Smith *et al.*, 1982a). In addition, DA recipients bearing long-term Lewis kidneys in lieu of a 14-day course of cyclosporine A at the time of transplantation made diabetic would accept Lewis islets, transplanted either intraportally (Gray *et al.*, 1983) or under the renal capsule (Reece-Smith *et al.*, 1982a), indefinitely without any additional immunosuppression.

The results obtained with cyclosporine A and islet transplantation in the model used by this group (Morris and associates at Oxford) are extremely interesting, but its applicability to other strain combinations has not been tested. Rynasiewicz *et al.* (1982) found that identical cyclosporine A protocols in the ACI-to-Lewis combination would not prevent rejection of immediately vascularized organ allografts. Accordingly, the latter group has focused on continuous administration of cyclosporine as a method of prevention rejection on islet allograft recipients. They found that the therapeutic ratio was narrow (Rynasiewicz *et al.*, 1982). Cyclosporine A 2.5 mg/kg per day nearly doubled islet allograft survival time when transplanted across a minor histocompatibility barrier (Fisher to Lewis). The 5 mg/kg per day prevented rejection indefinitely, but most of the recipients died after 7 weeks with functioning grafts (Rynasiewicz *et al.*, 1982). However, if cyclosporine A (1.25–2.5 mg/kg per day) was administered in combination with azathioprine (15–30 mg/kg per day), the low-dose combination was synergistic and resulted in indefinite survival (> 100 days) of 40% of the grafts. None were rejected in high-dose combinations, although again the rats died between 7 and 11 weeks after transplantation (Squifflet *et al.*, 1982b). In contrast, low-dose cyclosporine A and azathioprine could prevent the rejection of heart allografts indefinitely (Squifflet *et al.*, 1983a).

There is only one report of cyclosporine A being used for islet transplantation in a large animal model. DuToit *et al.* (1982b) administered cyclosporine A orally 25 mg/kg × 14 days to pancreatectomized diabetic dogs receiving dispersed pancreatic islet tissue prepared from one donor by a technique of Mirkovitch *et al.* (1976) into the spleen. The results are difficult to interpret because no animals became normoglycemic. The mean recipient survival time was extended from 13.0 days in nonimmunosuppressed animals to 28.1 days in cyclosporine-A-treated animals. Since DuToit *et al.* (1982c) subsequently showed that it is necessary to administer 40 mg/kg per day of cyclosporine A indefinitely to prevent rejection of pancreas allografts rejection in pancreatectomized recipients, the dosage and duration of treatment in the islet allograft recipients were probably inadequate to prevent ultimate rejection.

In summary, generalized immunosuppression has prolonged islet allograft survival or prevented rejection in some, but not all, animal models. In many of the experiments where an effect was not seen it is difficult to draw conclusions for a variety of reasons. In some experiments immunosuppression was aborted early. In others, only a small number of islets were transplanted, indeed normoglycemia was not achieved before rejection occurred in control animals and an effect of immunosuppression might have been seen if a larger number of islets had been transplanted. It is apparent that most generalized immunosuppression protocols are not as effective for preventing rejection of islets as for other types of allografts, and thus approaches in which specific allogeneic unresponsiveness to the donor or transplanted tissue might be induced are of supreme importance (Faustman *et al.*, 1982b).

3. Prevention of Rejection by Induction of Tolerance or Enhancement

Islet allografts will survive indefinitely in inbred rodents if immunological tolerance to the donor strain is induced by the classic technique of bone marrow injection in the neonatal period (Perloff *et al.*, 1980; Naji *et al.*, 1976, 1981a, 1982; Frangipane, 1977a). Lymph node cells are not effective (as they are not for skin) unless cardiac allografts (for which lymph node cells do induce split tolerance) are placed prior to and left in place at least initially after islet transplantation (Perloff *et al.*, 1983). Induction of specific immunological unresponsiveness is more difficult in adult animals and, at least for islet allografts, has never been achieved in large animal models.

In rodents a variety of manipulations can result in permanent acceptance of tissue allografts without, or with only a limited and temporary administration of, immunosuppressive agents and in which the unresponsiveness engendered is donor-specific with maintenance, or eventually recovery, of otherwise full immunocompetence (Fabri, 1982). Some of the manipulations are generally applicable while others may be effective only in certain donor–recipient strain combinations. An example of the latter might be the finding that spleen allografts from Wag rats are not rejected by Agus recipients and that such spleen transplants also permit the acceptance of Wag pancreas (Bitter-Suermann et al., 1979; Shah et al., 1980) or islet (Smith et al., 1983) allografts that would otherwise be rejected by at least 40% of Agus recipients. This phenomenon is associated with failure of the long-term islet allograft recipients to generate cytotoxic T cells in vitro to donor targets (Smith et al., 1983). On the other hand, Squifflet et al. (1982) found that donor spleen allografts did not prevent the rejection of Fisher pancreas allografts in human recipients. We have found (unpublished data) that combined spleen and pancreas allografts were rejected at the same time as pancreas allografts alone in dogs, so the immunosuppressive umbrage induced by Wag spleen allografts in Agus rats is probably a strain-restricted phenomena.

In only one report was possible tolerance to islet allografts from adult animals induced by active immunization of donor strain antigens without the use of concomitant immunosuppression, and without treatment of the islets by measures designed to reduce their immunogenicity. Faustman et al. (1982c) found that if B6(H-2^b) mice were injected with B10.BR(H-2^k) red blood cells (which do not express H-2 I-region-encoded Class II antigens) that had been treated with anti-Ia^k antiserum (to eliminate Ia $\pm$ contaminating leukocytes from the red blood cell preparation), 80% had B10.BR islets, transplanted 2–3 weeks later, survive indefinitely ($>$ 100 days). Only 20% of B10.BR islet allografts survived permanently in nontreated B6 and no islet mice allograft functioned for $>$ 2 weeks in B6 mice previously injected with B10.BR red blood cells not treated with anti-Ia^k antiserum. In previous experiments Faustman et al. (1981) had shown that fresh B10.BR islets treated with anti-Ia^k antiserum were not rejected in nonimmunosuppressed mice (which they attributed to reduction of islet immunogenicity by elimination of Ia $+$ passenger leukocytes necessary to induce an alloimmune response to the recipient). Faustman et al. (1982a) obtained some evidence that the long-term maintenance of the islets was associated with suppressor alloactivity, since administration of anti-I-J^b antiserum (putatively directed against suppressor cells) lowered the threshold for the number of donor strain spleen cells required to induce rejection of long-term islet allografts. Since the animals in the earlier experiment (Faustman et al., 1981) could mount an immune response to the donor strain, they were not fully tolerant, although they would tolerate nonimmunogenic islets unless an allogeneic response was induced by injection of immunogenic donor strain cells (Faustman et al., 1982b). This group has not reported whether islet allograft rejection can be induced in animals injected with anti-Ia-serum-treated donor strain red blood cells. This protocol allows islet allografts (at least in this particular donor–recipient strain combination) to be transplanted without any measure to alter graft immunogenicity and without the need for even limited duration of generalized immunosuppression of the recipient.

The combination of reduction of islet immunogenicity by tissue culture followed by administration of ultraviolet (UV)-irradiated donor spleen cells is also able to induce specific immunological unresponsiveness (Prowse et al., 1982a). In previous experiments, this group had demonstrated that approximately half of CBA mice carrying long-term Balb/C islet allografts rendered nonimmunogenic by prior tissue culture would reject the islet allografts if injected with donor spleen cells (Bowen et al., 1981). However, if the donor spleen cells system were first subjected to UV irradiation, rejection would not occur and subsequent injections of living spleen cells could also not induce rejection (Prowse et al., 1982a). This experiment, as well as the one of Faustman et al. (1982b), suggests that a form of tolerance can be induced in adult mice by certain manipulations which alter the way in which alloantigen is presented to the recipient, allowing long-term survival of islet allografts without the need for immunosuppression. There are no reports of such protocols being tested yet in other rodent or large animal models.

Passive and active immunological enhancement protocols effective in prolonging the survival of heart or kidney allografts have had variable effect on islet allografts (Sutherland, 1981b; Morris et al., 1980). Finch and Morris (1976, 1977a,b) found that the survival of DA adult islets in Lewis rats was increased from 2–5 days in untreated rats to 5–11 days in rats treated with anti-DA serum; in Lewis recipients of semiallogeneic (DA × Lewis) islets, normoglycemia was maintained for 12–16 days in three of five rats and for > 360 days in two rats. Garvey et al. (1980c) saw no prolongation of (DA × Lewis) fetal allografts in Lewis recipients treated with anti-DA serum with or without donor pretreatment with cyclophosphamide. Anti-Lewis serum of DA recipients of semiallogenic fetal pancreas was also ineffective (Morris et al., 1980). The same treatment protocols also had a minimal effect except in an occasional Lewis or DA recipient of adult (Lewis × DA) islets (Garvey et al., 1980c; Morris et al., 1980). Enhancing sera prolonged the survival of islet allografts to > 100 days in 4 of 10 rats in one experiment (Nash et al., 1977) and in 1 of 5 in another (Nash et al., 1978). Islet allograft survival was not prolonged after transplantation to rats bearing enhanced heart grafts (Nash et al., 1978). Active enhancement has been no more effective. Perloff et al. (1980) found that administration of donor-specific antigen and alloantiserum actually curtailed the survival of allogeneic islets, particularly if monoclonal antibody was used. The latter was also ineffective in prolonging the survival of heart allografts, unlike the crude antiserum (Perloff et al., 1981b). Reckard et al. (1981) found that the survival of allogeneic islets was only slightly prolonged in recipients bearing enhanced hearts from the same donor strain. The difficulties with enhancement protocols are not surprising, given the sensitivity of islets to destruction by some alloantiserum preparations (Naji et al., 1979a).

A variety of islet allograft experiments have been performed in which donor-specific tissue or antigens were injected into islet allograft recipients temporarily treated with generalized immunosuppressive agents. Allograft survival was prolonged over that achieved with generalized immunosuppression alone. The results of some of these experiments, particularly those in which antilymphocyte preparations were administered, and in which the islets had prolonged function but were ultimately rejected were described in the previous section (Nelken *et al.*, 1977; Vialettes *et al.*, 1978b; Panijayanond *et al.*, 1974; Finch and Morris, 1977b; Mullen, 1980). In other experiments, the islets survived indefinitely, but the animals were not tolerant in the classic sense, as shown by Selawry *et al.* (1981) in rats treated with donor strain blood and a limited course of ALS. These animals remained normoglycemic after islet allotransplantation even when subsequent donor strain skin grafts were rejected.

The most promising protocol for antigen pretreatment in association with limited immunosuppression is that adapted by Mullen (1981). Donor strain liver extract was injected at 3 weeks before the procarbazine at 1 day before and 1 day after and ALS at 1 and 4 days after transplantation of F344 fetal pancreas allograft to under the kidney capsule of diabetic Lewis recipients. Each treatment alone was associated with rejection within 14 days, while with the combined treatment the islet graft functioned indefinitely. Subsequent skin grafts exhibited a delayed rejection, and spleen cells from rats bearing long-term islet allografts adoptively transferred to otherwise untreated F334 rats were associated with prolongation of skin allograft survival (Mullen and Shintaku, 1982). The treatment was not effective for preventing rejection of F344 rats in Lewis recipients (Mullen, 1981), but prevented rejection for more than 1 year in 13 of 16 F334 recipients (Mullen and Shintaku, 1982). The fact that skin grafts were ultimately rejected suggests that skin expressed alloantigens not expressed in the islets. However, fetal pancreas grafts functioning for the long term in primary recipients retained their immunogenicity and susceptibility to rejection as evidenced by retransplant experiments and subsequent rejection in nonimmunosuppressed secondary F334 hosts (Mullen and Shintaku, 1982).

Zitron *et al.* (1981a) also obtained evidence of active suppression in the maintenance of rat pancreas and islet allografts rendered relatively nonimmunogenic by culture at 24°C for 1 week prior to transplantation to ALS-treated recipients. Rejection of the islet allografts could be induced by injection of donor strain lymphocytes, but subsequent noncultured islet allografts from the original donor strain were accepted even when third-party islets were not. Spleen cells from such recipients specifically inhibited the MLC response of normal animals of the recipient to the donor strain.

A temporary course (14 days) of cyclosporine A is able to prevent rejection of rat heart or kidney allografts indefinitely in some (Reece-Smith *et al.*, 1981a), but not in other (Rynasiewicz *et al.*, 1982) donor–recipient strain combinations. In the strain combination where this phenomenon does occur (Lewis to DA), Reece-Smith *et al.* (1982a) found that rats with long-term (>100 days) surviving renal allografts, in lieu of previous treatment of cyclosporine for 14 days of subsequently induced diabetes, could be permanently ameliorated by transplantation of islets from the donor strain to under the transplanted kidney capsule without the need for resumption of immunosuppression. The same results were obtained by intraportal transplantation to similarly conditioned rats, showing that the site of transplantation in this model was not important (Gray *et al.*, 1983). Lewis islets transplanted simultaneously with Lewis renal allografts to four DA rats treated with a temporary course of cyclosporine A were rejected (Reece-Smith *et al.*, 1981b,d, 1982a). Experiments to determine the minimal interval necessary for conditioning renal allograft recipients by a temporary course of cyclosporine A to permit acceptance of islet allografts without additional immunosuppression have not yet been reported. Reece-Smith *et al.* (1981b) have previously shown that allogeneic islets transplanted as a composite renal islet allograft to a secondary host were not rejected in recipients receiving a temporary course of cyclosporine A if the islets were in residence under the kidney capsule of the donor for at least 48 hr in the primary host (Reece-Smith *et al.*, 1981d). Experiments to elucidate the mechanisms by which a temporary course of cyclosporine A induces specific unresponsiveness in some donor–recipient rat strain combinations have not yet been reported, but the protocols employed are generally not effective in preventing rejection in large animals (Fabri, 1982) or even in rodents (Rynasiewicz *et al.*, 1982).

The only other immunosuppressive treatment that has been used in conjunction with administration of donor alloantigens is irradiation of the recipient, either whole-body, total lymphoid, or selective lymphoid. Kramp *et al.* (1975) made mice allogeneic radiation chimeras by injecting bone marrow after otherwise sublethal total body irradiation. In mice that did not die from graft-versus-host disease, diabetes induced by streptozotocin was ameliorated for at least 16 weeks in 7 of 13 recipients of allogeneic islets derived from the original bone marrow donor strain.

Total lymphoid irradiation followed by bone marrow administration can induce donor-specific unresponsiveness without the occurrence of graft-versus-host-disease in some donor–recipient rat or mice strain combinations (Slavin *et al.*, 1977, 1979). Graft-versus-host disease has occurred in other models and donor–recipient strain combinations following TLI and allogeneic bone marrow administration (Rynasiewicz *et al.*, 1981). Thus Rynasiewicz *et al.* (1980b) used TLI only for its generalized immunosuppressive effect in islet allograft recipients. Recently, however, two groups have been able to achieve permanent acceptance of isolated adult islet (Britt *et al.*, 1982) or fetal pancreas (Mullen and Shibukawa, 1982; Mullen *et al.*, 1983) allografts in rats made chimeric with fractionated TLI and donor bone marrow administration without the occurrence of graft-versus-host disease.

Britt *et al.* (1982) treated nondiabetic Lewis rats with 17 fractions of 200 rad each prior to administration of Wistar–Furth bone marrow. Diabetes was then induced, using half of the usual dosage of streptozoticin because of the extreme sensitivity of TLI-animals to any insult. The three animals that survived this protocol received Wistar-Furth islets intraportally and two were permanently ameliorated of diabetes without any further immunosuppression. Two of three animals who received TLI without bone marrow administration rejected the islets within 2 weeks.

Mullen and Shibukawa (1982) made Lewis rats diabetic prior to administration of TLI in fractionated doses of 200 rad each. They found that a low total dosage (1000 rad) and a low dosage of donor bone marrow (1×10^8 cells) were associated with indefinite survival of F344 fetal pancreas allografts transplanted across a minor barrier to under the kidney capsule. At least 2600 rad were required to achieve this effect with transplantation of semiallogeneic (Buffalo × Lewis) and 3000 rads with extended fields to include the pelvis and a higher dosage of bone marrow (3×10^8 cells) with fully allogeneic (Buffalo) fetal pancreas allografts transplanted across a major histocompatibility barrier. There was a relatively high morbidity (weight loss) and mortality associated with high-dose TLI and bone marrow administration, but the animals who survived the treatment and who achieved greater than 50% chimerism accepted fetal pancreas allografts permanently without any further immunosuppression (Mullen *et al.*, 1983).

The technique of selective lymphoid irradiation (SLI) with pallidum-109–hematoporphyrin combined with ALG administration (Reemstma *et al.*, 1981) can result in permanent (>100 days) acceptance of Wistar–Furth (WF) islet allografts in Lewis recipients even without administration of donor antigen in another form (5 of 10 animals). Subsequent WF allogeneic hearts were also not rejected in such animals while third-party hearts were (Hardy *et al.*, 1982).

Many of the experiments described in this section were performed under highly artificial conditions, and the animals were not even diabetic before an attempt was made to induce a tolerant state. Thus, the specific protocols may not be relevant to islet transplantation in diabetic humans. Nevertheless, specific immunological unresponsiveness is the most important concept in transplantation, and future efforts may lead to practical approaches for clinical application.

4. Prevention of Rejection by Alteration of Graft Immunogenicity

Passenger leukocytes or dendritic cells are thought to play a major role in sensitizing a host to an allograft (Lafferty, 1980; Steinmen, 1981). Their elimination, either by pretreatment of the donor before procurement of the graft *ex vivo* with agents that selectively damage or eliminate such cells, or by *in vitro* maintenance of the tissue in culture before transplantation, has been associated with prolonged survival of a variety of organ allografts (Lafferty *et al.*, 1983).

a. Effects of Pretransplant Culture on Islet Immunogenicity.   The initial attempts to apply tissue culture techniques to reduce immunogenicity and prevent or delay rejection of islet allografts gave variable results. Hegre *et al.* (1976a,b) found that fetal rat pancreatic tissue cultured in 95% oxygen for 10 days was rejected < 15 days after allotransplantation, although more recently this group found that neonatal rat islets isolated by an 8–17-day culture technique (Hegre *et al.*, submitted) functioned for 4–17 weeks as xenografts under the kidney capsule in nonimmunosuppressed diabetic mice (Serie *et al.*, 1983). Mandel and Higginbothum (1979) found that fetal mouse and Garvey *et al.* (1979b) that fetal rat pancreases cultured for 21 days in an ambient environment were rejected within 2 weeks after allotransplantation, only a very slight prolongation (Mandel *et al.*, 1980). More recently Mandel *et al.* (1982a), in histological studies only, reported that in 50–60% of cases fetal CBA islets cultured for 21–28 days in 90% O_2 and transplanted to Balb/C recipients were still essentially intact in spite of focal or periislet mononuclear cell infiltrates. Monkey islets cultured for 7–9 days by Jonasson *et al.* (1977) and adult mouse islets in Medium 199 cultured for 10 days by Andersson and Buschard (1977) were also rejected after allotransplantation. Recently Andersson (1982) has used RPMI 1640 to culture mouse islets for 4 weeks, and three of seven nonimmunosuppressed recipients of intrasplenic cultured islets transplants across a major histocompatibility barrier maintained normoglycemia for 3–17 weeks.

Simeonovic *et al.* (1980) found that 17 days of culture in 95% oxygen reduced the immunogenicity of Balb/C fetal mouse pancreas, while 10 days of culture did not; on the other hand, 7 days of culture were sufficient to prevent histological rejection of adult islets transplanted to nondiabetic histoincompatible CBA mice, unless donor strain peritoneal exudate cells were given to the recipient concomitantly with the islets. Since intact fetal pancreases associated with a large amount of lymphoid tissue that disappears only after a relatively long culture period (Prowse *et al.*, 1982a) and since fetal islet survival declines at > 17 days of culture, prejudicing the function even of isografts (Simeonovic and Lafferty, 1981), this group has more recently examined the immunogenicity of fetal mouse proislets isolated by 4 days of culture of collagenase-dispersed fetal tissue (Simeonovic and Lafferty, 1983). They found that after transplantation to nondiabetic allogeneic recipients histological evidence of rejection is seen in half of the recipients at 4 weeks (Prowse *et al.*, 1982a). For the same reason, this group has focused on culture of isolated adult islets as a method for reducing the immunogenicity of allogeneic islets before transplantation to diabetic recipients (Prowse *et al.*, 1982a), using a technique in which 50 islets are aggregated into a cluster and maintained in a 95% O_2–5% CO_2 atmosphere for 7 days (Bowen *et al.*, 1979). In their initial experiments, 300 Balb/C $(H-2^d)$ islets (6 clusters of 50) transplanted under the kidney capsule after a 7-day culture partially reversed the diabetes of two CBA $(H-2^k)$ mice with no evidence of rejection for > 100 days (Bowen and Lafferty, 1980). Recently, complete amelioration of the diabetic state has been demonstrated in eight of the eight CBA mice for > 100 days by transplantation of 350 Balb/C islets (seven clusters) cultured for 7 days (Prowse *et al.*, 1982a). In histological studies, 7-day cultured islet cultures remained histologically intact 28 days after transplantation to various allogeneic strains in 55–100% of the recipients, depending on the histocompatibility differences (Prowse *et al.*, 1982a).

Lacy *et al.* (1982a) adopted the technique of rat islet aggregation by 7-day culture in 95% oxygen for xenotransplantation to diabetic mice. The mean functional survival of 14–15 megaislets transplanted via the portal vein was only slightly prolonged (16.9 days vs. 7.4 days in recipients of fresh islets) and those transplanted via the spleen not at all (7.0 days), but those transplanted under the kidney capsule functioned for > 70 days in 4 of 11 recipient mice (mean of 52.1 days in all mice of this group, as opposed to 14.4 days for recipients of fresh islets). A single injection of antimouse and rat lymphocyte serum did not further improve the long-term or mean survival rates of xenogenetic megaislets transplanted under the kidney capsule, in contrast to the results of previous experiments with transplantation of isolated cultured islet allografts in rats where immunosuppression was required to show an effect of culture on reduction of islet immunogenicity (Lacy *et al.*, 1979c, 1980b).

In functional studies by another group, Kedinger *et al.* (1977) partially ameliorated diabetes in 11 of 13 recipients by direct injection into the liver of adult allogeneic islets cultured in an ambient environment for 4 days. Nine of the recipients maintained fasting normoglycemia for 90 days without immunosuppression, while recipients of noncultured allogeneic islets reverted to the diabetic state by a mean of 8.2 days after transplantation. These results are surprising because other groups have found that a much longer culture period is required to reduce immunogenicity of adult islets sufficiently to obviate resection in nonimmunosuppressed recipients. There are no other reports of successful transplantation of isolated rat islets by direct intrahepatic injection. For example Rabinovitch *et al.* (1982a) cultured Lewis rat islets for 7 days at 37°C before transplantation to WF rats given a single injection of ALS, and found that although the mean functional survival time (as determined by the duration glycosuria was reduced below pretransplant levels) was prolonged (27.0 days) over those in recipients of fresh islets (5.3 days), most recipients of cultured islets rejected the grafts.

Lacy *et al.* (1979a) found that culture of handpicked adult rat islets in 95% oxygen at 37°C for more than 5 days was associated with islet disintegration. For that reason they combined a shorter period of culture with other treatments. Handpicked islets obtained from donors pretreated with irradiation and intravenous silica were cultured at 95% oxygen in media containing ALS for 1–3 days before transplantation across a minor histocompatibility barrier to seven nonimmunosuppressed diabetic recipients. Five rats rejected the islets between 8 and 18 days (controls rejected at 4–10 days), but in two, transplanted islets functioned for > 200 days. Any of the measures alone did not significantly improve islet functional survival after allotransplantation.

In separate experiments, this same group found that handpicked rat islets cultured for 7 days at 24° (Lacy *et al.*, 1979c) or 37°C (Yasunami *et al.*, 1982a) in an ambient atmosphere did not disintegrate. They initially investigated the effect of pretransplant culture at 24°C on the survival of rat islet allografts (Lacy *et al.*, 1979c). According to their criterion (glycosuria at the same level as pretransplant was taken as the day of rejection, hence animals could be hyperglycemic and still not be considered to have rejection of the islets), cultured islets were not rejected during 100 days of observation after intraportal transplantation across a major histocompatibility barrier to diabetic rats immunosuppressed with a single injection of ALS. If ALS was not given, the rats rejected cultured as well as fresh islet allografts. In Lewis rats bearing long-term WF islet allografts, rejection could be induced by injection of peritoneal exudate cells (Lacy *et al.*, 1979b) or splenic T cells but not B cells (Zitron *et al.*, 1981b) obtained from the original donor strain. Spleen cells or (occasionally) peritoneal exudate cells of Buffalo origin also induced rejection (Zitron *et al.*, 1981b), possibly because of transplant antigen cross-reactivity of the third-party strain chosen with the original donor strain. This explanation cannot be excluded because of the incomplete characterization of rat major and minor histocompatibility complexes. These results show that culture at 24°C did not alter the immunological recognition of allogeneic beta cells, even though the immunogenicity of the islets was reduced.

This group has also used the 7-day 24°C rat islet culture technique for xenotransplantation to diabetic mice treated with a single intravenous dose of antimouse lymphocyte serum (Lacy *et al.*, 1980a). Fresh cultured islets were rejected at approximately the same time (mean of 49.0 and 59.5 days, respectively, compared to 8.8 days of immunosuppressed recipients of fresh islet xenografts). If the recipients were also given intravenous injection of antirat lymphocyte serum, 70% of the mice maintained graft function for greater than 100 days and 33% for greater than 200 days (Lacy *et al.*, 1981b). Unfortunately, a control group of fresh islets transplanted to animals given both antirat and antimouse lymphocyte sera were not included. Therefore, it is impossible to know if the period of culture reduced the xenoimmunogenicity of the rat islets, and they remained susceptible to rejection, as shown by recurrence of diabetes in mice bearing long-term grafts after injection of spleen cells of donor origin (Lacy et al., 1981b). The protocol of 7-day culture at 24°C before xenotransplantation of rat islets to diabetic mice treated with antimouse and antirat lymphocyte sera was much less effective when the spleen was used as the site for grafting (Janney et al., 1982b). But it was clear in this set of experiments that culturing of islets influenced results since fresh islets in mice injected intraperitoneally with both antirat and antimouse lymphocyte sera were rejected at a mean of 9.7 days, while cultured islets were rejected at 28.4 days in identically treated recipients, and at 35.8 days and 18.3 days in mice receiving either antimouse or antirat lymphocyte serum, respectively. Intravenous administration of both antirat and antimouse lymphocyte sera to recipient mice resulted in a mean functional survival of 38.0 days for 7-day 24°C-cultured rat islets transplanted intrasplenically (Janney et al., 1982b). This is much less than the 120.1-day mean survival seen in previous experiments with intraportal transplantation of similarly cultured islet xenografts to recipient mice (Lacy et al., 1981a,b).

This group has tested the effect of culture of rat islets at 37° in air and 5% CO_2 only in the diabetic mouse xenograft model (Yasunami et al., 1983). Fresh isolated islets were rejected at a mean of 7.0 days when transplanted intraportally and at 18.7 days when transplanted under the renal capsule. Cultured islets were rejected at means of 20.4 days and 46.1 days after transplantation to the portal vein and renal subcapsular sites, respectively, with 30% of the latter functioning for > 60 days (Yasunami et al., 1983a,b). Since this group (Lacy et al., 1981a; Janney et al., 1982b; Yasunami et al., 1982a, 1983a,b) did not treat any recipients of islets cultured at 37°C with ALS and treated all recipients of islets cultured at 24°C with ALS, it is uncertain whether the culture techniques differ in their effect on islet immunogenicity. Another group (Rabinovitch et al., 1982a) cultured rat islets for 7 days at either 25°C or 37°C before transplantation to nonimmunosuppressed recipients, and found that culture at 37° delayed the mean onset of islet allograft rejection (27.0 days) more than culture at 25°C (10.0 days) over that of fresh islets (3.3 days).

It appears from these experiments that culture alone cannot totally eliminate immunogenicity of rat islets, and that immunosuppression of the recipient is still required. This statement is consistent with the findings of Rabinovitch et al. (1982a) that tissue culture reduces, but does not altogether eliminate, Ia-antigen-bearing cells in rat islets. Morphological studies by Rabinovitch et al. (1982a) using peroxidase-labeled anti-Ia serum detected positive staining of macrophages and endothelial cells in fresh, but not in 7-day cultured islets; however, using a radioligand assay there was only a 45% decreased binding of anti-Ia serum to cultured rat islets. Nevertheless, the morphological findings indicate that Ia-bearing cells are reduced. Such a reduction probably accounts for the decreased immunogenicity most apparent when islet allograft or concordant xenograft recipients are given immunosuppression (Lacy et al., 1981a). It is possible that culture of mouse islets is more effective in reducing immunogenicity, since Parr et al. (1980a) have made observations similar to those of Rabinovitch et al. (1982a) on cultured mouse islets using an immunoferation anti-H-2 labeling technique for morphological studies. In the experiments with islet allografts (Prowse et al., 1982a) culture alone was sufficient to result in indefinite islet allograft survival without immunosuppression in some of the recipients, the effect depending in part on the donor–recipient strain combinations tested. The effect of islet culture on immunogenicity of islets from other species is uncertain, but morphological studies of cultured human fetal pancreases suggest that Ia-positive cells can be reduced with maintenance of β cell integrity (Thomson *et al.*, 1983).

The effect of culture on reduction of islet immunogenicity is not entirely reproducible from laboratory to laboratory; some examples were given in the first paragraph of this subsection. Other groups have also had some difficulty in prolonging islet allograft or xenograft survival by pretransplant islet culture (Reemtsma *et al.*, 1981; Hardy *et al.*, 1982). Reemtsma *et al.* (1981) transplanted handpicked WF islets intraportally to diabetic Lewis recipients; fresh islets were rejected at a mean of 3.3 days, while islets cultured for 7 days at 24°C and 95% O_2–5% CO_2 were rejected at a mean of 4.7 days in nonimmunosuppressed rats and at 27.3 days in rats treated with one dose of ALS (provided by P. E. Lacy) pretransplant. This protocol was nearly, but not entirely identical to that of Lacy *et al.* (1979). First, Reemstma *et al.* (1981) did not use the green-light technique (Finke *et al.*, 1979) for islet isolation, and the islets may have been less pure than those transplanted by Lacy *et al.* (1979c). Second, even though they cultured the islets at 24°C, they used a 95% O_2 environment instead of ambient atmosphere in which islets were cultured by Lacy *et al.* (1979c). Third, they used a more sensitive indicator of rejection (recurrence of hyperglycemia) then did Lacy *et al.* (1979c); the latter, at least in these particular experiments, defined the day of islet allograft rejection as the day glycosuria reached pretransplant levels, long after recurrence of diabetes. This is a conventional definition of rejection for most (Matas *et al.*, 1978a), but not all (Lacy *et al.*, 1979a; Rabinovitch *et al.*, 1982a), investigators. When Reemstma *et al.* (1981) reassessed their data by degree of glycosuria in islet allograft recipients, the survival of cultured islet allografts in the ALS-treated rats ranged from 60 to 100 days, but similar survival was seen in the ALS-treated recipients of fresh islets. In further experiments by this group (Hardy *et al.*, 1982) with WF islets cultured for 7 days at 24°C and 95% O_2–5% CO_2 before transplantation to Lewis recipients treated with either six doses of ALG posttransplant or two doses of selective lymphoid irradiation with palladium-109–hematoporphyrin pretransplantation, graft functional survival times were extended by the immunosuppressive treatment of the recipient. The results were similar whether the islets were fresh (3/8 functioned > 60 days) or cultured (4/8 functioned > 60 days) in ALG alone or ALG+palladium-109–hematoporphyrin-treated (8/10 fresh vs. 6/8 cultured islet grafts functioned < 60 days) recipients. Both cultured or uncultured study of islets were capable of inducing cytotoxic alloantibodies in Lewis recipients. Hardy *et al.* (1982) demonstrated the presence of endothelial cells in cultured islets and concluded that their islet isolation culture technique was unable to eliminate immunogenic cells from the grafts.

The divergence of results by various investigators, following transplantation of cultured allogeneic islets reflects in part the different models used, but also indicates that specific culture techniques are critical to success. The treatment of the recipient was also important and at least for transplantation across a major barrier, culture can reduce but not entirely eliminate immunogenicity. Nevertheless, if minimal immunosuppression is all that is necessary to ensure the survival of cultured islet allografts, it is possible that the need for generalized immunosuppression can be eliminated altogether if even more effective measures are developed to eliminate immunogenic cells from islet allografts.

b. In Vitro Treatment of Islet Allograft with Cytotoxic Agents Designed to Eliminate Immunostimulatory Cells Selectively. The presumed mechanism by which culture reduces the immunogenicity of islet (or other tissue) allografts is through the loss of passenger leukocytes or other immunostimulatory cells, with maintenance of viability of the desired parenchymal (beta) cells under the culture conditions chosen. If this theory is correct, it should be possible to treat islets *in vitro* with agents that are selectively toxic to non-beta immunogenic cells.

Toledo-Pereyra *et al.* (1982b) added horse antidog lymphocyte globulin to dispersed canine pancreatic allogeneic islet tissue immediately before intrasplenic transplantation to dogs minimally immunosuppressed with azathioprine. They observed a mean graft survival of 29.6 days, as compared to 11.0 days in immunosuppressed recipients of non-ALG-treated allogeneic islet tissue. Unfortunately, a control group in which an equivalent amount of ALG was given concomitantly with, but separate from, the islets was not included. Several investigators have found it difficult to achieve normoglycemia in transplantation of dispersed pancreatic allogenic islet tissue in the dog (Kretschmer *et al.*, 1979; DuToit *et al.*, 1981), and there are no confirmatory reports of the work by Toledo-Pereyra *et al.* (1982b). Zeigler *et al.* (1982) took another approach and attempted to eliminate passenger leukocytes in isolated rat islets by irradiation *in vitro*, but found that the manipulations damaged the beta cells sufficiently so that even with transplantation to syngeneic recipients, normoglycemia was only transiently achieved.

The most spectacular success with *in vitro* treatment of islets for reduction of immunogenicity has been achieved by Faustman *et al.* (1981) in a mouse islet allograft model. This group briefly incubated 550–750 B10.BR islets (H-2^k) derived from 20 donor pancreases per recipient with anti-I^k serum and complement before transplantation to C57BL/6J (H-2^b) diabetic mice (B6). They found that all islet allografts so treated functioned for > 200 days, while 80% of B6 mice rejected non-Ia-treated B10.BR islet allografts. They initially hypothesized that the loss of the Ia allostimulus was responsible for the loss of islet immunogenicity. However, subsequent experiments by Morrow *et al.* (1983a) showed that B10.AQR mice receiving islets from B10.T(6R) donors, with whom they were identical for *I* region (Class II) encoded antigens but disparate for H-2 K and D (Class I) antigen, could still reject the islets. These results indicate that removal of an allogenic Ia epitope itself is not required to eliminate immunogenicity, and, in fact, will not do so by itself; rather the immunostimulatory cells express Ia, but also stimulate an allogenic response by presenting Class I antigens. Thus the cells themselves must be inactivated to prevent an immune response, which is one of the hypotheses also entertained by Faustman *et al.* (1981).

Although treatment of mouse islets with anti-Ia sera reduces their immunogenicity, they remain susceptible to rejection, since injection of 5×10^7 spleen cells into mice bearing long-term anti-Ia-treated islet allografts is followed by recurrence of hyperglycemia (Faustman *et al.*, 1981). In further experiments Faustman *et al.* (1982a) showed that injection of recipient mice with a small number of donor splenocytes (5×10^4 cells) by itself was not sufficient to induce rejection of long-term surviving anti-Ia-treated islet allografts. If this dose of splenocytes were combined with administration of anti-I-J$^\kappa$ antiserum (specifically directed against recipient strain suppressor cells), rejection could be induced. They interpreted these data to indicate that the long-term tolerance to the anti-Ia-treated islet allografts depended on active immune mechanisms by the host. However, the mice were not tolerant to the donor strain in the classic sense, since a sufficient dose of splenocytes alone could cause rejection, and the anti-I-J^k sera (which by itself could not unmask an immune process leading to rejection) merely lowered the threshold by which splenocytes could induce an immune response. This threshold may not have been dependent upon the presence or absence of the anti-Ia-treated allogeneic islets. The important point of the experiments of Faustman *et al.* (1981, 1982a), however, is the demonstration that anti-Ia-treated islets are rendered nonimmunogenic. The most likely explanation, according to current theories of tissue immunogenicity (Minan and Shreffler, 1981; Lafferty *et al.*, 1983), is that the anti-Ia treatment eliminates only cells shown to express Ia antigens in mouse islets (the dendritic cells) which are immunogenic as long as Class I disparities with the recipient exist. This explanation is consistent with the observations of Morrow *et al.* (1983b) that islets from donor mice disparate for Class I (H-2 K+D) antigens only are immunogenic even though the *I*-region (Class II) antigens are identical between the donor and recipient, but that islets transplanted to mice that are *I*-region (Class II) disparate only are not susceptible to rejection (Morrow *et al.* 1983a). Treatment of islets from donors disparate for K+D only (which are rejected if no other measures are taken) with antisera to the donor *I*-region (Class II) antigens (identical to the recipient) before transplantation would test this hypothesis.

c. Effect of Donor Pretreatment with Cytolytic Agents on Islet Immunogenicity.

An alternative to removal of immunogeneic passenger or dendritic cells by treatment of the islets *in vitro* is to pretreat the donor with cytolytic agents that are selectively toxic to immunostimulatory but not parenchymal (beta) cells. Such treatment has been applied to various organ and tissue grafts, both experimentally and clinically, by a variety of protocols and with variable effects (Lafferty *et al.*, 1983), but only a few experiments have been reported on this approach in islet transplant models.

The additive effect of pretreatment of donor rats with silica and 1–3-day culture in 95% oxygen and ALS-containing media of islets derived from the donors on islet allograft survival was briefly summarized in the preceding section on islet culture (Lacy *et al.*, 1979a). This protocol actually combined all three methods to reduce islet immunogenicity; donor pretreatment, *in vitro* treatment with a cytolytic agent (ALG), and culture. However, even though transplantation was across a minor histocompatibility barrier most rats rejected the islet allografts in less than 3 weeks (Lacy *et al.*, 1979a).

Bowen *et al.* (1980) also combined donor pretreatment with islet culture prior to allotransplantation in mice, but their studies were histological only. Nevertheless, islets derived from cyclophosphamide-treated donors and cultured in clusters of 50 (megaislets) in 95% O_2 for 7–12 days were subjected to virtually no inflammatory response after allotransplantation, while noncultured islets derived from cyclophosphamide-treated donors were histologically rejected, even though the intensity of mononuclear cell infiltration was less than that observed in noncultured islets derived from normal donors. Since islet culture alone, using the megaislet technique developed by this group (Bowen *et al.*, 1980), is able to alter the islets sufficiently to prevent or delay rejection in some donor–recipient strain combinations (Prowse *et al.*, 1982a), it is apparent that the cyclophosphamide treatment of the donor had only a minimal effect on the immunogenicity of islets derived from the donors (Bowen *et al.*, 1980).

The minimal effect of cyclosphosphamide treatment on the immunogenicity of subsequently derived islets is also apparent from the results of experiments by Garvey *et al.* (1980c) in the DA and Lewis rat strains. Single or multiple doses of cyclophosphamide 24–96 hr before preparation of islets from either fetal or adult donors, did not prolong islet allograft survival in nonimmunosuppressed diabetic rat recipients.

Unless the recipients are immunosuppressed to at least some degree, however, an effect of donor pretreatment might be missed. For example, Schulak *et al.* (1980) irradiated (1200 rad) WF donor rats 24–72 hr prior to islet isolation and transplantation to ALS- or non-ALS-treated diabetic recipients. Irradiation alone barely had a minimal effect; mean survival of islets derived from nonirradiated donors was 5.0 days and from donors irradiated 72 hr before islet harvesting was 7.0 days in nonimmunosuppressed recipients. However, when islets derived from donors, irradiated 72 hr prior to harvesting, were transplanted to recipients given a single dose of ALS, mean islet allograft survival time was 45.6 days as opposed to 18.2 days in ALG-treated recipients of fresh islets. Thus, donor irradiation and recipient ALG treatment had a synergistic effect on islet allograft survival and the effect would have been missed had the recipients not been immunosuppressed.

The overall theme of the experiments summarized in this section indicate that the immunogenicity of islets can be altered by measures designed to eliminate certain cells selectively or semiselectively, such as dendritic or passenger leukocytes, that are more potent stimulators of the immune response than are beta or other parenchymal cells. Almost all of the experiments have been performed on rodents. It remains to be seen whether the various approaches can be successful with islet transplantation in large animals and whether the methods will be practical for clinical application. Even if the latter is not possible, however, the experimental islet allograft models are extremely useful for demonstrating the differences in immunogenicity and susceptibility to rejection of islets and of allogeneic tissue in general.

5. Prevention of Rejection by Immunomechanical Barriers

The results of transplantation of islet tissue enclosed in diffusion chambers have, in general, been poor or difficult to reproduce. Theoretically a semiporous membrane will exclude cells or molecules able to mediate rejection, while allowing flux of insulin and glucose. The composition, structure, and diffusion characteristics of several members and chambers and the problems with their use have been assessed by Theodorou and Howell (1981).

In addition, Scharp *et al.* (1982) have recently written a comprehensive review on the historical development and the use of hybrid artificial organs to provide immunoisolation to endocrine grafts, with emphasis on islets. The devices can be classified as extravascular diffusion chambers, intravascular infusion chambers, and intravascular ultrafiltration chambers. In addition, a new version of immunoisolation—microencapsulation of cells within cross-linked polymers—has recently been applied to islet grafts. The theoretical and practical considerations in the use of these devices, or limitations (such as clotting within the intravascular chambers) and the current approaches being employed to overcome the multiple problems in the use have also been reviewed by Scharp (1982), and will not be reiterated here. Instead, only a brief listing of the reported attempts at transplantation of islets within each category of immunoisolation devices is provided.

The results reported concerning inclusion of islets within diffusion chambers have been extremely divergent. Swenne *et al.* (1979) found that mouse islets survived in millipore chambers, but they could not reproduce the results of Strautz *et al.* (1970), and ob/ob mice receiving islets from lean littermates remained hypoglycemic after intraperitoneal implantation. Gates and Lazarus (1977) reported that streptozotocin-induced diabetes in rats was ameliorated by intraperitoneal implantation of neonatal rabbit pancreatic tissue enclosed in millipore chambers and that the diabetic state recurred after removal of the chamber. Garvey *et al.* (1979a) could not reproduce these results and found no viable tissue at the end of 6 weeks. Jolley *et al.* (1977) reported that transplantation of dog islets in protease-coated millipore chambers into the peritoneal cavity of alloxan-induced diabetic rats was followed by slow reversal of the hyperglycemic state, but they did not remove the chambers to see if the diabetes would recur, nor did they follow a control group of untreated diabetic rats. Chen *et al.* (in press) could not reproduce their results even with collagenase- or protease-coated chambers. On the other hand, Archer *et al.* (1980) reported that both šyngeneic and xenogeneic mouse islets enclosed in Amicon 50-K hollow fibers restored normoglycemia for several weeks in Chinese hamsters with mild streptozotocin-induced diabetes. Altman *et al.* (1982) have recently reported that rat islets enclosed in Amicon 50-K hollow fibers can reverse hyperglycemia after implantation in syngeneic diabetic rats. Araki *et al.* (1980) have also reported that neonatal rat pancreatic tissue encased in chambers with XM 100-A Amicon membranes reversed hyperglycemia after implantation in the omentum of totally pancreatectomized dogs, with recurrence of diabetes after their removal. These unbelievably spectacular results await confirmation by independent investigators.

In contrast to these reports, other investigators have not been able to produce a sustained reduction of hyperglycemia in insulinopenic diabetic animals treated by transplantation of membrane-enclosed syngeneic (Kemp *et al.*, 1973; Bushard, 1975; Theodorou *et al.*, 1980a; Scharp *et al.*, 1982a,b), allogeneic (Helmke *et al.*, 1975), or xenogeneic (Weber *et al.*, 1976, 1980b; Hardy *et al.*, 1982) islets. Theodorou *et al.* (1981) found that WAG rat islets enclosed in polycarbonate diffusion chambers did not elicit cytotoxic alloantibodies in Lewis recipients, but neither did they reverse diabetes. In previous experiments, Theodorou *et al.* (1980a) found that 1400 syngeneic islets, capable of reversing diabetes after intraportal transplantation, failed to ameliorate diabetes after intraperitoneal transplantation in polycarbonate diffusion chambers and no viable islet tissue could be recovered at the end of 12 weeks.

The problems with implantable membrane chambers include poor neovascularization, deposition of fibrous connective tissue, and inadequate flux of insulin and glucose between the chamber and the host.

A possible solution to some of these problems may be provided by microcapsulation of islets with cross-linked nontoxic polysaccharides, although such a technique presents an entirely new set of questions, including the durability of the capsules. Lim and Sun (1980) reported that isolated rat islets enclosed in polylysine alginate microcapsules reversed hyperglycemia after intraperitoneal transplantation to diabetic recipients. However, the results are difficult to interpret. Because hyperglycemia recurred between 6 and 8 days in recipients of unencapsulated islets and at 3 weeks in recipients of encapsulated islets, it was not clear from the report whether the islets were transplanted to syngeneic or allogeneic hosts. These results have not been confirmed by an independent group of investigators, but an associate of Sun (O'Shea *et al.*, 1982) reported that intraperitoneal transplantation of islets encapsulated within a modified semipermeable alginate poly-L-lysine membrane restored normoglycemia in diabetics rats for 15–20 days. Failure was stated to be due to an inflammatory response induced by one of the membrane components, but again the genetic relationship between the donors and recipients was not clear. Better-designed and better-reported experiments are needed for critical assessment of this new technique.

In attempts to improve the perfusion characteristics of islet-containing chambers, several groups have attached devices directly to the blood vessels of diabetic animals, with islets isolated on one side of a synthetic porous membrane or artificial capillary bundle and blood flowing on the other side (reviewed by Scharp *et al.*, 1982a,b). If the main conduit has only two connections (one arterial in flow, one arterial or venous outflow), insulin released can reach the circulation only by simple diffusion. However, if the main conduit has two arterial connections, the addition of a venous run-off improved the diffusion characteristics even further by ultrafiltration (Reach *et al.*, 1981; Scharp *et al.*, 1982). Almost all of the investigators have used rat pancreases as a source of islets for enclosure within the chambers. Since the devices are quite large, external vessel connectors have been used for *ex vivo* perfusion in rats, but intracavitary implantation is possible in larger animals. In actual practice, islet-containing intravascular diffusion chambers have lowered plasma glucose levels for only a short time (hours to a few days) in diabetic rats (Tze *et al.*, 1976a; Sun *et al.*, 1977; Chick *et al.*, 1979; Orsetti *et al.*, 1981; Reach *et al.*, 1981), dogs (Tze *et al.*, 1980; Scharp *et al.*, 1982a), and monkeys (Sun *et al.*, 1980), but normal glucose tolerance test results have been obtained (Sun *et al.*, 1980; Scharp *et al.*, 1982a) during the period that the devices could be maintained. Blood clotting and other complications have not allowed the devices to function for a long enough period to determine whether the theoretical objective of preventing rejection can be achieved. Some progress in solving the technical problems is being made (Scharp, 1982; Scharp *et al.*, 1982b). We, however, project that advances in immunology eventually will allow organs and tissues to be transplanted by standard techniques with absolutely reliable prevention of rejection by specific, nontoxic, immunosuppression and that such an advance will occur before the problems associated with the immunoisolation devices are solved.

6. Islet Xenografts

If rejection of tissues transplanted from animals to humans can be prevented, a major problem of organ procurement would be solved. It would facilitate the use of multiple donors, should this be necessary for islets. The general problems with xenotransplantation and the classification of xenografts into concordant and discordant types have been succinctly summarized by Kemp (1978). Unfortunately, xenografts between widely disparate species are usually rejected with unusual vigor, often within a few minutes of vascularization because of the preformed, complement-fixing heterophile antibodies. For this reason several investigators have enclosed islets within semipermeable membrane chambers for transplantation between discordant species. Although a positive effect was reported by some groups (Gates and Lazarus, 1977; Jolley *et al.*, 1977; Archer *et al.*, 1980; Araki *et al.*, 1980), attempts to reproduce some of these results failed (Garvey *et al.*, 1979a). The results of other experiments (Weber *et al.*, 1976, 1980b; Hardy *et al.*, 1982; Scharp *et al.*, in press b) were discouraging, as described in the previous section.

Xenografts between closely related (concordant) species, however, can function for a reasonable period of time even without immunosuppression. Fresh neonatal or adult rat islets transplanted to the peritoneal cavity of nonimmunosuppressed diabetic mice have reduced hyperglycemia (Weber *et al.*, 1976, 1980b) or restored normoglycemia (Frangipane *et al.*, 1977; Delmonico *et al.*, 1977) for up to 1 week.

In a series of experiments by one group of investigators, transplantation of 350–1000 fresh rat islets to nonimmunosuppressed diabetic mice resulted in functional graft survival times ranging from 7.4 to 8.8 days following intraportal injection (Lacy *et al.*, 1980a, 1981b, 1982a), from 11.2 to 18.7 days with placement under the kidney capsule (Bobzien *et al.*, 1983; Yasunami *et al.*, 1982), and from 5.1 days with intrasplenic (Janney *et al.*, 1982b) to 30.8 days with intratesticular (Bobzien *et al.*, in press) transplantation. In the latter set of experiments 3 of 12 intratesticular rat-to-mouse islets xenografts functioned > 60 days (Bobzien *et al.*, 1983). This constitutes one of the most convincing pieces of evidence that the testes may be in immunologically privileged sites since previous claims for such a phenomena have been based on histological studies only (Ferguson and Scothorne, 1973).

Administration of heterologous recipient-species-specific ALS is effective in delaying the rejection of rat-to-mouse islet xenografts. Mice treated with ALS after receiving adult adult rat islets intraperitoneally (1979a) remained normoglycemic for 9–21 days in the experiments by Frangipane *et al.* and for 2.5–8 weeks in experiments by Delmonico *et al.* (1977). The period of reduced blood glucose was extended from a median of 3 to 10 days by ALS treatment (Weber *et al.*, 1980b). A single dose of ALS at the time of rat-to-mouse islet transplantation resulted in mean survival time of 49.0

days for intraportal graft (Lacy *et al.*, 1981b), although the same ALS delayed the mean rejection time to only 9.7 days for intrasplenic grafts (Janney *et al.*, 1982b). The only other report on the use of a generalized immunosuppressive regimen in recipients of concordant islet xenografts is by Nakajima *et al.* (1982). Diabetic hamsters treated with 1200 rad (200 × 6) TLI (pretransplant) rejected intraportal rat islet xenografts at a mean of 30.3 days, compared to 2.9 days in nonimmunosuppressed recipients.

The survival time of concordant rat-to-mouse islet xenografts has also been extended by a period of pretransplant culture (Lacy *et al.*, 1981a) to reduce islet graft immunogenicity. The rat islets were cultured for 1 week in an ambient atmosphere at 24°C before transplantation. Diabetic mice recipients were also given heterologous antimouse (MALS) alone or antimouse antirat (RALS) lymphocyte sera (Lacy *et al.*, 1980a). With either protocol, after intraportal transplantation approximately 70% of the cultured islets functioned > 60 days, and with MALS alone 33% functioned > 200 days (Lacy *et al.*, 1981b). With intrasplenic transplantation, only 7% of cultured islets in the ALS treated rats functioned > 100 days, but mean survival times ranged from 18.3 to 38.0 days depending on whether MALS or RALS was given alone or in combination to the recipients. MALS was the most effective (Janney *et al.*, 1982b).

Rat islets cultured for 7 days at 37°C in ambient atmosphere by themselves is sufficient to delay their rejection after transplantation to diabetic mice (Yasunami *et al.*, 1982a). Cultured islets transplanted to the liver functioned for a mean of 20.4 days compared to those transplanted to under the kidney capsule which functioned for a mean of 46.1 days (Yasunami *et al.*, 1983).

Lacy *et al.* (1982a) also found that the megaislet 7-day culture technique in 95% oxygen was also effective in delaying rejection in the rat-to-islet xenograft model if the islets were placed under the kidney capsule (mean graft survival of 52.1 days vs. 14.4 days for uncultured islets) and that results were not enhanced by treatment of the recipients with a single dose of ALS. Seven-day cultured rat megaislets transplanted via the portal vein also had a slightly prolonged survival (16.9 days) compared to controls (8.7 days). Lymphoid reaction around the subrenal capsule or xenograft was primarily composed of T lymphocytes with a predominance of Ly2 cells except in the cultured xenografts, in which the percentage of Ly2 cells was decreased early. The studies suggest that the kidney is a more efficient site for xenotransplantation, and similar observations have been made in allograft models (Reece-Smith *et al.*, 1981a).

In experiments by another group (Serie *et al.*, 1983), xenotransplantation of 200–300 neonatal rat islets cultured for 8–17 days before transplantation to the kidney subcapsular site of nonimmunosuppressed mice functioned > 4 weeks in 6 of 13 recipients. They did not compare the graft survival times at different sites, and since then islet isolation technique depends on culture, they could not make a comparison to fresh islets.

Although the combination of islet culture and recipient immunosuppression can greatly prolong or even prevent the rejection of rat-to-mouse islet xenografts, the graft nevertheless remains susceptible to rejection, since Lacy *et al.* (1981a) found that injection of rat splenocytes 8 weeks after transplantation of cultured islet xenografts to ALS-treated recipients was promptly followed by recurrence of hyperglycemia. Frangipane *et al.* (1977) and Delmonico *et al.* (1977) had previously shown that recurrence of hyperglycemia could be prematurely precipitated in mouse recipients of intraperitoneal rat islet xenografts by injection of recipients with rat antimouse serum.

It appears that rat-to-mouse islet xenografts behave very similarly to rat-to-rat or mouse-to-mouse islet allografts. Thus this particular system may not be representative of the results that can be obtained in most xenograft systems, particularly those in which the donor and recipients are discordant species.

Discordant xenografts are usually rejected promptly. Eloy *et al.* (1979) found that islet-rich, 15-day (but not 18-day) chick embryo pancreas significantly improved diabetes in rats after direct implantation into the hepatic parenchyma. Weber *et al.* (1980b) and Hardy *et al.* (1982) could not reproduce these results in rats in immunosuppressed or nonimmunosuppressed mice. Weber *et al.* (1980a) found that neonatal rabbit, calf, or fish islets enclosed or not enclosed in cuprophine envelopes before intraperitoneal transplantation to diabetic rats lowered blood sugar levels for only 0–6 days. Bretzel *et al.* (1981c) found that cryopreserved pig islets transplanted intraportally to diabetic mice resulted in normoglycemia for < 4 days. On the other hand Lacy *et al.* (1982) found that beef islets isolated by the Velcro technique, and Yasumami *et al.* (1982b) found that neonatal pig islets prepared by the dispersed cell culture reaggregation technique, would reduce hyperglycemia for approximately 1 week after intraportal transplantation to diabetic mice. In the latter experiments the grafts functioned for a mean of 21.3 days in recipient mice given a dose each of antipig and antimouse ALS.

Except for these reports, discordant xenografts have been successfully engrafted only under very special circumstances, to thymic aplastic mutant nude (nu/nu) mice or nude (rnu/rnu) rats: animals that are genetically unable to reject allo- and xenografts (Povlsen *et al.*, 1974; Festing *et al.*, 1978). Reintgen *et al.* (1980a) restored normoglycemia in nude mice with streptozotocin-induced diabetes by subcutaneous transplantation of a hamster insulinoma. Mirkovitch *et al.* (1981) observed histological evidence of survival of dispersed canine, but not human, pancreatic islet tissue transplanted subcutaneously or intraperitoneally to nude mice.

Human islets can also survive after xenotransplantation to these unusual animals. Usadel *et al.* (1980b) transplanted human fetal pancreatic fragments (6–23 weeks' gestation) subcutaneously or into the mammary gland (Usadel *et al.*, 1981) of nondiabetic nude mice, or into a plastic-lined epigastric pouch in nondiabetic nude rats (Bastert *et al.*, 1981). Functional studies were not reported, but histological examination of the implants between 21 and 120 days after transplantation showed well-formed islets with all hormone cell types (Usadel, 1980a; Bastert *et al.*, 1981). Mandel *et al.* (1982a) also observed histological survival of fetal human islets transplanted to under the kidney capsule of nude mice. Partial amelioration of diabetes has also been observed after transplantation of human islets to nude mice with streptozotocin-induced diabetes (Lundgren *et al.*, 1977). Histological rejection of cultured human islet tumor tissue was observed after intramuscular concordant xenotransplantation to a monkey (Weber *et al.*, 1980b).

Application of discordant xenografts to clinical transplantation seems remote, although the results of some experiments indicate that the situation, at least for islets, is not hopeless. The observation that concordant rat xenogeneic islets can function for prolonged periods in immunosuppressed mice provides hope that transplantation of islets from subhuman primates to diabetic humans will someday be possible.

7. Future of Islet Allotransplantation

The major barriers to clinical application of islet transplantation are islet yield and allograft rejection. Early experiments suggested that islets were more susceptible to rejection than other tissues. Most recent experiments with transplantation of large numbers of highly purified islets suggest that such is not the case, and that islets are probably similar to other endocrine tissue in their immunogenicity and susceptibility to rejection. However, unless special preventive measures are taken, islets are rejected more readily than pancreas grafts in nonimmunosuppressed hosts. Nevertheless, a variety of immunosuppressive protocols have significantly prolonged islet allograft functional survival. The importance of transplanting a sufficient islet mass is now understood. The success with transplantation of allogeneic islets in animals underscores the potential for and the need to develop specific immunosuppressive techniques that will be applicable to human transplantation.

F. Preservation of Islet Tissue

A reliable technique for short-term preservation is necessary for clinical islet transplantation to be logistically practical. Long-term preservation would allow islets to be accumulated and transplanted in one procedure to a diabetic recipient selected on the basis of histocompatibility match or other factors.

Three methods of islet preservation have been investigated: (1) tissue culture, (2) cold storage, and (3) freezing. The technical aspects of islet culture and storage for transplantation have recently been reviewed (Gordon and Toledo-Pereyra, 1982). Numerous investigators have obtained *in vitro* evidence of islet function after storage by these methods. Reversal of diabetes after transplantation is a more critical test of viability, and experiments designed to make this test deserve to be emphasized.

1. Culture

Rodent islets maintained in culture for days or weeks can synthesize and secrete insulin in response to appropriate stimuli (Andersson and Buschard, 1977; Lacy *et al.*, 1976; Nakagawara *et al.*, 1978; Bretzel *et al.*, 1981a; Ziegler *et al.*, 1981; Collier *et al.*, 1982). In cultures of fetal or neonatal pancreas, islets preferentially differentiate (Hegre *et al.*, 1976b, 1981; Jonasson *et al.*, 1977; Lazarow *et al.*, 1973), and beta cells can replicate (Hegre *et al.*, 1976a, 1981). High oxygen concentrations may be detrimental to isolated islets (Lacy *et al.*, 1979a) unless they are protected by aggregation (Bowen *et al.*, 1980) or cultured at 24°C (Ono *et al.*, 1979).

Some of the experiments on transplantation of cultured islets were described in the preceding section on islet allografts and xenografts (Faustman *et al.*, 1982b; Kedinger *et al.*, 1977; Prowse, 1982a; Mandel *et al.*, 1982a; Andersson, 1982; Hegre *et al.*,

1981; Garvey *et al.*, 1980a; Yasunami *et al.*, 1983). These experiments were designed to test the ability of *in vitro* passage to alter islet immunogenicity, but their technical success depended upon preservation of viability.

Other experiments have been designed specifically to test the feasibility of culture for islet preservation. Scharp *et al.* (1974) found that the interval between intraportal transplantation and restoration of normoglycemia was delayed in diabetic rats receiving isologous adult islets stored in stationary tissue culture for 3 weeks, but other groups ameliorated diabetes promptly by intraportal transplantation of syngeneic islets cultured for 24–96 hr (Ziegler *et al.*, 1981), 7 days (Nakagawara *et al.*, 1978), or 5–18 days (Bretzel *et al.*, 1981a). Andersson *et al.* (1977) also restored normoglycemia to diabetic nude mice within 2 weeks by intraperitoneal transplantation of islets cultured for 10 days. Using a system designed to improve islet yield, Scharp *et al.* (1978) found that intraportal transplantation of rat islet pellets originally derived from the nine donor pancreas and aggregated by gyrorotational culture for 1 week reversed diabetes as well as fresh islets after transplantation, even though central necrosis was present in the aggregates.

Selawry *et al.* (1978) found that islets isolated from old rats lost the ability to bind concanvaline A *in vitro* and failed to ameliorate diabetes if transplanted immediately. A 48-hr period of tissue culture restored both conconavaline-A-binding activity and the ability to ameliorate diabetes after intraportal transplantation to syngeneic recipients.

Payne *et al.* (1979) successfully transplanted unpurified collagenase dispersed pancreatic islet tissue from D L-ethionine treated donor rats after storage for 24–48 hr. Tissue from one-third of a donor pancreas restored normoglycemia at the same rate as fresh tissue. Culture of adult pancreatic tissue from dogs (Matas *et al.*, 1976c) and monkeys (Jonasson *et al.*, 1977) for 24–48 hr results in reduction of exocrine enzyme content, but transplants to diabetic hosts were only partially successful (Matas *et al.*, 1977e,f; Jonasson *et al.*, 1977).

Diabetes in rats was reversed after intraperitoneal (Weber *et al.*, 1975) or intramuscular (Axen *et al.*, 1982) transplantation of collagenase-dispersed neonatal pancreatic tissue stored at 37°C for 24 hr (Weber *et al.*, 1975) or 6 days (Axen *et al.*, 1982). Hegre *et al.* (1976a,b,c) maintained intact neonatal rat pancreases from 10 to 25 donors in organ culture for 2–9 days before collagenase dispersal and reversed diabetes within 2–8 weeks following intraperitoneal transplantation. Using the nonenzymatic technique of neonatal islet preparation for periods of 8–17 days was followed by reversal of diabetes within 2 weeks of transplantation to the renal subcapsule of diabetic recipients (Serie *et al.*, 1983). They found that intact fetal rat pancreases cultured for 8 days reversed diabetes after transplantation to under the kidney capsule (Hegre *et al.*, 1981).

Other groups have primarily been interested in culture of intact fetal pancreases to affect immunogenicity, but they first have had to examine the metabolic efficiency of transplantation of cultured pancreases to syngeneic diabetic recipients. In the initial experiments of Mandel *et al.* (1980), intact fetal mouse pancreases cultured for 21 days only reduced hyperglycemia after intrasplenic transplantation to syngeneic diabetic mice. They later found that the results were better if the grafts were cultured in medium with a low rather than a high glucose concentration (Collier *et al.*, 1982). Short-term insulin treatment of the recipient did not improve the results of transplantation of cultured fetal pancreases, although such treatment did improve the long-term function of uncultured single fetal pancreas intrasplenic isografts (Hoffman *et al.*, 1981). Mandel *et al.* (1982a) also examined the effect of high ambient O_2 concentrations on fetal pancreases maintained in tissue culture, and found some detrimental effects of high O_2 concentrations, more pronounced for human and mouse fetal pancreas. However, the high O_2 concentration was more effective at reducing immunogenicity, but at the expense of functional viability. Simeonovic and Lafferty (1981) also studied the effect of organ culture in 95% O_2–5% CO_2 on the function of fetal mouse pancreases transplanted under the kidney capsule of syngeneic diabetic recipients. They found that the function deteriorated after 17 days of culture, the minimal period necessary to affect immunogenicity; nevertheless, isotransplantation of two 20-day cultured fetal pancreases would reverse diabetes, although not as rapidly as a single uncultured fetal pancreas isograft.

At this point, culture is only a means of islet storage or a method to reduce immunogenicity. No pure beta cell lines have been established to provide a continuous source of insulin-producing tissue for transplantation. Rodent islets can be stored for at least 3 weeks before transplantation. The relatively sophisticated equipment and fastidious conditions required for maintenance of islets in tissue culture, however, makes it difficult to store the quantities necessary for transplantation in large animal models.

2. Cold Storage

Storage in the cold is the simplest preservation method and requires the least amount of equipment. *In vitro* studies have defined some of the parameters that may be important in maintaining short- (Tellez-Yudilevich *et al.*, 1977) or long-term islet viability (Frankel *et al.*, 1976). However, *in vitro* function does not always correlate with *in vivo* function and assessment of preservation techniques in a transplantation is essential (Sutherland *et al.*, 1983b).

Matas *et al.* (1977d, 1978b,c) reversed diabetes in rats by intraportal transplantation of collagenase-dispersed neonatal pancreatic islet tissue stored for up to 63 hr (1977d) in a small amount up to 101 hr and (1978c) in a large amount of culture medium 199 at 4°C. In follow-up experiments islets stored at 4°C up to 146 hr in GIB media reversed diabetes after transplantation (Sutherland *et al.*, 1983b). In addition, Matas *et al.* (1978b) found that an *in situ* pancreatic ischemia period of 1 hr at 37°C, 3 hr at room temperature, and 7 hr at 7°C was tolerated with (Matas *et al.*, 1978b) or without (Matas *et al.*, 1977c) a 48-hr period of storage at 4°C after collagenase dispersal; 35 of 39 transplants in the combined group were successful (Sutherland *et al.*, 1983b). In complementary studies, Henriksson *et al.* (1977c) successfully transplanted adult rat islets isolated from donor pancreases after 40 min of warm ischemia.

In follow-up to the successful preservation of dispersed neonatal rat pancreatic islet tissue by cold storage (Sutherland *et al.*, 1983b), similar experiments were performed by Morrow *et al.* (1982) using dispersed tissue prepared from DL-ethionine-treated adult rat donors for intraportal transplantation to syngeneic diabetic recipients. A large media/pancreas ratio (15:1) was used, and the media was changed at 24 and 48 hr for storage times > 24 hr. Normoglycemia, however, occurred in only 50%, 25%, and

17% of recipients of tissue stored for 36, 48, and 72 hr, respectively, although 100% of recipients were ameliorated of diabetes following transplantation of tissue stored for 6 and 24 hr. The functional results correlated with the tissue insulin content of liver in animals sacrificed 4 weeks after transplantation. The results showed a progressive loss of viability, at least in terms of engraftment of adult rat islet tissue stored for longer than 24 hr. It thus appears that adult rat islets may be more sensitive than neonatal islets to the detrimental effects of cold.

Short-term cold storage of impure islets has been applied with moderate success for transplantation in dogs. Sutherland *et al.* (1977) found that 8 of 16 and Schulak and Reckard (1978) found that 5 of 5 dogs became normoglycemic after intrasplenic transplantation of autologous islet tissue stored at 4°C for 24 but not those stored for 48 hr. The latent period between transplantation and normoglycemia was prolonged and glucose tolerance was impaired in the study of Sutherland *et al.* (1977), but not in that of Schulak and Reckard (1978). This may relate to differences in storage techniques as recently discussed (Sutherland *et al.*, 1983b).

In summary, both rat and dog pancreatic islets have been successfully transplanted after storage in the cold. If the reliability of this technique is improved and if the period of storage can be increased in a large-animal model, this method should be suitable as a practical means for short-term preservation of human islet tissue before transplantation.

3. Cryopreservation

A variety of cells or tissue fragments can be frozen and stored at $-196°C$ for months or years without evident loss of viability (Karow, 1981). Several investigators have used *in vitro* tests to determine the optimal conditions for freezing and thawing of adult islets (Rajotte *et al.*, 1977; Bank *et al.*, 1979; Bank and Reichard, 1981) or fetal rat pancreas (Mazur *et al.*, 1976). Critical factors include the cooling and warming rates, the concentration and penetration of agents added to protect against intracellular ice crystal formation, and the osmotic changes that occur during removal of the cryoprotectant (Karow, 1981; Gordon *et al.*, 1982).

Mazur *et al.* (1976) found that 17.5-day fetal rat pancreases suspended in 2 M dimethyl sulfoxide (DMSO), cooled to $-8°C$ nucleated with an ice crystal, frozen at $0.3°C/min$ to $-78°C$, thawed at room temperature, and then slowly diluted in 0.75 M sucrose solution to preclude osmotic shock, could synthesize protein and insulin *in vitro*. Kemp *et al.* (1978) used this technique to store fetal pancreases for 13 weeks at $-196°C$, prior to transplantation under the kidney capsule of rats with renal–portal-vein shunts and reversed diabetes within 30 days.

Similar experiments have been carried out using isolated adult rat islets. Banks *et al.* (1977) found that freezing in 1 M DMSO at 75°C/min gave optimal viability by *in vitro* parameters, and that a two-step method was preferred (Bank *et al.*, 1981). Rajotte *et al.* (1981) found different conditions to be optimal: stepwise suspension in 2 M DMSO, seeding with ice at $-7.5°C$, freezing to $-75°C$ at $0.25°C/min$, storage at $-196°C$, and warming at 7.5°C/min. Islets frozen at one center by this technique and transported and thawed at another center ameliorated diabetes after intraportal transplantation to syngeneic rats (Rajotte *et al.*, 1981). Bretzel *et al.* (1980a,b) have also normalized blood glucose in diabetic rats with isologous islets frozen in 1 M DMSO at 2°C/min and stored for 4 weeks at −196°C before rapid thawing and intraportal transplantation. They have also applied this protocol to porcine islets (Bretzel *et al.*, 1981a). Nakagawara *et al.* (1981) used a similar protocol, except that the islets were frozen in 20% DMSO, but they ameliorated diabetes in only four of six by intraportal transplantation of frozen islets and found that recovery from the diabetes took much longer than in recipients of fresh islets.

Sandler and Andersson (1982a,d) have assessed the effect of DMSO on pancreatic islet β cell function *in vitro* and found that a 1-M but not 0.25-M concentration decreased glucose-stimulated insulin and protein biosynthesis. They have applied these principles to preserve mouse pancreatic islets successfully at −196°C, followed by thawing and tissue culture for 1 week before intrasplenic transplantation to diabetic mice (Sandler and Andersson, 1980).

Payne *et al.* (1978) used a protocol similar to that of Rajotte *et al.* (1981) to freeze neonatal rat pancreatic fragments to −70°C. Fragments were thawed at room temperature, dispersed by collagenase digestion, and transplanted intraportally to syngeneic diabetic rats. Only half of the rats receiving no further treatment were ameliorated of diabetes, but 12 of 13 rats treated with insulin for 1–2 weeks became permanently normoglycemic. These results suggest that freeze–thaw-induced injury is compounded by the diabetic state, but that the injury is reversible if the effect of diabetes is blunted by temporary administration of insulin.

There is very limited experience with cryopreservation of islets prepared from large-animal pancreases. Toledo-Pereyra *et al.* (1981a,b) cooled dispersed canine pancreatic islet tissue in 1.5 M DMSO to −196°C. The tissue was either thawed immediately or after 24 hr of storage and then transplanted to the spleen of totally pancreatectomized immunosuppressed allogeneic dogs. Diabetes was temporarily ameliorated in some recipients. The difficulties with interpretation of results in the canine pancreatic islet allograft model require that these experiments be repeated by independent investigations in an autograft model before the validity is accepted.

In summary, standard cryogenic techniques, appropriately modified, allow rat or mouse islets to be preserved before transplantation. Human fetal pancreatic fragments have been evaluated by *in vitro* studies after freezing and thawing (Brown *et al.*, 1980; Sandler *et al.*, 1981), but more work needs to be done in large animal models to assess the reliability of the cryopreservation techniques for possible clinical application.

Some efforts along these lines, as well as further refinements in cryopreservation of islets before transplantation in the rodents, were the subjects of a special symposium of the Society for Cryobiology, the proceedings of which were published in the June, 1983, issue of *Cryobiology*.

4. Transplantation after Preservation of Intact Pancreas

Recent work has shown that pancreas grafts can be reliably preserved by either cold storage or pulsatile perfusion for up to at least 24 hr. It would thus be reasonable to expect that viable islets could also be isolated from preserved pancreases for transplantation. Surprisingly, there is only one report of an attempt to apply this principle (Toledo-Pereyra *et al.*, 1980a). In this experiment, the entire pancreas was removed from dogs and subjected to hypothermic pulsatile perfusion. Six of 10 dogs receiving 24-hr perfused islet cells and 4 of 10 receiving 48-hr perfused islets cells became normoglycemic after intrasplenic autotransplantation. The success rate is similar to that achieved with segmental pancreas transplantation alone using hypothermic pulsatile perfusion. Again, independent confirmation of these observations is needed.

IV. EFFECT OF TRANSPLANTATION ON SECONDARY LESIONS IN EXPERIMENTAL DIABETES

One of the most exciting aspects of experimental pancreas and islet transplantation has been the demonstration that the renal and other lesions associated with induced diabetes in animals are secondary to the diabetic state and the finding that early, but established, lesions either regress or stabilize following correction of the metabolic abnormalities by transplantation.

The renal lesions that develop in diabetic animals are similar, in some respects, to those associated with diabetes in humans (Steer-Olson *et al.*, 1966; Mauer *et al.*, 1972; 1981). In rats with streptozotocin- or alloxan-induced diabetes urinary albumin excretion increases, there is a progressive increase in mesangial matrix volume and in basement membrane thickness, tubular vacuolization and hyalinization of arterioles are present, and immunoglobulin and other macromolecules are deposited within the mesangium, a process that is accelerated by unilateral nephrectomy (see review by Mauer *et al.*, 1981). Lee *et al.* (1974) provided proof that these lesions are not a direct result of the agent inducing diabetes, but are truly secondary to the abnormal metabolic environment to which the kidney is exposed. Kidneys transplanted from normal rats to diabetic rats developed lesions identical to those occurring in the diabetic recipient's own kidneys; conversely, lesions in diabetic rats kidneys disappeared or failed to progress after transplantation to normal rats (Lee *et al.*, 1974). The secondary nature of those lesions has also been inferred by their failure to develop in rats or mice receiving pancreas (Weil *et al.*, 1975; Bell *et al.*, 1980) or islet (Mauer *et al.*, 1974; Gray and Watkins, 1976; Slater *et al.*, 1978; Howard *et al.*, 1979; Weber *et al.*, 1979, 1980a; Federlin and Bretzel, 1980; Mandel *et al.*, 1981a) transplants soon after the induction of diabetes.

The influence of islet transplantation on established renal glomerular lesions has been shown in a series of experiments in diabetic rats by Mauer *et al.* (1974, 1975, 1978) and Steffes *et al.* (1979, 1980, 1982). After islet transplantation to rats with diabetes of more than 6 months' duration, light microscopic lesions present at the time of transplantation either failed to progress or there was an actual decrease in mesangial matrix material (Mauer *et al.*, 1974). Immunoglobulin and complement progressively disappeared (Mauer *et al.*, 1975) as the metabolic abnormalities were corrected (Mauer *et al.*, 1978), while in untreated diabetic rats, the renal lesions continued to progress. Quantitative electron microscopic morphometric studies confirmed that the increased glomerular and mesangial matrix and cellular volume in rats with diabetes of 9 months' duration decreased after successful islet transplantation (Steffes *et al.*, 1980). The increased proportion of glomerular capillary surface and glomerular basement membrane–epithelium interface juxtaposed to the mesangium also declined after transplantation. In separate experiments (Steffes *et al.*, 1979), the increase in basement membrane thickness in rats 7 months after induction of diabetes did not decline over a 6-month observation period after islet transplantation. Failure to reverse this, but not other morphologic lesions, may be due to the slow turnover of basement membrane in rats. However, the basement membrane lesion may be relatively unimportant, since Mauer *et al.* (1978) found that the urinary albumin excretion rate declines to normal following amelioration of long-standing diabetes by islet transplantation, even though mesangial, but not basement membrane, thickness declined. Gotzsche *et al.* (1981) also found that glomerular basement membrane accumulation was irreversible even though the renal hypertrophy of experimental diabetes in rats regressed following successful islet transplant. Interestingly, in uninephrectomized rats, a maneuver which accelerates the development of both functional and morphological changes of diabetic nephropathy, Steffes *et al.* (1982) found that even the increase in mesangial cellular and matrix volumes did not decline by 2 months after transplantation, although IgG deposits and albumin did decrease, reinforcing the dichotomy between basement membrane thickness and this functional parameter. The experiments of Steffes *et al.* (1982) also support the concept that the hemodynamic state of the glomerulus influences the rate at which diabetic glomerular lesions develop, and suggest that more advanced diabetic glomerulopathy in rats is resistant to reversal by successful islet transplantation.

Quantitative studies of glomerular lesions in rats with diabetes of 3–6 months' duration have also been performed by Bretzel *et al.* (1979) and Federlin and Bretzel (1981). Four months after islet transplantation there was a reduction of mesangial space, absence of IgG, and a decrease in complement deposition in the mesangium; a rewidening of the capillary lumen; and a decrease in the proportion of abnormal glomeruli. These results are consistent with those of Koesters *et al.* (1977) who found that islet transplantation in diabetic rats restored phagocytic and clearance function of mesangial cells. Functional studies by Bretzel *et al.* (1981d) showed a return of increased urinary alanine aminopeptidase excretion rates to normal following correction of diabetes by islet transplantation, and the results correlated with reduction of periodic-acid-Schiff-positive material in renal tubules. The increased renal glucosyltransferase activity in diabetic rats also decreases to normal following correction of hyperglycemia by islet transplantation (Bretzel *et al.*, 1981b). The serum levels of 7-S collagen and laminin P-2 decreased as well (Bretzel *et al.*, 1982).

There are a few reports on the effect of islet transplantation on the nerve (Orloff *et al.*, 1975; Macedo *et al.*, 1981; Schmidt and Sharp, 1982; Schmidt *et al.*, 1983) and eye (Gray *et al.*, 1976; Worthen *et al.*, 1976; Krupin *et al.*, 1979) lesions that develop in diabetic rats. Gray *et al.* (1976) found that new vessel formation and retinal capillary dilation did not develop in rats transplanted within a month of induction of diabetes. Worthen *et al.* (1976) obtained very similar results in rats treated with whole-pancreas transplantation soon after the induction of diabetes. Actual regression of eye pathology in diabetic rats was shown by Krupin *et al.* (1979) using ocular fluorophotometry. In diabetic rats, fluorescein accumulation in the vitreous and anterior chamber was twice-normal 1 hr after injection. Two weeks after islet transplantation the integrity of the blood–ocular barrier was restored and the values returned to baseline.

In regard to nerve lesions, Macedo *et al.* (1981) found that diabetic rats developed glucogen deposits in the axons on the sciatic nerve, but that depositions could be prevented by pancreas transplantation performed within a week of induction of diabetes. On the other hand, Schmidt and Sharp (1982) and Schmidt *et al.* (1983) were not able to identify lesions in the peripheral nerve of diabetic rats, but did find autonomic neuropathy of unmyelinated axons of the extrinsic innervation of the small bowel. This is a possible explanation for the dilated alimentary track observed in diabetic rats. Schmidt and Sharp (1982) and Schmidt *et al.* (1983) showed that the lesions were not secondary to streptozotocin since their development was prevented by islet transplantation soon after induction of diabetes. However, they also showed that after 6 months of diabetes, when the iliomesentery nerves showed marked dilation of both axons and subcellular organelles, the lesions were reversed within 3 months of restoration of normoglycemia by islet transplantation. The reversal of diabetes was also associated with restoration of a normal bowel pattern.

A variety of other abnormalities can be demonstrated in animals with experimental diabetes and the effect of islet transplantation on some of these has been studied. For example, Korec (1981) observed that the high incidence of fetal abnormalities seen in the offspring of female diabetic rats was reduced following correction of diabetes by islet transplantation, but effect was not completely abolished until after two generations, suggesting that streptozotocin also played a role in their generation. Noack *et al.* (1982) performed studies of pregnant rats cured of streptozotocin-induced diabetes by islet transplantation. Islet transplantation did not completely restore the increased insulin release that occurs during pregnancy, but glucose homeostasis was maintained and the islet transplantation was sufficient to compensate for the additional needs during pregnancy. Finally, alterations in immune function have been observed in mice with streptozotocin-induced diabetes, and these are also corrected by islet cell transplantation (Handwerger *et al.*, in press).

In summary, the secondary nature of renal, neural, and eye, as well as other lesions, in experimental diabetes is well established. The demonstration that pancreas and islet transplantation can stabilize or induce regression of early lesions provides an impetus and a rational basis for pursuing such an approach in humans.

V. CLINICAL TRANSPLANTATION: A BRIEF SUMMARY

An International Human Pancreas and Islet Transplant Registry was organized a few years ago (Sutherland, 1980) to supercede the defunct ACS/NIH Organ Transplant Registry. As of November, 1982, the Registry had information on 247 pancreas transplants performed in 231 diabetic patients since 1966. Interest in the application of pancreas transplantation has increased in recent years (Sutherland, 1982). One hundred eighty-seven of the transplants were reported to the Registry between July, 1977, and November 20, 1982, 54 in 1981, and 57 in 1982. Forty-three patients currently have functioning pancreas grafts and are insulin-independent, 17 for greater than 1 year, the longest for 4.5 years.

Although islet transplantation remains an area of intense experimental activity, as summarized in this chapter, only three clinical attempts at islet allotransplantation have been reported to the Registry since 1980 (Sutherland, 1983). All 3 were unsuccessful, and of the 76 cases included in the Registry data there are only 4 in which the recipients were able to survive without exogenous insulin after transplantation (Sutherland, 1981b). Only one of these cases was documented as a Type 1 insulin-dependent diabetic pretransplant, and none were insulin-independent as of November, 1982 (Sutherland, 1982). All of the islet allotransplantation attempts to date have been made using relatively unsophisticated techniques and the recent innovations in experimental islet allotransplantation reviewed here have not yet been applied clinically.

Although the success rate of clinical pancreas transplantation is much lower than that of kidney transplantation, the results are improving. Technical advances are partially responsible. Pancreaticoduodenal transplants are no longer done (Lillehei et al., 1970), and 186 of the transplants performed since 1977 have either been of whole (seven cases) or segmental pancreas. The pancreatic exocrine secretions present the major technical problem, and various methods for treatment of the pancreatic duct have been employed.

Of the pancreas transplants performed since 1977, 0 of 2 with ductocystostomy, 1 of 2 with ductoureterostomy (3 months), 0 of 9 with duct ligation, 3 of 16 with open duct into the peritoneal cavity (36–52 months), 11 of 38 with pancreaticoenterostomy (1–15 months), and 28 of 119 with polymer injection into the pancreatic duct (1–39 months) are functioning. Better patient selection has also contributed to the improved results, even though most of the recipients have still had diabetic nephropathy and far-advanced lesions of diabetes mellitus. Of the pancreases transplanted since 1977, 22 of 84 performed simultaneous with, 13 of 51 after, 0 of 2 before, and 8 of 49 not associated with kidney transplants are currently functioning. Even though the pancreas graft survival rate is approximately the same for those done simultaneously or subsequent to a kidney transplant, the patient survival is much higher in those who have had a pancreas transplant performed subsequent to rather than simultaneous with a kidney transplant (Sutherland, 1982). Of the 177 patients who have received pancreas transplants since July 1, 1977, 30 (17%) died within the first 3 months, but 124 (70%) were alive as of November, 1982.

Another factor that may be responsible for the improvement of results of pancreas transplantation is advances in immunosuppression. Of the pancreas allograft performed since July 1, 1977, 24 of 68 treated with cyclosporine A (35%) and 19 of 116 treated with azathioprine and other conventional agents (16%) are functioning.

Only a few institutions have active pancreas transplant programs, including the University of Zurich (Baumgartner et al., 1983), Cambridge (McMaster et al., 1982; Calne and White, 1982), Stockholm (Groth et al., 1982), Lyon, France (Dubernard et al., 1983), and the University of Minnesota (Sutherland et al., 1982, 1983). The University of Minnesota has the largest experience, with 75 total cases of pancreas transplantation. Nineteen of 56 Minnesota recipients of pancreas grafts since 1977 have functioning grafts and are insulin-independent, the longest for 4.5 years, and histological lesions of diabetic nephropathy in a previous transplant kidney have regressed in the latter patient (observations by Mauer and Steffes).

Pancreas transplantation has gradually become safer and more frequently successful, but further improvements in techniques and advances in immunosuppression are needed. The current role of pancreas transplantation is in the treatment of patients whose complications of diabetes are, or predictably will be, more serious than the potential side effects of chronic immunosuppression.

VI. SUMMARY AND PROSPECTS

Current evidence favors the concept that the secondary complications of diabetes will be prevented or their progression halted if homeostatic control of carbohydrate metabolism can be provided, ideally by functioning islet tissue. Pancreas and islet transplantation have achieved this objective in animals.

The experimental studies reviewed in this chapter show the potential for both pancreas and islet tranplantation to achieve these objectives. There are relative advantages and disadvantages to both approaches. Currently, pancreas transplantation is more efficient since only one donor is required. Islet transplantation in most experimental models, requires multiple donors, although more efficient techniques of islet preparation are being developed and the potential exists for one pancreas to be the source of islets for more than one recipient.

Islet isolation is a complicated procedure, and pancreas transplantation is much simpler for the transplant team. Nevertheless, islet transplantation is a smaller operation for the recipient.

Pancreas grafts appear to be less susceptible to rejection, while islets are very sensitive to rejection effector mechanisms. On the other hand, islets do not appear to be very immunogenic and islets can also be manipulated *in vitro* to reduce immunogenicity before transplantation. The current techniques of islet isolation and *in vitro* treatment are impractical for clinical application, but the fact that generalized immunosuppression is currently needed to prevent pancreas rejection provides a strong stimulus to pursue the approach of islet allograft pretreatment. However, pancreas transplantation is currently clinically applicable and successful, while clinical attempts at islet transplantation have failed and the latter procedure is currently only experimental.

We are optimistic that the immunological and oither problems associated with both pancreas and islet transplantation will be solved and that pancreas and islet transplantation ultimately will be applied to diabetic patients before the development of end-stage complications. Methods will then be needed to identify patients whose diabetes cannot be adequately controlled by exogenous insulin and who are at high risk to develop secondary complications. Rosenbloom *et al.* (1981) found that certain features, such as limited joint mobility in childhood, are predictive in this regard.

An adequate number of donors for the diabetic patients who could potentially benefit from pancreas transplantation should be available. Approximately 5000 kidney transplants are done per year in the United States. The incidence of new cases of Type 1 diabetes in the United States is approximately 10,000 per year, of which less than half develop serious complications (West, 1978). Only a small proportion of potential donors is currently used (Bart *et al.*, 1981), but there are no inherent reasons why procurement of other organs should be any different than procurement of kidneys for transplantation. A sufficient number of pancreases should be available for the patients who are most likely to benefit from pancreas or islet transplantation.

ACKNOWLEDGMENTS.   Appreciation is expressed to Janet Sanders for preparation of this manuscript.

REFERENCES

Abri, O., Wolff, H., Lorenz, D., Lippert, H., Kuhn, F., and Corfei, G., 1982, Endocrine function and histology of allogeneic pancreatic segmental grafts after duct occlusion (Ethibloc or neoprene) in comparison with open-duct technique, *Eur. Surg. Res.* **14**:130–131.

Acquino, C., Ruiz, J. O., Schultz, L. S., and Lillehei, R. D., 1973, Pancreatic transplantation without the duodenum in the dog, *Am. J. Surg.* **125**:240–244.

Agnes, S., Castagneto, M., and Castiglioni, G. C., 1980, Segmental pancreatic transplantation in the pig: Comparative study of different techniques, *Transplant. Proc.* **12**(Suppl. 2):129–134.

Agostino, M., Prowse, S. J., and Lafferty, K. J., 1982, Resistance of established islet allografts to rejection by antibody and complement, *Aust. J. Exp. Biol. Med. Sci.* **60**(Pt. 2):219–222.

Alejandro, R., Rabinovitch, A., Severyn, W., Hajek, S., Miller, J., and Mintz, D. A., 1982a, Expression of DR antigens on human islets, *Diabetes* **3**(Suppl. 2):65A.

Alejandro, R., Shienvold, F. L., Hajek, S. V., Ryan, U., Miller J., and Mintz, D. H., 1982b, Immunocytochemical localization of HLA-DR in human islets of Langerhans, *Diabetes* **31**(Suppl. 4):17–22.

Altman, J. J., Houlbert, D., Bruzzo, F., Desplanque, N., Manonx, A., and Galletti, P., 1982, Implantation of semi-permeable hollow fibers to prevent immune rejection of transplanted pancreatic islets, *Horm. Metab. Res.* **12**(Suppl.):43–44.

Amamoo, D. G., Woods, J. E., Halley, K. E., 1975, Effect of intrahepatically implanted islets of Langerhans on hepatic function in the rat, *Mayo Clin. Proc.* **50**:416–419.

Andersson, A., 1979, Islet implantation normalizes hyperglycemia caused by streptozotocin induced insulin, *Lancet* **1**:581–584.

Andersson, A., 1982, Reversal of hyperglycemia by intrasplenic transplantation of 4-week-cultured allogeneic mouse islets, *Diabetes* **15**(Suppl. 4):55–59.

Andersson, A., and Buschard, F., 1977, Culture of isolated pancreatic islets: Its application for transplantation purposes, *Trans. Am. Soc. Artif. Intern. Organs* **23**:342–345.

Andersson, A., Eriksson, U., Petersson, B., Reibring, L., and Swenne, I., 1981, Failure of successful intrasplenic transplantation of islets from lean mice to cure obese-hyperglycaemic mice, despite islet growth, *Diabetologia* **20**:237–241.

Araki, Y., Yoshida, T., Watanabe, A., Kanda, T., Inui, R., Yamamoto, M., Yoshioka, K., and Kondo, M., 1979, Pancreatic islet allotransplantation in the total pancreatectomized dog, *J. Kyoto Pref. Univ. Med.* **88**:541–552.

Araki, Y., Inoue, Y., Yoshioka, K., Nakamura, Y., Yoshida, T., and Kondo, M. 1980, Normalization of blood glucose in totally pancreatectomized dogs by use of pancreatic chambers, *Endocrinol. Jpn.* **27**(2):157–161.

Archer, J., Kaye, R., and Mutter, G., 1980, Control of streptozotocin diabetes in Chinese hamsters by cultured mouse islet cells without immunosuppression: A preliminary report, *J. Surg. Res.* **28**:77–85.

Ashida, E. R., Johnson, A. R., and Lipsky, P. E., 1981, Human endothelial cell-lymphocyte interaction: endothelial cells functioning as accessory cells necessary for mitogen induced human T-lymphocyte activity *in vitro*, *J. Clin. Invest.* **67**:1490–1491.

Axen, K. V., and Pi-Sunyer, F. X., 1981, Long-term reversal of streptozotocin-induced diabetes in rats by intramuscular islet implantation, *Transplantation* **31**:439–441.

Baekkeskov, S., Lernmark, A., and Klareskog, L., 1980, Presence of transplantation antigens in pancreatic islets, *Diabetologia* **19**:255, 1980.

Baekkeskov, S., Kanatsuna, T., Klareskog, L., Nielsen, D. A., Peterson, P. A., Rubenstein, A. H., Steiner, D. F., and Lernmark, A., 1981, Expression of major histocompatibility antigens on pancreatic islet cells, *Proc. Natl. Acad. Sci. USA* **78**:6456–6460.

Ballinger, W. F., and Lacy, P. E., 1972, Transplantation of intact pancreatic islets in rats, *Surgery* **72**:175–186.

Bank, H. L., A high yield method for isolating rat islets of Langerhans using differential sensitivity to freezing, *Cryobiology* **20**:237–244.

Bank, H. L., and Reichard, L., 1981, Cryogenic preservation of isolated islets of Langerhans: Two step cooling, *Diabetologia* **18**:489–496.

Bank, H. L., Davis, R. F., and Emerson, D., 1979, Cryogenic preservation of isolated rat islets of Langerhans: Effect of colling and warming rates, *Diabetologia* **16**:195–199.

Banks, I. G., Sloan, J. M., and Buchanan, K. D., 1981, A histological study of intrasplenic transplanted neonatal rat pancreas and of adjacent adipose tissue proliferation, *Diabetologia* **22**:128–133.

Barker, C. F., Reckard, C. K., Ziegler, M. M., Naji, A., 1975, The liver as an immunologically privileged site for rat pancreatic islet allografts. *Diabetes* **24** (Suppl. 2):418.

Barker, C. F., Frangipane, L. G., Silvers, W. K., 1977, Islet transplantation in genetically determined diabetes, *Ann. Surg.,* **186**:401–410.

Barker, C. F., Naji, A., Silvers, W. K., 1980, Immunologic problems in islet transplantation, *Diabetes* **29**(Suppl. 1):86–92.

Barker, C. F., Naji, A., Perloff, L. J., Dafoe, D. C., and Bartlett, S., 1982a, Invited commentary: An overview of pancreas transplantation—biologic aspects, *Surgery* **92**:133–137.

Barker, C. F., Naji, A., Perloff, L. J., Dafoe, D. C., and Bartlett, S., 1982b, Animal models of diabetes and immunological problems with islet allografts, Trans. *Am. Soc. Artif. Intern. Organs* **28**:691–699.

Bart, K. J., Macon, E. J., Whittier, F. C., Baldwin, P. J., and Blaunt, J. H., 1981, Cadaveric kidneys for transplantation: A paradox of shortage in the face of plenty, *Transplantation* **31**:379–382.

Bastert, G., Eichholz, H., Usadel, K. H., Althoff, P. H., Schwedes, U., Steinau, U., Klempa, I., and Fortmeyer, H. P., 1981, Xenografts of benign and malignant endocrine tissues in thymusaplastic nude mice and rats: Development and function, in: *Thymus-Aplastic Nude Mice and Rats in Clinical Oncology,* (G. B. A. Bastert, ed.), pp. 383–407. Gustav Fischer Verlag, Stuttgart, New York.

Baumgartner, D., Sutherland, D. E. R., Heil, J., Hustad, J., and Najarian, J. S., 1980a, Effect of systemic venous drainage and denervation of the pancreas on glucose tolerance after partial pancreatectomy in dogs, *Diabetes* **29**(Suppl. 2):19A.

Baumgartner, D., Sutherland, D. E. R., Heil, J., Zweber, B., Awad, E. A., and Najarian, J. S., 1980b, Machine preservation of canine segmental grafts, *Surg. Forum* **31**:352–354.

Baumgartner, D., Sutherland, D. E. R., Heil, J. E., and Najarian, J. S., 1980c, Cold storage of segmental canine pancreatic grafts for 24 hours, *J. Surg. Res.* **29**:248–257.

Baumgartner, D., Sutherland, D. E. R., and Najarian, J. S., 1980d, Studies on segmental autotransplantation in dogs, *Transplant. Proc.* **12**(No. 4, Suppl. 2):163–171.

Baumgartner, D., Sutherland, D. E. R., Heil, J. E., and Najarian, J. S., 1981, Long-term canine seegmental pancreas transplants with the duct left open, neoprene injected duct and pancreaticoureterostomy: A comparative study, *Transplant. Proc.* **13**(1):163–171.

Baumgartner, D., Largiader, F., Uhlschmid, G., and Binswanger, U., 1983, Rejection episodes in recipients of simultaneous pancreas and kidney transplants, *Transplant. Proc.* **15**(1):1330–1331.

Bell, P. R. F., Wood, R. F. M., Peters, M., and Nash, J. R., 1980, Comparison of various methods of chemical immunosuppression in islet cell transplantation, *Transplant. Proc.* **12**:241–243.

Bell, R. N., Fernandez-Cruz, L., Brimm, J. E., Sayers, H., and Orloff, M. J., 1980, Prevention of glomerular basement membrane thickening in alloxan-diabetes, *Surgery* **88**:31–40.

Bellgran, D., Naji, A., Silvers, W. K., Markmann, J. F., and Barker, C. F., 1982, Spontaneous diabetes in BB rats: Evidence for T-cell defect, *Diabetologia* **23**:359–364.

Berlatsky, Y., Munda, R., Jonung, M., Murphy, R. F., Brackett, K., Joffe, S. N., and Alexander, J. W., 1982, Hormonal and metabolic effects of vascularized segmental pancreatic autotransplants, *Eur. Soc. Surg. Res.* **14**:129–131.

Berthoud, H. R., Trimble, E. R., Siegel, E. G., Bereiter, D. A., and Jeanrenaud, B., 1980, Cephalic phase insulin secretion in normal and pancreatic islet-transplanted rats, *Am. J. Physiol.* **238**:E36–E340.

Bewick, M., 1976, Pancreatic allotransplantation in dogs and its relevance to the treatment of diabetes mellitus in man. Thesis, M. Chir., University of Cambridge.

Bewick, M., Mundy, A. R., Eaton, B., and Watson, F., 1981a, The endocrine function of the heterotopic pancreatic allotransplant in dogs: I. The immediate posttransplant period, *Transplantation* 31:19–22.

Bewick, M., Mundy, A. R., Eaton, B., and Watson, F., 1981c, The endocrine function of the heterotopic pancreatic allotransplant in dogs: II. The cause of hyperinsulinema, *Transplantation* 31:23–25.

Bewick, M., Mundy, A. R., Eaton, B., and Watson, F., 1981b, The endocrine function of the heterotopic pancreatic allotransplant in dogs: III. Normal and rejection, *Transplantation* 31:15–18.

Bewick, M., Gonzales-Carello, M., Argoustis, A., Miller, B. H. R., Compton, F. J., and Eaton, B., 1983, Canine pancreatic endocrine function after interruption of pancreatic exocrine drainage, *Transplantation*, 36:246–251.

Beyer, M. M., and Friedman, E. A., 1979, Histocompatibility-dependent long-term islets of Langerhans survival induced by antithymocyte globulin, *Transplant. Proc.* 11:1436–1439.

Beyer, M. M., Lane, F. C., and Friedman, E. A., 1981, Dissociation of skin and islet allograft rejection in antithymocyte globulin treated rats, *Transplant. Proc.* 13:815–818.

Bitter-Suermann, J., and Save-Soderberg, J., 1978, The course of pancreas allografts in rats conditioned by spleen allografts, *Transplantation* 26:28–34.

Bitter-Suermann, H., Brynger, H., Wikstrom, I., Gabel, H., Save-Soderberg, J. S., and Gelin, L. E., 1979, A new technique of orthotopic en bloc transplantation of the porcine liver and duct ligated pancreas, *J. Surg. Res.* 27:105–113.

Blanc-Brunat, N., Dubernard, J. M., Touraine, J. L., Neyra, P., Dubois, P., Paulin, C., and Traeger, J., Pathology of the pancreas after intraductal neoprene injection in dogs and diabetic patients treated by pancreatic transplantation, *Diabetologia* in press.

Bobzien, B., Yasunami, Y., Majercik, M., Lacy, P. E., and Davie, J. M., 1983, Intratesticular transplants of islet xenografts (rat to mouse), *Diabetes* 32:213–216.

Bowen, K. M., and Lafferty, K. J., 1980, Reversal of diabetes by allogeneic islet transplantation without immunosuppression, *Aus. J. Exp. Biol. Med.* 58:441–447.

Bowen, K. M., Andrus, L., and Lafferty, K. J., 1980, Successful allotransplantation of mouse pancreatic islets to nonimmunosuppressed recipients, *Diabetes* 29(Suppl. 2):98–104.

Bowen, K. M., Prowse, S. J., and Lafferty, K. J., 1981, Reversal of diabetes by islet transplantation: Vulnerability of the established allograft, *Science* 213:1261–1262.

Brekke, I. B., Gullesen, F., Refsum, S. B., and Flotmark, A., 1980a, Long-term endocrine function of duct-ligated pancreatic allografts in rats, *Eur. Surg. Res.* 12:167–178.

Brekke, I. B., Hostmark, A. T., and Flaten, O., 1980b, Long-term effect of heterotopic pancreas transplantation on plasma lipids in diabetic rats, *Transplant. Proc.* 12(Suppl. 2):154–156.

Brekke, I. B., Oyasaeter, S., and Vidnes, J., 1982, Long-term effect of pancreas transplantation on diabetic hyperglucagonemia, *Eur. Surg. Res.* 14:211–220.

Bretzel, R. G., Breidenbach, C., Hoffman, J., Schwemmle, K., Pfeiffer, E. F., and Federlin, K. I., 1979, Islet transplantation in experimental diabetes of the rat. III. Role of regulation in diabetic kidney lesions after isogeneic islet transplantation: Quantitative measurements, *Horm. Metab. Res.* 11:200–207.

Bretzel, R. G., Merforth, K., Leferink, H., Beule, B., and Federlin, K., 1980a, Morphological and functional restoration of cryopreserved islets in vitro culture, *Diabetologia* 19:254.

Bretzel, R. G., Schneider, J., Dobroschke, J., and Kederlin, K., 1980b, Islet transplantation in experimental diabetes of the rat VII. Cryopreservation of rat and human islets. Preliminary report, *Horm. Metab. Res.* 12:274–275.

Bretzel, R. G., Beule, B., and Federlin, K., 1981a, Function and morphology of adult rat islets after culture and transplantation, in: *Islet Isolation, Culture, and Preservation* (K. Federlin and R. G. Bretzel, eds.), pp. 96–110, Thieme-Stratton, New York.

Bretzel, R. G., Menden, A., Richardt, M., Brocks, D. G., Draeger, K. E., and Federlin, K., 1981b, Renal collagen glycosyltransferase activity following islet transplantation in streptozotocin-diabetic rats, *Diabetologia* 21:428–429.

Bretzel, R. G., Schneider, J., Zekorn, T., and Federlin, K., 1981c, Cryopreservation of rat, porcine and human pancreatic islets for transplantation, in: *Islet Isol., Cul. and Cryopres.* (K. Federlin and R. C. Bretzel, eds.), pp. 152–160, Thieme Stratton, New York.

Bretzel, R. G., Schneider, J., Zimmerman, I., Kuppers, B., Weise, M., and Federlin, K., 1981d, Urinary excretion of alanine aminopeptidase and total proteinuria in experimental diabeties mellitus before and after islet transplantation, *Contrib. Nephrol.* **24**:153–164.

Bretzel, R. G., Lefesmk, K. H., Timpl, R., and Federlin, K., 1982, Serum levels of basement fragments in diabetic and islet transplanted rats: New markers of diabetic microangiopathy? *Diabetes* **31**(Suppl. 2):11a.

Britt, L. D., and Scharp, D. W., 1980, Formation of pseudo-islets from neonatal pig pancreas, *Surg. Forum* **31**:359–360.

Britt, L. D., Stojeba, P. C., Scharp, C. R., Greider, M. H., and Scharp, D. W., 1981, Neonatal pig pseudo-islets: A product of selective aggregation, *Diabetes* **30**:580–583.

Britt, L. D., Scharp, D. W., Lacy, P. E., and Slavin, S., 1982, Transplantation of islet cells across major histocompatibility barriers after total lymphoid irradiation and infusion of allogeneic bone marrow cells, *Diabetes* **15**(Suppl. 4):63–68.

Broe, P. J., Zuidema, G. D., and Cameron, J. L., 1982, The role of ischemia in acute pancreatitis: Studies with an isolated perfused canine pancreas, *Surgery* **91**:337–382.

Brooks, J. R., and Gifford, G. H., 1959, Pancreatic homotransplantation, *Transplant. Bull.* **6**:100–103.

Brown, J., Clark, W. R., Molnar, G., and Mullen, Y. S., 1976, Fetal pancreas transplantation for reversal of streptozotocin-induced diabetes in rats, *Diabetes* **25**:56–64.

Brown, J., Clark, W. R., Makoff, R. K., Weisman, H., Kemp, J. A., and Mullen, Y., 1978, Pancreas transplantation for diabetes mellitus, *Ann. Intern. Med.* **89**:951–965.

Brown, J., Muller, Y., Clark, W. I., and Molnar, I. G., 1979, Importance of hepatic portal circulation for insulin action in streptozotocin-diabetic rats transplanted with fetal pancreases, *J. Clin. Invest.* **64**:1688–1694.

Brown, J., Kemp, J. A., Hurt, S., and Clark, W. R., 1980, Cryopreservation of human fetal pancreas, *Diabetes* **29**(Suppl. 1):70–73.

Brown, J., Heininger, D., Kuret, J., and Mullen, Y., 1981, Islet cells grow after transplantation of fetal pancreas and control of diabetes, *Diabetes* **30**:9–13.

Brown, J., Heininger, D., Kuret, J., and Mullen, Y., 1982, Normal response to pregnancy in rats cured of streptozotocin diabetes by transplantation of one fetal pancreas, *Diabetologia* **22**:273–275.

Brownlee, M., and Cahill, G. F., 1979, Diabetic control and vascular complications, in: *Atherosclerosis Reviews*, Vol. 4 (R. Paoletti, and A. M. Gatto, eds.), pp. 29–70, Raven Press, New York.

Brundstedt, J., 1980, Rapid isolation of functionally intact pancreatic islets from mice and rats by Percoll® gradient centrifugation, *Diab. Metab.* **6**:87.

Brynger, H., 1975, Twenty-four-hour preservation of the duct ligated canine pancreatic allograft, *Eur. Surg. Res.* **7**:341–354.

Brynger, H., Bermark, J., and Claes, G., 1975, The function of the duct ligated pancreatic allograft, *Eur. Surg. Res.* **7**:212–229.

Brynger, H., Mjornstedt, L., and Olausson, M., 1980, Heterotopic grafting of pancreas to the neck in the rat—An experimental model, *Transplant. Proc.* **12**(Suppl. 2):148–149.

Buitrago, A., Gylfe, E., Henriksson, C., and Pertoft, H., 1977, Rapid isolation of pancreatic islets from collagenase digested pancreas by sedimentation through Percoll® at unit gravity. *Biochem. Biophys. Res. Commun.* **79**:823–828.

Buschard, K., 1975, Cultivation of islets of Langerhans in Millipore chamber in vivo, *Horm. Metab. Res.* **7**:441–442.

Butcher, G. H., and Howard, J. C., 1982, Genetic control of transplant rejection, *Transplantation* **34**:161–166.

Calne, R. Y., and White, D. J. G., 1982, The use of cyclosporine in clinical organ grafting, *Ann. Surg.* **196**:330–337.

Calne, R. Y., McMaster, P., Rolles, K., and Duffy, T. J., 1980, Technical observations in segmental allografting: Observations on pancreatic blood flow, *Transplant. Proc.* **12**(Suppl. 2):51–57.

Castellanos, J., Manifacio, G., Toledo-Pereyra, L. H., Shatney, C. H., and Lillehei, R. C., 1975, Consistent protection from pancreatitis in canine pancreas allografts treated with 5-fluorouracil, *J. Surg. Res.* **19**:305–311.

Champault, G., Michel, F., Callard, P., Garnier, M., Legoult, J., Soulier, Y., Burnichon, J., Mannoux, A., and Patel, J. C., 1978, Transplantation pancreatique: Implantation d'auto et d'allogreffes pancreatiques dans la paroi gastrique du lapin diabetique, *J. Chir. (Paris)* 115(4):233–242.

Chen, Y., Mason, N. S., Scharp, D. W., Ballinger, W. F., and Sparks, R. E., Collagenase immobilized on millipore membranes, in: *Symposium on Morphology, Structural and Interactions of Biomaterials,* in press.

Chiba, T., Taminato, T., Kadowaki, S., Chihara, K., Matsukura, S., Nozawa, M., Seino, Y., and Fujita, T., 1981, Reversal of increased gastric somatostatin in streptozotocin-diabetic rats by whole pancreas transplantation, *Diabetes* 30:724–727.

Chick, W. L., Perris, J. J., Lauris, V., Low, D., Callett, P. M., Panol, G., Whittemore, A. D., Like, A. L., Cotton, C. K., and Lysaght, M. J., 1977a, Artificial pancreas using living beta cells: Effect on glucose homeostasis in diabetic rats, *Science* 197:780–782.

Chick, W. L., Warren, S., Chute, R. N., Like, A. A., Lauris, V., and Kitchen, K. C., 1977b, A transplantable insulinoma in the rat, *Proc. Natl. Acad. Sci. USA* 74:628–632.

Choudhury, A., 1973, The pancreas as a transplantable organ, *Ann. R. Coll. Surg.* 53:218–236.

Cobb, L., Horaguchi, A., and Merrell, R., 1982, Canine islet isolation in ethionine pancreatitis, *Surg. Forum* 33:356–358.

Coleman, D. L., 1978, Obese and diabetes: Two mutant genes causing diabetes–obesity syndromes in mice, *Diabetologia* 14:141–148.

Collier, S. A., Mandel, T. E., Hoffman, L., and Caruso, G., 1981, Organ culture of fetal mouse pancreas. The effect of culture conditions on insulin and glucagon secretion, *Diabetes* 30:804–812.

Collier, S. A., Mandel, T. E., and Carter, W. M., 1982, Detrimental effect of high medium glucose concentration on subsequent endocrine function of transplanted organ-cultured foetal mouse pancreas. *Aust. J. Exp. Biol. Med. Sci.* 60(Pt. 4):437–445.

Collin, J., 1978, Current state of transplantation of the pancreas, *Ann. R. Coll. Surg.* 60:21–27.

Collin, J., Taylor, R. M. R., Johiston, I. D. A., 1980, Portal or systemic venous drainage for pancreatic transplantation? A physiological study, *Ann. R. Coll. Surg.,* 62:326.

Cook, K., Sollinger, H. W., Warner, T., and Belzer, F. O., 198X, Pancreaticocystostomy: An alternative method for exocrine drainage of segmental pancreatic allografts, *Transplantation* 35:634–636.

Cowing, C., Schwartz, B., and Dickler, H., 1978, Macrophage Ia antigens, I. Macrophage populations differ in their expression of Ia antigens, *J. Immunol.* 120:378–384.

Daar, A. S. Fuggle, S. V., Hart, D. N., Dalchau, R., Fabre, J. W., Ting, A., and Morris, P. J., 1983, Demonstration of phenotypic characterization of HLA-DR positive interstitial denditric cells widely distributed in human connective tissues, *Transplant. Proc.* 15(1):311–315.

DaFoe, D., Naji, A., and Barker, C. F., 1980, Susceptibility to diabetogeneic virus: Host versus pancreatic factors, *J. Surg. Res.* 28:338–347.

DaFoe, D., Naji, A., and Barker, C. F., 1981, Susceptibility to murine viral diabetes: Host versus intrinsic pancreatic factors, *Transplant. Proc.* 13(1):829–831.

DaFoe, D., Moore, C., Naji, A., Gadzik, J., and Barker, C., 1983, Pancreas transplantation fails to cure genetic diabetes caused by extrapancreatic factors, *Transplant. Proc.* 15:1359–1361.

Danilovs, J. A., Hofman, F. M., Taylor, C. R., and Brown, J., 1982, Expression of HLA-DR antigens in human fetal pancreas tissue, *Diabetes* 131(Suppl. 4):23–28.

DeGruyl, J., Westbroek, D. L., Diijkhuis, C. M., Vriesendorp, H. M., MacDicken, I., Elien-Geritsen, W., Verschoor, L., Hukmans, H. A. M., and Aurcher, P., 1973, Influence of DLA matching, ALS and 24 hours preservation on isolated pancreas allograft survival, *Transplant. Proc.* 5:755–759.

DeGruyl, J., Westbroek, D. L., Macdicken, I., Ridderlice, E., Verschur, L., and van Strik, X., 1977, Cryoprecipitated plasma perfusion preservation and cold storage preservation of duct-ligated pancreatic allografts, *Br. J. Surg.* 64:490–493.

DeJode, L. R., and Howard, J. M., 1962, Studies in pancreaticoduodenal homo-transplantation, *Surg. Gynecol. Obstet.* 114:553–558.

Delmonico, F. L., Chase, C. M., and Russell, P. S., 1977, Transplantation of rat islets of Langerhans into diabetic mice. *Transplant. Proc.* 9:367–369.

Devonec, M., Faure, J. L., Blanc-Brunat, N., Dubernard, J. M., and Traeger, J., 1980, Effects of pancreatic intraductal injection of a radioisotope in dogs, *Transplant. Proc.* 12(Suppl. 2):141–144.

Dickerman, R. M., Twiest, M. W., Crudup, J. W., and Turcotte, J. G., 1975, Transplantation of the pancreas into a retroperitoneal jejunal loop, *Am. J. Surg.* **129**:48–54.

Dixit, P. K., Bauer, G. E., Younoszai, R., and Hegre, O., 1982, Reversal of diabetes by the isotransplantation of nicotinamide-streptozotocin-induced islet adenoma in rats, *Transplantation* **33**:163–167.

Downing, R., Scharp, D. W., and Ballinger, W. F., 1980, An improved technique for the isolation and identification of mammalian islets of Langerhans, *Transplantation* **29**:79–83.

Dubernard, J. M., Traeger, J., Neyra, P., Touraine, J. L., Traudiant, D., and Blanc-Brunat, N., 1978, A new method of preparation of segmental pancreatic grafts for transplantation: Trials in dogs and in man, *Surgery* **84**:633–639.

Dubernard, J. M., Traeger, J., Neyra, P., Touraine, J. L., Blanc, N., and Devonec, M., 1979, Long term effect of neoprene injection in the canine pancreatic duct, *Transplant. Proc.* **11**:1448–1499.

Dubernard, J. M., Traeger, J., Pozza, G., Bosi, E., Gelet, A., Martin, X., Beutel, H., Touraine, J. L., Cardoyo, C., Da Ponte, F., Cantrovich, D., Elyafi, S., Diab, N., Sechia, A., and Pontrioli, A. E., 1983, Clinical experience with 31 pancreatic transplants in man, *Transplant. Proc.* **15**(1):1318–1321.

DuToit, D. F., Reece-Smith, H., McShane, P., Denton, T., and Morris, P. J., 1980, Intraportal embolization of fragments during intrasplenic pancreatic autotransplantation in dogs, *Transplantation* **30**:389–391.

DuToit, D. F., Reece-Smith, H., McShane, P., Denton, T., and Morris, P. J., 1981, A successful technique of segmental pancreatic autotransplantation in the dog, *Transplantation* **31**:395–396.

DuToit, D. F., Reece-Smith, H., McShane, P., Denton, T., and Morris, P. J., 1982a, Citrate flushing and 24-hour cold storage of segmental canine pancreatic autografts. *Transplantation* **33**:202–204.

DuToit, D. F., Reece-Smith, H., McShane, P., Denton, T., and Morris, P. J., 1982b, Effect of cyclosporin A on allotransplanted pancreatic fragments to the spleen of total pancreatectomized dogs, *Transplantation* **33**:302–307.

DuToit, D. F., Reece-Smith, H., McShane, P., Denton, T., and Morris, P. J., 1982c, Prolongation of segmental pancreatic allografts in dogs receiving cyclosporin A, *Transplantation* **33**:432–437.

DuToit, D. R., Heydenrych, J. J., Louw, G., Zuurmond, T., and Els, D., 1983, Intraperitoneal transplantation of vascularized segmental pancreatic autografts without duct ligation in the primate, *Surgery* **94**:471–477.

Eloy, R., Kedinger, M., Garaud, J. C., Jaffer, K., Launay, J. F., Moody, J., Clendinnen, G., Grenier, A. F., 1977, Intrahepatic transplantation of pancreatic islets in the rat. *Horm. Metab. Res.* **9**:40–46.

Eloy, R., Haffen, K., Kedinger, M., and Grenier, A. F., 1979, Chick embryo pancreatic transplants reverse experimental diabetes of rats, *J. Clin. Invest.* **64**:361–373.

Fabri, J. W., 1982, Rat kidney allograft model: Was it all too good to be true? *Transplantation* **34**:223–225.

Fabri, P. J., Weber, C. J., Gorver, W. R., and Reemtsma, K., 1983, Hypogastrinemia in streptozotocin diabetes with islet transplantation. *J. Surg. Res.* **34**:432–437.

Fairbrother, B. J., Boyle, P., Slater, D. N., George, J., Nolan, M. S., and Fox, M. S., 1980a, Long term results of transplantation of the duct ligated pancreas in the rat, *Transplant. Proc.* **12**(Suppl. 2):150–153.

Fairbrother, B. J., Boyle, P. F., Slater, D. N., George, J., Nolan, M. S., and Fox, M., 1980b, The effect of ischemia on the duct-ligated pancreatic transplant in the rat, *Transplant. Proc.* **12**(Suppl. 2):172–175.

Faure, J. L., Devonec, M., Martin, X., Eloy, R., Margonari, J., and Dubernard, J. M., 1980, Local irradiation of rat pancreas by intraductal injection of Erbium-169: Short-term effects, *Transplant. Proc.* **12**(Suppl. 2):145–147.

Faustman, D., Hauptfeld, V., Davie, J. M., Lacy, P. E., and Shreffler, D. C., 1980, Murine pancreatic B-cells express H-2K and H-2D but not Ia antigens, *J. Exp. Med.* **151**:1553–1568.

Faustman, D., Hauptfeld, V., Lacy, P., and Davie, J., 1981, Prolongation of murine islet allograft survival by pretreatment of islets with antibody direct to Ia determinants, *Proc. Natl. Acad. Sci. USA* **78**:5156–5159.

Faustman, D., Hauptfeld, V., Lacy, P., and Davie, J., 1982a, Demonstration of active tolerance in maintenance of established islet of Langerhans allografts, *Proc. Natl. Acad. Sci. USA* **79**:4153–4155.

Faustman, D., Lacy, P. E., and Davie, J. W., 1982b, Transplantation without immunosuppression, *Diabetes* **31**(Suppl. 4):11–14.

Faustman, D., Lacy, P., Davie, J., and Hauptfeld, V., 1982c, Prevention of allograft rejection by immunization with donor blood depleted of Ia-bearing cells, *Science* **217**:157–158.

Faustman, D., Lacy, P. E., Davie, J. M., and Hauptfeld, V., 1983, Allograft prolongation by immunizations with donor blood depleted of Ia-bearing cells, *Transplant. Proc.* **15**(1):1341–1343.

Federlin, K. F., and Bretzel, R. G., 1980, The metabolic and hormonal status of animals in experimental diabetes after islet transplantation and its effect upon microvascular and other diabetic complications, in: *Proceedings 10th Congress of the International Diabetes Federation* (H. Waldhausen, ed.), Excerpta Medica, pp. 237–242.

Federlin, K. F., and Bretzel, R. G., 1981, Reversibility of diabetic glomerulopathy by islet transplantation in experimental animals, *Pediatr. Adolesc. Endocrinol.* **9**:326–332.

Feldman, S. D., Dodi, G., Hard, K., Scharp, D. W., Ballinger, W. F., and Lacy, P. E., 1977, Intrasplenic islet isografts, *Surgery* **82**:386–394.

Feldman, S. D., Scharp, D. W., Lacy, P. E., and Ballinger, W. F., 1980, Fetal pancreas isografts cultured and uncultured to reversive streptozotocin induced diabetes mellitus, *J. Surg. Res.* **29**:309–318.

Ferguson, J., and Scothorne, R J., 1973, The survival of transplanted isolated pancreatic islets in the omentum and testis, *Br. J. Surg.* **60**:907.

Festing, M. F. W., May, D., Conners, J. A., and Lovell, D., 1978, An athymic nude mutation in the rat. *Nature* **274**:365.

Finch, D. R. A., and Morris, P. J., 1976, Passive enhancement of isolated pancreatic islet allografts, *Transplantation* **22**:508–512.

Finch, D. R. A., and Morris, P. J., 1977a, The effect of increasing islet numbers on survival of pancreatic islet allografts in immunosuppressed diabetic rats, *Transplantation* **23**:104–106.

Finch, D. R. A., and Morris, P. J., 1977b, Failure to demonstrate a syngergistic effect between enhancing serum and ALS in recipients of pancreatic islet allograft, *Transplantation* **23**:386–388.

Finch, D. R. A., Wise, P. H., Morris, P. J., 1977, Successful intrasplenic transplantation of syngeneic and allogeneic isolated pancreatic islets, *Diabetologia* **13**:195–199.

Finke, E. H., Lacy, P. E., and Oho, J., 1979, Use of reflected green light for specific identification of islets in vitro after collagenase isolation, *Diabetes* **28**:612–613.

Florack, G., Sutherland, D. E. R., Heil, J. E., and Squifflet, J. P., 1982a, Endocrine function of heterotopic segmental pancreas grafts, *Diabetes* **31**:(Suppl. 2):159A.

Florack, G., Sutherland, D. E. R., Heil, J., Zweber, B., and Najarian, J. S., 1982b, Long-term preservation of segmental pancreas autografts, *Surgery* **92**:260–269.

Florack, G., Sutherland, D. E. R., Squifflet, J. P., Heil, J., Rabe, F., and Najarian, J. S., 1982c, Effect of graft denervation, systemic venous drainage and reduction of beta cell mass on insulin levels after heteroptopic pancreas transplantation in dogs, *Surg. Forum* **33**:351–353.

Florack, G., Sutherland, D. E. R., Heil, J. E., Squifflet, J. P., and Najarian, J. S., 1983a, Preservation of canine segmental pancreatic autografts: Cold storage versus pulsatile machine perfusion, *J. Surg. Res.* **34**:493–504.

Florack, G., Sutherland, D. E. R., Squifflet, J. P., Morrow, C. E., and Najarian, J. S., 1983b, Preservation of segmental pancreatic autografts by pulsatile machine perfusion, *Transplant Proc.* **15**:(1):1314–1317.

Florack, G., Sutherland, D. E. R., Morrow, C. E., Zweber, B., and Najarian, J. S., 1983, Warm ischemia tolerance of the pancreas for transplantation, *Surg. Forum*, in press.

Frangipane, L. G., Barker, C. F., Silvers, W. K., 1977a, Importance of weak histocompatibility factors in survival of pancreatic islet transplants, *Surg. Forum* **28**:294–296.

Frangipane, L. G., Poole, T. W., Barker, C. F., and Silvers, W. K., 1977b, Vulnerability of allogeneic and xenogeneic pancreatic islets to antisera, *Transplant. Proc.* **9**:371–373.

Frankel, B. J., Gylfe, E., Hellman, B., and Idahl, L. A., 1976, Maintenance of insulin release from pancreatic islets stored in the cold for up to 5 weeks, *J. Clin. Invest.* **57**:47–52.

Franklin, W. A., Schulak, J. A., and Reckard C. R., 1979, The fate of pancreatic islets in the rat, *Am. J. Pathol.* **94**:95.

Garvey, J. F. W., Morris, P. J., and Finch, D. R. A., 1979a, Experimental pancreas transplantation, *Lancet* **1**:971–972.

Garvey, J. F. W., Morris, P. J., and Millard, P. R., 1979b, Early rejection of allogenic fetal rat pancreas, *Transplantation* **27**:342–344.

Garvey, J. F. W., Klein, C., Millard, P. R., and Morris, P. J., 1980a, Rejection of organ-cultured allogeneic fetal rat pancreas, *Surgery* **87**:157–163.

Garvey, J. F. W., McShane, P., Poole, M. D., Millard, P. R., and Morris, P. J., 1980b, The effect of Cyclosporin A on experimental pancreas allografts in the rat, *Transplant. Proc.* **12**:266–269.

Garvey, J. F. W., Millard, P. R., and Morris, P. J., 1980c, Experimental transplantation of fetal pancreas and isolated islets in the rat: Studies on donor pretreatment and recipient immunosuppression, *Transplant. Proc.* **12** (No. 4, Suppl. 2):186–189.

Gates, R. J., Hunt, M. I., Smith, R., and Lazarow, M. R., 1972, Return to normal of blood-glucose, plasma insulin, and weight gain in New Zealand obese mice after implantation of islets of Langerhans. *Lancet* **2**:567–570.

Gates, R. J., Hunt, M. I., and Lazarus, M. R., 1974, Further studies on the amelioration of the characteristics of New Zealand obese (NZO) mice following implantation of islets of Langerhans, *Diabetologia* **10**:401–406.

Gates, R. J., and Lazarus, N. R., 1977, Reversal of streptozotocin-induced diabetes by intraperitoneal implantation of encapsulated neonatal rabbit pancreatic tissue, *Lancet* **2**:1257–1259.

Gebhardt, C., and Stolte, M., 1978, Pankreasgang-okklusion durch Injektion einer schnellhartenden Aminosäurelosung, *Langenbecks Arch. Chir.* **346**:149–166.

Georgakais, A., 1979, Experimental pancreatic islet transplantation, *Ann. R. Col Surg.* **59**:231–235.

Germain, M., Gremillet, C., Arci, C., Da Cunha, X., Lesec, G., and Levy, J. R., 1979, Transplantation du pancreas avec donneur vivant a l'aide de techniques microchirurgicales, *Chirurgie* **105**:358–362.

Gliedman, M. L., Gold, M., Whittaker, J., Rifkin, H., Soberman, R., Freed, S., Tellis, V., and Veith, F. J., 1973, Pancreatic duct to ureter anastomosis in pancreatic transplantation, *Am. J. Surg.* **125**:245–252.

Gooszen, H. G., van Schilfgaarde, R., and Terpstra, J. L., 1983, The arterial blood supply of the left lobe of the canine pancreas. II. Electromagnetic flow measurements in unmodified and duct-obliterated left pancreatic segments, *Surgery* **93**:549–553.

Gordon, D. A., MacKenzie, G. H., and Toledo-Pereyra, L. H., 1981, Efficient pancreatic islet cell preparation utilizing a new tissue chopper prior to transplantation, *Diabetologia* **20**:79–80.

Gordon, D. A., Toledo-Pereyra, L. H., and MacKenzie, G. H., 1982, Preservation for transplantation: A review of techniques of islet cell culture and storage, *J. Surg. Res.* **32**:182–193.

Gotzsche, O., Fundersen, H. J. G., and Osterby, R., 1981, Irreversibility of glomerular basement membrane accumulation despite reversibility of renal hypertrophy with islet transplantation in early experimental diabetes, *Diabetes* **30**:481–485.

Gray, B. N., and Watkins, E., 1974, Prolonged relief from diabetes after syngeneic or allogeneic transplantation of isolated pancreatic islets in rats, *Surg. Forum* **25**:382–384.

Gray, B. N., and Watkins, E., 1976, Prevention of vascular complications of diabetes by pancreatic islet transplantation, *Arch. Surg.* **111**:254–257.

Gray, B. N., Carusco, G., Alford, F., and Chisholm, D., 1979, Insulin and glucagon response of transplanted intrasplenic islets, *Arch. Surg.* **114**:96–99.

Gray, D. W. R., Reece-Smith, H., Fairbrothers, B., McShane, P., and Morris, P. J., 1983, Is the survival of pancreatic islets in allogeneic rats already tolerant to kidney allografts of the same donor strain dependent on the site of transplantation? *Transplant. Proc.* **15** (1):**1338–1340.**

Griffith, R. C., Scharp, D. W., Hartman, B. K., Ballinger, W. F., and Lacy, P. E., 1977, A morphologic study of intrahepatic portal vein islet isografts, *Diabetes* **26**:201–214.

Groth, C. G, Lundgren, G., Klintman, G., Gunnarsson, R., Colste, H., Wilczek, H., Ringden, O., and Ostman, J., 1982, Successful outcome of segmental diversion after modifications in technique, *Lancet* **2**:522–524.

Hadji-Georgopoulos, A., Broe, P., Mehigan, D., Kowarski, A., and Cameron, J. L., 1982, Endocrine and exocrine function of intrasplenic pancreatic autografts, *Surgery* **91**:210–216.

Hammerling, G., S., Mauve, B., Goldberg, E., and McDermott, H. O., 1975, Tissue distribution of Ia antigens, *Immunogenetics* **1**:428–437.

Handwerger, B. S., Brown, D. M., and Sutherland, D. E. R., 1984, Alterations in immunological function in streptozotocin-induced murine diabetes: Correction by islet cell transplantation, *Diabetes*, in press.

Hanson, S. L., Sutherland, D. E. R., Field, M. J., and Najarian, J. S., 1981, Comparison of techniques for pancreatic islet transplantation in dogs, *Surg. Forum.* **32**:383–385.

Hardy, M. A., Sataki, K., Fawwaz, R., Nowygrod, R., and Reemtsma, K., 1982, Experimental islet allografts and xenografts as a potential diabetic cure, in: *Diabetic–Renal Retinal Syndrome: Prevention and Management,* 2nd Ed., (E. Friedman and S. A. L'Esperance, eds.), pp. 503–518, Grune & Stratton, New York.

Hart, D. N. J., and Fabres, J. W., 1981, Demonstration and characterization of Ia-positive dendritic cells in the interstitial connective tissues of rat heart and other tissues, but not brain, *J. Exp. Med.* **153**:347–361.

Hegre, O. D., Leonard, R. J., Erlandson, S. L., McEvoy, R. C., Parsons, J. A., Elde, R. P., and Lazarow, A. 1976a, Transplantation of islet tissue in the rat, *Acta Endocrinol.* **83** (Suppl. 205):257–278.

Hegre, O. D., Leonard, R. J., Rusin, J. R., and Lazarow, A., 1976b, Growth of islet issue following organ culture and subsequent allo and isotransplantation, *Anat. Rec.* **185**:209–222.

Hegre, O. D., Leonard, R. J., Schmitt, R. V., and Lazarow, A., 1976c Isotransplantation of organ-cultured neonatal pancreas: Reversal of alloxan diabetes in the rat. *Diabetes* **25**:180–189.

Hegre, O. D, and Lazarow, A., 1977, Islet cell transplantation, in: *The Diabetic Pancreas,* B. W. Volk and K. R. Wellman, eds., p. 517–550, Plenum Press, New York.

Hegre, O. D., Schmitt, R. V., and McEvoy, R. C., 1979, Syngeneic transplantation of the fetal rat pancreas. IV. Dissociated versus whole organ implantation, *Metabolism* **18**:157–169.

Hegre, O. D., Schmitt, R. V., and McEvoy, R. C., 1979, Syngeneic transplantation of the fetal rat pancreas. IV. Dissociated versus whole organ implantation, *Metabolism* **18**:157–169.

Hegre, O. D., Schulte, J. A., Parsons, J. A., and Erlandsen, S. L., 1981, The preservation isolation of perinatal islet tissue utilizing in vitro techniques, in: *Proceedings of 1980 Geissen Workshop on Islet Isolation, Culture and Cryopreservation* (K. Federlig and R. G. Bretzel, eds.), pp. 83–95, Georg Thieme Verlag, Stuttgart, and Thieme-Stratton, New York.

Hegre, O. D., Marshall, S., Schulte, B. A., Hickey, G. E., Williams, F., Sorenson, R. C., and Serie, J. R. Non-enzymatic in vitro isolation of perinatal islets of Langerhans, *In Vitro,* in press.

Helmke, K., Slijepcevic, M., and Federlin, K. 1975, Islet transplantation in experimental diabetes of the rat, II. Studies in allogeneic pancreatectomized rats, *Horm. Metab. Res.* **7**:210–214.

Henriksson, C., 1978, Isolation and transplantation of islets of Langerhans, *Acta Chir. Scand.* **483**(Suppl.): 5–21.

Henriksson, C., 1978, Repeated isologous transplantation of islets of Langerhans in the diabetic rat, *Acta Chir. Scand.* **144**:137–140.

Henriksson, C., Bergmark, J., and Claes, G., 1977a, Metabolic response to isologous transplantation of small numbers of isolated islets of Langerhans in the rat, *Eur. Surg. Res.* **9**:411–418.

Henriksson, C., Bergmark, J., and Claes, G., 1977b, Use of trypsin for isolation of islets of Langerhans in the rat, *Eur. Surg. Res.* **9**:427–431.

Henriksson, C., Claes, G., and Pehrsson, N. G., 1977c, Viability of the islets of Langerhans after warm ischemia as judged by isologous transplantation, *Acta Chir. Scand.* **143**:323–328.

Hess, W. N., and Root, K. W., 1938, Study of the pancreas of white rats of different age groups, *Am. J. Anat.* **63**:489–498.

Hinshaw, D. B., Jolley, W. B., Knierim, K. H., and Hinshaw, D. B., 1981, Nonenzymatic method for isolation of functional pancreatic islets, *Surg. Forum* **32**:381–383.

Hirschberg, H., Bergh, O. S., and Thorsby, E., 1980, Antigen-presenting properties of human vascular cells, *J. Exp. Med.* **152**:244–255.

Hoffman, L., Martin, F. I. R., Carter, W., Mandel, T. E., and Campbell, D. G., 1981, Effect of short-term insulin treatment on the reversal of diabetes after transplantation of syngeneic cultured or uncultured fetal mouse pancreas, *Transplantation* **32**:342–345.

Hoffman, L., Mandel, T. E., and Carter, W., 1982, Insulin content of fetal mouse pancreas in organ culture and after transplantation, *Diabetes* **31**:826–829.

Homan, W. P., Fabre, J. W., William, K. A., Millard, P. R., and Morris, P. J., 1980, Studies in the immunosuppressive properties of cyclosporin A in rats receiving renal allografts, *Transplantation* **29**:361–366.

Horaguchi, A., and Merrell, R. G., 1981, Preparation of viable islet cells from dogs by a new method, *Diabetes* **30**:455–458.

Howard, R. J., Balfour, H. H., Matas, A. J., Najarian, J. S., and Sutherland, D. E. R., 1979, Encephalomyocarditis virus induced diabetes mellitus treated by islet transplantation, *Transplantation* **27**:200–202.

Idezuki, Y., Feemster, J. A., Dietzman, R. H., and Lillehei, R. C., 1968a, Experimental pancreaticoduodenal preservation and transplantation. *Surg. Gynecol. Obstet.* **126**:1002–1014.

Idezuki, Y., Goetz, F., Kaufman, S. E., and Lillehei, R. C., 1968b, In vitro insulin productivity of preserved pancreas: A simple test to assess the viability of pancreatic allografts, *Surgery* **64**:940–947.

Idezuki, Y., Goetz, F. C., and Lillehei, R. C., 1969, Late effect of pancreatic duct ligation on beta cell function, *Am. J. Surg.* **117**:33–39.

Janney, C. G., Davie, J. M., Lacy, P. E., and Finke, E. H., 1982a, Characterization of lymphocytes from rejected and nonrejected islet xenografts, *Transplantation* **33**:585–587.

Janney, C. G., Lacy, P. E., Finke, E. H., and Davie, J. M., 1982b, Prolongation of intrasplenic islet xenograft survival, *Am. J. Pathol.* **107**:1–5.

Jolley, W. B., Hinshaw, D. B., Call, T. W., and Alverd, L. S., 1977, Xenogeneic pancreatic islet transplantation in proteolytic enzyme bonded diffusion chambers in diabetic rats, *Transplant. Proc.* **9**:363–365.

Jolley, W. B., Knierim, K., Hinshaw, D. B., Ham, J. M., and Hinshaw, D. B., 1982, Successful allografts of pancreatic islets in diabetic rabbits after donor-specific blood transfusion and antilymphocyte serum treatment, *Transplant. Proc.* **14**:413–414.

Jonasson, O., Reynolds, W. A., Snyder, G., 1977, Experimental and clinical therapy of diabetes by transplantation, *Transplant. Proc.* **9**:223–232.

Kadowaki, S., Taminato, T., Chiba, T., Goto, Y., Nozawa, M., Seino, Y., Matsukura, S., and Fujita, T., 1980, Reversal of the enhanced somatostatin release from the isolated, perfused diabetic rat pancreas after the amelioration of diabetes by whole pancreas transplantation, *Diabetes* **29**:742–746.

Karow, A. M., 1981, Biophysical and chemical considerations in cryopreservation, in: *Organ Preservation for Transplantation* (A. W. Karow and D. E. Pegg, eds.) pp. 113–142, Marcel Dekker, New York.

Kedinger, M., Haffen, K., Grenier, J., and Elroy, R., 1977, In vitro culture reduces immunogenicity of pancreatic endocrine islets, *Nature* **270**:736–738.

Kemp, C. B., Knight, M. J., Sharp, D. W., Ballinger, W. F., and Lacy, P. E., 1973a, Effect of transplantation site on the results of pancreatic isografts in diabetic rats, *Diabetologia* **9**:486–491.

Kemp, C. B., Scharp, D. W., Knight, M. J., Ballinger, W. F., and Lacy, P. E., 1973b, Importance of implantation site of pancreatic islet isografts in the treatment of experimental diabetes, *Surg. Forum* **24**:297–299.

Kemp, E., 1978, *Xenografting: The Future of Organ Transplantation,* Odense University Press, Copenhagen.

Kemp, J. A., Mullen, Y., Weissman, H., Heininger, D., Brown, J., and Clark, W. R., 1978, Reversal of diabetes in rats using fetal pancreases stored at −196°C, *Transplantation* **26**:260–264.

Kiviluoto, T., Schroder, T., Taskinen, M. R., and Lempinen, M., 1982, Autotransplantation of pancreatic fragments to the portal vein: A new isolation technique for the pig and human, *Eur. Soc. Surg. Reg.* **14**:128.

Klein, J., 1975, in: *The Biology of the Mouse Histocompatibility-2 Complex,* p. 454, Springer Verlag, New York.

Klempnauer, J., Kasahara, K., White, D. J. G., and Calne, R. Y., 1982a, Differential susceptibility to cyclosporin A immunosuppression of fully allogenic vascularized heart and pancreas transplants in the rat, *Eur. Soc. Surg. Res.* **14**:128–129.

Klempnauer, J., Pegg, D. E., Taylor, M. J., and Diaper, M. P., 1982b, Hypothermic preservation of the rat pancreas, in: *Organ Preservation. Basic and Applied Aspects* (D. E. Pegg, I. A. Jacobsen, and N. A. Halasz, eds.), pp. 191–197, MTP Press, Lancaster, U.K.

Klempnauer, Wonigeit, K., Gunther, E., and Pichlmayr, R., 1983, Pancreas whole organ transplantation in the rat. Differential effect of MHC subregions. *Transplant. Proc.* **15**:1308–1310.

Koesters, W., Seelig, H. P., and Stauch, M., 1977, Reversibility of function and morphologic glomerular lesions by islet transplantation in long-term diabetic rats, *Diabetologia* **13**:409.

Kolb, E., Ruchert, R., and Largiader, F., 1977, Intraportal and intrasplenic autotransplantation of pancreatic islets in the dog, *Eur. Surg. Res.* **9**:419–426.

Kolb, E., Urfer, K., and Largiader, F., 1979, Early rejection of allotransplanted pancreatic islets in the dog, *Transplant. Proc.* **11**:543–548.

Koncz, L., Davidoff, F., DeLellis, R. A., Selby, M., and Zimmerman, C. E., 1976, Quantitative aspects of the metabolic response to pancreatic islet transplantation in rats with severe ketotic diabetes, *Metabolism* **25**:147–156.

Korec, R., 1977, The cure of streptozotocin diabetes in rats by homotransplantation of isolated intraportally injected Langerhans islets or by renal-subcapsular transplantation of neonatal pancreases, *Diabetologia* **13**:409–410.

Korec, R., 1981, Observations on the progeny of alloxan- or streptozotocin-diabetic rats cured by pancreatic transplantation, *Diabetologia* **20**:678.

Kortz, W. J., Reiman, T. H., Bollinger, R. R., Eisenbarth, G. S., 1982, Identification and isolation of rat and human islet cells using monoclonal antibodies, *Surg. Forum* **33**:354–356.

Kramp, R. C., and Burr, I. M., 1981, Subcutaneous, isogeneic transplantation of duct-ligated pancreas in streptozotocin-diabetic mice. Relationships between carbohydrate tolerance and hormone content in transplant or host pancreas, *Diabetes* **30**:857–864.

Kramp, R. C., Congdon, C. C., and Smith, L. H., 1975, Isogeneic and allogeneic transplantation of duct-ligated pancreas in streptozotocin diabetic mice, *Eur. J. Clin. Invest.* **5**:249–258.

Kramp, R. C., Cuche, R., Renold, A. E., Gonet, J. C., 1976, Subcutaneous isogeneic transplantation of either duct-ligated pancreas or isolated islets in streptozotocin diabetic mice, *Endocrinology* **99**:1161–1167.

Kretschmer, G. J., Sutherland, D. E. R., Matas, A. J., Cain, T. L., and Najarian, J. S., 1977a, The dispersed pancreas: Transplantation without islet purification in totally pancreatectomized dogs, *Diabetologia* **13**:495–502.

Kretschmer, G. J., Sutherland, D. E. R., Matas, A. J., and Najarian, J. S., 1977b, Autotransplantation of pancreatic islets without separation of exo- and endocrine tissue in totally pancreatectomized dogs, *Surgery* **82**:74–81.

Kretschmer, G. J., Sutherland, D. E. R., Matas, A. J., Payne, W. D., and Najarian, J. S., 1978, Autotransplantation of pancreatic fragments to the portal vein and spleen of totally pancreatectomized dogs, *Ann. Surg.* **187**:79–86.

Kretschmer, G. J., Sutherland, D. E. R., Matas, A. J., and Najarian, J. S., 1979, Preliminary experience with allotransplantation of pancreatic fragments to the spleen of totally pancreatectomized dogs, *Transplant. Proc.* **11**:537–542.

Krupin, T., Waltman, S. R., Scharp, D. W., Oestrich, C., Feldman, S. D., Becker, B., Ballinger, W. F., and Lacy, P. E., 1979, Ocular fluorphotometry in streptozotocin diabetes mellitus in the rat: Effect of pancreatic islet isografts, *Invest. Ophthamol. Vis. Sci.* **18**:1185–1190.

Kyriakides, G. K., Arora, V. K., Lifton, J., Nuttal, F., and Miller, J., 1976, Porcine pancreatic transplantation. I. Autotransplantation of duct ligated pancreatic segments, *J. Surg. Res.* **20**:451–460.

Kyriakides, G. K., Sutherland, D. E. R., Olson, L., Miller, J., and Najarian, J. S., 1979a, Segmental pancreatic transplantation in dogs. *Transplant. Proc.* **11**:530–532.

Kyriakides, G. K., Nuttall, F. W., and Miller, J., 1979b, Segmental pancreatic transplantation in pigs, *Surgery* **85**:154–158.

Kyriakides, G. K., Olson, L., Rabinovitch, A., Mintz, D., Flaa, C., Severyn, W., and Miller, J., 1981a, Immunologic effect of cyclosporin A on beagle recipients of free-draining pancreatic segmental allografts, *Surg. Forum* **32**:355–357.

Kyriakides, G. K., Rabinovitch, A., Mintz, D., Olson, L., and Rapaport, F. T., 1981b, Long-term study of vascularized free-draining intraperitoneal pancratic segmental allografts in beagle dogs, *J. Clin. Invest.* **67**:292–303.

Kyriakides, G. K., Rabinovitch, A., Olson, L., Mintz, O., Rapaport, F. T., and Miller, J., 1981c, Intraperitoneal segmental pancreatic allografts with unligated duct in dogs: The role of histocompatibility for long term survival, *Transplant. Proc.* **13**:(1):810–811.

Kyriakides, G. J., Miller, J., Olson, L., Flaa, C., Rabinovitch, A., and Mintz, D., 1982, Effects of Cyclosporin A in stimultaneous canine pancreatic and renal allografts, *Diabetes* **31**:(Suppl. 2):153A.

Lacy, P. E., Walker, M. M., and Fink, C. E. J., 1972, Perfusion of isolated rat islets in vitro, *Diabetes* **21**:987–998.

Lacy, P. E., Finke, E. H., Conant, S., and Naber, S., 1976, Long-term perfusion of isolated rat islets in vitro, *Diabetes* **25**:484–493.

Lacy, P. E., Davie, J. M., Finke, E. H., and Scharp, D. W., 1979a, Prolongation of islet allograft survival, *Transplantation* **27**:171–174.

Lacy, P. E., Davie, J. M., and Finke, E. H., 1979b, Induction of rejection of successful allografts of rat islets by donor peritoneal exudate cells, *Transplantation* **28**:415–420.

Lacy, P. E., Davie, J. M., and Finke, E. H., 1979c, Prolongation of islet allograft survival following in vitro cultured (24°C) and a single injection of ALS, *Science* **204**:312–313.

Lacy, P. E., Davie, J. M., and Finke, E. H., 1980a, Prolongation of islet xenograft survival without immunosuppression, *Science* **209**:283–285.

Lacy, P. E., Davie, J. M., and Finke, E. H., 1980b, Effect of culture on islet rejection, *Diabetes* **29**:93–97.

Lacy, P. E., Davie, J. M., and Finke, E. H., 1981a, Transplantation of insulin producing tissue, *Am. J. Med.* **70**:589–594.

Lacy, P. E., Davie, J. M., and Finke, E. H., 1981b, Prolongation of islet xenograft survival (rat to mouse), *Diabetes* **30**:285–291.

Lacy, P. E., Finke, E. H., Janney, C. G., and Davie, J. M., 1982a, Prolongation of islet xenograft survival by in vitro culture of rat megaislets in 95% O_2, *Transplantation* **33**:588–592.

Lacy, P. E., Lacy, E. T., Finke, E. H., and Yasunami, Y., 1982b, An improved method for the isolation of islets from the beef pancreas, *Diabetes* **31**(Suppl. 4):109–111.

Lafferty, K. J., 1980, Immunogenicity of foreign tissue, *Transplantation* **29**:179–182.

Lafferty, K. J., and Woolnough, J., 1977, The origin and mechanism of the allograft rejection, *Immunol. Rev.* **35**:231–262.

Lafferty, K. J., Prowse, S. J., Agostino, M., and Simeonovic, C. J., 1983, Modulation of tissue immunogenicity, *Transplant Proc.* **15**:(1):1366–1370.

Land, W., Gebhardt, Ch, Gall, F. P., and Weitz, H., 1980, Pancreatic duct obstruction with prolamine solution, *Transplant. Proc.* **12**(Suppl. 2):72–75.

Largiader, F., Lyons, G. W., Hidalgo, F., Dietzman, R. H., and Lillehei, R. C., 1967, Orthotopic allotransplantation of the pancreas, *Am. J. Surg.* **113**:70–76.

Lazarow, A., Wells, L. J., Carpenter, A. M., Hegre, O. D., Leonard, R. J., and McEvoy, R. C., 1973, Islet differentiation, organ culture, and transplantation, *Diabetes* **22**:413–428.

Lee, C. S., Mauer, S. M., Brown, D. M., Sutherland, D. E. R., Michael, M. F., and Najarian, J. S., 1974, Renal transplantation in diabetes mellitus in rats, *J. Exp. Med.* **139**:793–800.

Lee, S., Tung, K. S. K., Koopmans, H., Chandler, J. G., and Orloff, M. J., 1972, Pancreaticoduodenal transplantation in the rat, *Transplantation* **13**:421–425.

Leonard, R. J., Lazarow, A., and Hegre, O., 1973, Pancreatic islet transplantation in the rat, *Diabetes* **22**:413–428.

Leonard, R. J., Lazarow, A., McEvoy, R. C., and Hegre, O. D., 1974, Islet cell transplantation, *Kidney Int.* **6**(Suppl. 1):169–178.

Lillehei, R. C., Simmons, R. L., Najarian, J. S., Weil, R., III, Uchida, H., Ruiz, J. O., Kjellstrand, C. M., and Goetz, F. C., 1970, Pancreaticoduodenal allotransplantation. Experimental and clinical experience, *Ann. Surg.* **172**:405–436.

Lillehei, R. C., Ruiz, J. O., Acquino, C., and Goetz, F. C., 1976, Transplantation of the pancreas, *Acta Endocrinol.* **83**(Suppl. 205):303–320.

Lim, F., and Sun, A. M., 1980, Microencapsulated islets as bioartificial endocrine pancreas, *Science* **20**:908–910.

Lindall, A. W., Steffes, M. W., and Sorenson, R., 1969, Immunoassayable content of subcellular fractions of rat islets, *Endocrinology* **85**:218–223.

Liquori, L., Campione, O., Reversi, C. A., DiNino, G. F., Melotti, R., Masiello, G., Cavicchi, A., Stano, R., Petrone, F., and Marrano, D., 1979, Valutazioni metaboliche nel trapianto sperimentale di pancreas, *Il Policlinico Sez. Chirurgica* **87**:292–298.

Long, J. A., Britt, L. D., Olack, B. J., and Scharp, D. W., 1983, Autotransplantation of isolated canine pancreatic islet cells, *Transplant. Proc.* **15**(1):1332–1337.

Lorenz, D., Petermann, J., Beckert, R., Rosenbaum, K. D., Ziegler, M., and Dorn, A., 1975, Transplantation of isologous islets of Langerhans in diabetic rats, *Acta Diabetol. Lat.* **12**:30–40.

Lorenz, D., Lippert, J., Tietz, W., Worm, V., Hahn, H.-J., Dorn, A., Koch, G., Ziegler, M., and Rosenbaum, K. D., 1979a, Transplantation of isolated islets of Langerhans in diabetic dogs. I. Results after allogeneic intraportal islet transplantation, *J. Surg. Res.* **27**:181–192.

Lorenz, D., Lippert, J., Hahn, H.-J., Panzig, E., Kohler, H., Dorn, A., Koch, G., Tietz, W., Worm, V., and Ziegler, M., 1979b, Transplantation of isolated islets of Langerhans in diabetic dogs. II. The influence of histocompatibility, *J. Surg. Res.* **27**:193–204.

Lorenz, D., Lippert, H., Panzig E., Kohler, J., Koch, G., Tietz, W., Hahn, H. J., Dorn, A., Worm, V., and Ziegler, M., 1979c, Transplantation of isolated islets of Langerhans in diabetic dogs. III. Donor selection by mixed lymphocyte reaction and immunosuppressive treatment, *J. Surg. Res.* **27**:205–213.

Louis-Sylvestre, J., 1978, Relationship between two stages of prandial insulin release in rats, *Am. J. Physiol.* **235**:E103–111.

Lum, C. T., Sutherland, D. E. R., Eckhardt, J., Matas, A. J., and Najarian, J. S., 1979, Effect of an adenosine deaminase inhibitor on survival of mouse pancreatic islet allografts, *Transplantation* **27**:355–357.

Lum, C. T., Sutherland, D. E. R., Payne, W. D., Gorecki, P., Matas, A. J., and Najarian, J. S., 1980, Prolongation of mouse and rat pancreatic islet cell allografts by adenosine deaminase inhibitors and adenine arabinoside, *J. Surg. Res.* **28**:44–48.

Lundgren, G., Andersson, A., Borg, H., Groth, C. G., Gunnarsson, R., Hellerstrom, C., Petersson, B., and Ostman, J., 1977, Structural and functional integrity of isolated human islets of Langerhans maintained in tissue culture for 1–3 weeks, *Transplant. Proc.* **9**:237–240.

MacDonald, M. J., 1980, Inexpensive modification of a polytron for rapid mincing of pancreases for islet isolation, *Anal. Biochem.* **108**:419–421.

Macedo, A. R., Skivolocki, W. P., Thompson, K. R., Lee, S., and Orloff, M. J., 1981, Morphometric electron microscopic study of the effect of whole pancreas transplantation on alloxan diabetic neuropathy, *Surg. Forum* **32**:379–380.

Maki, T., Sakar, A., Pettrrossi, O., and Kountz, S. L., 1977, En bloc transplantation of the liver, pancreas, duodenum, spleen, and kidney in the rat, *Transplantation* **24**:25–62.

Mandel, T. E., and Higginbotham, L., 1979, Organ culture and transplantation of fetal mouse pancreatic islets, *Transplant. Proc.* **11**:1505–1506.

Mandel, T. E., Collier, S., and Carter, W., 1980, Effect of vitro glucose concentration on fetal mouse pancreas cultures used as grafts in sygeneic diabetic mice, *Transplantation* **30**:231–233.

Mandel, T. E., Hoffman, L., and Carter, W. M., 1981a, Long-term isografts of cultured fetal mouse pancreatic islets, *Am. J. Pathol.* **104**:227–236.

Mandel, T. E., Hoffman, L., Collier, S., Carter, W. M., de Moore, G., Martin, F. I. R., and Campbell, D., 1981b, Organ cultured fetal pancreas: A source of islets for transplantation in diabetic mice, *Transplant. Proc.* **13**:832–836.

Mandel, T. E., Hoffman, L., Collier, S., Carter, W. M., and Koulmanda, M., 1982a, Organ culture of fetal mouse and fetal human pancreatic islets for allografting, *Diabetes* **15**(Suppl. 4):39–47.

Mandel, T. E., Jack, I., and Tait, B. D., 1982b, HLA-DR typing of fetal human spleen and liver lymphoblastoid cells transformed by Epstein–Barr virus, *Transplantation* **34**:50–53.

Mandel, T. E., Hoffman, L., Carter, W. M., and Koulmanda, K., 1983, Proliferation of cultured and isografted fetal mouse pancreatic islets, *Transplant. Proc.* **15**:(1):1362–1365.

Mangnall, Y., Smythe, A., Slater, D. N., Milner, R. D. G., Taylor, C. B., and Fox, M., 1977, Neonatal islet cell transplantation in the diabetic rat: Effect on hepatic enzyme activity and glucose homeostasis, *J. Endocrinol.* **74**:231–241.

Markowitz, J., 1959, *Experimental Surgery*, Williams and Wilkins, Baltimore.

Marliss, E. B., Nakhooda, A. F., Poussier, P., and Sima, A. A. F., 1982, The diabetic syndrome of the "BB" Wistar rat: Possible relevance to Type 1 (insulin-dependent) diabetes in man, *Diabetologia* **22**:225–232.

Marner, B., Lernmark, A., Egeberg, J., Donhowe, J. M., and Steffes, M. W., Functioning allografted or isografted pancreatic islets exhibit different population proportions of a-cells, *Science*, in press.

Marquet, R. L., and Heystek, G. A., 1975, The effect of immunosuppressive treatment on the survival of allogeneic islets of Langerhans in rats, *Transplantation* **20**:428–431.

Martin, X., Faure, J. L., Amiel, J., Eloy, R., Margonair, J., and Dubernard, J. M., 1980, Systemic versus portal drainage of segmental pancreatic transplants in dogs, *Transplant. Proc.* **12**(Suppl. 2):138–140.

Martin, X., Faure, J. L., Eloy, R., Margonari, J., Amiel, J., Gelet, A., and Dubernard, J. M., 1980, Long-term survival of pancreatic isografts in rats, *Transplant. Proc.* **12**(Suppl. 2):126–128.

Matas, A. J., Sutherland, D. E. R., Steffes, M. W., and Najarian, J. S., 1976a, Islet transplantation using neonatal rat pancreata: Quantitative studies, *J. Surg. Res.* **20**:143–147.

Matas, A. J., Sutherland, D. E. R., Steffes, M. W., and Najarian, J. S., 1976b, Minimal collagenase digestion: Amelioration of diabetes in the rat with transplantation of one dispersed neonatal pancreas, *Transplantation* **22**:71–73.

Matas, A. J., Sutherland, D. E. R., Steffes, M. W., and Najarian, J. S., 1976c, Short-term culture of adult pancreatic fragments for purification and transplantation of islets of Langerhans, *Surgery* **80**:183–191.

Matas, A. J., Payne, W. D., Grotting, J. C., Sutherland, D. E. R., Steffes, M. W., Hertel, B. F., and Najarian, J. S., 1977a, Portal versus systemic transplantation of dispersed neonatal pancreas, *Transplantation* **24**:333–337.

Matas, A. J., Sutherland, D. E. R., Payne, W. D., Eckhardt, J., and Najarian, J. S., 1977b, A mouse model of islet transplantation using neonatal donors, *Transplantation* **24**:389–393.

Matas, A. J., Sutherland, D. E. R., Payne, W. D., Kretschmer, G. J., Steffes, M. W., and Najarian, J. S., 1977c, Islet transplantation. The critical period of donor ischemia in neonatal rats, *Transplantation* **23**:295–298.

Matas, A. J., Sutherland, D. E. R., Payne, W. D., Steffes, M. W., Kretschmer, G. J., and Najarian, J. S., 1977d, Successful transplantation of neonatal rat islet tissue preserved for up to 63 hours, *Trans. Am. Soc. Artif. Intern. Organs* **23**:347–351.

Matas, A. J., Sutherland, D. E. R., Steffes, M. W., and Najarian, J. S., 1977e, Islet transplantation, *Surg. Gynecol. Obstet.* **145**:757–772.

Matas, A. J., Sutherland, D. E. R., Kretschmer, G. J., Steffes, M. W., and Najarian, J. S., 1977, Pancreatic tissue culture: Depletion of exocrine enzymes and purification of islets for transplantation, *Transplant. Proc.* **9**:337–339.

Matas, A. J., Sutherland, D. E. R., Payne, W. D., and Najarian, J. S., 1978a, On the interpretation of islet allograft and xenograft results, *Transplantation* **25**:281–283.

Matas, A. J., Sutherland, D. E. R., Payne, W. D., and Najarian, J. S., 1978b, Transplantation of neonatal rat islet tissue after in situ and cold ischemia, *Diabetes* **27**(Suppl. 2):440.

Matas, A. J., Sutherland, D. E. R., Steffes, M. W., and Najarian, J. S., 1978c, Transplantation of neonatal rat islets after cold preservation, *Ann. R. Coll. Phys. Surg. Canada* **11**:40.

Mauer, S. M., Michael, A. F., Fish, A. J., and Brown, D. M., 1972, Spontaneous immunoglobulin and complement deposition in glomeruli in diabetic rats, *Lab. Invest.* **27**:488–494.

Mauer, S. M. Sutherland, D. E. R., Steffes, M. W., Leonard, A. J., Najarian, J. S., Michael, A. F., and Brown, D. M., 1974, Pancreatic islet transplantation: Effects on the glomerular lesions of experimental diabetes in the rat, *Diabetes* **23**:748–753.

Mauer, S. M., Steffes, M. W., Sutherland, D. E. R., Najarian, J. S., Michael, A. F., and Brown, D., 1975, Studies on the rate of regression of the glomerular lesions in diabetic rats treated with pancreatic islet transplantation, *Diabetes* **24**:280–285.

Mauer, S. M., Brown, D. M., Matas, A. J., and Steffes, M. W., 1978, Effects of pancreatic islet transplantation on the increased urinary albumin excretions rates in intact and uninephrectomized rats with diabetes mellitus, *Diabetes* **27**:959–964.

Mauer, S. M., Steffes, M. W., and Brown, D. M., 1981, The kidney in diabetes, *Am. J. Med.* **70**:603–612.

Mazur, P., Kemp, J. A., and Miller, R. H., 1976, Survival of fetal rat pancreases frozen to −78 and −196° *Proc. Natl, Acad. Sci. USA* **78**:4105–4109.

McEvoy, R. C., and Hegre, O. D., 1978, Syngeneic transplantation of fetal pancreas. II. Effect of insulin treatment on the growth and differentiation of pancreatic implants fifteen days after transplantation, *Diabetes* **27**:988–995.

McEvoy, R. C., and Hegre, O. D., 1979, Syngeneic transplantation of fetal rat pancreas. III. Effect of insulin treatment on the growth and differentiation of the pancreatic implants after reversal of diabetes, *Diabetes* **28**:141–146.

McEvoy, R. C., Schmitt, R. V., and Hegre, O. D., 1978, Syngeneic transplantation of fetal rat pancreas. I. Effect of insulin treatment on the reversal of diabetes, *Diabetes* **27**:982–987.

McMaster, P., Gibby, O. M., Calne, R. Y., Evans, D. B., Thirn, S., Rolles, K., Bevan, R., and Smith, J., 1982, Pancreatic transplantation, *J. R. Soc. Med.* **75**:47–51.

McMaster, P., Procyshyn, A., Calne, R. Y., Valdes, R., Rolles, K., and Smith, D., 1980a, Prolongation of canine pancreas allograft survival with cyclosporin A, *Br. Med. J.* **240**:444–445.

McMaster, P., Procyshyn, A., Calne, R. Y., Valdes, R., Rolles, K., and Smith, D., 1980b, Prolongation of canine pancreas allografts with cyclosporin A, *Transplant. Proc.* **12**:275–277.

Mehigan, D. G., Ball, W. R., Zudema, G. D., Eggleton, J. G., and Cameron, J. L., 1980a, Disseminated intravascular coagulation and portal hypertension following pancreatic islet autotransplantation *Ann Surg.* **191**:287–293.

Mehigan, D., Zuidema, G. D., Eggleston, J. C., and Cameron, J. L., 1980b, Pancreatic islet autotransplantation: Results in dogs with chronic cut ligation, *Am. J. Surg.* **139**:170–174.

Mehigan, D. G., Zuidema, G. D., and Cameron, J. L., 1981, Pancreatic islet transplantation in dogs: Critical factors in technique, *Am. J. Surg.* **141**:208.

Meister, R., Schwille, P. O., Engelhardt, W., Paul, K. J., Walter, G., and Gall, F. P., 1981, Short term results on intravenous glucose tolerance and blood concentration of islet hormones following isologous pancreas transplantation in the rat, *Horm. Metab. Res.* **13**:468–469.

Mendez-Picon, G., and McGeorge, M., 1983, Effect of total lymphoid irradiation and pretransplant blood transfusion on pancreatic islet allograft survival in the rat, *J. Surg. Res.* **34**:427–431.

Mennini., G., Longo, R., Soriani, M., Minervini, S., and Speranza, V., 1978, Transplantations of islets of Langerhans in diabetic rats: Techniques and prospectives, *Il Policlinico Sez. Chirurgica* **85**:341–349.

Merkel, F. K., Kelly, W. D., Goetz, F. C., and Maney, J. W., 1968, Irradiated hetertopic segmental canine pancreatic allografts, *Surgery* **63**:291–297.

Merrell, R., Cobb, L., Horaguchi, A., Marincola, F., and Maeda, M., 1982, Islet function following subtotal pancreatectomy in dogs, *Surg. Forum* 33:216–217.

Merrell, R., Scharp, D. W., Gingerich, R., Feldmeier, M., Greider, M., and Downing, R., 1979, New approaches to the separation of islet cells, *Surg. Forum* **30**:303–305.

Metzgar, R. S., 1980, Pancreas-specific alloantigens, *Transplant. Proc.* **12**(No. 3, Suppl. 1):123–128.

Mieny, C. J., and Smit, J. A., 1978, Autotransplantation of pancreatic tissue in totally pancreatectomized baboons, *S. Afr. J. Surg.* **16**:19–21.

Millard, P. R., Garvey, J. F. W., Jeffery, E. L., and Morris, P. J., 1980, The grafted fetal rat pancreas: Features of development and rejection, *Am. J. Pathol.* **100**:209–219.

Millard, P. R., Reece-Smith, H., Clark, A., Lafferty, E. L., McShane, P., and Morris, P. J., 1983, The long-term allografted rat islet: A histologic and immunohistologic study, *Am. J. Pathol.* **111**:166–173.

Miller, J., Rabinovitch, A., Fuller, J., Kyriakides, G., Severyn, W., Noel, J., Flaa, C., and Mintz, D., 1981, Responses of canine lymphocytes to allogeneic and autologous islets of Langerhans in mixed cell cultures, *Transplant. Proc.* **13**:807–809.

Minan, I. M., and Shreffler, D. C., 1981, Ia positive stimulator cells are required in primary, but not in secondary, mixed leukocyte reactions against H-2 K and H-2 D differences, *J. Immunol.* **126**:1774–1779.

Mirkovitch, V., and Campiche, M., 1976, Successful intrasplenic autotransplantation of pancreatic tissue in totally pancreatectomized dogs, *Transplantation* **21**:265–269.

Mirkovitch, V., and Campiche, M., 1977, Intrasplenic autotransplantation of canine pancreatic tissues; Maintenance of normoglycemia after total pancreatectomy, *Eur. Surg. Res.* **9**:173–190.

Mirkovitch, V., Winistorfer, B., and Campiche, M., 1979a, Total and immediate pancreatectomy as the mandatory requirement for the ultimate function of autotransplanted islets in dogs, *Transplant. Proc.* **11**:1502–1504.

Mirkovitch, V., Campiche, M., Moisman, F., Macarone-Palmier, R., and Blanc, D. 1979b Auto- and allotransplantation of canine pancreatic tissue, *Helv. Chir. Acta* **46**:225–229.

Mirkovitch, V., Mosimann, F., and Winistorfer, B., 1981, Letter to the Editor, *Ann. Surg.* **194**:664.

Molnar, G. D., Taylor, W. F., and Ho, M. M, 1972, Day to day variation of continuously monitored glycaemia: A further measure of diabetes instability, *Diabetologia* **8**:342–348.

Morris, P. J., Finch, D. R., Garvey, J. F., Poule, M. D., and Millard, P. R., 1980, Suppression of rejection of allogenic islet tissue in the rat, *Diabetes* **29**(Suppl. 1):107–112.

Morrow, C. E., Sutherland, D. E. R., Squifflet, J. P., Monda, L., Mukai, K., and Najarian, J. S., 1982, Cold storage of rat pancreatic islets prior to transplantation, *Trans. Am. Soc. Artif. Intern. Organs* **28**:240–244.

Morrow, C. E., Sutherland, D. E. R., Steffes, M. W., Bach, F., and Najarian, J. S., 1983a, Effect of isolated H-2 K, D, and I region encoded histocompatibility antigen differences in mouse islet allograft rejection, *J. Surg. Res.* **34**:358–366.

Morrow, C. E., Sutherland, D. E. R., Steffes, M. W., Najarian, J. S., and Bach, F. H., 1983b, The isolated effects of H-2, K, D and I region encoded histocompatibility antigens on mouse pancreatic islet allograft rejection. *Science* **219**:1337–1339.

Moskalewski, S., 1965, Isolation and culture of the islets of Langerhans of the guinea pig, *Gen. Comp. Endocrinol.* **5**:342–353.

Mullen, Y., 1980, Specific immunosuppression for fetal pancreas allografts in rats, *Diabetes* **29**(Suppl. 1):113–120.

Mullen, Y., 1981, Permanent reversal of experimental diabetes in rats by allogeneic fetal pancreases across minor histocompatibility loci: Effects and characteristics of immunosuppression induced by alloantigen, PCH, and ALS treatment, *Transplant. Proc.* **13**:823–828.

Mullen, Y., and Shintaku, I. P., 1980, Fetal pancreas allografts for reversal of diabetes in rats. I. Allograft survival in nonimmunosuppressed recipients, *Transplantation* **29**:35–42.

Mullen, Y., and Shibukawa, R. L., 1982, Use of total lymphoid irradiation in transplantation of rat fetal pancreases, *Diabetes* **15**(Suppl. 4):69–74.

Mullen, Y., and Shintaku, I. P., 1982, Fetal pancreas allografts for reversal of diabetes in rats. Induction of life-term specific unresponsiveness to pancreas allografts across nonmajor histocompatibility complex barriers, *Transplantation* **33**:3–11.

Mullen, Y. S., Clark, W. R., Molnar, I. G., and Brown, J., 1977a, Complete reversal of experimental diabetes in rats by a single fetal pancreas transplant, *Science* **195**:68–70.

Mullen, Y. S., Clark, W. R., Kemp, J., Molnar, I. G., and Brown, J., 1977b, Reversal of experimental diabetes by fetal rat pancreas. II. Critical procedures for transplantation, *Transplant Proc.* **9**(1):329–332.

Mullen, Y., Gottrib, M., and Shibukawa, R. L., 1983, Reversal of diabetes in rats by foetal pancreas allografts following TLI, *Transplant. Proc.* **15**:1355–1358.

Najarian, J. S., Sutherland, D. E. R., Steffes, M. W., 1975, Isolation of human islets of Langerhans for transplantation. *Transplant Proc.* **7**:611–613.

Naji, A., Reckard, C. R., Ziegler, M. M., Barker, C. F., 1975, Vulnerability of pancreatic islets to immune cells and serum, *Surg. Forum* **26**:459–461.

Naji, A., and Barker, C. F., 1978, Differential susceptibility of endocrine tissues to humoral immunity, *Surg. Forum* **29**:349–351.

Naji, A., Barker, C. F., and Silvers, W. K., 1979a, Relative vulnerability of isolated pancreatic islets, parathyroid, and skin allografts to cellular and humoral immunity, *Transplant. Proc.* **11**:560–562.

Naji, A., Silvers, W. K., Polkins, S. E., Defoe, D., and Barker, C. F., 1979b, Successful islet transplantation in spontaneous diabetes, *Surgery* **86**:218–26.

Naji, A., Frangipane, L., Barker, C. F., and Silvers, W. K., 1981a, Survival of H-Y-incompatible endocrine grafts in mice and rats, *Transplantation* **31**:145–147.

Naji, A., Silvers, W. K., and Barker, C. F., 1981b, Islet transplantation in spontaneously diabetic rats, *Transplant. Proc.* **13**:826–828.

Naji, A., Silvers, W. K., Dellgrau, D., Anderson, A. O., Plotkin, S., and Barker, C. F., 1981c, Prevention of diabetes in rats by bone marrow transplantation, *Ann. Surg.* **194**:328–338.

Naji, A., Silvers, W. K., Bellgrau, D., and Barker, C. F., 1981d, Spontaneous diabetes in rats: Destruction of islets is prevented by immunological tolerance, *Science* **213**:1390–1392.

Naji, A., Bellgrau, D., Anderson, A., Silvers, W. K., and Barker, C. F., 1982, Transplantation of islets and bone marrow cells to animals with immune insulitis, *Diabetes* **31**:(Suppl. 4):84–89.

Naji, A., Bellgrau, D., Silvers, W. K., Kimura, H., Bellgran, D., Anderson, A. O., and Barker, C. F., 1983, Correction of the peripheral T-cell functional and microenvironmental defects in BB rats by transplantation, *Transplant. Proc.* **15**:1424–1426.

Nakagawara, G., Yamasaki, G., Kimura, S., Kojima, Y., and Miyazaki, I., 1978, Insulin-releasing activity and successful transplantation of pancreatic islets preserved by tissue culture, *Surgery* **83**:188–193.

Nakagawara, G., Kojima, Y., Mizukami, T., Ono, S., and Miyazaki, I., 1981, Transplantation of cryopreserved pancreatic islets into the portal vein, *Transplant. Proc.* **13**:1503–1507.

Nakajima, Y., Nakano, H., Nakagawa, K., Segawa, M., and Shiratori, T., 1982, Effect of total lymphoid irradiation on pancreatic islet xenografts survival in rats, *Transplantation* **34**:98–100.

Nash, J. R., and Bell, P. R., 1979, Effect of macrophage suppression on the survival of islet allografts, *Transplant. Proc.* **11**:986–988.

Nash, J. R., Peters, M., and Bell, P. R. F., 1977, Comparative survival of pancreatic islets, heart, kidney, and skin allografts in rats, with and without enhancement, *Transplantation* **24**:70–73.

Nash, J. R., Peters, M., and Bell, P. R. F., 1978, Studies on the enhancement of rat islet allografts, *Transplantation* **25**:180–181.

Nash, J. R., Smit, J. A., Myburgh, M. A., and Bell, P. R. F., 1981, The effect of total lymphoid irradiation (TLI) and donor bone marrow (BM) on islet transplantation in baboons, *Transplant. Proc.* **13**:458–459.

Natali, P. G., DeMartino, C., Quaranta, V., Nicotra, M. R., Frezza, F., Pellegrino, M. A., and Ferrone, S., 1981a, Expression of Ia-like antigens in normal human nonlymphoid tissues, *Transplantation* **31**:75–78.

Natali, P. G., Quaranta, V., Nicotra, R., Apollonj, C., Pellegrino, M. A., and Ferrone, S., 1981b, Tissue distribution of Ia-like antigens in different species: Analysis with monoclonal antibodies, *Transplant. Proc.* **13**:1026–1029.

Nelken, D., Friedman, E. A., Morse, S. I., and Beyer, W. M., 1977, Islets of Langerhans allotransplantation in the rat, *Transplant. Proc.* **9**:333–336.

Noack, S., Ziegler, B., Kloting, I., Besch, W., Reiher, K., and Hahn, H. J., 1982, Enhanced insulin release during pregnancy in transplanted streptozotocin-diabetic rats, *Diabetologia* **23**:188–189.

Noel, J., Rabinovitch, A., Olson, L., Kyriakides, G., Miller, J., and Mintz, D., 1982, A method for large-scale, high-yield isolation of canine pancreatic islets of Langerhans, *Metabolism* **31**:184–187.

Nolan, M. S., Lindsay, N. J., Savas, C. P., Herold, A., Slater, D. N., and Fox, M., 1980, Pancreatic transplantation in the rat: Long-term study following different methods of management of exocrine drainage, *Diabetologia* **22**:391.

Nolan, M. S., Lindsey, N. J., Savas, C. P., Slater, D. N., and Fox, M., 1982, Pancreatic transplantation in the rat. A simplified method using aortic interposition and cuff techniques, *Transplantation* **33**:327–329.

Nolan, M. S., Lindsey, N. J., Ingram, N. P., Herold, A., Slater, D. N., and Fox, M., 1983, Hypothermic preservation of the pancreas: Comparison of three infusion media, *Transplant. Proc.* **15**:1311–1313.

Nozawa, M., Weil, R., McIntosh, R., and Reemtsma, K., 1974, Vascularized transplantation of the rat pancreas without duodenum, *Transplantation* **17**:137–140.

Oakes, P. D., Spees, E. K., Annable, C. A., and Reckard, C. R., 1978, Acute hepatocellular damage following intraportal transplantation of pancreatic islets in rats, *J. Surg. Res.* **24**:182–187.

Ono, J., Lacy, P. E., Michael, H. E. B., and Grieder, M. H., 1979, Studies of the functional and morphological status of islets maintained at 24C for four weeks in vitro, *Am. J. Pathol.* **97**:489–498.

Orloff, M. J., Lee, S., Charters, A. C., Grambort, D. E., Storck, G., and Knox, D., 1975, Long-term studies of pancreas transplantation in experimental diabetes mellitus, *Ann. Surg.* **182**:198–206.

Orsetti, A., Bouhaddioni, N., Crespy, S., and Perez, R., 1981, Analyse critique de la valeur fonctionnelle d'un pancreas bio-artificiel (modèle a fibres creusés), *C. R. Soc. Biol. (Paris)* **175**(2):221–230.

O'Shea, G. M., Van Rooy, H., Wood, A., and Sun, A. M., 1982, Reversal of diabetic symptoms by transplantation of microencapsulated islets of Langerhans, *Diabetes* **31**(Suppl. 2):51A.

Outzen, H. C., and Leiter, E. H., 1981, Transplantation of pancreatic islets into cleared mammary fat pads, *Transplantation* **32**:101–105.

Panijaynond, P., Soroff, H. S., and Monaco, A. P., 1973, Pancreatic islet isografts in mice, *Surg. Forum* **24**:329–331.

Panijayanond, P., and Monaco, A. P., 1974, Enhancement of pancreatic islet allograft survival with ALS and donor bone marrow, *Surg. Forum* **25**:379–381.

Papachristou, D. N., and Fortner, J. G., 1979, Duct ligated versus duct obliterated canine pancreatic autografts: Early postoperative results. *Transplant. Proc.* **11**:522–526.

Papachristou, D. N., and Fortner, J. G., 1980, A simple method of pancreatic transplantation in the dog, *Am. J. Surg.* **139**:344–347.

Parr, E. L., 1979, The absence of H-2 antigens from mouse pancreatic B-cells demonstrated by immunoferritin labeling, *J. Exp. Med.* **150**:1–9.

Parr, E. L., Bowen, K. M., and Lafferty, K. J., 1980a, Cellular changes in cultured mouse thryoid and islets of Langerhans, *Transplantation* **30**:135–141.

Parr, E. L., Lafferty, K. J., Bowen, K. M., and McKenzie, I. F., 1980b, H-2 complex and Ia antigens on cells dissociated from mouse thyroid glands and islets of Langerhans, *Transplantation* **30**:142–148.

Parr, E. L., Oliver, J. R., and King, N. J. C., 1982, The surface concentration of H-2 antigens on mouse pancreatic B-cells and islet cell transplantation, *Diabetes* **31**(Suppl. 4):1–8.

Payne, W. D., Sutherland, D. E. R., Matas, A. J., and Najarian, J. S., 1978, Cryopreservation of neonatal rat islet tissue, *Surg. Forum* **29**:347–349.

Payne, W. D., Sutherland, D. E. R., Matas, A. J., and Najarian, J. S., 1983a, Successful long-term cryopreservation of neonatal rat islet tissue, *Cryobiology*, **20**:226–229.

Payne, W. D., Drath, W. D., and Kahan, D. D., 1983b, Streptozotocin-induced abnormalities in diabetic rat neutrophil oxygen metabolism, *J. Surg. Res.*, in press.

Payne, E. D., Sutherland, D. E. R., Matas, A. J., Gorecki, P., and Najarian, J. S., 1979, DL-ethionine treatment of adult pancreatic donors: Amelioration of diabetes in multiple recipients with tissue from a single donor, *Ann Surg.* **189**:248–256.

Pegg, D. E., Klempnauer, J., Diaper, M. P., and Taylor, M. J., 1982, Assessment on hypothermic preservation of the pancreas in the rat by a normothermic perfusion assay. *J. Surg. Res.* **33**:194–200.

Perloff, L. H., Naji, A., and Barker, C. F., 1980, Whole pancreas versus isolated islet transplant on an immunological comparison, *Surgery* **88**:222–230.

Perloff, L. J., Naji, A., and Barker, C. F., 1981a, Islet sensitivity to humoral antibody, *Surg. Forum* **32**:390–391.

Perloff, L. J., Naji, A., Silvers, W. K., McKearn, T. J., and Barker, C. F., 1981b, Enhancement of whole pancreas and islet allografts, *Transpl. Proc.* **13**:1423.

Perloff, L. J., Barker, C. F., and Naji, A., 1983, Further studies on split tolerance. *Transplant. Proc.* **15**:841–844.

Piegari, V., Parmeggiani, U., Canonico, S., Barbarisi, A., Gentile, A., Procaccini, E., Bifani, M., and Cardamone, B., 1981, Physiopathological problems and comparison of different technical solutions in pancreas transplantation. Experimental research on the dog, *New Trends* **1**:15–29.

Pipeleers-Marichal, M., Pipeleers, D. G., Cutler, J., Lacy, P. E., and Kipnis, D., 1976, Metabolic and morphologic studies in intraportal islet transplanted rats, *Diabetes* **25**:1041–1051.

Pipeleers, D. G., Pipeleers-Marichal, M. A., Karl, I. E., and Kipnis, D. M., 1978, Secretory capability of islets transplanted intraportally in the diabetic rat, *Diabetes* **27**:817–824.

Pi-Sunyer, F. K., Woo, R., Weber, C., Hardy, M. A., and Reemstma, K., 1979, Selection of a practical method of pancreatic islet transplantation in the rat, *Surg. Forum* **30**:301–303.

Povlsen, C. O., Skakkebaek, N. E., Rygaard, J., Jensen, G., 1974, Heterotransplantation of human fetal organs to the mouse mutant nude, *Nature* **248**:247–249.

Prowse, S. J., Lafferty, K. J., Simeonovic, C. J., Agostino, M., Bowen, K. M., and Steele, E. J., 1982a, The reversal of diabetes by pancreatic islet transplantation, *Diabetes* **31**(Suppl. 4):30–37.

Prowse, S. J., Steel, E. J., and Lafferty, K. J., 1982b, Reversal of insulitis associated and spontaneous diabetes in nonimmunosuppressed mice by islet allografts, *Aust. J. Exp. Biol. Med. Soc.*, in press.

Rabinovitch, A., Muller, W. A., Vastutic, F., Malaisse-Lagae, G., and Mintz, D. H., 1976, Pancreatic isotransplantation. Influence of severity of diabetes in the recipient, *Diabetologia* **12**:415.

Rabinovitch, A., Fuller, L., Mintz, D., Severyn, W., Noel, J., Flaa, C., Kyriakides, G. J., and Miller, J., 1981, Responses of canine lymphocytes to allogeneic and autologous islets of Langerhans in mixed cell cultures, *J. Clin. Invest.* **67**:1507–1516.

Rabinovitch, A., Alejandro, R., Noel, J., Brunschwig, J. P., and Ryan, U. S., 1982a, Tissue culture reduces Ia antigen-bearing cells in rat islets and prolongs islet allograft survival, *Diabetes* **15**(Suppl. 4):48–54.

Rabinovitch, A., Russel, T., Sheinwald, F., Noel, J., Files, N., Patel, Y., and Ingram, M., 1982b, Preparation of rat islet B-cell enriched fractions by light-scatter flow egtometry, *Diabetes* **31**:939–943.

Rajotte, R. B., Stewart, H. L., Voss, W. A. G., Shnitka, T. K., and Dossetor, J. B., 1977, Viability studies on frozen-thawed rat islets of Langerhans, *Cryobiology* **14**:116–120.

Rajotte, R. B., Scharp, D. W., Downing, R., Preston, R., Ballinger, W. F., and Molnar, G. D., 1981, Pancreatic islet banking: Transplantation of frozen thawed islets transplanted between centers, *Cryobiology* **18**:357–369.

Rausis, C., Choudhury, A., and Ogata, Y., 1970, Influence of pancreatic duct anastomosis and function of autotransplanted canine pancreatic segments, *J. Surg. Res.* **10**:551–557.

Rayfield, E. J., and Seto, Y., 1978, Viruses and the pathogenesis of diabetes mellitus, *Diabetes* **27**:1126–1142.

Reach, G., Poussier, P., Sausse, A., Assan, R., Itoh, M., and Gerich, J. E., 1981, Functional evaluation of a bioartificial pancreas using isolated islets perifused with blood ultrafiltrate, *Diabetes* **30**:296–301.

Reckard, C. R., Zeigler, M. M., and Barker, C. F., 1973, Physiological and immunological consequences of transplanting isolated pancreatic islets, *Surgery* **74**:91–99.

Reckard, C. R., Franklin, W., and Schulak, J. A., 1978, Intrasplenic vs. intraportal pancreatic islet transplantation: Quantitative, qualitative and immunological aspects, *Trans. Am. Soc. Artif. Intern. Organs* **24**:232–234.

Reckard, C. R., Stuart, F. P., and Schulak, J. A., 1979, Immunologic comparison of isolated pancreatic islets and whole-organ allografts, *Transplant. Proc.* **11:563–566.**

Reckard, C. R., Stuart, F. P., Clayman, J. L., Buckingham, F., and Schulak, J. A., 1981, Differential susceptibility of segmental and isolated islet allografts of rat pancreas to rejection and enhancement, *Transplant. Proc.* **13**(1):819–822.

Reece-Smith, H., DuToit, D. R., McShane, P., and Morris, P. J., 1981a, Prolonged survival of pancreatic islet allografts transplanted beneath the renal capsule, *Transplantation* **31**:305–306.

Reece-Smith, H., DuToit, D. F., McShane, P., and Morris, P. J., 1981b, Effect of cyclosporin A on rejection of pancreatic islets transplanted under the renal capsule, *Transplantation* **32**:333–334.

Reece-Smith, H., Homan, W. P., DuToit, D. F., McShane, P., and Morris, P. J., 1981c, A technique for transplanting pancreatic islets as a vascularized graft and prevention of rejection with cyclosporin A, *Transplantation* **31**:442–444.

Reece-Smith, H., Homan, W. P., DuToit, D. F., McShane, P., and Morris, P. J., 1981d, How quickly does "vascularization" of isolated adult pancreatic islets occur? *Transplantation* **32**:341–342.

Reece-Smith, H., DuToit, D. F., McShane, P., Morris, P. J., 1981e, Effect of silica pretreatment and cyclosporin A therapy in isolated islet allografts in the rat, *Transplantation* **31**:484–485.

Reece-Smith, H., Homan, W. P., McShane, P., and Morris, P. J., 1982a, Indefinite survival of isolated pancreatic islets in rats rendered immunologically unresponsive to renal allografts, *Transplantation* **33**:452–453.

Reece-Smith, H., McShane, P., and Morris, P. J., 1982b, Glucose and insulin changes following a renoportal shunt in streptozotocin diabetic rats with pancreatic islet isografts under the kidney capsule, *Diabetologia* **23**:343–346.

Reece-Smith, H., Fairbrother, B. J., McShane, P., and Morris, P. J., 1983, Composite kidney/islet allografts: Effect of immunosuppression and the diabetic status of the intermediate host, *Transplant. Proc.* **15**(1):1347–1348.

Reemtsma, K., Oluwole, S., Fawwaz, R., and Hardy, M. A., 1981, Pancreatic islet allograft prolongation by selective lymphoid irradiation (SLI), culture techniques, and ALG, *Transplant. Proc.* **13**:801–806.

Reintgen, D., Feldman, J., Vervaerti, C., and Seigler, H. F., 1980a, Transplantation of insulinoma into the diabetic Syrian hamster, *Ann. Surg,* **191**:105–113.

Reintgen, D., Croker, B., Vervaerti, C., Feldman, J., and Seigler, H. G., 1980b, Immunological consequences of transplanting rat insulinomas, *Transplantation* **30**:16.

Rosenbloom, A. L., Silverstein, J. H., Lezotte, D. C., Richardson, K., and McCallum, R. N., 1981, Limited joint mobility in childhood diabetes mellitus indicates increased risk (or microvascular disease), *N. Engl. J. Med.* **305**:191–194.

Roversi, C. A., Campione, O., Liguori, L., Spighi, M., Nicoli Aldini, N., Torchi, B. M., Petrone, F., Melotti, R., Rossi, M., and Marrano, D., 1979, Experimental model of isolated pancreas isothermic perfusion. Preliminary study, *Il Policlinico Sez. Chirurgica* **86**:293–298.

Ruiz, J. O., Uchida, J., Schultz, L. S., and Lillehei, R. C., 1972, Function studies after auto- and allotransplantation and denervation of pancreaticuduodenal segments in dogs, *Am. J. Surg.* **123**:236–242.

Rumpf, D. Lohlein, D., and Pichalmayr, R., 1977, Multiple transplantation of islets of Langerhans, *Eur. Surg. Res.* **9**:403–410.

Rynasiewicz, J. J., Sutherland, D. E. R., Kawahara, K., Gorecki, P., and Najarian, J. S., 1980a, Cyclosporin A prolongation of segmental pancreatic and islet allograft function in rats, *Transplant. Proc.* **12**:270–274.

Rynasiewicz, J. J., Sutherland, D. E. R., Kawahara, K., and Najarian, J. S., 1980b, Total lymphoid irradiation: Prolongation of pancreas and islet allografts in rats, *Surg. Forum* **31**:359–360.

Rynasiewicz, J. J., Sutherland, D. E. R., Ferguson, R. M., Squifflet, J. P., Morrow, C. E., Goetz, F. C., and Najarian, J. S., 1982, Cyclosporin A for immunosuppression: Observations in rat heart, pancreas, and islet allograft models and in human renal and pancreas transplantation, *Diabetes* **31**:92–107.

Sandler, S., and Andersson, A., 1980, Successful transplantation of cryopreserved mouse pancreatic islets, *Diabetologia* **19**:312.

Sandler, S., and Andersson, A., 1981, Islet implantation into diabetic mice with pancreatic insulitis, *Acta Pathol. Microbiol. Scand. [A]* **89**:107–112.

Sandler, S., and Andersson, A., 1982a, Short- and long-term effects of dimethyl sulfoxide on mouse pancreatic islet B-cell function in vitro, *Cryobiology* **19**:299–305.

Sandler, S., and Andersson, A., 1982b, Survival of intrasplenically implanted islets in mice with experimental insulitis and hyperglycemia, *Diabetes* **31**(Suppl. 4):78–82.

Sandler, S., Nelsson, B., Pelesson, B., Hellerstrom, C., and Andersson, A., 1982c, Functional characteristics of cryopreserved mouse islets, *Horm. Metab. Res.* **12**:71–74.

Sandler, S., Andersson, A., Hellerstrom, C., Petersson, B., Swenne, I., Bjorken, C., and Groth, C. G., 1982d, Preservation of morphology, insulin biosynthesis and insulin release of cryopreserved human fetal pancreas, *Diabetes* **31**:238–241.

Satake, K., Nowygrod, R., Oluwole, S., Todd, G. J., Hardy, M. A., and Reemtsma, K., 1979, Free duct pancreatic transplantation in rats, *Surg. Forum* **30**:308–309.

Satake, K., Hardy, M. A., Nagorsky, M. J., Wolff, M., Reemtsma, K., and Nowygrod, R., 1983, Comparison of exocrine and endocrine function of islet grafts, and "duct-ligated" and "free duct" whole pancreas transplants in diabetic rats, *J. Surg. Res.*, in press.

Savas, C. P., Lindsey, N. J., Nolan, M. S., Slater, D. N., and Fox, M. 1981, Rejection patterns following different methods of dealing with the exocrine drainage of the rat pancreas utilizing a new simplified technique of vascular anastomosis, *Diabetologia* :**21**:513.

Scharp, D. W., 1981, Rejection of islet "isografts" in a strain of Lewis rats. *Transplantation* **31**:229–230.

Scharp, D. W., 1982, Hybrid artificial pancreas. *Trans. Amer. Soc. Artif. Intern. Organs* **28**:642–643.

Scharp, D. W., Kemp, C. B., Knight, M. J., Ballinger, W. F., and Lacy, P. E., 1973, The use of Ficoll in the preparation of viable islets of Langerhans from the rat pancreas, *Transplantation* **16**:686–689.

Scharp, D. W., White, D. J., Ballinger, W. F., and Lacy, P. E., 1974, Transplantation of intact islets of Langerhans after tissue culture, *In Vitro* **9**:364 (abstract).

Scharp, D. W., Murphy, J. J., Newton, W. T., Ballinger, W. F. and Lacy, P. E., 1975, Transplantation of islets of Langerhans in diabetic Rhesus monkeys. *Surgery* **77**:100–105.

Scharp, D. W., Merrell, R. C., Feldman, S. D., Downing, R., Lacy, P. E., and Ballinger, W. E., 1978, The use of gyrotation cultures for the preservation of isolated islets, *Surg. Forum* **29**:100–102.

Scharp, D. W., Downing, R., Merrell, R. C., Greider, M., 1980, Isolating the elusive islet, *Diabetes* **29**(Suppl. 1):19–30.

Scharp, D. W., Downing, R., Merrell, R. C., Nunnelly, S., Kiske, D., and Greider, M. H., 1981, New approaches in the methods for isolating mammalian islets of Langerhans utilizing the dog pancreas, in: *Islet Isolation, Cultures, and Cryopreservations* (K. Federlin and R. G. Bretzel, eds.), pp. 9–28, Thieme-Stratton, New York.

Scharp, D. W., Hirshberg, G., and Long, J., 1982, The effect of islet dosage and time on rat portal vein isografts, *Diabetes* **31**(Suppl. 2):162a.

Scharp, D. W., Feldman, S. D., Finley, T., Mason, N. S., and Ballinger, W. F., 1982a, An intravascular transplantation chamber for immuno-isolation of islets of Langerhans, *Trans. Am. Soc. Artif. Intern. Organs* **28**:229–231.

Scharp, D. W., Mason, N. S., and Sparks, R. E. 1982b, The use of hybrid artificial organs to provide immuno-isolation to endocrine grafts, *Trans. Amer. Soc. Artif. Intern. Organs* **28**:642–643.

Schmidt, R. E., and Scharp, D. W., 1982, Axonal Dystrophy in experimental diabetic autonomic neuropathy, *Diabetes* **31.**:761–770.

Schmidt, R. E., Santiago, B. P., Olack, B. J., and Scharp, D. W. 1983, The effect of pancreatic islet transplantation and insulin therapy on experimental diabetic autonomic neuropathy, *Diabetes* **32**(6):532–540.

Schulak, J. A., Franklin, W., and Reckard, C. R., 1977, Morphological and functional changes following intraportal islet allograft rejection: Irreversibility with steroid pulse therapy, *Surg. Forum* **28**:296–299.

Schulak, J. A., and Reckard, C. R., 1978, Experimental transplantation of pancreatic islet allografts, *J. Surg. Res.* **25**:562–571.

Schulak, J. A., Stuart, F. P., and Reckard, C. R., 1978, Physiologic aspects of intrasplenic autotransplantation of pancreatic fragments in the dog after 24 hours of cold storage, *J. Surg. Res.* **24**:125–131.

Schulak, J. A., and Reckard, C. R., 1979, Intrasplenic islet function in the dog following distal splenorenal shunts, *Surg. Forum* **29**:340–343.

Schulak, J. A., Clayman, J. L., Stuart, F. P., and Reckard, C. R., 1980, Synergistic effect of donor irradiation and antilymphocyte serum on isolated pancreatic islet allograft survival, *Surg. Forum* **31**:361–362.

Schulak, J. A., Franklin, W., Buckingham, F., Stuart, F. P., and Reckard, C. R., 1981, Warm ischemia in pancreas transplantation: A functional and histologic evaluation, *Surg. Forum* **32**:392–393.

Schulak, J. A., Franklin, W. A., Stuart, F. P., and Reckard, C. R., 1983, The effect of warm ischemia on segmental pancreas transplantation in the rat, *Transplantation* **35**:7–11.

Scott, J., Steffes, M. W., and Lernmark, A., 1982, Islet transplantation in mice differing in the I and S subregions of the H-2 complex. Effects of presensitization with skin allografts, *Scand. J. Immunol.* **16**:9–15.

Selawry, H., Harrison, J., Patipa, M., and Mintz, D. H., 1978, Pancreatic islet isotransplantation: Effects of age and organ culture of donor islets on reversal of diabetes in rats, *Diabetes* **27**:625–631.

Selawry, H. P., Cohen, H. L., and Mui M. M., 1981, The effect of donor strain blood and ALS therapy on pancreatic islet allograft survival in the rat, *Diabetes* **30**:947–950.

Sells, R. A., Calne, R. Y., Hadjiyanakis, V., and Marshall, V. C., 1972, Glucose and insulin metabolism after pancreatic transplantation, *Br. Med. J.* **3**:678–681.

Serie, J. R., Hegre, O. D., Hickey, G. E., and Schmitt, R. V., Prolongation of xenograft survival with culture-isolated neonatal islets without the use of immunosuppression, *Transplantation,* **36**:6–10.

Severyn, W., Olson, L., Miller, J., Kyriakides, G., Rabinovitch, A., Flaa, C., and Mintz, D., 1982, Studies on the survival of simultaneous canine renal and segmental pancreatic allografts, *Transplantation* **33**:606–612.

Shah, K. H., Bitter-Suermann, H., and Save-Soderber, J., 1980, Morphologic finding in duct-ligated pancreas grafts in the rat. An analysis of isografts, allografts and long standing allografts in hosts conditioned by previous spleen allografts, *Transplantation* **30**:83–89 in press.

Shibata, A., Ludviggen, C. W., Naber, S. P., McDaniel, M. L., and Lacy, P. E. 1976, Standardization of a digestion filtration method for isolation of pancreatic islets, *Diabetes* **25**:667–672.

Shienvold, F., Alejandrom, Hajek, S., and Mintz, S., 1982, Immunocytochemical localization of HLA-DR in the human islets of Langerhans, *Diabetes* **31**(Suppl. 2):47a.

Silberberg, K., Hirshberg, G. E., and Lesker, P., 1977, Enzymes studies in the articular cartilage of diabetic rats and of rats bearing transplanted pancreatic islets, *Diabetes* **26**:732–735.

Siegel, E. G., Trimble, E. R., Berthoud, H.-R., Bereiter, D. A., and Renold, A. E., 1980a, Effect of absence of early insulin response on oral glucose tolerance in islet-transplanted rats, *Transplant. Proc.* **12**(Suppl. 2):192–194.

Siegel, E. G., Trimble, E. R., Renold, A. E., and Berthoud, H. R., 1980b, Importance of preabsorptive insulin release on oral glucose tolerance: Studies in pancreatic islet transplanted rats, *Gut* **21**:1002–1009.

Silvers, W. K., Fleming, H. L., Naji, A., and Barker, C. F., 1982, The influence of removing passenger cells on the fate of skin and parathyroid allografts. Evidence for major histocompatibility complex restriction in transplantation immunity, *Diabetes* **15**(Suppl. 4):60–62.

Simeonovic, C. J., Bowen, K. M., Kotlavsk, I., and Lafferty, K. J., 1980, Modulation of tissue immunogenicity by organ culture: Comparison of adult islets and fetal pancreas, *Transplantation* **30**:174–179.

Simeonovic, C. J., and Lafferty, K. J., 1981, Effect of organ culture on function of transplanted foetal pancreas, *Aust. J. Exp. Biol. Med. Sci.* **59** (Pt. 6):707–712.

Simeonovic, C. J., and Lafferty, K. J., 1982, Immunogenicity of isolated foetal mouse proislets, *Aust. J. Exp. Biol. Med. Soc.* **60**:391–395.

Slater, D., Mangnall, Y., Smythe, A., and Fox, M., 1976, The rejection of islets of Langerhans following intrahepatic transplantation in the rat, *Acta. Endocrinol.* **83**:295–302.

Slater, D. N., Mangnall, Y., Smythe, A., Ward, A. M., and Fox, M., 1978, Neonatal islet cell transplantation in the diabetic rat: Effect on the renal complication, *J. Pathol.* **124**:117–124.

Slavin, S., Strober, S., Fuks, Z., and Kaplan, J. S., 1977, Induction of specific tissue transplant tolerance using fractionated total lymphoid irradiation in adult mice: Long term survival of bone marrow and skin grafts, *J. Exp. Med.* **146**:34–48.

Slavin, S., Strober, S., Fuks, Z., and Kaplan, H. S., 1979, Immunosuppression and organ transplantation tolerance using total lymphoid irradiation, *Diabetes* **29**:121–123.

Slijepcevic, M., Helmke, K., and Federlin, K., 1975, Islet transplantation in experimental diabetes in the rat. III. Studies in allogeneic streptozotocin-treated rats, *Horm. Metab.* **7**:456–461.

Smith, J. P., Pennline, J., Edwards, M. G., Dobersen, M. J., and Bitter-Suermann, H., 1983, Survival of islet allografts in specifically tolerant hosts, *Transplant. Proc.* **15**:1349–1354.

Sopwith, A. M., Hutton, J. C., Naber, S. P., Chick, W. L., and Hales, C. N., 1981, Insulin secretion by a transplantable rat islet cell tumor, *Diabetologia* **21**:224–229.

Spence, R. K., Perloff, L. J., and Barker, C. F., 1979, Fetal pancreas in treatment of experimental diabetes in rats, *Transplant. Proc.* **11**:533–536.

Squifflet, J. P., Sutherland, D. E. R., Morrow, C. E., Braunwarth, J., and Najarian, J. S., 1982a, Physiologic comparison between segmental pancreas and islet cell transplants in rats, *Diabetes* **31**(Suppl. 2):160A.

Squifflet, J. P., Sutherland, D. E. R., Rynasiewicz, J. J., Field, J., Heil, J., and Najarian, J. S., 1982b, Combined immunosuppression therapy with cyclosporin A and azathioprine: A synergistic effect in three of four experimental models, *Transplantation* **34**:315–318.

Squifflet, J. P., Sutherland, D. E. R., Field, J., Rynasiewicz, J. J., and Heil, J., 1983a, Synergistic immunosuppressive effect of cyclosporin A (CYA) and azathioprine (AZA), *Transplant. Proc.* **15**:520–522.

Squifflet, J. P., Sutherland, D. E. R., Morrow, C. E., Florack, G., Field, J., and Najarian, J. S., 1983b, Comparison of rejection of intraportal islet versus immediately vascularized segmental pancreatic allografts in rats in relation to beta cell mass engrafted, *Transplant. Proc.* **15**(1):1344–1346.

Squifflet, J.-P., Sutherland, D. E. R., Rynasiewicz, J. J., Bentley, F. R., Florack, G., and Najarian, J. S., 1982a, Technical aspects of segmental pancreatic grafting in rats, *J. Microsurg.* **4**:61–66.

Squifflet, J. P., Sutherland, D. E. R., Florack, G., and Najarian, J. S., 1983b, The course of combined pancreas and spleen allografts in rats, *Transplantation* **34**:302.

Steen-Olson, T., Orskov, H., and Lundbaek, K., 1966, Kidney lesions in rats with severe long term alloxan diabetes, comparison with human diabetic glomerular lesions, *Acta Pathol. Microbiol. Scand.* **66**:1–12.

Steffes, M. W., Sutherland, D. E. R., Mauer, S. M., Leonard, R. J., Najarian, J. S., and Brown, D. M., 1974, Plasma insulin and glucose levels in diabetic rats prior to and following islet transplantation, *J. Lab. Clin. Med.* **85**:75–81.

Steffes, M. W., Brown, D. M., Basgen, J. M., and Mauer, S. M., 1979, Glomerular basement membrane thickness following islet transplantation in the diabetic rat, *Lab. Invest.* **41**:116–118.

Steffes, M. W., Brown, D. M., Basgen, J. M., and Mauer, S. M., 1980, Amelioration of mesangial volume and surface alteration following islet transplantation in rats, *Diabetes* **29**:509–515.

Steffes, M. W., Nielsen, O., Dyrberg, T., Baekkeskov, S., Scott, J., and Lernmark, A., 1981, Islet transplantation in mice differing in the I and S subregions of the H-2 complex, *Transplantation* **31**:476–479.

Steffes, M. W., Vernier, R. L., Brown, D. M., Basgen, J. M., and Mauer, M. S., 1982, Diabetic glomerulopathy in the uninephrectomized rat resists amelioration following islet transplantation, *Diabetologia* **23**:347–353.

Steinman, R. M., 1981, Dendritic cells, *Transplantation* **31**:151–155.

Strautz, R. L., 1970, Studies of hereditary-obese mice (ob/ob) after implantation of pancreatic islets in Millipore filter capsules, *Diabetologia* **6**:306–312.

Streilein, J. W., Toews, G. B., and Bergstresser, P. R., 1979, Corneal allografts fail to express Ia antigens, *Nature* **282**:326–327.

Strubbe, J. H., 1982, Effects of pancreas transplantation on insulin secretion in the rat during ingestion of varying glucose loads, *Diabetologia* **22**:354–357.

Strubbe, J. H., and van Wachem, P., 1981, Insulin secretion by the transplanted neonatal pancreas during food intake in fasted and fed rats, *Diabetologia* **20**:228–236.

Sun, A. M., Parisius, W., Healy, G. M., Vacek, I., and Macmorine, H. G., 1977, The use in diabetic rats and monkeys of artificial capillary units containing cultured islets of Langerhans, *Diabetes* **26**:1136–1139.

Sun, A. M., Parisius, W., Macmorine, H., Sefton, M., and Stone, R., 1980, An artificial endocrine pancreas containing cultured islets of Langerhans, *Artif. Organs* **4**:275–278.

Sutherland, D. E. R., 1980, International human pancreas and islet transplant registry tabulation, *Transplant. Proc.* **12**(No. 4, Suppl. 2):229–236.

Sutherland, D. E. R., 1981a, Pancreas and islet transplantation. I. Experimental studies, *Diabetologia* **20**:161–185.

Sutherland, D. E. R., 1981b, Pancreas and islet transplantation. II. Clinical trials, *Diabetologia* **20**:435–450.

Sutherland, D. E. R., 1982, Report of International Human Pancreas and Islet Transplantation Registry cases through 1981, *Diabetes* **31**(Suppl. 4):112–116.

Sutherland, D. E. R., 1983, Current status of pancreas transplantation: Registry statistics and an overview, *Transplant. Proc.* **15**(1):1303–1307.

Sutherland, D. E. R., Steffes, M. W., Mauer, S. M., and Najarian, J. S., 1974, Isolation of human and porcine islets of Langerhans and islet transplantation in pigs, *J. Surg. Res.* **16**:102–111.

Sutherland, D. E. R., Kretschmer, G. J., Matas, A. J., and Najarian, J. S., 1977, Experience with auto and allotransplantation of pancreatic fragments to the spleen of totally pancreatectomized dogs, *Trans. Am. Soc. Artif. Intern. Organs* **23**:723–725.

Sutherland, D. E. R., Frenzel, E., Payne, W. D., Matas, A. J., and Najarian, J. S., 1979a, Transplantation of adult islet tissue in rats: Spleen vs. portal vein site, *Surg. Forum* **30**:305–307.

Sutherland, D. E. R., Goetz, F. C., and Najarian, J. S., 1979b, Intraperitoneal transplantation of immediately vascularized segmental grafts without duct ligation: A clinical trial, *Transplantation* **28**:485–491.

Sutherland, D. E. R., Baumgartner, D., and Najarian, J. S., 1980a, Free intraperitoneal drainage of segmental pancreas grafts: Clinical and experimental observations on technical aspects, *Transplant. Proc.* **12**(No. 4, Suppl. 2):26–32.

Sutherland, D. E. R., Rynasiewicz, J. J., Kawahara, K., Gorecki, P., and Najarian, J. S., 1980b, Rejection of islets versus immediately vascularized pancreatic allografts: A quantitative comparison, *J. Surg. Res.* **29**:240–247.

Sutherland, D. E. R., Matas, A. J., Goetz, F. C., and Najarian, J. S., 1980c, Transplantation of dispersed pancreatic islet tissue in humans, *Diabetes* **29**(Suppl. 1):31–41.

Sutherland, D. E. R., Goetz, F. C., Elick, B. A., and Najarian, J. S., 1982, Experience with 49 segmental pancreas transplants in 49 diabetic patients, *Transplantation* **34**:330–338.

Sutherland, D. E. R., Goetz, F. C., Elick, B. A., and Najarian, J. S., 1983a, Pancreas transplantation for diabetics: Clinical experience and metabolic studies in 54 recent cases at the Univesity of Minnesota, *Transplant. Proc.* **15**(1):1322–1325.

Sutherland, D. E. R., Morrow, C. E., Florack, G., Kretschmer, G. J., Baumgartner, D. Matas, A. J., and Najarian, J. S., 1983b, Cold storage preservation of islet and pancreas grafts as assessed by in vivo function after transplantation to diabetic hosts, *Cryobiology* **20**:245–255.

Swenne, I., Reibring, L., Petersson, B., and Andersson, A., 1979, Growth of pancreatic islets of normal mice after transplantation into obese hyperglycemic mice littermates, *Acta Endocrinol.* **227**(Suppl.):70–71.

Tchobroutsky, G., 1978, Relation of diabetic control to development of microvascular complications, *Diabetologia* **15**:143–152.

Tellez-Yudilevich, M., Tyhurati, M., Howell, S. L., and Sheldon, J., 1977, Secretory capacity and ultrastructure of rat pancreatic islets after preservation of pancreas in different conditions, *Transplantation* **33**:217–221.

Tersigni, R., Toledo-Pereyra, L. H., Palestini, M., Cavellini, M., Capua, G., Caramin, F., and Stipa, S., 1980, Effect of ex vivo hypothalamic irradiation of duct-ligated pancreas allografts in dogs: functional, histological and ultrastructural findings, *The American Surgeon* **46**:713–721.

Theodorou, N. A., and Howell, S. L., 1981, An assessment of diffusion chambers for use in pancreatic islet transplantation, *Transplantation* **27**:350–353.

Theodorou, N. A., Vrbova, H., Tyhurst, M., and Howell, S. L., 1980a, Problems in the use of polycarbonate diffusion chambers for syngeneic pancreatic islet transplantation in rats, *Diabetologia* **18**:313–317.

Theodorou, N. A., Tyhurst, M., Vrbova, H., and Howell, S., 1980b, Advantages of pilocarpine pretreatment of donors before pancreatic islet transplantation in rats, *Diabetologia* **19**:320.

Theodorou, N. A., Easterbrook, P., Tyhurst, M., and Howell, S. L., 1981, Islets of Langerhans implanted in diffusion chambers do not initiate antibody production, *Transplantation* **31**:89–90.

Thomson, N. M., Hancock, W. W., Lafferty, K. J., Kraft, N., and Atkins, R. C., 1983, Organ culture reduces Ia-positive cells present within the human foetal pancreas before and after prolonged organ culture, *Transplant. Proc.* **15**(1):1373–1376.

Toledo-Pereyra, L. H., 1981, Organ preservation. I. Kidney and pancreas, *J. Surg. Res.* **30**:165–180.

Toledo-Pereyra, L. H., and Castellanos, J., 1979, Role of pancreatic duct ligation for segmental pancreas autotransplantation, *Transplantation* **28**:469–475.

Toledo-Pereyra, L. H., Castellanos, J., Lampe, E. W., Lillehei, R. C., and Najarian, J. S., 1975, Comparative evaluation of pancreas transplantation techniques, *Ann. Surg.* **182**:567–571.

Toledo-Pereyra, L. H., Castellanos, J., Manifacio, G., and Lillehei, R. C., 1979a, Basic requirements of pancreatic mass for transplantation, *Arch. Surg.* **114**:1058–1062.

Toledo-Pereyra, L. H., Chee, M., Condie, R. M., Najarian, J. S., and Lillehei, R. C., 1979b, Forty-eight hours hypothermic storage of whole canine pancreas allografts, improved preservation with a colloid hyperosmolar solution, *Cryobiology* **16**:221–228.

Toledo-Pereyra, L. H., Gordon, D. A., and MacKenzie, G. H., 1981, Cryopreservation of islets of Langerhans, *Cryobiology* **18**:483–488.

Toledo-Pereyra, L. H., Gordon, D. A., and MacKenzie, G. H., 1981, Cryopreservation of whole pancreas versus islet cells, *Trans. Am. Soc. Artif. Intern. Organs.* **27**:259–262.

Toledo-Pereyra, L. H., Gordon, D. A., and MacKenzie, G. H., 1982a, Current research review. Organ freezing, *J. Surg. Res.* **32**:75–84.

Toledo-Pereyra, L. H., Gordon, D. A., and MacKenzie, G. H., 1982b, Prolongation of pancreatic islet cell allograft survival by graft pretreatment with antilymphoblast globulin (ALG), *Horm. Metab. Res.* **12**(Suppl.):141–144.

Toledo-Pereyra, L. H., Valjee, K. D., Chee, M., and Lillehei, R. C., 1979c, Preservation of the pancreas for transplantation, *Surg. Gynecol. Obstet.* **148**:57–61.

Toledo-Pereyra, L. H., Valjee, K. D., Chee, M., and Castellanos, J., 1980a, 24–48 hour pancreas preservation by hypothermic pulsatile perfusion prior to islet cell transplantation, *Arch. Surg.* **115**:95.

Toledo-Pereyra, L. H., Valjee, L. H., Zammitt, H. M., 1980b, Important factors in islet cell transplantation: The role of pancreatic fragments size, pH, potassium concentration and length of intraportal infusion, *Eur. Surg. Res.* **12**:72–78.

Toledo-Pereyra, L. H., Zammit, M., Cromwell, P. W., and Malcom, S. E., 1980c, Improvement of islet cell transplant survival with reduced number of islet cells after donor pretreatment with methylprednisolone and glucagon, *J. Surg. Res.* **29**:302–308.

Traeger, J., Dubernard, J. M., Touraine, J. L., Neyra, P., Malik, M. C., Pelissard, C., and Ruitton, A., 1979, Pancreatic transplantation in man: A new method of pancreas preparation and results on diabetes correction, *Transplant. Proc.* **11**:331–335.

Traverso, L. W., Abou-ZamZam, A. M., and Tompkins, R. K., 1978, Effect of an elemental diet on canine pancreatic autografts, *Surg. Forum* **29**:378–379.

Trimble, E. R., Vassutine, I., Delray-Sachs, M., and Renold, A. E., 1979, Long term survival of pancreatic islets transplanted without immunosuppression across weak histompatibility barriers, *Transplant. Proc.* **11**:1995–1999.

Trimble, E. R., Karakash, C., Malaisse-Lagae, F., Vissatine, I., Orci, L., and Renold, A. E., 1980a, Effects of intraportal islet transplantation on the transplanted tissues and the recipient pancreas. I. Functional studies, *Diabetes* **29**:341–347.

Trimble, E. R., Siegel, E. G., Berthoud, H. R., and Renold, A. E., 1980b, Intraportal islet transplantation: Functional assessment in conscious unrestrained rats, *Endocrinology* **106**:791–797.

Trimble, E. R., Berthoud, H. R., Siegel, E. G., Jeanrenaud, B., and Renold, A. E., 1981, Importance of cholinergic innervation of the pancreas for glucose tolerance in the rat, *Am. J. Physiol.* **241**:E337–41, 1981.

Tze, W. J., and Tai, J., 1982a, Effect of body weight on islet isolation in rats, *Transplantation* **34**:68.

Tze, W. J., Wong, F. C., and Tingle, A. J., 1976b, The use of hypaque ficoll in the isolation of pancreatic islets in rats, *Transplantation* **22**:201–205.

Tze, W. J., and Tai, J., 1982b, Preparation of pseudoislets for morphological and functional studies, *Transplantation* **34**:228–231.

Tze, W. J., Wong, F. C., Chen, L. M., and O'Young, 1976a, Implantable artificial endocrine pancreas unit used to restore normoglycaemia in the diabetic rat, *Nature* **264**:466–476.

Tze, W. J., Tai, J., Wong, F., and Davis, H., 1980, Studies with implantable artificial capillary units containing rat islets on diabetic dogs, *Diabetologia* **19**:541–545.

Uchida, J., Ruiz, O., Catlefranchi, P. L., Schultz, L. S., and Lillehei, R. C., 1971, New technique of one stage heterotopic pancreaticoduodenal autotransplantation in the dog, *Surgery* **70**:604–608.

Umeyama, K., Hashimoto, H., Shim, K., and Satake, K., 1980, Ultrastructural studies on the allotransplanted pancreas in dogs, *Transplantation* **26**:373–381.

Ungar, R. H., 1982, Meticulous control of diabetes: Benefits, risks and precautions, *Diabetes* **31**:479–483.

Usadel, K. H., Schwedes, U., Leuacher, U., and Schoffling, K., 1974, Development of isologous transplants of cell suspensions of the fetal pancreas in the rat, *Acta Endocrinol.* **184**(Suppl.):97.

Usadel, K. H., Schwedes, U., Bastert, G., Fassbinder, W., Klempa, I., and Schoffling, K., 1980a, Fetal pancreatic transplantation, in: *Proceedings of the 10th International Congress of the Diabetes Federation* (W. K., Waldhausl, ed.), pp. 243–245, Excerpta Medica, Amsterdam.

Usadel, K. H., Schwedes, U., Bastert, G., Steinan, U., Klempa, I., Fassbinder, W., and Schoffling, K., 1980b, Transplantation of human fetal pancreas: Experience in thymusaplastic mice and rats and in a diabetic patient, *Diabetes* **29**(Suppl. 1):74–77.

Usadel, K. H., Schwedes, U., Maitland, J., and Turtle, J., 1981, Precultivation of human fetal pancreas prior to xenotransplantation, in: *Islet Isolation Culture and Cyropreservation* (K. Federlin and R. G., Bretzel, eds.), pp. 111–114, Thieme Stratton, New York.

van Hoorn, W. A., Vinik, A. I., and van Hoorn-Hickman, R., 1978, A comparison of two methods of orthotopic pancreas transplantation in the pig, *Transplantation* **26**:287–291.

van Schilfgaarde, R., Gooszen, H. G., Overbosch, E., and Terpstra, J. L., 1983, The arterial blood supply of the left lobe of the canine pancreas. I. Anatomical variations relevant to segmental pancreatic transplantation, *Surgery*, **93**:545–548.

Verschoor, L., Hulsmans, H. A. M., deGruyl, J., Westbroek, D. L., and MacDicken, I., 1975, Endocrine function of the canine pancreas: The effect of duct ligation and transplantation of the total duct ligated pancreas, *Acta Endocrinol.* **80**:302–318.

Vesely, D. L., Selawry, H., and Levey, G., 1979, Correction of decreased granylate cyclase activity in diabetic rats by pancreatic islet transplantation, *Transplantation* **27**:403–405.

Vialettes, B., Sutherland, D. E. R., Matas, A. J., Payne, W. D., and Najarian, J. S., 1978a, Quantitative studies of yield and efficiency of islet transplantation in rats. Comparison of isolated adult islets and dispersed neonatal pancreas, *Diabetologia* **14**:278.

Vialettes, B., Sutherland, D. E. R., Payne, W. D., Matas, A. J., and Najarian, J. S., 1978b, Synergistic effect of donor specific soluable membrane antigen injection and antilymphocyte globulin administration on the survival of islet allografts in rats, *Transplantation* **25**:336–338.

Vialettes, B., Lassmann, V., Vagre, P., and Simon, M. C., 1979a, Islet transplantation in diabetic rats. Long term followup of glucose tolerance, *Acta Diabet. Lat.* **16**:1–8.

Vialettes, B., Simon, M. C., Lassmann, V., Vague, P. H., 1979b, Prolonged survival of allotransplanted islets of Langerhans after cyclosporin A treatment in rats, *Transplantation* **28**:435–436.

Vialettes, B., Sutherland, D. E. R., Matas, A. J., Payne, W. D., and Najarian, J. S., 1979c, Amelioration of streptozotocin induced diabetes in rats: Effect of islet isografts on plasma lipids and other metabolic abnormalities according to donor source and site of transplantation, *Metabolism* **28**:489–494.

Vrbova, H., Theodorosa, N. A., Tyhurst, M., and Howell, S. E., 1979, Transplantation of islets of Langerhans from pilocarpine treated rats: A method of enchancing islet yield, *Transplantation* **28**:433–435.

Warnock, G. L., Rajotte, R. V., and Procyshyn, A. W., 198X, Normoglycemia after reflux of islet-containing pancreatic fragments into the splenic vasular bed in dogs, *Diabetes* **32**:452–459.

Wayand, W., Pattermann, M., and Umlauft, M., 1980, Transplantation of Ethibloc-occluded pancreas in pigs, *Transplant. Proc.* **12**(Suppl. 2):135–137.

Weber, C., Weil, R., McIntosh, R., and Reemtsma, K., 1975a, Transplantation of pancreatic islets from neonatal to adult rats, *Transplantation* **19**:442–444.

Weber, C., Lerner, R., Hardy, M., and Reemtsma, K., 1976a, Hyperinsulinemia and hyperglucagonemia following pancreatic islet transplantation in diabetic rats, *Diabetes* **25**:944–948.

Weber, C., Zatrigi, A., Weil, R., McIntosh, R., Hardy, M. A., and Reemtsma, K., 1976, Pancreatic islet isografts, allografts and xenografts: Comparison of morphology and function, *Surgery* **79**:144–151.

Weber, C. J., Silva, F. G., Hardy, M. A., Pirani, C. L., and Reemtsma, K., 1979, Effects of islet transplantation on renal function and morphology of short- and long-term diabetic rats, *Transplant. Proc.* **11**:549–556.

Weber, C. J., Zatugi, A., Weil, R., Hardy, M. A., and Reemtsma, K., 1980a, Towards xenografts in human diabetics, in: *Diabetic Renal Retinal Syndrome* (E. Friedman and F. L'Esperance, eds.), pp. 419–433, Grune and Stratton, New York.

Weber, C. J., Silva, F. G., Hardy, M. A., and Reemtsma, K., 1980b, Islet transplants and nephropathy, in: *Diabetic Renal Retinal Syndrome* (E. Friedman, and F. L'Esperance, eds.), pp. 373–402, Grune and Stratton, New York.

Weil, R., Nozawa, M., Koss, M., Weber, C., Reemtsma, K., and McIntosh, R. M., 1975, Pancreatic transplantation in diabetic rats: Renal function, morphology ultrastructure and immunhistology, *Surgery* **78**:142–148.

Weir, G. C., and Bonner-Weir, S., 1982, Insulin secretion after partial pancreatectomy: Evidence for B cell "exhaustion," *Diabetes* **31**(Suppl. 2):35A.

Weiser, R. K., Tellis, V. A., Wilk, P. J., Veith, F. J., Mohadevia, P. S., and Gliedman, M. L., 1980, Comparison of methods for elimination of exocrine pancreatic function for transplantation, *Surg. Forum* **31**:357–359.

Weisman, H., Mullen, Y., and Brown, J., 1980, Insulin released from fetal rat pancreases transplanted into normal and diabetic animals during perfusion, *Diabetes* **29**:566–570.

West, K. M., 1978, *Epidemiology of Diabetes and Its Vascular Lesions*, Elsevier, New York.

Westbroek, D. L., de Gruyl, J., Dijkhjuis, C. M., McDicken, I., Drop, A., Scholte, A., and Hulmans, H. A. M., 1974, Twenty-four-hour hypothermic preservation perfusion and storage of the duct ligated canine pancreas with transplantation, *Transplant. Proc.* **6**:319–322.

White, D. C., Sutherland, D. E., and Najarian, J. S., 1981a, Endocrine function and histology of the canine pancreas after exocrine ablation by ductal injection of silicone rubber adhesive, *J. Surg. Res.* **31**:371–374.

White, D. C., Sutherland, D. E. R., Zweber, B., and Najarian, J. S., 1981b, Pancreatic endocrine function following exocrine ablation with silicone rubber polymers, *Trans. Am. Soc. Artif. Intern. Organs* **27**:254–258.

Wojcikowski, C. Z., and Arendarczyk, W., 1982, A long-term study of the function of transplantable rat pancreatic islets, *Diabetologia* **23**:210.

Woo, R., and Xavier-Pi Sunyer, F., 1982, Normal responses of rats with transplanted neonatal islets to stress, epinephrine, and cortisol, *Diabetes* **31**:856–861.

Worthen, D. M., Lee, S., Nakaji, N. T., Sayers, H. J., Orloff, M. J., 1976, Effect of whole pancreas transplantation eye lesion of alloxan diabetes, *Surg. Forum* **27**:544–546.

Yasunami, T., Lacy, P. E., Davie, J. M., and Finke, E. H., 1982a, Prolongation of islet xenograft survival (rat to mouse) by in vitro culture at 37°C, *Diabetes* **31**(Suppl. 2):151a.

Yasunami, Y., Lacy, P. E., Scharp, D. W., and Britt, L. D., 1982b, Isolation and transplantation of islet cells from the neonatal rat pancreas, *Surg. Forum* **33:**359–361.

Yasunami, Y., Lacy, P. E., Davie, J. M., and Finke, E. H., 1983a, Prolongation of islet xenograft survival (rat to mouse) by in vitro culture at 37°C, *Transplantation* **35:**281–284.

Yasunami, Y., Lacy, P. E., Davie, J. M., and Finke, E. H., 1983b, Use of in vitro culture at 37°C to prolong islet xenograft survival (rat to mouse), *Transplant. Proc.* **15**(1):1371–1372.

Younoszai, R., Sorenson, R. L., and Lindall, A. W., 1970, Homotransplantation of isolated pancreatic islets (abstract), *Diabetes* **19**(Suppl.):406.

Zammit, M., Valijee, K., and Toledo-Pereyra, L. H., 1979, Comparative study of different pancreas transplantation modalities: Islet cell vs. organ pancreas transplantation in pancreatectomized dogs, *J. Surg. Res.* **26:**308–313.

Ziegler, M. M., Reckard, C. R., and Barker, C. F., 1974, Long term metabolic and immunologic considerations in transplantation of pancreatic islets, *J. Surg. Res.* **16:**575–781.

Ziegler, M. M., Reckard, C. R., Naji, A., and Barker, C. F., 1975, Extended function of isolated pancreatic islet isografts and allografts, *Transplant. Proc.* **7:**743–745.

Ziegler, B., Lorenz, D., Lippert, H., Butter, R., Ziegler, M., and Hahn, H. J., 1981, Reversal of diabetes by isogeneic transplantation of cultured pancreatic islets, *Endokrinologie* **77:**346–352.

Ziegler, B., Heinzmann, D., Jahr, H., Besch, W., Nadrowtiz, R., Schmidt, W., and Hahn, H. J., 1982, Limited effectiveness of irradiated rat islets as grafts despite complete recovery of B cell function after culture, *Diabetologia* **23:**211.

Zitron, I. M., Ono, J., Lacy, P. E., and Davie, J. M., 1981a, Active suppression in the maintenance of pancreatic islet allografts, *Transplantation* **32:**156–158.

Zitron, I. M., Ono, J., Lacy, P. E., and Davie, J. M., 1981b, The cellular stimuli for the rejection of established islet allografts, *Diabetes,* **30:**242–246.

II

Clinical Diabetes

8

Antibodies to Insulin and Insulin Receptors: Mechanisms of Insulin Resistance

C. Ronald Kahn

I. INTRODUCTION

Insulin resistance is said to exist whenever normal concentrations of insulin produce a less-than-normal biological response (Kahn, 1978). In humans, insulin resistance is usually defined by the presence of hyperinsulinemia in the face of normal or elevated blood sugar or by resistance to exogenous insulin. Insulin resistance may occur in a large number of different disease states. The most frequent causes of mild to moderate insulin resistance are obesity and maturity-onset, insulin-independent diabetes (Olefsky, 1981). This chapter will consider two of the rare forms of insulin resistance: the syndrome of insulin resistance due to antireceptor antibodies and insulin resistance due to insulin antibodies. In both of these the patients are severely insulin-resistant and frequently fail to respond to 10 or even 1000 times or more the normal therapeutic dose of insulin.

The ability of insulin to regulate the level of blood glucose is a complex, integrated process involving synthesis and secretion of insulin, its transport in the bloodstream, and its action at the target cell level. Insulin resistance may occur as a result of any process that alters the transport of insulin in the bloodstream (such as the development of antiinsulin antibodies) or alters insulin action at the target cell level (such as development of antireceptor antibodies). In a hormone-resistant state, both the maximal response and the dose-response may be changed, and it is important to distinguish these possibilities if one is to understand the possible mechanisms. In general,

C. Ronald Kahn • Joslin Diabetes Center, and Department of Medicine, Brigham and Women's Hospital, Harvard Medical School, Boston, Massachusetts 02115.

alterations in both availability of insulin due to antibodies and in receptor concentration or affinity will produce decreased insulin sensitivity, whereas alterations at postreceptor steps will produce decreased responsiveness (Kahn, 1978).

II. INSULIN RESISTANCE DUE TO ANTIINSULIN ANTIBODIES

The mainstay of treatment for almost all patients with juvenile-onset (Type I) diabetes mellitus and many patients with maturity-onset (Type II) diabetes mellitus is insulin. Since insulin is a polypeptide hormone obtained by acid-ethanol extraction of animal pancreas, it is not surprising that administration of insulin to diabetic patients or to normal persons regularly evokes some immune response. In almost all patients who have taken insulin for longer than 2 months, levels of circulating antibodies to insulin can be measured by assays *in vitro*. Although in most patients the immune response is clinically insignificant, many insulin-taking diabetic patients will at sometime present a clinical problem related to chronic exposure to this foreign protein; the exact nature of the clinical manifestation will depend on which pathway in the immune system shows the major activation (Kahn and Rosenthal, 1979).

A. Structure and Antigenicity of Insulin

Insulin is a polypeptide hormone of molecular weight 5900 composed of two chains joined by two disulfide bonds between cystine molecules (Fig. 1). The A chain has 21 amino acids, the B chain has 30. A number of insulin molecules of different species, from the most primitive vertebrate (North Atlantic hagfish) to humans, have been completely sequenced. In general, the insulin molecule has been well conserved in evolution, although up to 35% of the amino acid residues are altered in primitive vertebrates (Blundell *et al.*, 1972). When one compares the structures of mammalian insulins, it is apparent that major variations occur in two regions of the molecule: in the region between the intrachain disulfide bridge of the A chain (A8,9,10) and in the carboxy-terminal region of the B chain, particularly the B 30 residue (Fig. 1). Human and porcine insulin are identical except for substitution of alanine for threonine at position 30 of the B-chain, whereas beef insulin differs from human insulin in positions 8 and 10 of the A chain. It is not surprising, therefore, that, of the various animal species used routinely for therapeutic purposes, pork insulin is probably the least antigenic (Berson and Yalow, 1966; Andersen, 1973). In the United States, however, standard commercial insulin is a combination of beef and pork insulins in a ratio of about 2:1.

Until recently, commercial insulin in the United States (USP insulin) was simply purified by repeated crystallization and, therfore, was contaminated with small amounts of other peptides (Table 1). Although proinsulin (the single chain precursor of insulin), proinsulin intermediates, and C peptide are relatively minor contaminants of insulin preparations, these molecules have many more variations in amino acid sequence between different species and, thus, may provide more potent antigenic stimuli than the intact insulin molecule itself (Chance *et al.*, 1976). Older insulin preparations also contained a small amount of high-molecular-weight, biologically inactive material (A component) (Fig. 2), and studies in animals suggest that this high-molecular-weight

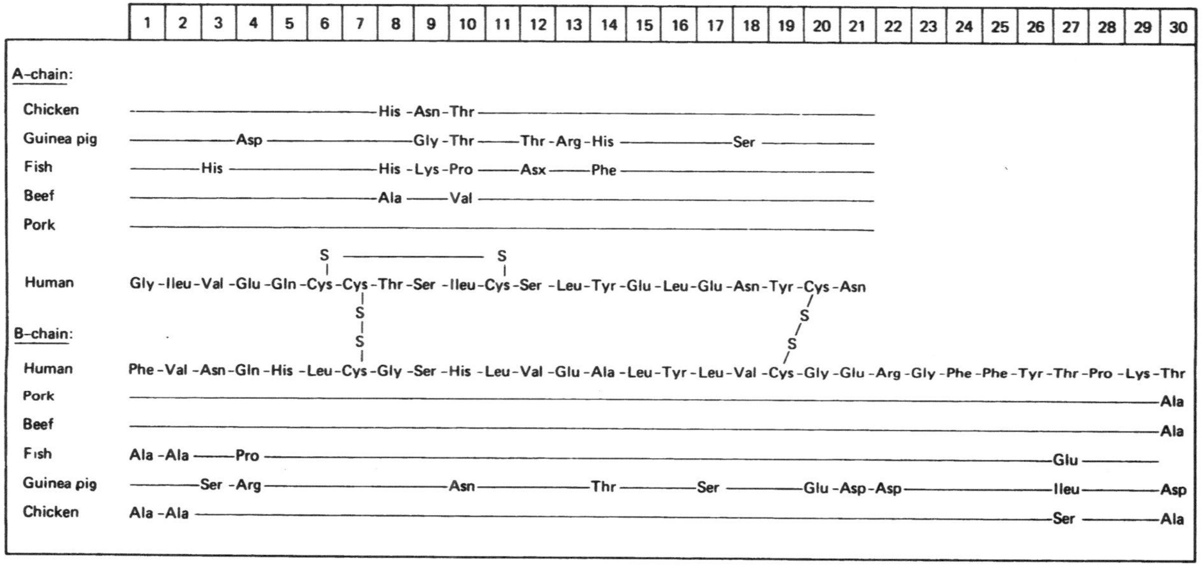

	1	2	3	4	5	6	7	8	9	10	11	12	13	14	15	16	17	18	19	20	21	22	23	24	25	26	27	28	29	30

A-chain:

- Chicken: ——————— His - Asn - Thr ———————
- Guinea pig: ——— Asp ——— Gly - Thr ——— Thr - Arg - His ——— Ser ———
- Fish: ——— His ——— His - Lys - Pro ——— Asx ——— Phe ———
- Beef: ——— Ala ——— Val ———
- Pork: ———————————
- Human: Gly - Ileu - Val - Glu - Gln - Cys - Cys - Thr - Ser - Ileu - Cys - Ser - Leu - Tyr - Glu - Leu - Glu - Asn - Tyr - Cys - Asn

B-chain:

- Human: Phe - Val - Asn - Gln - His - Leu - Cys - Gly - Ser - His - Leu - Val - Glu - Ala - Leu - Tyr - Leu - Val - Cys - Gly - Glu - Arg - Gly - Phe - Phe - Tyr - Thr - Pro - Lys - Thr
- Pork: ——————————— Ala
- Beef: ——— Ala ——— Val ——— Ala
- Fish: Ala - Ala ——— Pro ——— Glu ———
- Guinea pig: ——— Ser - Arg ——— Asn ——— Thr ——— Ser ——— Glu - Asp - Asp ——— Ileu ——— Asp
- Chicken: Ala - Ala ——————— Ser ——— Ala

Figure 1. Amino acid sequences of insulins from different species.

Table 1.   Potential Antigens in Commercial Insulin

Insulin (and its derivatives)
Proinsulin and proinsulin intermediates
Other hormones
    Glucagon
    Somatostatin
    Pancreatic polypeptide
    Vasoactive intestinal peptide
Protamine (and its contaminants)

contaminant may be the most antigenic component of all. In addition, many insulin preparations made by recrystallization were contaminated with other peptide hormones, including glucagon, human pancreatic polypeptide, vasoactive intestinal peptide, and somatostatin. Antibodies to these noninsulin contaminants, especially pancreatic polypeptide, have been identified in a significant number of insulin-treated patients but are of no known clinical significance (Bloom *et al.*, 1979).

Over the past several years, attempts have been made to increase the purity of commercial insulin preparations using chromatographic and ion-exchange processes, in the hope of eliminating most of the noninsulin contaminants. This has resulted in "single-peak" insulin, that is, insulin that behaves as molecules of uniform size when subjected to get filtration procedures and "monocomponent" or "single component" insulin, which behaves as uniform by both size and charge criteria.

Another important factor affecting immunogenicity of insulin may be the pharmaceutical form used. Protamine zinc insulin (PZI) and neutral protamine Hagadorne (NPH) insulin are both mixtures of zinc, insulin, and the basic protein protamine. The protamine decreases insulin solubility and thus delays its peak of action. Lente insulins, which are made using a higher zinc concentration and an acetate rather than a

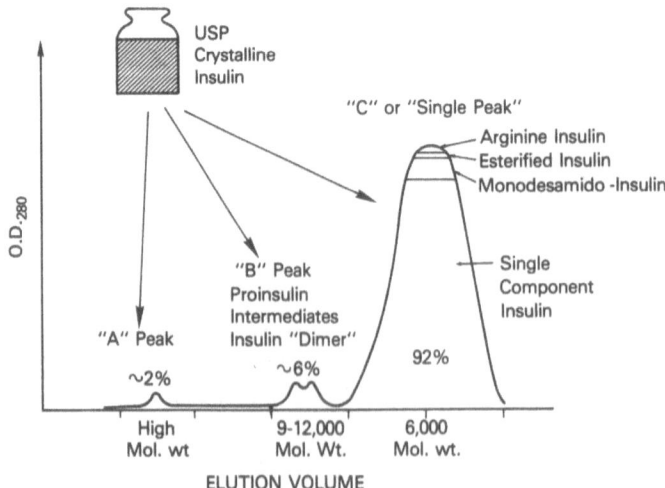

Figure 2.   Gel filtration pattern on Sephadex G-50 1 of USP grade insulin.

phosphate buffer, also have delayed absorption without the addition of protamine. In general, it is found that regular crystalline insulin is less immunogenic than the lente or NPH forms (Galloway and Bressler, 1978; Reeves, 1980; Andersen, 1973).

B. Genetics of the Immune Response

Recent studies in both humans and animals suggest that the immune response to insulin, like the immune response to other antigens, is under genetic control (Chapter 2). Thus, inbred strain 2 and 13 guinea pigs both respond to immunization with beef and pork insulin by developing antigen-specific T cells and by producing circulating antibodies. T cells from the strain 2 animals, however, respond to the alterations in residues 8, 9, and 10 of the A chain, while strain 13 guinea pigs respond to the determinants in the amino terminal region of the B chain. Similarly, in the mouse, H-2^b mice are A chain responders, whereas H-2^d mice are B chain responders. H-2^b mice do not develop an immune response to insulin, although they will make insulin antibodies when immunized with proinsulin. Studies in humans suggest that a stronger immune reponse to insulin is associated with HLA-DR4, B15, and Cw3 than with HLA DR3, B8 (Bertrams et al., 1976; Ludvigsson et al., 1977; Schernthaner et al., 1977). Individuals who have a combination of HLA A2, Bw44, and DR7 also show a marked increase in relative risk of an exaggerated immune response (Kahn et al., 1982).

The role of protamine in the development of insulin allergy or resistance remains unclear. In experimental animals, it is possible to demonstrate that highly charged molecules such as protamine may act as an adjuvant and make an animal that would normally be a genetic nonresponder to an antigen become a responder, presumably because such molecules bind the antigen electrostatically and help present it to the macrophage (schlepper phenomenon) (Green et al., 1966). Such individuals also have an increased frequency of HLA-DR7 (Mann, D., personal communication), one of the HLA antigens associated with an increased immune response to insulin treatment.

The most direct measurement of the offending antigen in a patient or animal with insulin allergy is the effect of insulin or its contaminants on the T cell mitogenic response (Rosenthal, 1978). In recent studies (Kahn and Rosenthal, 1979) we found that about 50% of patients with insulin allergy show an increased mitogenic response to insulin or proinsulin. In most individuals, beef insulin is more antigenic than pork, and proinsulin is frequently even more antigenic (Fig. 3, left). About 20% of patients with insulin allergy and insulin antibodies have lymphocytes that failed to show a response to insulin when tested in vitro. In some of these cases, dramatic responses to protamine were observed (Fig. 3, right), suggesting that in these patients protamine serves as an adjuvant or schlepper that allows insulin allergy to develop in an individual who would have been a genetic nonresponder.

C. Clinical Measurements of Insulin Antibodies

All five major classes of immunoglobulins are found in insulin-taking diabetic patients (Patterson et al., 1973a, deShazo, 1978). Quantitatively, the most significant and the first antibodies demonstrated were those of the IgG class. In addition, IgM antibodies

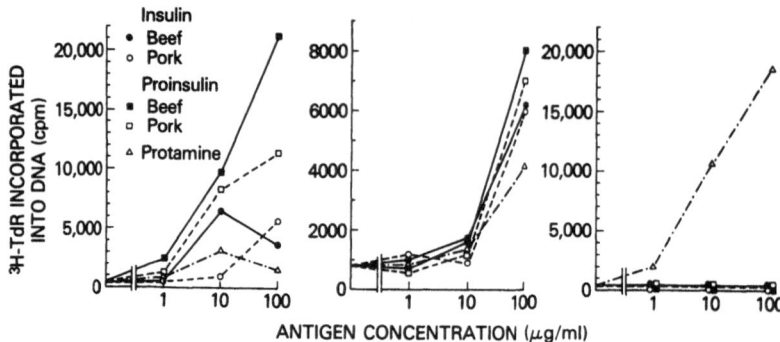

Figure 3. Stimulation of DNA synthesis in human lymphocytes by insulins, proinsulins, and protamine. Each panel represents cells derived from a single insulin-taking diabetic (Rosenthal, A.S. and Kahn, C.R., unpublished data).

were evident early after initiation of insulin treatment and in patients with insulin resistance; IgD was found in some patients with insulin resistance as well. IgA and, especially, IgE have been demonstrated in patients with allergy to insulin.

IgG antibodies are readily demonstrated after a brief incubation of the plasma with ^{125}I-labeled insulin, followed by an appropriate separation of the antibody-bound (B) and free (F) insulin. A number of methods have been used for this purpose, including paper and starch block electrophoresis, paper chromatoelectrophoresis, paper chromatography, gel filtration, precipitation by addition of a second antibody, or precipitation by polyethylene glycol or alcohol. Alternatively, the bound and free insulin may be separated using an agent that will preferentially absorb the free insulin, such as charcoal or silicates. Quantitative analysis of antibody concentration is usually carried out by preparing a series of incubation tubes containing variable concentrations of unlabeled insulin and constant amounts of the labeled insulin and antibody. With increasing concentrations of insulin, the ratio of bound (B) to free (F) of the labeled ligand decreases (Fig. 4A). This corresponds to an increasing amount of insulin bound to antibody, and, from such curves, it is possible to calculate both the affinity and the binding capacity of the antibody using the Scatchard plot as described by Berson and Yalow (1959) (Fig. 4B). In general, such studies reveal heterogeneous classes of antibodies. These can be divided into a class of high affinity-low capacity and low affinity-high capacity antibodies. Most insulin-treated patients have insulin-binding capacities of less than 10 U/liter and, since the space of distribution of antibody in humans is about 6 liters, a total insulin-binding capacity of about 60 U. In patients with insulin resistance, the titer of antiinsulin bodies is usually significantly higher (Fig. 5).

D. Insulin Resistance due to Antiinsulin Antibodies

In an insulin-taking diabetic, insulin resistance may be said to exist whenever the insulin requirement exceeds the normal pancreatic output (~0.5 U/kg body weight). For practical purposes, however, most physicians do not consider insulin resistance significant unless the total daily dose exceeds 200 U or 2.5 U/kg body weight.

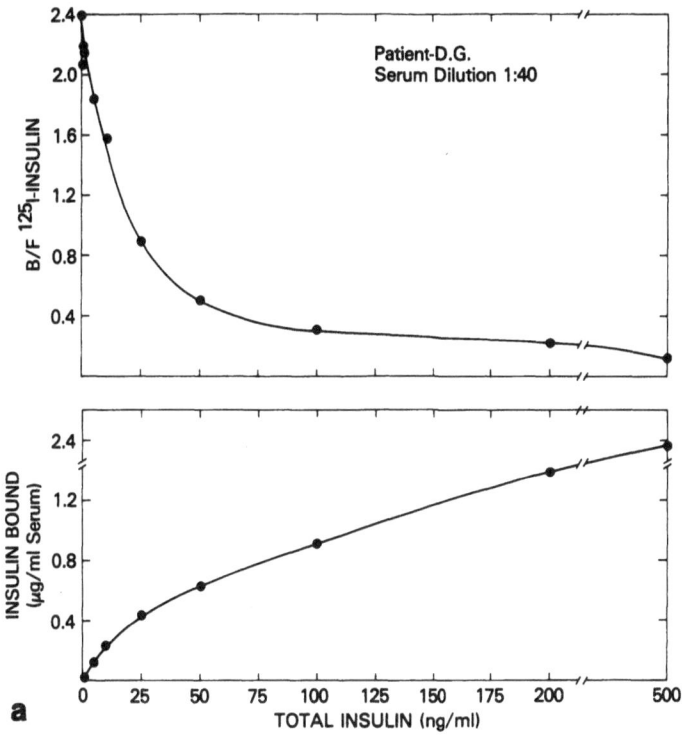

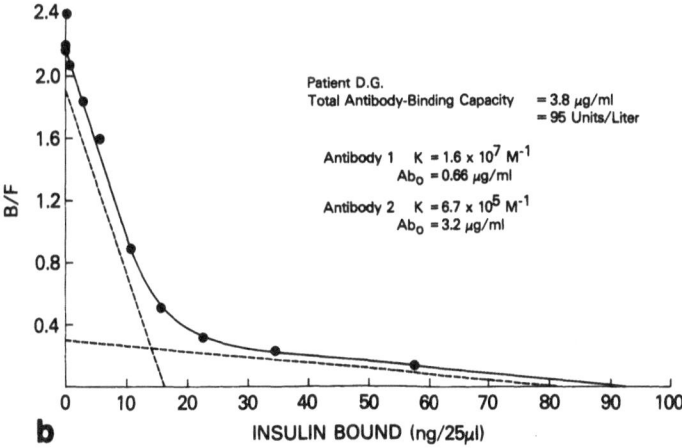

Figure 4. (A) Determination of insulin antibody titer using $[^{125}I]$insulin and various concentrations of unlabeled insulin. (B) Scatchard analysis of the data (from Kahn and Rosenthal, 1979).

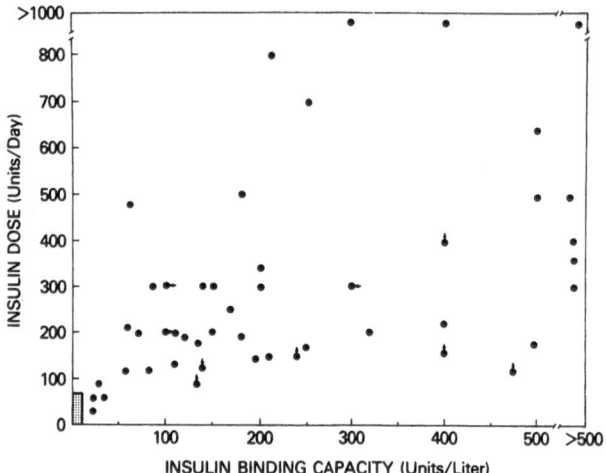

Figure 5. IgG insulin-binding capacity in insulin-taking diabetics. The shaded area represents the range for non-insulin-resistant patients. The individual dots show data on insulin-resistant patients (adapted from Berson and Yalow, 1959).

Insulin resistance caused by the development of high-titer antiinsulin antibodies is a relatively rare complication of diabetes. At the Joslin Diabetes Center, about 0.01% of all patients seen between 1940 and 1960 were insulin-resistant (Shipp *et al.*, 1967). Insulin resistance was observed in diabetic patients of all ages (from 4 to 84), although about 75% were 40 or older at the time of onset of the resistance. There is no sex preponderance. The duration of insulin treatment before the onset of insulin resistance ranges from 1 month to 15 years; about two-thirds of the patients have received insulin for less than 1 year. Commonly, there is a history of intermittent or interrupted insulin treatment. In general, the onset of insulin resistance is gradual, occurring over weeks to months, although occasional patients present in ketoacidosis when insulin resistance is a result of antiinsulin antibodies. The precise incidence of concomitance of insulin allergy and insulin resistance is not known, but it is probably in the range of 25 to 35% (Shipp *et al.*, 1967). It is not clear, however, if the patients with insulin allergy are at increased risk to develop insulin resistance. In some cases, the development of insulin resistance occurs at a time when insulin allergy is diminishing, suggesting that the IgG may block the IgE effect (Patterson *et al.*, 1973b).

The amount of insulin required for treatment may be very high. About half of the patients require 1000 or more units per day. Patients needing more than 25,000 U per day of insulin have been reported, although most of them probably represent the rare forms of insulin-resistant diabetes associated with target cell defects in insulin action or antireceptor antibodies rather than insulin resistance due to antiinsulin antibodies.

The exact reason for insulin resistance in patients who have insulin antibodies is unclear, since one would predict that after a short time of increased insulin treatment a new steady state would be reached. Assuming that such antigen-antibody complexes are cleared by the spleen and reticuloendothelial system with a half-life of 2–3 days,

Berson and Yalow (1970) calculated that insulin-resistant diabetic patients might lose between 100 and 1000 U of insulin per day. No direct measurements of the increased clearance rate of insulin, however, have been made.

E. Therapy

Immunologic insulin resistance tends to be a self-limited disorder that spontaneously remits in about 60% of patients within 6 months (Shipp *et al.*, 1967). Treatment, therefore, should be directed at prevention of the severe metabolic problems of the patient without placing the patient in any significant risk. Three general approaches in therapy have been used. The first is to substitute a less antigenic form of insulin for that which the patient is receiving (Boshell *et al.*, 1964; Kahn and Rosenthal, 1979). Since the insulin antibodies in the sera of most patients with insulin resistance show a higher affinity for beef than for pork insulin (Fig. 6), changing the patient to pork single-peak or monocomponent insulin should be the first therapeutic maneuver attempted. The latter results in at least some decrease in the requirement for insulin in about 50% of the patients. Other, less antigenic insulins, such as fish insulin, desalanine-pork insulin (in which the single amino acid different from human insulin has been removed), and human insulin have also been used (Akre *et al.*, 1964). Preliminary studies with both the biosynthetic and semisynthetic human insulins, however, suggest that once antibodies are formed, most cross-react with human, as well as beef and pork insulins. Sulfated insulin, a chemically modified form of beef or pork insulin that contains an average of six sulfate groups per molecule combines less avidly with antibodies to beef and pork insulin (Fig. 6); consequently, it is a good substitute, when available, for the patient who has immunological insulin resistance. On average, patients with insulin resistance, when switched to sulfated insulin, will require only 15% of their former insulin dosage, and this will fall even further as the antigenic stimulus is removed and the antibody titer falls (Little and Arnott, 1966; Davidson and DeBra, 1978).

In the patient who does not respond to more porcine, less antigenic insulins, treatment with glucocorticoids has been used (Shipp *et al.*, 1967). The patient should be

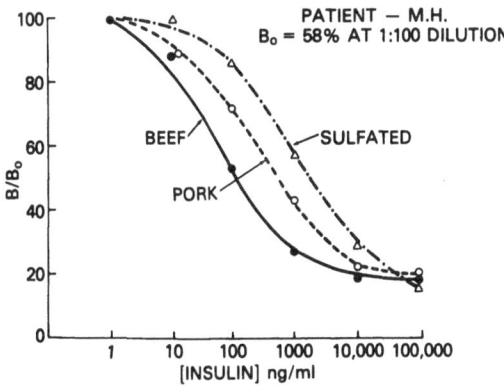

Figure 6. Comparative affinity of insulin antibody for beef, pork, and sulfated insulin (from Kahn and Rosenthal, 1979).

started on high dosages (60–80 mg prednisone per day), and this will result in a decreased insulin requirement in up to 75% of patients. The latter effect will occur rapidly, frequently within a few days. The exact mechanism of the effect, however, is unclear, since in a significant number of patients antibody titers do not fall during the early phase of treatment. Further, the effect is somewhat paradoxic, since glucocorticoids frequently induce a state of insulin resistance when given to normal individuals or to non-insulin-resistant diabetic patients. The individual response is erratic and unpredictable, however, and side effects from steroid treatment are prominent. Thus, the dosage should be tapered as rapidly as possible (usually in 2–3 weeks) and discontinued when the patient is no longer resistant to insulin. Cytotoxic drugs, such as cyclophosphamide and 6-mercaptopurine, have also been used; however, since the disease is self-limited and alternative methods of treatment are available, such aggressive therapy is rarely warranted. Desensitization has also been used in patients with insulin resistance, especially when combined with insulin allergy, and is effective in about 50% of cases (Galloway and Bressler, 1978; Patterson et al., 1973b).

III. THE INSULIN RECEPTOR

The first step in the action of insulin at the cellular level is binding to specific receptors on the surface of target cells. The interaction of insulin with its receptor has been extensively studied (Kahn et al., 1981). These studies have revealed that this reaction is complex. Evidence has been presented for cooperative interactions between receptors, multiple classes of binding sites, compartmentalization of receptor bound hormone, and both receptor-mediated and non-receptor-mediated pathways of insulin degradation (DeMeyts et al., 1976; Gorden et al., 1980; Freychet et al., 1972).

The insulin receptor retains both insulin-binding and immunological reactivity when solubilized in neutral detergents such as Triton X-100 and in this form has been characterized by gel filtration and gel electrophoresis. The estimated Stokes radius of the insulin receptor in Triton is 68–72 Å (Ginsberg et al., 1976; Lang et al., 1980). Depending on the assumptions made regarding shape and detergent binding, this corresponds to an estimated molecular weight of 300,000–1,000,000. Under some conditions an active receptor of a smaller size can be detected. This smaller active receptor has a Stokes radius of 38–40 Å (mol. wt. 75,000–125,000) and is dissociated from the larger complex in the presence of high concentrations of insulin (Ginsberg et al., 1976).

Using antireceptor antibodies, we have developed methods to study the subunits of the insulin receptor after either surface labeling or biosynthetic labeling (Van Obberghen et al., 1981; Kasuga et al., 1981; Hedo et al., 1982). In brief, cultured human IM-9 are radioactively labeled and either biosynthetically or by surface labeling and the proteins extracted with Triton X-100. The glycoprotein fraction is then concentrated and purified by chromatography on wheat germ agglutinin agarose, and the insulin receptors specifically precipitated by antireceptor antibodies upon addition of second antibody or staphlococcal protein A. Analysis of the immune precipitates of sodium dodecyl-sulfate-polyacrylamide gel electrophoresis under reducing conditions followed by autoradiography revealed specific precipitation on two major bands with

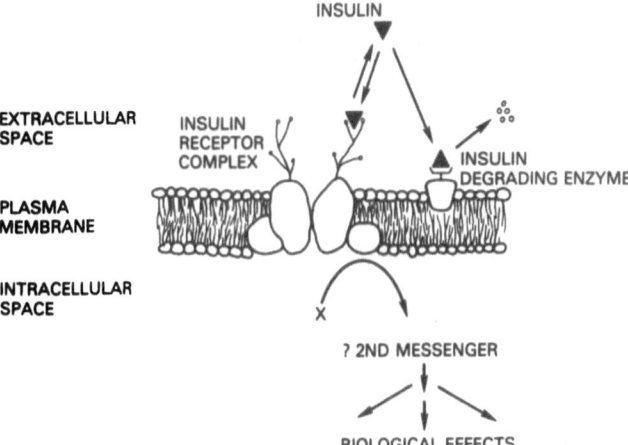

Figure 7. Model of insulin receptor in the cell membrane.

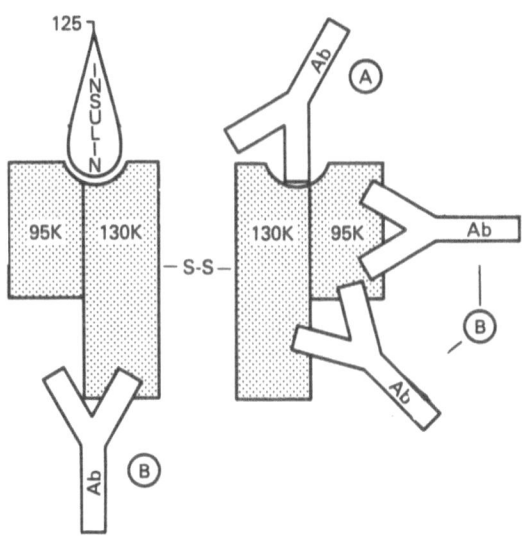

Figure 8. Model of insulin receptor based on SDS-polyacrylamide gel electrophoresis. Antireceptor antibodies may bind near the insulin binding site (A) or at sites distant from the insulin binding site (B).

molecular weights of about 135 K and 95 K. These have been termed the α and β subunits (Figs. 7 and 8).

When the receptor is labeled using affinity labeling techniques (Massague *et al.*, 1980; Yip *et al.*, 1980), the majority of the label is on the α subunit suggesting that this subunit contains the insulin binding site. The β subunit, on the other hand, may be the effector site, since this subunit is transmembrane and undergoes phosphorylation in response to insulin binding (Kasuga *et al.*, 1982). The insulin receptor is subject to rapid changes in both affinity and concentration. This modulation of the receptor is under the influence of a number of physiological and pathologic factors. A major factor regulating receptor concentration is insulin itself (Gavin *et al.*, 1974). Thus, in several states in which insulin levels are elevated (obesity, maturity-onset diabetes, insulinoma), receptor concentration is reciprocally decreased leading to a state of insulin resistance (Kahn *et al.*, 1977a; Olefsky, 1981). In other insulin-resistant states, such as glucocorticoid excess, the major effect is to reduce receptor affinity. Recently, a new class of disorders of the insulin receptor has been described in which the resistance is due to circulating autoantibodies which alter insulin receptor function (Flier *et al.*, 1975; Kahn *et al.*, 1976).

A. Clinical Syndrome Associated with Antibodies to the Insulin Receptor

Since their initial discovery (Flier *et al.*, 1975) antibodies to the insulin receptor have been found in the sera of about 25 patients. Most of the patients fit into a clinical syndrome termed the syndrome of insulin resistance and acanthosis nigricans, type B (Kahn and Harrison, 1980), the features of which are summarized in Table 2. In most cases the presenting features have been insulin resistance and glucose intolerance. Features of a more generalized autoimmune disease have been found in virtually all patients, although only about one-third have a clinically recognizable autoimmune syndrome such as lupus erythematosus or Sjogren's syndrome. Despite the evidence of generalized autoimmune disease, there has been a paucity of findings of organ-specific autoimmunity. Several patients with ataxia telangiectasia, an autosomal recessive disorder characterized by neurological degeneration, cutaneous telangiectasia, and humoral and cellular immune deficiency, have also been found to have antibodies to the

Table 2.   *Clinical Features of Patients with Antiinsulin Receptor Antibodies*

Sex ratio: 2 female, 1 male
Age range: 12–70 years
Race: 60% black, 30% caucasian, 10% oriental

Clinical features
  Abnormal glucose tolerance and insulin resistance
  Usually severe, but may vary
  Patients have received up to 10,000 units/hr of insulin
  Some patients develop hypoglycemia and two cases have had hypoglycemia

Acanthosis Nigricans
  Present in about 80% of cases
  Often severe
  Tends to follow clinical course of glucose tolerance abnormalities

Immunological features
  1/3 have a classic "autoimmune" syndrome (SLE, Sjogren's syndrome, ataxia telangiectasia)
  Approximately 100% of cases have ↑ erythrocyte sedimentation rate, ↑ γ-globulins, + ANA, antiDNA, leukopenia
  Less frequently: alopecia, proteinuria, organ-specific antibodies

---

insulin receptor (Bar et al., 1978; Harrison et al., 1979a). Antireceptor activity has also been found in the sera of insulin-resistant New Zealand obese (NZO) mice (Harrison and Itin, 1980).

B. Methods for Detecting Antibodies to the Insulin Receptor

At least six methods have been shown to be of some potential use in the detection of antireceptor antibodies, although in practice only two have been given much attention and use. These are the binding-inhibition assay and the immunoprecipitation assay which are shown schematically in Fig. 9.

The binding-inhibition assay (Flier et al., 1975) is the simplest assay and the most frequently performed. The assay depends on the ability of the antibody to inhibit insulin binding and can be performed using any cell that possess insulin receptors, such as cultured human lymphocytes or rat adipocytes. Some of the antireceptor antibodies cross-react with nonmammalian species, although in most cases with a lower titer (Muggeo et al., 1979a).

The immunoprecipitation assay was developed using a modification of the technique employed to detect antibodies to the acetylcholine receptor (Harrison et al., 1979b) (Fig. 9). This assay is more tedious and difficult to perform but has the ability to detect antibodies to sites on the insulin receptor other than the insulin-binding site (Fig. 8).

Of the antireceptor antibodies characterized thus far, most have been IgG in nature, and polyclonal (Flier et al., 1976). Antireceptor activity has also been found in the high-molecular-weight IgM in one patient with the type B syndrome (Flier et al., 1976), and in low-molecular-weight IgM in some of the patients with ataxia telangiectasia (Harrison et al., 1979a).

C. Effects of Antireceptor Antibodies on Insulin Binding

Exposure of cells to antibodies to the insulin receptor results in a decrease in insulin binding due, in most cases, to a decrease in receptor affinity. This is evident in both in vitro studies (Flier et al., 1977) and when insulin binding is studied using cells freshly isolated from the affected individual (Fig. 10) (Bar et al., 1980). Thus, most of the antireceptor antibodies behave as "competitive" antagonists of insulin binding. Cells isolated from patients with antireceptor antibody show increased rates of dissociation of insulin from its receptor; when treated with antibody in vitro, however, the major effect is on the association rate of insulin with the receptor. Most of the antireceptor antibodies bind to the receptor in some way so as to inhibit the negatively cooperative interactions (Flier et al., 1977).

Using one high-titer antibody to the insulin receptor, we were able to show direct competition of insulin for labeled antibody binding, suggesting that both bind to the same site, or nearly the same site, on the receptor (Jarrett et al., 1976). This antireceptor antibody appears to bind to the insulin-binding subunit of the receptor as determined by radiation inactivation studies (Harmon et al., 1980). All antireceptor antibodies studied thus far appear to be able to immunoprecipitate both subunits of the insulin receptor, but since they are probably covalently linked via disulfide bonds, this provides little direct evidence of the antibody-binding domain.

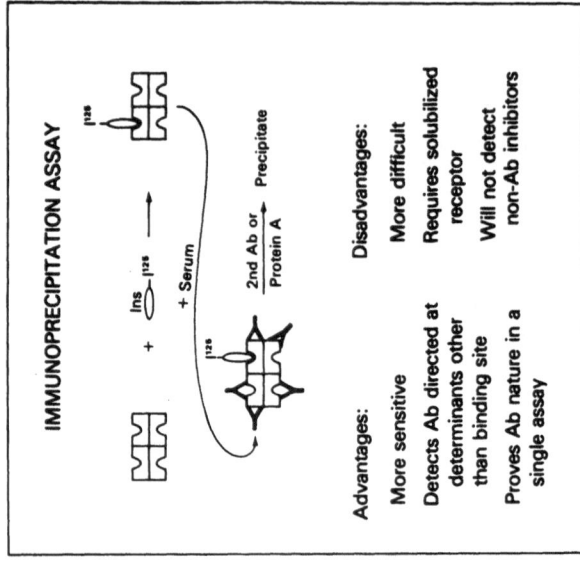

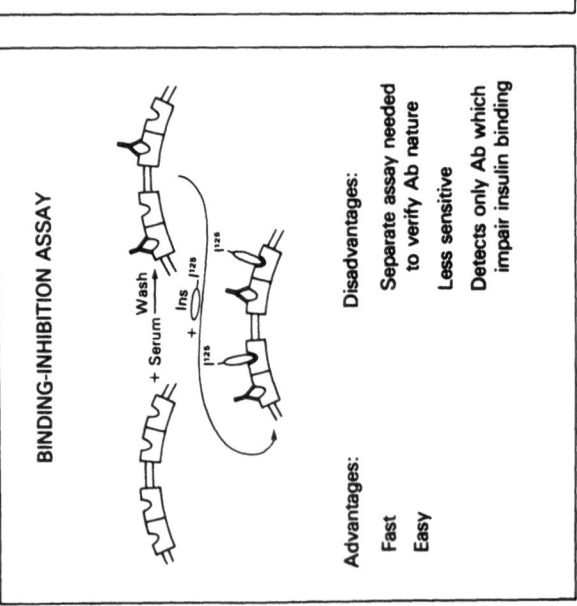

Figure 9. Assays for antibodies to insulin receptors.

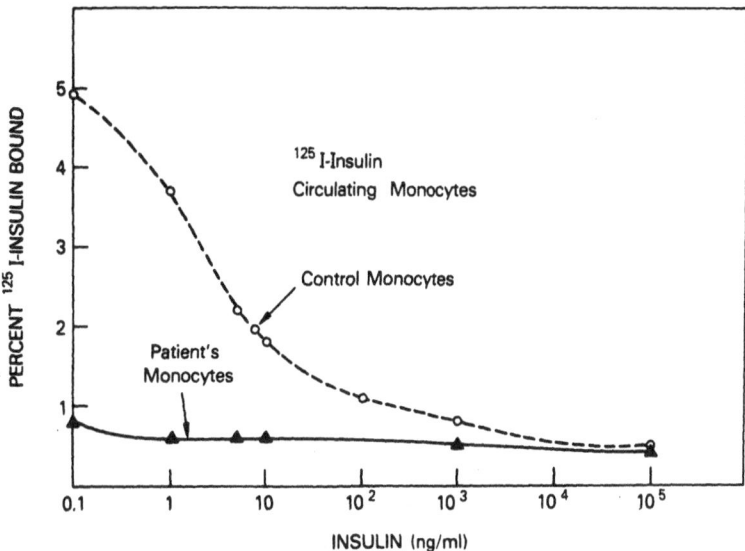

Figure 10. Effect of antiinsulin receptor antibodies on insulin binding. Insulin binding to menocytes isolated from a patient with antireceptor antibodies; a similar defect in binding can be produced by exposing cultured human lymphocytes with normal insulin receptors to serum from this patient.

It is likely that most, if not all, of the antireceptor antisera contain multiple antireceptor antibodies which bind to different sites on the receptor. When the IgG from a single patient is fractionated by diethylaminoethyl (DEAE) chromatography, antirecptor activity is found in all fractions. Furthermore, the ratio of binding inhibitory activity to immunoprecipitating and biological activity varies from fraction to fraction, suggesting populations of antibodies that bind to different sites on the receptor (Kahn *et al.*, 1980).

D. Mechanisms of Insulin Resistance in Patients with Antibodies to Insulin Receptors

The clinical picture and the observation that the antibodies to the receptor impair insulin binding suggested that the antibodies would be antagonists of insulin action; however, this was not found to be the case. The acute effect of the antibodies in most *in vitro* systems is to mimic the actions of the insulin. This has been most extensively studied in isolated rat adipocytes. In these cells, antibodies to the insulin receptor stimulate glucose transport and metabolism, inhibit lipolysis, activate glycogen synthase in the presence and absence of glucose, inhibit epinephrine-stimulated phosphorylase, stimulate leucine incorporation into protein, stimulate pyruvate dehydrogenase and acetyl CoA carboxylase, and mimic the effects of insulin on protein phosphorylation (Kahn *et al.*, 1977b; Kasuga *et al.*, 1978; Lawrence *et al.*, 1978; Belsham *et al.*, 1980). The antibodies also mimic the effect of insulin in the 3T3-L1 preadipocyte, isolated muscle preparations, and isolated hepatocytes. Interestingly, the antireceptor an-

Table 3.   Titers of Antireceptor Antibodies (1 per Titer)

| | Immunoprecipitation assay in human placenta | Binding-inhibition assay | | Bioassay in rat adipocyte |
		Human lymphocyte	Rat adipocyte	
B2	6000	2000	41000	4000
B5	4500	2000	450	1700
B4	1000	300	90	500
B6	400	80	10	17
B3	400	50	20	200
B1	25	3	5	<2

tibodies do *not* mimic the ability of insulin to stimulate thymidine incorporation into DNA in fibroblasts (King *et al.*, 1980). The titer of the antisera with respect to insulinlike activity is usually higher than the titer by binding inhibition, suggesting that some of the antireceptor antibodies that bind to the receptor and mimic insulin action are binding to sites other than the insulin-binding site (Table 3). When the IgG itself is further fractioned in DEAE in exchange chromatography, subpopulations of antibody with varying activity may be obtained (Fig. 11).

   The biological activity of the antireceptor antibody, in contrast to the inhibition of insulin binding, appears to require antibody bivalency (Kahn *et al.*, 1978). Purified IgG and F(ab')^2 inhibit insulin binding and mimic the activity of insulin with equal efficacy (Fig. 12). Monovalent Fab' or Fab antibody fragments, on the other hand, inhibit insulin binding, but are without biological effect. The biological activity of the monovalent antibody fragment can be restored by addition of a second antibody. This has led to the conclusion that cross-linking of receptors or receptor aggregation is important in antibody action. Whether this is also true in insulin action remains uncertain. In some cases antiinsulin antibodies can be shown to enhance the action of insulin (Kahn *et al.*, 1978; Shechter, 1979). Both insulin and receptor antibody have also been shown to induce patching and capping of insulin receptors or cultured lymphocytes (Schlessinger *et al.*, 1980). The monovalent receptor antibody provides a competitive antagonist of insulin at the receptor level, since it blocks insulin binding, but is without intrinsic activity (King *et al.*, 1980).

   The apparent discrepancy between the *in vitro* finding that the receptor antibodies are insulinlike and the fact that the patients are insulin-resistant appears to be explained by differences between acute and more chronic effects of the antibody. When 3T3-L1 cells are exposed to antireceptor antibody, they show stimulation of acute biological effects similar to those seen in adipocytes. This insulinlike effect, however, is transient, reaching a maximum at 30 min to 1 hr and then decreasing (Karlsson *et al.*, 1979). After 6 hr of exposure, the cells have returned to a normal basal activity, and at this time demonstrate resistance to insulin action. This change in action occurs without any further change in insulin binding and appears to be due to two separate mechanisms: first, the antibody blocks insulin binding, shifting the dose–response curve for insulin action to the right and, secondly, there is a decrease in maximal insulin re-

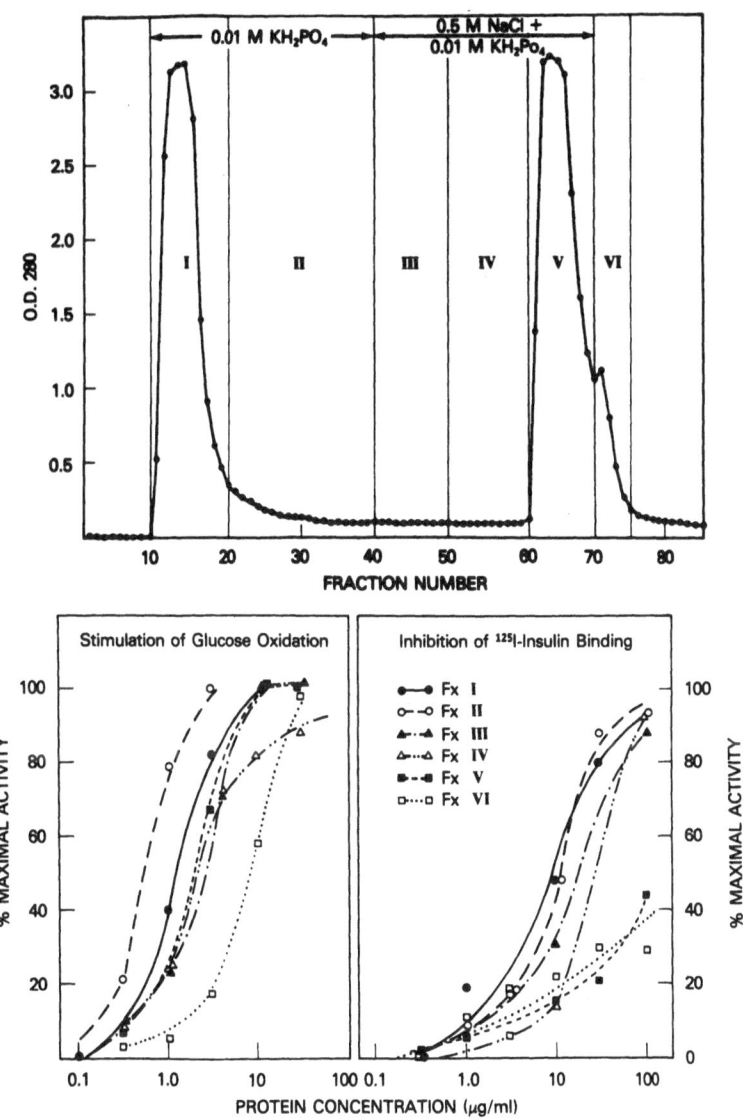

Figure 11.   Effect of various fractions of IgG from DEAE column (top panel) on insulin binding and action in isolated rat adipocytes (bottom panel).

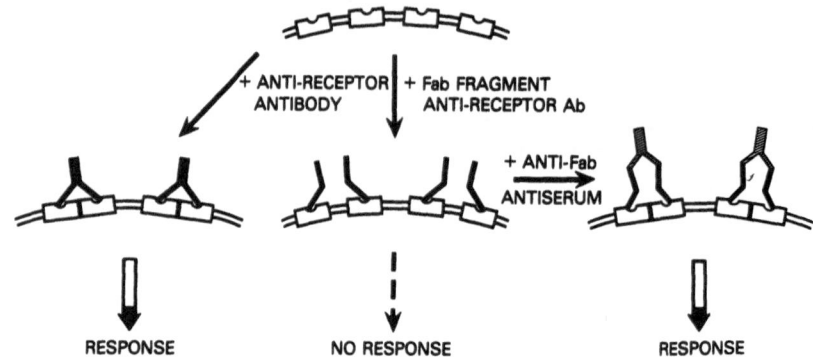

Figure 12.   Cross-linking of insulin receptors by antireceptor antibodies in biological responses.

sponse termed "desensitization" which appears to be due to an alteration in insulin action at some site beyond insulin binding.

The exact site and mechanism of desensitization are not yet clear (Grunfeld *et al.*, 1980). The site appears to be at some step postreceptor but relatively early in the pathway, since the insulinlike effects of spermine and vitamin K_5 activity are unaltered. The desensitized cell will not, however, respond fully to concanavalin A or to addition of more antireceptor antibody. Like the other biological effects of the antibody, desensitization appears to require antibody bivalence. In addition, the medium must contain a source of energy, such as glucose or pyruvate or a glucose derivative capable of being phosphorylated. There is no effect of antimicrotubular, antimicrofilament, or antilysosomal agents on this process.

E. Is the Underlying Receptor Normal?

It is important in patients with circulating antibodies to the insulin receptor, as in all patients with autoimmune disease, to determine the cause of the antibody development. Did antibodies develop because of an underlying defect in the receptor? Or did they develop due to some defect in the immune system? All the currently available data point to a defect in the immune system. Thus, in virtually all patients with antireceptor antibodies, there is a more generalized autoimmune disorder. In addition, the underlying receptor appears to be normal by several criteria (Table 4) (Muggeo *et al.*,

Table 4.   Evidence That the Underlying Receptor is Normal

Reproduction of the defect *in vitro* by antibody treatment of normal cells
Elution of cell-bound antibodies from patients' cells
Exposure to acid wash
Effect of plasma exchange
Studies of patients in remission
Studies of cells in culture

1979b,c). Obviously, none of these criteria is absolute evidence that no minor change in chemical structure of the receptor exists. Such studies await complete purification of the receptor.

Although antibodies to insulin receptors have been produced in rodents injected with antiinsulin antibodies (Serge and Pedersen, 1978), and even in rodents injected with insulin (Shechter *et al.*, 1982), suggesting these may be antiidiotypes to antiinsulin antibodies; this does not appear to be an important factor in humans. Most patients with antireceptor antibodies have only low titers of antiinsulin antibodies, and some patients have not received insulin treatment.

F. Therapy of Patients with Antireceptor Antibody

Since most of the data suggest that the underlying receptor is normal, treatment of the insulin resistance should be directed at lowering the titer of the antibodies. Several patients have received immunosuppressive therapy with glucocorticoids and/or immuran. In at least two cases this has produced a lowering of antibody titer and a remission of the insulin resistance (Kawanishi *et al.*, 1977; Flier *et al.*, 1978). Plasma exchange has also been used as therapy in two cases. In one case, there was a lowering of antibody titers and an improvement in the diabetic state (Muggeo *et al.* 1979b). This partial remission, however, was transient, since the antibody titer rapidly rose after cessation of the exchange therapy. In the other case, there was no improvement in the insulin resistance and the symptoms related to the lupus erythematosus, particularly the skin rash, actually got worse.

As in most autoimmune disease, evaluation of therapy is also confused by the variable nature of the disease. At lease one patient has had a complete spontaneous remission, and others have shown improvement without therapy in only a few years of follow-up. Several other patients have gone from a state of marked insulin resistance to hypoglycemia during follow-up. In one case, this was associated with a marked increase in receptor numbers, usually without a major change in antibody titer (Flier *et al.*, 1978). In most of the cases the hypoglycemia has been profound and in several patients ultimately fatal.

REFERENCES

Akre, P. R. Kirtley, W. R., and Galloway, J. A., 1964, Comparative hypoglycemic response of diabetic subjects to human insulin or structurally similar insulins of animal sources, *Diabetes* 13:135–143.

Andersen, O. O., 1973, Insulin antibody formation. II. The influence of species difference and method of administration, *Acta Endocrinol. (Copenh.)*, 72:33–45.

Bar, R. S., Levis, W. R., Rechler, M. M., Siebert, C. W., Podskalny, J. M., Roth, J., and Muggeo, M., 1978, Extreme insulin resistance in ataxia telangiectasia: Defect in affinity of insulin receptors. *N. Engl. J. Med.* 298:1164–1171.

Bar, R. S., Muggeo, M., Kahn, C. R., Gorden, P., and Roth, J., 1980, Characterization of the insulin receptors in patients with the syndromes of insulin resistance and acanthosis nigricans, *Diabetologia* 18:209–216.

Belsham, G. J., Browney, R. W., Hughes, W. A., and Denton, R. M., 1980, Anti-insulin receptor antibodies mimic the effects of insulin on the activities of pyruvate dehydrogenase and acetyl CoA carboxylase and a specific protein phosphorylation in rat epididymal fat cells, *Diabetologia* 18:307–312.

Berson, S. A., and Yalow, R. S., 1959, Quantitative aspects of reaction between insulin and insulin-binding antibody, *J. Clin. Invest.* **38**:1996–2016.

Berson, S. A., and Yalow, R. S., 1966, Insulin in blood and insulin antiobodies, *Am. J. Med.* **40**:676–690.

Berson, S. A., and Yalow, R. S., 1970, Insulin "antagonists" and insulin resistance. *Diabetes Mellitus: Theory and Practice* (M. Ellenberg and H. Rifkin, eds.), pp 388–422, McGraw-Hill, New York.

Bertrams, J., Jansen, F. K., Gruneklee, D., Reis, H. E., Drost, H., Beyer, J., Gries, F. A., and Kuwert, E., 1976, HLA antigens and immunoresponsiveness to diabetes mellitus, *Tissue Antigens* **8**:13–19.

Bloom, S. R., Adrian, T. E., Barnes, A. J., and Polak, J. M., 1979, Autoimmunity induced by hormonal contaminants of insulin, *Lancet,* **1**:14–17.

Blundell, T. L., Dodson, G. C., Hodgkin, D. C., and Mercola, D. A., 1972, Insulin: Structure in the crystal and its reflection in chemistry and biology, *Adv. Protein Chem.* **26**:279–402.

Boshell, B. R., Barrett, J. C., Witensky, A. S., and Patton, T. B., 1964, Insulin resistance: Response to insulin from various animal sources including human, *Diabetes* **13**:144–152.

Chance, R. E., Root, M. A., and Galloway, J. A., 1976, The immunogenicity of insulin preparations, *Acta Endocrinol. (Copenh.)* 83 (Suppl. 205):185–196.

Davidson, J. K., and De Bra, D. W., 1978, Immunologic insulin resistance, *Diabetes* **27**:307–318.

DeMeyts, P., Bianco, A. R., and Roth, J., 1976, Site-site interactions among insulin receptors: Characterization of the negative cooperativity, *J. Biol. Chem.* **251**:1877–1888.

deShazo, R. D., 1978, Insulin allergy and insulin resistance. Two immunologic reactions, *Postgrad. Med.* **63**:85–92.

Flier, J. S., Kahn, C. R., Roth, J., and Bar, R. S., 1975, Antibodies that impair insulin receptor binding in an unusual diabetic syndrome with severe insulin resistance, *Science* **190**:63–65.

Flier, J. S., Kahn, C. R., Jarrett, D. B., and Roth, J., 1976, Characterization of anti-insulin receptor antibodies: A cause of insulin resistant diabetes in man, *J. Clin. Invest.* **548**:1442–1449.

Flier, J. S., Kahn, C. R., Jarrett, D. B., and Roth, J., 1977, Autoantibodies to the insulin receptor: Effect on the insulin–receptor interaction in IM-9 lymphocytes, *J. Clin. Invest.* **60**:784–794.

Flier, J. S., Bar,f R. S., Muggeo, M., Kahn, C. R., Roth, J., and Gorden, P., 1978, The evolving clinical course of patients with insulin receptor antibodies: spontaneous remission or receptor proliferation with hypoglycemia, *J. Clin Endocrinol. Metab.* **47**:985–995.

Freychet, P., Kahn, C. R., Roth, J., Neville, D. M., Jr.,1972, Insulin interactions with liver plasma membranes: Independence of binding and degradation, *J. Biol. Chem.* **247**:3953–3961.

Galloway, J. A., and Bressler, R., 1978, Insulin treatment in diabetes. *Med. Clin North Am.,* **62**:663–680.

Gavin, J. R., III, Roth, J., Neville, D. M., Jr., DeMeyts, P., and Buell, D. N., 1974, Insulin-dependent regulation of insulin receptor concentrations: A direct demonstration in cell culture, *Proc. Natl. Acad. Sci. USA,* **71**:84–88.

Ginsberg, B. H., Kahn, C. R., Roth, J., and DeMeyts, P., 1976, Insulin-induced dissociation of its receptor into subunits: possible molecular concomitant of negative cooperativity, *Biochem. Biophys. Res. Commun.* **73**:1068–1074.

Gorden, P., Carpentier, J. L., Freychet, P., and Orci, L., 1980, Internalization of polypeptide hormones: Mechanism, intracellular localization and significance, *Diabetologia* **18**:263–274.

Green, I., Paul, W. E., and Benacerraf, B., 1966, The behavior of hapten-poly-L-lysine conjugates as complete antigens in genetic responder and as haptens in nonresponder guinea pigs, *J. Exp. Med.* **123**:859–879.

Grunfeld, C., Van Obberghen, E., Karlsson, F. A., and Kahn, C. R., 1980, Antibody-induced desensitization of the insulin receptor: Studies of the mechanism of desensitization in 3T3-L1 fatty fibroblasts, *J. Clin. Invest.* **66**:1124–1134.

Harmon, J. T., Kahn, C. R., Kempner, E. J., and Schlegel, W., 1980, Characterization of the insulin receptor in its membrane environment by radiation inactivation, *J. Biol. Chem.* **255**:3412–3419.

Harrison, L. C., and Itin, A., 1979, A possible mechanism for insulin resistance and hyperglycemia in NZO mice, *Nature (Lon.)* **279**:334–336.

Harrison, L. C., Muggeo, M., Bar, R. S., Flier, J. S., Waldman, T., and Roth, J., 1979a, Insulin binding defects induced by a serum globulin factor in ataxia telangectasia, *Clin. Res.* **27**:252A.

Harrison, L. C., Flier, J. S., Roth, J., Karlsson, F. A., and Kahn, C. R., 1979b, Immunoprecipitation of the insulin receptor: A sensitive assay for receptor antibodies and a specific technique for receptor purification, *J. Clin. Endocrinol. Metab.* **48**:59–65.

Hedo, J., Kasuga, M., Van Obberghen, E., Roth, J., and Kahn, C. R., 1981, Direct demonstration of glycosylation of insulin receptor subunits by biosynthetic and external labeling: Evidence for heterogeneity, *Proc. Natl. Acad. Sci., USA* **78**:4791–4795.

Jarrett, D. B., Roth, J., Kahn, C. R., and Flier, J. S., 1976, Direct method for detection and characterization of cell surface receptors for insulin by means of ^{125}I-anti-receptor autoantibodies. *Proc. Natl. Acad. Sci. USA* **73**: 4115–4119.

Kahn, C. R., 1978, Insulin resistance, insulin insensitivity and insulin unresponsiveness: A necessary distinction, *Metabolism* **27**(suppl. 2): 1893–1902.

Kahn, C. R., and Harrison, L. C., 1980, Insulin receptor antibodies, in: *Carbohydrate Metabolism and its Disorders* (P. J. Randle, D. F. Steiner, and W. J. Whelan, eds.), pp. 279-330, Academic Press, London.

Kahn, C. R., and Rosenthal, A. S., 1979, Immunologic reactions to insulin: Insulin allergy, insulin resistance and the automimmune insulin syndrome, *Diabetes Care* **2**:283–295.

Kahn, C. R., Flier, J. S., Bar, R. S., Archer, J. A., Gorden, P., Martin, M. M., and Roth, J., 1976, The syndromes of insulin resistance and acanthosis nigricans: Insulin receptor disorders in man, *N. Engl. J. Med.* **294**:739–745.

Kahn, C. R., Megyesi, K., Bar, R. S., Eastman, R. C., and Flier, J. S., 1977a, Receptors for peptide hormones: New insights into the pathophysiology of disease states in man, *Ann. Intern. Med.* **86**:205–219.

Kahn, C. R., Baird, K. L., Flier, J. S., and Jarrett, D. B., 1977b, Effect of autoantibodies to the insulin receptor on isolated adipocytes: Studies of insulin binding and insulin action, *J. Clin. Invest.* **60**:1094–1106.

Kahn, C. R., Baird, K. L., Jarrett, D. B., and Flier, J. S., 1978, Direct demonstration that receptor cross-linking or aggregation is important in insulin action, *Proc. Natl. Acad. Sci. USA* **75**:4209.

Kahn, C. R., Harrison, L. C., Flier, J. S., Muggeo, M., Van Obberghen, E., Grunfeld, C., Karlsson, F. A., King, G. L., and Roth, J., 1980, Antibodies to the insulin receptor and insulin resistant diabetes, in: *Autoimmune Aspects of Endocrine Disorders* (A. Pinchera, D. Domach, G. F. Fenzi, and L. Baschieri, eds.), pp. 275–280, Academic Press, London.

Kahn, C. R., Baird, K. L., Flier, J. S., Grunfeld, C., Harmon, J. T., Harrison, L. C., Karlsson, F. A., Kasuga, M., King, G. L., Lang, U. C., Podskalny, J. M., and Van Obberghen, E. M., 1981, Insulin receptors, receptor antibodies, and the mechanism of insulin action, *Rec. Prog. Horm. Res.* **37**: 477–532.

Kahn, C. R., Mann, D. L., Rosenthal, A. S., Galloway, J. A., Johnson, A. H., and Mendell, N., 1982, The immune response to insulin in man. Interaction of HLA alloantigens and the development of the immune response, *Diabetes* **31**:716–723.

Karlsson, F. A., Van Obberghen, E., Grunfeld, C., and Kahn, C. R., 1979, Desensitization of the insulin receptor at an early post-receptor step by prolonged exposure to anti-receptor antibody, *Proc. Natl. Acad. Sci. USA* **76**:809–813.

Kasuga, M., Akanuma, U., Tsushima, T., Suzuki, K., Kosaka, K., and Kibata, M., 1978, Effects of anti-insulin receptor autoantibody in the metabolism of rat adipocytes, *J. Clin. Endocrinol. Metab.* **47**:66–77.

Kasuga, M., Kahn, C. R., Hedo, J. A., Van Obberghen, E., and Yamada, K. M., 1981, Insulin-induced receptor loss in cultured human lymphocytes is due to accelerated receptor degradation, *Proc. Natl. Acad. Sci. USA* **78**:6917–6921.

Kasuga, M., Karlsson, F. A., and Kahn, C. R., 1982, Insulin stimulates the phosphorylation of the 95,000-dalton subunit of its own receptor, *Science* **215**:185–187.

Kawanishi, K., Kawamura, K., Nishina, A. G., Okada, S., Ishide, T., Ohiji, T., Kahn, C. R., and Flier, J. S., 1977, Successful immunosuppressive therapy in insulin resistant diabetes caused by anti-insulin receptor autoantibodies, *J. Clin. Endocrinol. Metab.* **44**:15–21.

King, G. L., Kahn, C. R., Rechler, M. M., and Nissley, S. P., 1980, Direct demonstration of separate receptors for growth and metabolic activities of insulin and multiplication stimulating activity (an insulin-like growth factor) using antibodies to the insulin receptor, *J. Clin. Invest.* **66**:130–140.

Lang, U. C., Kahn, C. R., and Chrombach, A., 1980, Characterization of the insulin receptor and insulin-degrading activity from human lymphocytes by quantitative polyacrylamide gel electrophoresis, *Endocrinology* **106**:40–49.

Lawrence, J. C., Jr., Larner, J., Kahn, C. R., and Roth, J., 1978, Autoantibodies to the insulin receptor activate glycogen synthase in rat adipocytes, *Mol. Cell. Biochem.* **22:**153–158.

Little, J. A., and Arnott, J. H., 1966, Sulfated insulin in mild, moderate, severe, and insulin-resistant diabetes mellitus, *Diabetes* **15:**457–465.

Ludvigsson, J., Safwenberg, J., and Heding, L. G., 1977, HLA-types, C-peptide and insulin antibodies in juvenile diabetes, *Diabetologia* **13:**13–17.

Massague, J., Pilch, P. F., and Czech, M. P., 1980, Electrophoretic resolution of three major insulin receptor structures with unique subunit stiochiometries, *Proc. Natl. Acad. Sci. USA* **77:**7137–7141.

Muggeo, M., Ginsberg, B. H., Roth, J., Neville, D. M., Jr., DeMeyts, P., and Kahn, C. R., 1979a, The insulin receptor is functionally more conserved during evolution than insulin itself, *Endocrinology* **104:**1393–1402.

Muggeo, M., Flier, J. S., Abrams, R. A., Harrison, L. C., Deisseroth, A. B., and Kahn, C. R., 1979b, Treatment by plasma exchange of a patient with autoantibodies to the insulin receptor, *N. Engl. J. Med.* **300:**477–480.

Muggeo, M., Kahn, C. R., Bar, R. S., Rechler, M. M., Flier, J. S., and Roth, J., 1979c, The underlying insulin receptor in patients with antireceptor antibodies: Demonstration of normal binding and immunological properties, *J. Clin. Endocrinol. Metab.* **49:**110–119.

Olefsky, J. M., 1981, Insulin resistance and insulin action: An in vitro and in vivo perspective, *Diabetes* **30:**148–162.

Patterson, R., O'Rourke, J., Robert, M., and Suszko, I., 1973a, Immunologic reactions against insulin. I. IgG anti-insulin and insulin resistance, *J. Immunol.* **110:**1126–1134.

Patterson, R., Mellies, C. J., and Roberts, M., 1973b, Immunologic reactions against insulin. II. IgE anti-insulin, insulin allergy and combined IgE and IgG immunologic insulin resistance, *J. Immunol.* **110:**1135–1145.

Reeves, W. G., 1980, Immunology of diabetes and insulin therapy, *Recent Adv. Clin. Immunol.* **2:**183–220.

Rosenthal, A. S., 1978, Determinant selection and macrophage function in genetic control of the immune response, *Immunol. Rev.* **40**136–152.

Schernthaner, G., Ludwig, H., Mayr, W. R., and Frish, H., 1977, Evidence for genetic control of anti-insulin immunity in juvenile onset diabetes mellitus, *Diabetes Metab.* **3:**117–121.

Schlessinger, J., Van Obberghen, E., and Kahn, C. R., 1980, Insulin and antibodies against the insulin receptor cap on the membrane of cultured human lymphocytes, *Nature* **286:**729–731.

Serge, K., and Peterson, P. A., 1978, Use of anti-idiotypic antibodies as cell-surface receptor probes, *Proc. Natl. Acad. Sci. USA,* **75:**2443–2447.

Shechter, Y., Chang, K. J., Jacobs, S., and Cuatrecas, P., 1979, Modulation of binding and bioactivity of insulin by anti-insulin antibody: Relation to possible role of receptor self-aggregation in hormone action, *Proc. Natl. Acad. Sci. USA* **76:**2720–2724.

Shechter, Y., Maron, R., Elias, D., and Cohen, I. R., 1982, Autoantibodies to insulin receptor spontaneously develop as anti-idiotypes in mice immunized with insulin, *Science* **216:**542–544.

Shipp, J. C., Cunningham, R. W., Russell, R. O., and Marble, A., 1967, Insulin resistance: Clinical features, natural course and effects of adrenal steroid treatment, *Medicine* **44:**165–186.

Van Obberghen, E., Kasuga, M., Lelam, A., Hedo, J. A., Itin, A., and Harrison, L. C., 1981, Biosynthetic labeling of insulin receptor: Studies of subunits in cultured human IM-9 lymphocytes, *Proc. Natl. Acad. Sci. USA* **78:**1052–1056.

Yip, C., Yeung, C. W. T., and Mark, M. L., 1980, Photoaffinity labeling of insulin receptor proteins of liver plasma membrane preparations, *Biochemistry* **19:**70–76.

9

Genetic Basis of Type I (Insulin-Dependent) Diabetes

A. G. Cudworth[†] and Eva Wolf

I. INTRODUCTION

It is now widely accepted that Type I (insulin-dependent) diabetes is etiologically distinct from the more common Type II (non-insulin-dependent) diabetes. However, it must be acknowledged that at times it is not always possible to draw a clear clinical distinction between these two major forms of the disease. Generally, Type I diabetes presents mainly in childhood or adolescence and Type II diabetes mainly in middle or later life. This is by no means a rigid phenomenon and almost certainly there is considerable heterogeneity in both Type I and Type II diabetes. Circumstantial evidence indicates that virus(es) may initiate an immune-mediated destructive process of the pancreatic islet B (insulin-producing) cells in early onset Type I diabetes (Type IA). In addition, there may be a more primary autoimmune form of the disease (Type IB) which has a later age of onset and exhibits a number of other striking characteristic features as discussed later. There is increasing evidence that the immunogenetic characteristics of Type IA and IB diabetes overlap considerably. However, there is no evidence that such immunological factors are operating in Type II diabetes, illustrating that this disease has an entirely different underlying pathogenesis.

There has been considerable confusion concerning the genetics of diabetes because both types show a striking familial aggregation. This is far more impressive in Type II diabetes and particularly in the relatively rare so-called MODY (maturity onset diabetes of the young) families. (Tattersall, 1974; Tattersall and Fajans, 1975). This sort of evidence together with observations in identical twins (Barnett *et al.,* 1981) suggests genetic heterogeneity in diabetes. However, arguments still persist that there

A. G. Cudworth and Eva Wolf • Department of Diabetes and Immunogenetics, St. Bartholomew's Hospital Medical College, London, England.

could be a common genetic mechanism operating in both types of diabetes. It is worth emphasizing that it is not diabetes *per se* which is inherited but the suceptibility to develop the disease. Which factors convert the underlying predisposition into overt diabetes remain open to speculation. But as discussed later, there is increasing evidence that in Type I diabetes there is a slow immune-mediated destruction of islet B cells initiated perhaps by different viruses.

An important fact is that Type I diabetes is predominantly a Caucasoid disease being relatively rare in blacks and Mongoloids. To what extent this reflects genetic heterogeneity or variability in the role of environmental triggering factors is not known. In contrast, Type II diabetes is a worldwide phenomenon, being particularly prevalent in those ethnic groups exposed to rapid changes in food supply and the impact of western habits in general (Zimmet, 1982). This fascinating changing pattern of Type II diabetes may reflect the existence of a metabolic genotype which was more appropriate to our ancestors of the "hunter and gatherer" era. It has been argued (Neel, 1976) that the Western world has had more time genetically to adjust to the impact of environmental changes, particularly in relation to the amount and type of food availability compared with other ethnic groups. Certainly it would have to be acknowledged that a powerful genetic influence of this type is unlikely to be deleted from a population very rapidly. Therefore, because Type II diabetes is so common, it is quite likely that a "Type II diabetes gene or genes" will occur in some Type I diabetic families to produce a difficult and confusing picture. To what extent such admixture of genetic factors actually happens is unknown but there is no convincing evidence that the same underlying mechanisms are operating in these two clinically distinct forms of glucose intolerance.

Even though there is a strong inherited component in Type II diabetes, no genetic markers are known. Leslie and Pyke (1978) suggested that the phenomenon of chlorpropamide alcohol flushing was strongly associated with both MODY and Type II diabetes in general, particularly in the presence of a strong family history of Type II diabetes. However, many attempts have failed to confirm these findings (Köbberling *et al.*, 1980).

There are preliminary data on the human insulin gene polymorphism suggesting that the homozygous *UU* genotype defined by restriction fragment length could be a genetic marker for Type II diabetes (Owerbach and Nerup, 1982). More work needs to be done to clarify this very interesting proposal.

HLA studies carried out in caucasoid Type II diabetics showed no differences of HLA-A,B,C, and DR antigens compared to healthy controls (Cudworth 1978; Rotter and Rimoin 1979). In the Xhosas, a black tribe living in South Africa, a slight but not significant increase in A2 has been found (Briggs *et al.*, 1980). An increase of A2 ($r = 2.2$) has also been reported in the Pima Indians, who are American Indians of Mongoloid origin, and show a very restricted HLA polymorphism and a high degree of homozygosity. Only six alleles are detectable at the *B* locus and only four at the *A* locus of which *A2* and *AW24* are the most frequent ones. It was suggested that the *A2* allele or a gene closely linked to the *A* locus contributes to an earlier onset of the disease in this population, as almost all the younger diabetics were *A2*-positive and half of them were homozygous for this antigen (Williams *et al.*, 1981). Two reports also found a slight increase in BW61, which is a subgroup of B40, in Asian Indians, who are Caucasoids, living in Fiji (Serjeantson et al., 1981) and in South Africa (Asmal et al., 1981). A trend for B40 to be more frequent in black West Indian diabetics with a later onset was also reported (Wolf et al., 1981a). More studies are needed to verify these weak HLA associations with Type II diabetes especially as those antigens which are otherwise frequent in these populations, such as A2 in the Pimas and BW61 in the Asian Indians, are raised. It is highly unlikely that there is a strong HLA-linked susceptibility factor operating in Type II diabetes in these different ethnic groups.

II. THE SIZE OF THE PROBLEM

The incidence and prevalence rates of the different types of diabetes have been reviewed by West (1978), and in relation to Type I diabetes specifically by Spencer and Cudworth (1982). The most informative studies have been carried out in Europe and certain parts of the United States. In 1972, the British Diabetic Association (BDA) initiated a Register of newly diagnosed patients under the age of 16 years. This has been a most successful enterprise providing information on approximately 1200 new cases each year. The minimum annual incidence was reported to be 7–8/100,000 (Bloom et al., 1975), but unfortunately the ascertainment varies from one region to another and makes definitive conclusions difficult. Nevertheless there is a remarkable uniformity in the overall incidence rate and seasonal variability from year to year. Available information would suggest that in the "better" reporting areas, the incidence rate is of the order of 14/100,000 per year. This is of interest because it compares well with the 13.7/100,000 per year incidence rate reported by Christau et al., (1977) from Denmark. Although the age range considered was up to 30 years at diagnosis and the number of cases was much smaller compared with the BDA study, the Danish data have the advantage of achieving a virtual complete ascertainment. Therefore, if the incidence figure of 13–14/100,000 per year is taken as being reasonably accurate for a northern European population, the calculated prevalence by the age of 16 years if of the order of 0.22%, that is, 1:500 schoolchildren will be an insulin-dependent diabetic by the age of 16 years. However, the situation is not quite so simple. First, there is increasing evidence of differences in incidence and prevalence rates in different European countries, with a steady increase in rates from southern Europe to the highest values observed in Sweden and Finland. Secondly, there is teasing evidence from cohort studies of a real increase in the incidence rate in recent years. A recent study in Scotland (Patterson et al., 1981) has suggested a doubling of the number of new cases over the past decade. However, more studies of this type need to be carried out before firm conclusions can be reached.

As indicated above, Type I diabetes is seen mainly in Caucasoids, although there is increasing evidence that the same immunogenetic features are seen in true insulin dependent-diabetic patients from Japan and also in black patients (Svejgaard et al., 1980). Existing problems relate to the absence of any substantial data on incidence and prevalence rates of Type I diabetes in non-Caucasoid populations, and the definition of insulin dependence. This tends to be a variable feature in some ethnic groups. We have noticed this particularly in West Indian diabetics, irrespective of age of onset, who tend to be relatively ketosis-resistant.

A similar problem can be seen in relation to Caucasoid patients who eventually turn out to have Type IB diabetes. The dependence on insulin may be a relatively insidious development and there is little doubt that a number of patients who are well-maintained on diet and oral antidiabetic drugs possibly have underlying autoimmune diabetes. The accurate classification of such patients is probably only of academic interest, because obviously treatment has to be fashioned to the needs of each individual patient. Unacceptable hyperglycemia in a Type II diabetic may warrant insulin therapy, but of course this is not the same as insulin dependence. However, it is useful to know whether or not a middle-aged patient presenting with a difficult clinical picture is actually developing Type I diabetes. In this context, an accurate family history should be taken with particular reference to the type of diabetes, which may be present in close relatives, and also for a positive family history of related autoimmune organ-specific endocrinopathies. In addition, access to a laboratory which undertakes screening for islet cell antibodies (ICA), particularly complement-fixing ICA, will help to clarify many of these cases. This has some practical importance, because certain patients can then be observed more critically for the development of insulin dependence.

The coexistence of Type I diabetes with other autoimmune endocrine diseases such as Addison's disease and Graves' disease suggests that there may be a widespread immune-mediated destruction of endocrine organs. However, Type I diabetes also occurs more frequently than expected in the close relatives of patients with rheumatoid arthritis and vice versa. These important clinical associations not only provide strong suggestive evidence for an immune basis to these diseases, but may also offer important clues to the type and mechanisms of immune response involved in the pathogenesis of disease in apparently widely differing types of target organs and tissues.

Both major types of diabetes may lead to similar complications such as proliferative retinopathy, kidney failure, and neuropathy. Although there is increasing evidence that excessive glycosylation of basement membrane proteins by inappropriate and sustained poor blood glucose control may be the primary factor in the development of such crippling complications, it is also widely acknowledged that other factors are likely to be involved. This review will also attempt to assess the role of HLA genetic factors which have been suggested to play a role in the etiology of basement membrane disease, particularly in patients with Type I diabetes.

In the past 50 years there have been many attempts to examine the genetic basis of diabetes based mainly on analyses of familial aggregation and the assumption that the "disease susceptibility gene" behaves according to simple dominant or recessive modes of inheritance (for reviews on this see Clarke, 1966; Cudworth and Wolf, 1982). Many of the earlier investigators recognized that there must be heterogeneity in diabetes in order to explain the familial aggregation data. Incomplete penetrance, both genetic and environmental, was frequently invoked and still remains one of the most confounding factors in considering the different genetic models. Penetrance has often wrongly been assumed to be of the order of 50% based on the observations in identical twins. However, almost certainly this represents a gross overestimation because of the considerable bias towards ascertainment of concordant pairs.

Estimates of the incidence of affected siblings vary from about 6 to 14% up to age 30 years (Pincus and White, 1933; Simpson, 1962; Dengbol and Green, 1978; Gorsuch *et al.*, 1982a). A lower frequency of affected parents (approximately 3–10%) has usually been found. This very low frequency of affected siblings and parents excludes all forms of single-gene controlling susceptibility unless the prevalence is taken as less than 10%. If the frequency of the disease in siblings or dizygotic twins is less than one-quarter of that in monozygotic twins then a single gene hypothesis of any form can be rejected (Thomson, 1980). The data from carefully ascertained family studies tend to implicate a much lower order of penetrance than anticipated. This might be compatible with the concept that the initiating environmental factor is relatively rare, or alternatively, B cell loss is the result of cumulative damage from the same or different pancreatotropic agents.

It is now widely accepted that the major genetic susceptibility to Type I diabetes is conferred by a gene or genes operating at a locus or loci closely linked to the HLA complex. Before discussing the evidence in detail, it is important to consider one or two fundamental principles relating to the HLA system in order to appreciate the significance of the population and family studies.

III. THE HLA SYSTEM

The HLA system is located on the short arm of chromosome 6 and contains a number of major histocompatibility loci (*A,B,C,D,* and *DR*) which are closely linked (Fig. 1). Also situated in the same region are loci at which genes operate to control certain complement factors (e.g., C2 and C4 of the "classical" pathway and Bf of the "alternative" complement pathway). Recently a new locus between *GLO* (Glyoxalase 1) and *DR* coding for "secondary B cell" antigens (SB), which are identified by primed lymphocyte typing, has been described (Shaw *et al.*, 1981). Although no solid evidence exists in humans, it seems most likely that immune response (*IR*) genes are also present within the HLA complex, analagous to the situation now well-established

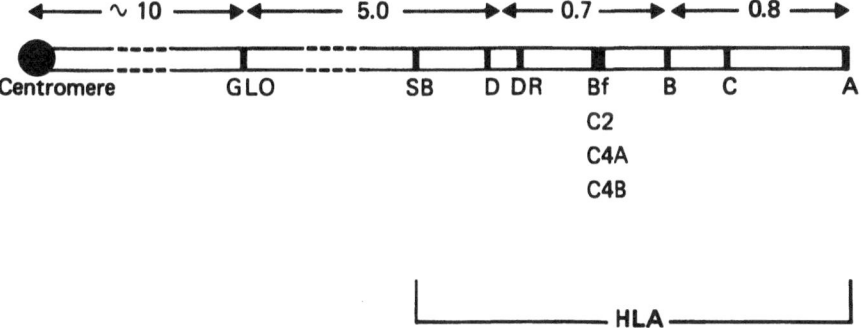

Figure 1. The major histocompatibility locus and the locus for red cell glyoxalase 1 (GLO) are shown in relation to the centromere. The distances between the different loci are given in centimorgans.

in mice and other animals. *IR* gene function has been shown to control susceptibility to certain viruses (e.g., lymphochorioimeningitis virus) and other agents in mice. If similar genes exist in humans, then they are more likely to be situated near the *HLA-D/DR* region and probably control the major susceptibility to several diseases.

HLA-A,B,C antigens are found on virtually all cells in the body except mature red cells, whereas the HLA-D and DR antigens are found only on B lymphocytes, monocytes, macrophages, endothelial cells, Langerhan cells, and sperm. They are very likely not expressed on islet B cells. A,B,C and DR antigens are serologically defined whereas the D specificities are detected by mixed lymphocyte culture techniques using homozygous typing cells.

Chemically, A,B,C antigens are glycoproteins consisting of a heavy chain with a molecular weight of 43,000, which carries the polymorphic specificity and is coded for by chromosome 6, and a light chain with a molecular weight of 12,000, which is β2 microglobulin and coded for by chromosome 17. DR antigens are also glycoproteins consisting of two noncovalently associated polypeptide chains with a molecular weight of 28,000 and 33,000, respectively; there might possibly be a third chain of 30,000 daltons. A,B,C and DR antigens are inserted into the lipid bilayer of the cell membrane. Their exact function is unknown. DR antigens probably play a key role in initiating the immune response by presenting foreign antigen to activated T cells. Theoreticlaly they could also act as "receptors" for viruses or other foreign agents to produce neoantigen on the cell surface.

Recombination or crossover during meiosis occurs with a very low frequency within the HLA region. It is less than 2% between *A* and *D/DR*. HLA antigens coded for by genes of the different loci are nearly always inherited "en bloc" from each parent. By HLA genotyping parents and offspring it is possible to identify the precise combination of these HLA antigens, referred to as haplotypes.

This has important implications for disease studies because it enables the investigator to determine whether or not the disease segregates with a particular haplotype in families, and thereby provide strong evidence for linkage with the putative susceptibility gene. Linkage disequilibrium is not unique to the HLA region, but this phenomenon can best explained in relation to this unique part of the human genome. For example, it is well-established that certain antigens tend to occur more frequently on the same haplotype than expected from the known gene frequencies for the antigens concerned. One of the best examples of this linkage disequilibrium in the HLA system is the A1-CW7-B8-DW3-DR3 haplotype which is particularly common in northern European populations. There are many other examples of linkage disequilibrium and it is of interest that the antigens involved can vary in different racial groups. The usual explanation for an association between a certain HLA antigen or antigens and a disease in a well-characterized population of patients is that there is a gene operating at a nearby locus, which is in linkage disequilibrium with the HLA antigen found to be increased in frequency in the disease group, and that the HLA antigen concern is merely acting as an "indirect" marker for the putative susceptibility gene. The possible cause and reasons for the persistence of linkage disequilibrium have been extensively discussed (Svejgaard *et al.*, 1975; Thomson and Bodmer, 1977, 1979). The most plausible theory emanates from the idea that there has been some selective advantage for these groups of interrelated genes and that their persistence in linkage disequilibrium provided protection against diseases or environmental hazards in the past. It is conceivable that these gene combinations are not disadvantageous in producing an inappropriate immune response to "new" environmental agents (Cudworth, 1981). It is interesting to speculate that in this context Type I diabetes and rheumatoid arthritis may be relatively new diseases in terms of our evolution.

Selective advantage may also provide the explanation for the unique polymorphic nature of the HLA complex. There are many different alleles operating at each locus to determine the known cell surface HLA antigens. At least 17 different officially recognized antigens can be defined at the A locus, 8 at the C locus, 33 at the B locus, 12 at the D locus, and 10 at the DR locus, but there is evidence for additional specificities particularly at the very polymorphic B locus. HLA antigens are a very good anthropological marker as the frequencies of these antigens vary in different ethnic groups, and some antigens only occur in certain populations, for example, BW54 in Mongoloids. This antigen, which is a subgroup of BW22, was reported to be increased in frequency in Japanese Type I diabetics (Wakisaka et al., 1976) and this provides a good example of the possibility that the same disease susceptibility gene may be in linkage disequilibrium with different HLA specificities in different populations. Whatever the explanation for the existence and persistence of linkage disequilibrium, the latter is an important concept for our understanding of HLA and disease associations.

An alternative view for the haplotype associations with certain diseases such as Type I diabetes is that there are multiple HLA-linked genes operating to influence susceptibility. This, a gene closely linked to the HLA A locus might be involved in T-cell recognition of foreign antigens, a gene closely linked to the B locus might control T-cell–B-cell interaction, and a gene or genes closely linked to the D/DR loci might control the specific immune responsiveness. An important question which is difficult to resolve is whether these "super" haplotypes are uniquely associated with a particular disease. Thomson and Bodmer (1979) have discussed the problem of these higher-order interactions and have pointed out that it is very difficult to identify complex haplotype associations with a disease, particularly if a strong association of the disease with an HLA antigen exists. One of the problems that continually hampers resolution of this question is the lack of adequate data concerning these "super" haplotypes in healthy families. Although higher-order interactions are difficult to calculate mathematically the comparison of disease and healthy families from the same geographical and ethnic background would help to resolve the question of particular patterns of linkage disequilibrium are more strongly associated with certain diseases.

A. Population Studies

In 1974, simultaneous studies in Copenhagen and Liverpool provided evidence for an association of juvenile-onset Type I (insulin-dependent) diabetes with B8 and B15, the major component of which is now referred to as BW62. No association was found with Type II (non-insulin-dependent) diabetes (Nerup et al., 1974; Cudworth and Woodrow, 1975). These findings provided scientific evidence for the existence of genetic heterogeneity between these two major forms of diabetes. Singal and Blajchman

(1973) had already reported an increase of B15 in Type I diabetics in Toronto and many reports were soon to follow confirming the increase of B8 and BW62 in Caucasoid Type I diabetics. It is of interest however that in southern Europe, the strongest association was found with B18 (Seignalet *et al.*, 1975). A weaker association with B40, which consists of the two subgroups BW60 and BW61, was also demonstrated in Type I diabetics in England (Cudworth, 1978). Most studies also showed a striking reduction of B7. The wide spread of relative risk from two to three times increased for HLA-B8, BW62, and B18 to less than 0.5 for B7 led to the idea that there could be a single susceptibility gene in varying linkage disequilibrium with all the HLA *B* locus alleles (Cudworth and Woodrow, 1976), which is preferentially found on haplotypes containing the "high-risk" alleles. It was also realized at this stage that Type I diabetics, who possessed both B8 and BW62, had an approximate additive risk compared with the risk seen with B8 or BW62 alone. This led to the hypothesis that there may be two separate susceptibility genes acting in an interactive manner. This was supported by the fact that there did not appear to be any increase in B8 or BW62 homozygotes although insufficient data were available at the time to resolve this issue.

The advent of techniques to identify the HLA *D* locus specificities soon led to the finding that in patients with Type I diabetes there was a stronger association of DW3 and DW4, in linkage disequilibrium with B8 and BW62 respectively (Thomsen *et al.*, 1975). It was elegantly demonstrated that the association with DW3 and DW4 formed the strongest or primary association with the disease (Svejgaard and Ryder, 1977) and that the *B* locus association was purely secondary.

From then on attention has been focused on the D-related (DR) antigens which are coded for at a locus or loci closely linked to HLA-D. The DR antigens are serologically defined and much easier determined than the D specificities which are detected by mixed lymphocyte culture reactions. Recently Platz *et al.* (1981) found that 14 out of 88 Type I diabetic patients (15.9%) were negative for DW4, but positive for DR4. In 7 out of 89 patients (8%) the definition of DW3 and DR3 was discordant. This indicates that the DR antigens are better markers for Type I diabetes than the DW antigens.

Many studies have been published analyzing the DR *phenotype* frequencies found in unrelated Type I diabetics. All these studies had the disadvantage that homozygosity had to be assumed if only one DR antigen was detectable. This is not necessarily true since unknown antigens might exist at the *DR* locus. We want to describe the population association found in Type I diabetes with the DR antigens taking our *genotyped* probands from the Barts-Windsor family study, which is discussed in detail later (Wolf *et al.*, 1982a). These probands are unrelated and represent a typical group of classic juvenile-onset Type I diabetics. An important advantage is that the exact rate of homozygosity for DR3 and DR4 was established in all the probands by genotyping. In Type I diabetes there is a strong association with both DR3 and DR4. The gene frequencies for DR3 and DR4 are 38.9 and 41.4%, the phenotype frequencies for DR3 and DR4 are 71% and 78%, respectively, in our genotyped Type I diabetic probands. Almost 98% of patients possess one of these antigens and approximately 51% had both DR3 and DR4. Similar findings using phenotype frequencies were found in many other countries (Ryder *et al.*, 1979). Recent reports from Denmark (Platz *et al.*, 1981), France (Deschamps *et al.*, 1980), and America (Rotter *et al.*, personal communication) are in accordance with our results. Among the Basques (DeMouzon-Cambon *et al.*, 1982) the phenotype frequency of DR3 was higher (90%) than in all other Caucasoid Type I diabetics studied. DRW9 and DRW10, which are two rare antigens of the *DR* locus, and MT1, MT2 and MT3, which might belong to a second *DR* locus (Tosi *et al.*, 1978) had not been defined in any of these studies. DRW9 and DRW10 showed no increase in our Type I diabetic patients and, as expected, MT2, which is associated with DR3, DR5, DRW6, and DRW8, and MT3, which is associated with DR4, DR7, and DRW9 showed a significant increase in Type I diabetics ($r = 2.6$ and 3.3, respectively). MT1, which is associated with DR1, DR2, DRW6, and DRW10, was decreased in our study.

An association of Type I diabetes with DR4 was also found in American blacks (Rodey *et al.*, 1979), in African blacks and in the Japanese, (Svejgaard *et al.*, 1980), in whom the disease is much rarer than in Caucasoids. DR3 was found to be associated with Type I diabetes in African and American blacks and in Chinese (Maeda *et al.*, 1980), but in the Japanese where DR3 and B8 are virtually absent (less than 1%), an increase of DRW8 was found (Svejgaard *et al.*, 1980).

Several possible conclusions result from these studies. First, the strong association with both DR3 and DR4, at least in Caucasoid populations, suggests that there are two separate susceptibility genes, each in linkage disequilibrium with DR3 and DR4 respectively operating at the same or different loci closely linked to the HLA *D/DR* loci. The very high frequency of DR3, DR4 heterozygotes lends powerful support to this interpretation. There is an approximate additive relative risk for DR3,DR4 (14.3) compared with the relative risk observed for DR3 or DR4 considered separately (5.0 and 6.8, respectively). If it was the same susceptibility gene in linkage disequilibrium with both DR3 and DR4, then it would be expected that a double dose of susceptibilty would also occur in DR3 and DR4 homozygotes. In marked contrast, out of 122 genotyped Type I diabetics we observed only 8 DR3 homozygotes and 6 DR4 homozygotes. Thus, there is no increase in the relative risk for homozygosity of these particular antigens which argues strongly against a single-gene concept. However, it must be pointed out that different interpretations of these data have been put forward (Rubinstein *et al.*, 1981).

The importance of the potential interactive effect of possessing both DR3 and DR4 in enhancing the susceptibility can be highlighted by examining the different parental matings in our 122 genotyped families. We have compared the number of DR3,DR4 heterozygous offspring with the expected number in families, where one or both parents possess these antigens. For example, in 120 children from 40 families in whom there was a potential DR3,DR4 combination 48 (40%) inherited both DR3 and DR4 compared with the expected 25%. Furthermore, 39 (81%) of these were Type I diabetics and only 9 (19%) were healthy sibililngs. In 26 families, where the chance was 50% that an offspring was DR3,DR4 heterozygous due to the parental DR combinations, 43 out of 64 children (67%) were positive for both DR3 and DR4. Twenty-four (56%) were Type I diabetics and 19 (44%) were healthy siblings. We have also observed a similar trend in Type I diabetic identical twins. There are twice as many concordant pairs (i.e., both twins diabetic) who are DR3,DR4 heterozygous (58%) compared with discordant pairs (i.e., only one twin diabetic more than 5 years after diagnosis) in whom the frequency of DR3,DR4 heterozygosity was 27% (Johnston *et al.*, 1982). Thus, the concordance rate in identical twins appears to be influenced by the coexistence of both DR3 and DR4.

There was a significant decrease in the frequency of DR7 in the genotyped probands (gene frequency 2.9 compared with 19.7 in healthy controls) and in the discordant twins (phenotype frequency 16% compared with 36% in healthy controls). DR7 was absent in the concordant twins.

The most striking negative association reported by several groups is with DR2 (gene frequency 2.0 compared with 15.3 in healthy controls). This is very much in accordance with the earlier data which showed a significant low frequency of B7 in Type I diabetes. B7 is in linkage disequilibrium with DR2 in healthy Caucasoid populations and therefore a reduced frequency of DR2 was anticipated. However, the situation may be more complicated because in our own data we have found no linkage disequilibrium between B7 and DR2 in the Type I diabetic probands. Thus, out of 16 B7-positive Type I diabetic probands only one was DR2-positive. There were however another four probands with DR2 and it is of great interest that in all five DR2-positive patients the alternative DR allele was either DR3 or DR4.

It is very difficult to establish that a low frequency of an allele at a particular locus infers a significant negative biological effect. However, the extremely low frequency of DR2 in Type I diabetes raises the argument that there may be a gene or genes in linkage disequilibrium with DR2 which confer(s) protection against islet B cell damage. One interpretation of the HLA DR data in Type I diabetes is that there are several mechanisms of immune response to pancreatotropic agents. The risk of developing the disease is considerably enhanced in DR3,DR4 heterozygotes and virtually absent in subjects who possess DR2. A perhaps more speculative idea is that these DR antigens might themselves be involved in the initial immune-mediated B-cell damage. The observation that less than 3% of Type I diabetic children do not possess DR3 or DR4 might lend support to this concept.

B. Family Studies

As explained earlier, HLA genotyping in families provides accurate information on the four different parental haplotypes and their inheritance by the offspring. It also provides a much more powerful method for studying the genetics of a disease. The probabilities of any pair of siblings being HLA-identical (inheriting the same HLA haplotypes), HLA haploidentical (inheriting one haplotype in common), or being HLA nonidentical (having neither haplotype in common) is 25%, 50%, and 25% respectively. In families with two or more Type I diabetic siblings, there is a very marked disturbance in the observed distribution of haplotypes in the diabetic children compared with the expected. Almost identical patterns of HLA haplotype identity in multiplex families have been found by several groups in northern Europe, Scandanavia, and the United States (for combined data see Gorsuch *et al.*, 1982b). Thus, 57% of pairs of affected siblings are HLA identical, 38% are HLA haploidentical, and only 5% are HLA nonidentical.

The haplotypes found in Type I diabetics are mostly made up of those antigens which have been found to be increased in the populations studied. The

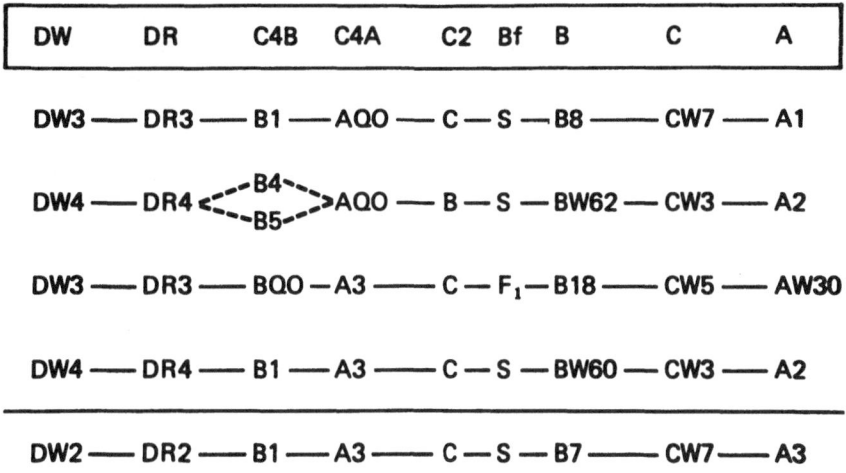

DW	DR	C4B	C4A	C2	Bf	B	C	A

Figure 2. The four major HLA haplotypes, which are increased in frequency in Type I diabetes, and the haplotype, which is decreased.

A1,CW7,B8,DR3 and the *A2,CW3,BW62,DR4* haplotype are common in Type I diabetic probands, and, dependent on the population studied, also the *AW30,CW5,B18,DR3* haplotype (Fig. 2). But often haplotypes are found segregating with the disease in multiplex families which are not made up "high-risk" antigen combinations, but of antigens that are not increased in frequency in the population data. As emphasized earlier, family studies provide evidence for linkage of the putative susceptibility gene and the various *HLA* genes.

The HLA haplotype distribution data in multiplex families provides conclusive evidence for the existence of an HLA-linked susceptibility gene or genes in Type I diabetes. This provides a unique rationale for long-term prospective studies in order to compare and contrast immunogenetic and environmental factors in healthy siblings who, on the basis of haplotype concordance with the proband, can be considered as potentially genetically susceptible and nonsusceptible, respectively. It can be reasonably assumed that in order for a second sibling to develop the disease the child has to inherit at least one haplotype in common with the proband. In 1978 the Barts-Windsor prospective family study was initiated. Basically, this study comprises approximately 200 families each with a Type I diabetic child and at least one unaffected sibling under the age of 20 years, ascertained from a geographical area of approximately 1500 km^2 in East Berkshire, England. All these families are visited every 3–4 months and have been HLA genotyped. Regular screening for autoantibodies including islet cell antibodies is carried out. So far six siblings and two parents have developed Type I diabetes (Gorsuch *et al.*, 1981).

An unresolved question arising from the multiplex family results is whether we are dealing with one or more susceptibility genes and the likely mode of inheritance. As already discussed evidence from the population studies is in favor of two genes. Certainly the haplotype data are not compatible with a single gene behaving in a dominant fashion and, as discussed by Walker and Cudworth (1980), a recessive mode of inheritance is also unlikely. The latter would have to allow for a relatively high gene frequency (0.35) and an extremely low penetrance (<2%). However, it must be conceded that a single gene model cannot be completely excluded and, as argued by Spielman *et al.* (1980), the data could be compatible with a gene dosage effect in which there is a greater risk (penetrance) in siblings who inherit two doses of the susceptibility gene (71% penetrance) compared with siblings who inherit a single gene dose (6.5% penetrance). It is also possible that, if there are two major susceptibility genes operating, one may be acting in a simple dominant fashion and the other in a recessive manner. However, it seems increasingly unlikely that the creation of more and more complex mathematical models based on family haplotype data will resolve this problem.

One question that does appear to have been answered is whether "familial" cases are different from so-called "sporadic" cases. Certainly the HLA characteristics of probands from families with one affected child do not show any significant differences from the probands of multiplex families (Cudworth and Walker, 1980), nor is there any difference in age of onset (Gamble, 1980). However, as elegantly demonstrated by Gamble (1980) there is a significantly shorter discordance time in the development of Type I diabetes in sib pairs compared with the calculated expected discordance interval. In 26% of a large number of pairs analyzed the discordance time was less than 12 months and less than 6 months in 18% of pairs. This observation underlines the importance of a possible simultaneous environmental factor initiating the disease in susceptible siblings.

In the 5% of sib pairs who are HLA A,B,C nonidentical, we have not found any evidence that these families differ in any way genetically or immunologically from the majority, although information on *DR* genotypes in multiplex families is relatively limited.

Rubinstein *et al.* (1976) reported an increased rate of recombination (16%) in diabetic families, but this could not be confirmed in combined data from Denmark and the United Kingdom (Platz *et al.*, 1978). A group in Australia also reported an increased recombination rate of 16% in Type I diabetic families (Dornan *et al.*, 1979). In our own family study we found an A–C recombination frequency of 1.9% based on 214 informative meioses and a B–DR recombination rate of 1.9% based on 210 informative meioses. All meioses which could have had hidden recombinations due to homozygosity at one of the loci had been excluded.

IV. POSSIBLE EVIDENCE FOR NON-HLA SUSCEPTIBILITY

Whereas undoubtedly the major genetic susceptibility is controlled by a gene or genes in the *HLA* chromosomal region, part of the underlying predisposition may be determined by genes at loci on different chromosomes. Thomson (1980) has put forward a good argument for the existence of a two-locus effect in order to explain the results observed in Type I diabetes.

Red cell glyoxalase 1 (GLO) is coded for by a locus with two alleles located on chromosome 6 near the centromere approximately 5 centimorgans from the HLA *D/DR* region and is linked to HLA. There seems to be no association between the three GLO phenotypes (GLO1-1, GLO2-1, and GLO2-2) and Type I diabetes (Kirk *et al.*, 1979a; Moens *et al.*, 1980; DeMouzen-Cambon *et al.*, 1982) even though McCann *et al.* (1981), reported an increase in GLO1-1 in 28 Type I diabetic patients. Linkage between GLO and Type I diabetes measured by lod scores was found (Hodge *et al.*, 1981).

Vague *et al.* (1978) reported an increased Lewis-negative (Lea-, b-) phenotype in both Type I and Type II diabetic subjects and this was cited as a possible example for a non-HLA-linked effect. In contrast no disturbance in the frequences of the Lewis phenotypes was observed in diabetic identical twins (Leslie and Pyke, 1979).

More recently, two better possibilities have emerged. It was shown by Bodansky *et al.* (1981) that there is a significant association of the fast acetylator phenotype with Type I diabetes ($r = 2.0$) based on a combination of data from three studies in northern European Caucasoids. Similar results have also been found in a study from Australia (Shenfield *et al.*, 1982). The site of the locus controlling the acetylator dimorphism is not known.

A third possible example of a non-HLA effect is provided by the finding of linkage measured by lod scores with the Kidd blood group system (JK) (Hodge *et al.*, 1981). No allelic association with the Kidd blood group was found in the 41 diabetic families who gave a positive lod score for Kidd and the distribution of positive and negative lod scores found in these families was independent of HLA. Barbosa *et al.* (1982) found an excess of the JKb allele with a relative risk of 1.5. The Kidd blood group system is located on chromosome 2 and it is of interest that the locus coding for the light chain of the immunoglobulin (*Km*) is next to it.

Also, the genes coding for the heavy chain of the immunoglobulin (*Gm*), which are not linked to the HLA system and are situated on chromosome 14, have been implicated in Type I diabetes. Nakao *et al.* (1981), found that the *Gm* phenotype 1,2,13,15,16,21 was increased in Japanese Type I diabetic patients with antiinsulin antibodies whereas Type I diabetic patients without antiinsulin antibodies had a normal distribution of *Gm* phenotypes. The *Gm* system is very polymorphic and like the HLA system it is a good anthropological marker as the phenotypes varies in different populations. Therefore, correlation with the Japanese data is difficult. In our own data there is a slight excess of the *Gm* haplotype 3,5,10 and a higher rate of homozygosity for this haplotype in Type I diabetics. We could not find a correlation with antiinsulin antibodies.

V. GENETIC HETEROGENEITY

Evidence for genetic heterogeneity in Type I diabetes is seen in relation to the distribution of organ specific autoantibodies in the healthy siblings of Type I diabetic probands. Thus, it has been shown that the distribution of these antibodies is quite independent of the inherited susceptibility to the disease (Gorsuch *et al.*, 1980; MacLaren, personal communication). A similar pattern was observed in relation to conventional islet cell antibody (ICA). This implies that there is a separate genetic control of autoantibody production in Type I diabetic families. In contrast, complement-fixing islet cell antibodies (CF-ICA) have so far only been found in HLA-identical or HLA-haploidentical healthy siblings. Since the beginning of our Barts-Windsor prospective family study 4 years ago, no one developed complement-fixing islet cell antibodies. It is of interest that all diabetic probands, healthy parents, and siblings who have complement-fixing islet cell antibodies already had them at entry to the study and although only 29 were tested they all carried the *Gm* haplotype *3,5.10*. If autoantibodies play a role in the pathogenesis of Type I diabetes then they might provide evidence for the existence of genetic heterogeneity in Type I diabetes, but for now it is reasonable to invoke only the simplest models compatible with the observations.

Perhaps one of the more clear-cut examples of heterogeneity in Type I diabetes is the characterization of a relatively small subgroup of patients who appear to have a more primary autoimmune form of the disease (Type IB). The majority of cases of Type I diabetes (Type IA) present in childhood or adolescence and there is a slight male preponderance (12–20%) in this group. In contrast, a number of cases (perhaps 10–20%) of Type I diabetics present in later life, often with a more insidious onset, in whom there is a strong female preponderance, a strong family history of autoimmune endocrinopathy, and a higher prevalence of organ-specific autoantibodies. These patients often have persistence of ICA whereas in the vast majority of Type IA diabetics both conventional and complement-fixing ICA tend to disappear very rapidly after diagnosis. Persistence of ICA, after 5 years of Type IA diabetes is also associated with many of the features described for typical IB diabetes, suggesting that these subjects are potential autoimmune polyendocrine patients (Bottazzo *et al.*, 1978). Addison's disease and autoimmune thyroid disease are the two most common conditions to be seen in association with Type I diabetes. In patients with coexistent Type I diabetes and Graves' disease and patients with coexistent Type I diabetes and primary myxedema the relative risk for B8 was found to be more than additive compared with the relative risk found for each disease considered independently. This suggests that separate HLA-linked immune response genes control the susceptibility to these different diseases. As might be expected they also show a stronger association with B8 and DR3 (Farid and Bear, 1981; Cudworth and Wolf, 1982). However, not all combinations of Type I diabetes with other autoimmune endocrinopathies show a consistent pattern of association with the HLA system, particularly subjects with coexistent Type I diabetes and pernicious anaemia (Doniach *et al.*, 1982).

Type I diabetes also occurs sometimes in association with nonendocrine autoimmune conditions such as myasthenia gravis, celiac disease, and systemic lupus erythematosus. These are not frequent problems and whether or not they coexist more frequently than might be expected remains to be confirmed. The possible coexistence of Type I diabetes with coeliac disease is of interest, although DR3 is the major association in both diseases, there is also an increase in the frequency of DR7 particularly in younger onset cases with celiac disease. In contrast we have found a signficant reduction of DR7 in our juvenile-onset Type I diabetic probands. We have studied a small group (16) of patients with coexistent Type I diabetes and celiac disease; many of these patients were female and had a late age of onset for both diabetes and the celiac disease, which suggested that in some cases the enteropathy might have a primary autoimmune basis.

The best validated example of an association with a nonendocrine autoimmune disorder is with rheumatoid arthritis (Thomas *et al.*, 1982). Approximately 12% of Type I diabetics have a close relative with rheumatoid arthritis, and a similar proportion of patients with well-characterized rheumatoid disease have a first- or second-degree relative with Type I diabetes. No familial aggregation was found with Type II diabetes and no increased frequency of Type I diabetes in the close relatives of patients with osteoarthritis was found. The association of Type I diabetes and rheumatoid arthritis is of potential interest because DW4-DR4, which is part of the major HLA association with Type I diabetes, is also the major HLA susceptibility factor in patients with rheumatoid arthritis. Thus, one possible implication is that there is a common immune response mechanism determined by a gene in linkage disequilibrium with DR4 which plays a major role in influencing immune-mediated damage in two entirely different tissues.

Many attempts to identify genetic heterogeneity have been made, mainly by trying to relate some clinical or immunological aspect of the disease with B8 and BW62 or DR3 and DR4, respectively (Rotter and Rimoin, 1978). This has often been based on conflicting data leading to unclear conclusions. An important point to be considered is that, where a strong association between the underlying disease and a particular HLA antigen already exists, it is statistically difficult to show an "extra" significant association with that particular antigen and some secondary aspect of the disease, unless very large numbers of well-characterized patients are compared with a similar number of subjects who are identical in all respects except for the particular issue under scrutiny. Another important factor is that some clinical features of the disease such as season of onset, acuteness of presentation, and similar phenomena are very imprecise and difficult to identify in order to make a meaningful analysis. In the light of these difficulties it is perhaps not too surprising that there is lack of agreement in relation to the question of HLA genetic heterogeneity. There does appear to be uniformity of opinion concerning the association of B8 with a low or absent antibody response to insulin (see Cudworth and Bodansky, 1982, who combined the available data on this issue).

In contrast, the possible association of HLA factors with age of onset and the presence or absence of specific diabetic complications remains unsolved. With regard to age of onset, DR4 may be associated with a younger age of onset, based on accumulated data from the 8th International Histocompatibility Workshop (Svejgaard *et al.*, 1980). We have not been able to confirm this in our own studies except there was a higher frequency of DR3, DR4 heterozygous diabetics with an age of onset less than 10 years (Cudworth *et al.*, 1981).

The question of a possible HLA influence on the development of certain diabetic complications is even less clear. Initially, it was argued that there may be an association with either B8 or BW62 and proliferative retinopathy (for review see Cudworth and Bodansky, 1982). Further controversy now exists concerning the possible association of DR4 with microvascular disease. An increase of DR4 with proliferative retinopathy has been reported by Bertrams *et al.* (1980), Schernthaner (1980), and Dornan *et al.* (1982), but disputed by others (Bodansky *et al.*, 1982).

No significant difference of A,B,C, DR antigens and Bf factors has been found in Type I diabetic patients with nephropathy (Walton *et al.*, 1981), although one report

(Christy *et al.*, 1981) indicated that there was a decrease in DR3,DR4 heterozygosity in a small group of patients with diabetic nephropathy. These findings will need to be confirmed. In collaboration with Drs. Ward and Boulton in Sheffield, England, we have done A,B,C and DR typing in a small group of Type I diabetic patients with well-characterized diabetic neuropathy. No additional increase of any HLA antigens was found. It can probably be safely concluded that if the HLA system does play any role in the etiopathogenesis of complications or determining age of onset of Type I diabetes, this effect is relatively minor and perhaps unimportant.

VI. COMPLEMENT FACTORS

Complement is a complex system of different proteins, the many components of which react in sequence usually after stimulation by antigen–antibody complexes and play an important role in inflammation and clearance of foreign substances. Genes coding for the complement factors Bf,C2, and C4 are situated in the HLA complex between the HLA *B* and *D* locus and these complement factors are in linkage disequilibrium with certain HLA antigens. No recombination has yet been reported between these four different complement loci (*Bf, C2, C4A, C4B*). *Bf, C2,* and *C4* are all C3 convertase in the active state.

A. Bf

Four main allelic products can be identified of properdin factor B(Bf) of the alternative complement pathway by immunofixation electrophoresis: two common alleles (*BfS* and *BfF*) and two less common variants *BfF1* and *BfS1*. Seven additional rare variants have also been identified. All these *Bf* variants have equal functional activity and no individual with homozygous *Bf* deficiency has yet been found and only very few subjects with partial factor B deficiency have been described (for review see Rittner and Bertrams, 1981).

In 1977 Cudworth *et al.* described a significant increase of *BfS* in Type I diabetics. *BfF1* was not tested in this study. This was confirmed by Budowle *et al.* (1982) in American Caucasoid Type I diabetic patients, but has not been found in all the studies mentioned below. In a recent analysis of 75 diabetic probands genotyped for HLA *A,B,C,* and *Bf,* all *B8*-positive haplotypes, 94% of the *BW62*-positive, and 25% of the *B18*-positive, *CW5* negative haplotypes were *BfS*-positive (Wolf *et al.*, 1982b).

Most studies of the Bf system in Type I diabetes have focused on the rare allele *BfF1,* which was found to be significantly increased in Type I diabetics (Raum *et al.*, 1979; Bertrams *et al.*, 1979a). This has been confirmed in reports from Australia (Kirk *et al.*, 1979a), France (Deschamps *et al.*, 1979), and Canada (Dornan *et al.*, 1980; Walsh *et al.*, 1982). It has also been suggested that *BfF1* may be associated with a younger age of onset (Kirk *et al.*, 1979b; Barbosa *et al.*, 1979; Bertrams *et al.*, 1979b) although this has been disputed (Wolf *et al.*, 1982; Walsh *et al.*, 1982). *BfF1* is in strong linkage disequilibrium with several HLA antigens and forms part of the haplotype *AW30-CW5-B18-BfF1-DR3,* which is particularly frequent in southern Europe (DeMouzon *et al.*, 1979) and in ethnic groups who have migrated from this area. The strength of the linkage disequilibrium between B18 and *BfFl* is greater in Type I diabetic subjects than in healthy controls (Raum *et al.*, 1979; Bertrams *et al.*, 1979b).

A significant decrease in *BfF* and a significant increase in a newly described variant *BfFl* was found in Japanese Type I diabetics (Tokunaga *et al.*, 1981) and also in American black Type I diabetic patients (Budowle *et al.*, 1982) in whom *BfFl* and *BfSl* were significantly increased. It is interesting to note that Suciu-Foca *et al.* (1980) found evidence for the existence of a possible *Bf* 'null' allele in a Type 1 diabetic with a maternal *B-D* crossing over.

B. C2

There are three variants in the *C2* system which are detected by isoelectric focusing with subsequent complement-dependent lysis in a *C2*-deficient overlay. $C2C\ (C2^1)$ is the most common allele, $C2B\ (C2^2)$ is rare, and $C2A\ (C2^3)$ is extremely rare. About 95% of European people are *C2C*-positive, about 5% are heterozygous for *C2BC*, and only 0.2% are homozygous for *C2B*. There might also be silent genes at this locus and there is some circumstantial evidence that the *C2B* allelic product may be functionally less efficient (Alper, 1976). Even though *C2* deficiency is the most common deficiency within the complement system, the frequency for $C2^0$ gene (null allele) might be less than 0.001 (Lachmann and Hobart, 1978). The $C2^0$ gene is almost exclusively associated with the rare HLA haplotype *A25-CWX-B18-DR2* and *C2*-deficient individuals are homozygous for this haplotype.

C2B is in linkage disequilibrium with BW62, CW3, BfS, and DR4, an antigen combination which is increased in Type I diabetes. Bertrams *et al.* (1980), reported an increased incidence of the rare *C2* allele *C2B* in Type I diabetic patients with severe proliferative retinopathy. This was not confirmed in other studies (Bodansky *et al.*, 1982).

In our own study (Wolf *et al.*, 1981b) of 112 Type I diabetic probands, *C2B* was only found in 12 patients, seven of whom were also positive for BW62 and CW3, whereas five were negative for these two antigens. There was no association between *C2* alleles in Japanese Type I diabetics (Tokonuga *et al.*, 1981) and there are no data available in black populations.

C. C4

Two closely linked *C4* loci—*C4A(F)* and *C4B(S)* —code for the most polymorphic of the complement factors and are detected by immunofixation electrophoresis. The nomenclature of the *C4* system is very confusing as different authors use different symbols for *C4* pheno- and genotypes. There are at least 10 alleles at the *C4A* locus and 15 at the *C4B* locus and a high proportion of "silent" alleles ($C4*AQO$ = f^0 and $C4*BQO$ = S^0) have to be assumed at each locus, which might be responsible for partial *C4* deficiency. Only four patients with complete *C4* deficiency have been described (for review see Rittner and Bertrams, 1981).

Evidence for an association of the *C4* system with Type I diabetes was reported by Lamm *et al.* 1980 in 64 Type I diabetics from Denmark. The relative risk for *C4Bl*(S)* was 3.1 and for *C4*B4+B5(g)* was 5.5. The rare allele *C4*B4* was found with a frequency of 26% and *C4*B2* with a frequency of 22% in Type I diabetics (Bertrams *et al.*, 1982). In our series of 24 Type I probands genotyped for HLA *A,B,C,DR,* and *C4,* the haplotype *C4*AQO* was increased and was found to be in linkage disequilibrium with *B8* and *DR3. BW62* was associated with *C4*B3,B4* and *B5. B18* was in linkage disequilibrium with *C4*BQO,* which has been previously reported in Basques (DeMouzon *et al.*, 1979), where *C4*BQO* was found in 75% of Type I diabetics compared to 36% in controls. In Basque Type I diabetic patients, the silent allele was particularly frequent in those diabetics with an onset of the disease under the age of 20 years (r=4.9) (DeMouzon-Cambon *et al.*, 1982). It is of interest that the only *C4* variant *C4*A6* which has been found to be functionally inactive (Teisberg *et al.*, 1980) does not seem to be associated with Type I diabetes. In our own study and in the Basques (DeMouzon-Cambon *et al.*, 1982), the haplotype *A1,CW6,BW57, BfS,C4*A6B1,DR7* has never been found in a Type I diabetic even though in our study this haplotype was found with a frequency of 3% in 211 "healthy" parental haplotypes.

Since *C4* is known to be important in neutralizing viruses (Daniels *et al.*, 1969; Leddy *et al.*, 1977) it would be of great interest to determine whether or not plasma levels of *C4* are related to particular *C4* haplotypes. So far in our own study we found that 39% of diabetic probands and their first-degree relatives, who inherited two silent alleles, showed low levels of *C4.* The up-to-date pattern of HLA and complement haplotypes important in Type I diabetes is shown in Fig. 2.

In summary, it is interesting to note that Type I diabetes is associated most strongly with the rare alleles of the complement loci *Bf* and *C2.* If those *C4* haplotypes, which carry silent alleles, really lead to partial *C4* deficiency and if they could be shown to be increased in Type I diabetes, then this might be important in the pathogenesis of the disease as suggested by Hauptman (1980).

VII. CONCLUSIONS

The genetic basis of Type I (insulin-dependent) diabetes is quite different from the underlying predisposition to Type II (non-insulin-dependent) diabetes. Whereas very little is known about the genetic factors and mechanisms involved in the etiology of Type II diabetes, it is now firmly established that the major susceptibility to Type I diabetes is determined by a gene or genes operating at a locus or loci in the HLA chromosomal region. Population studies indicate that the primary association is with HLA *DR3* and *DR4* and that all the reported increases in antigens encoded by genes at the other HLA loci, and also the associations with certain complement factors, are purely secondary because of linkage disequilibrium within the HLA system. Nearly 98% of Type I diabetics possess either HLA DR3 or DR4, or both of these antigens. The high frequency of DR3,DR4 heterozygotes and the lack of an increase in homozygosity for these antigens strongly supports the concept that there are two separate disease susceptibility genes acting synergistically.

Studies of families with two or more affected siblings show a marked disturbance in the zygotic assortment of HLA haplotypes compared with the expected distribution.

These data provide conclusive evidence that the putative susceptibility genes are linked to the HLA complex and probably are situated in or near the *D/DR* region. However, the exact mode of inheritance of these genes remains unresolved. Although there can be little argument that the major genetic predisposition is HLA-linked, other genetic factors outside the *HLA* region may also be contributing to the overall susceptibility.

Late-onset Type IA diabetic patients possess the same immunogenetic characteristics as those seen in classic juvenile-onset cases. Some 10–15% of Type I diabetics tend to show many characteristics suggestive of a more primary autoimmune form of disease, including a striking female preponderance, a strong family history of autoimmune endocrine disease, and a high prevalence of organ-specific autoantibodies (Type IB).

The evidence for HLA genetic heterogeneity in relation to different aspects of Type I diabetes, such as microvascular complications and insulin immunogenicity, remains controversial. The mode of action of the HLA-linked genes is quite unknown. The very strong association of HLA DR3 and DR4 with Type I diabetes could be compatible with the idea that these DR antigens are themselves involved in initiating the immune-mediated destruction of the pancreatic islet B cells. A speculative view of the possible sequence of events is shown in Fig. 3. Viral interaction with a specific membrane receptor resulting in neoantigen formation evoking an immune response involving the HLA "supergene" and both humoral and cell-mediated immune mechanisms seems likely.

ACKNOWLEDGMENTS.   We would like to acknowledge Drs. A. N. Gorsuch and K. M. Spencer for the excellent field work in the Barts-Windsor family study and Dr. J. Lister for permission to investigate these families. We would also like to thank Drs. C.

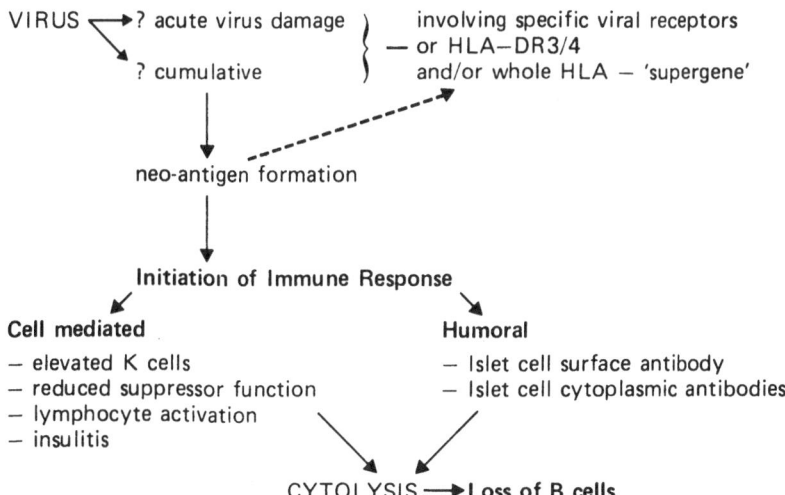

Figure 3.   A speculative view of the sequence of pathologic events involved in the destruction of the pancreatic islet B cells.

Johnston and D. A. Pyke (Kings College Hospital) for allowing us to quote the results obtained from our collaborative studies in identical twins, and also Drs. A. Boulton and J. D. Ward (Royal Hallamshire Hospital, Sheffield) for allowing us to study their patients with diabetic neuropathy. We would also like to express our thanks to Dr. G. F. Bottazzo and Professor Deborah Doniach for their support and close collaboration. Valuable technical assistance has been provided by Dr. B. Dean and Miss J. V. McNally regarding the autoantibody studies, Miss V. Drummond, Miss M. van Dam, Miss B. Watson, and Miss V. Algar for the HLA typing, and Miss P. Matharu for secretarial assistance.

This work has been financially supported by the Medical Research Council, the British Diabetic Association, the Juvenile Diabetes Foundation, and The Joint Research Board of St. Bartholomew's Hospital.

REFERENCES

Alper, C. A., 1976, Inherited structural polymorphism in human C2. Evidence for genetic linkage between C2 and Bf, *J. Exp. Med.* **144:**1111–1115.

Asmal, A. C., Dayal, B., Jialal, I., Leary, W. P., Omar, M. A. K., Pillay, N. L., and Thandroyen, F. T., 1981, Non-insulin dependent diabetes mellitus with early onset in Blacks and Indians, *S. Afr. Med. J.* **60:**93–96.

Barbosa, J., Weitkamp, L., Guttormsen, S., Johnson, S., and Szalapski, E., Jr., 1979, BF in early-onset insulin-dependent diabetes, *Lancet* **2:**1239–1240.

Barbosa, J., Rich, S. S., Dunsworth, T., and Swanson, J., 1982, Linkage disequilibrium between insulin-dependent diabetes and the Kidd blood group JKb allele, *J. Clin. Endocrinol. Metab.,* in press.

Barnett, A. H., Eff, C., Leslie, R. D. G., and Pyke, D. A., 1981, Diabetes in identical twins. A study of 200 pairs, *Diabetologia* **20:**87–93.

Bertrams, J., Baur, M. P., Gruneklee, D., and Gries, F. A., 1979a, Association of BfF1, HLA-B18 and insulin-dependent diabetes mellitus, *Lancet* **2:**98.

Bertrans, J., Sodomann, P., Gruneklee, D., and Gries, F. A., 1979b, Bf in early-onset insulin-dependent diabetes, *Lancet* **2:**1240.

Bertrans, J., Hintzen, U., Schlicht, V., and Schoeps, S., 1982, C4: Another marker for Type 1 diabetes, *Lancet* **1:**41.

Bertrams, J., Dewald, G., Spitznas, M., and Rittner, C., 1980, HLA-A,B,C, DR, Bf and C2 alleles in insulin-dependent diabetes mellitus with proliferative retinopathy, *Immunobiology* **158:**113–118.

Bloom, A., Hayes, T., and Gamble, D. R., 1975, Register of newly diagnosed diabetic children, *Br. Med. J.* **3:**580–583.

Bodansky, H. J., Drury, P. L., Cudworth, A. G., and Price Evans, D. A., 1981, Acetylator phenotypes in Type 1 (insulin-dependent) diabetics with microvascular disease, *Diabetes* **30:**907–910.

Bodansky, H. J., Wolf, E., Cudworth, A. G., Dean, B. M., Nineham, L. J., Bottazzo, G. F., Matthews, J. A., Kurtz, A. B., and Kohner, E. M., 1982, Genetic and immunologic factors in microvascular disease in Type 1 insulin-dependent diabetes, *Diabetes* **31:**70–74.

Bottazzo, G. F., Cudworth, A. G., Moul, D. J., Doniach, D., and Festenstein, H., 1978, Evidence for a primary autoimmune type of diabetes mellitus (Type Ib), *Br. Med. J.* **2:**1253–1255.

Briggs, B. R., Botha, M. C., Jackson, W. P. U., and DuToit, E. D., 1980, The histocompatibility (HLA) antigen distribution in South African Blacks (Xhosa), *Diabetes* **29:**68–70.

Budowle, B., Reitnauer, P. J., Barger, B. O., Go, R. C. P., Roseman, J. M., and Acton, R. T., 1982, Properdin factor B in Black Type 1 (insulin-dependent) diabetic patients, *Diabetologia* **22:**483–485.

Christau, B., Kromann, H., Ortved Andersen, O., Christy, M., Buschard, K., Arnung, K., Hojland Kristensen, I., Peitersen, B., Steinrud, J., and Nerup, J., 1977, Incidence, seasonal and geographical patterns of juvenile-onset insulin-dependent diabetes mellitus in Denmark, *Diabetologia* **13:**281–284.

Christy, M., Andersen, A., Parving, H. H., Nerup, J., Platz, P., Ryder, L., Thomsen, M., Morling, N., and Svejgaard, A., 1981, Genetics of late diabetic complications—HLA D/DR and diabetic nephropathy, *Diabetologia* **21**:82 (abstract).

Clarke, C. A., 1966, Genetic aspects of diabetes, in: *Diabetes Mellitus* (L. J. P. Duncan, ed.), pp. 104–113, Pfizer Medical Monographs.

Cudworth, A. G., 1978, Type 1 diabetes mellitus, *Diabetologia* **14**:281–291.

Cudworth, A. G., 1981, Types of diabetes and their pathogenesis, in: *Carbohydrate Metabolism and its Disorders*, (P. J. Randle, D. F. Steiner, and W. J. Whelan, eds.) pp. 229–277, Academic Press, London.

Cudworth, A. G., and Bodansky, J. H., 1982, Genetic and immunological factors in relation to the prevalence and severity of diabetic complications, in: *Complications of Diabetes*, 2nd edition (H. Keen and J. Jarrett, eds.), pp. 1–12, Year Book Medical, Chicago.

Cudworth, A. G., and Wolf, E., 1982, The genetic susceptibility to Type 1 (insulin-dependent) diabetes mellitus, in: *Clinics in Endocrinology and Metabolism*, vol. 11, No. 2, *New Aspects of Diabetes* (K. G. M. M. Alberti, ed.), pp. 389–408, Saunders, Eastbourne, Sussex.

Cudworth, A. G., and Woodrow, J. C., 1975, HL-A system and diabetes mellitus, *Diabetes* **24**:345–349.

Cudworth, A. G., and Woodrow, J. C., 1976, Genetic susceptibility in diabetes mellitus: analysis of the HLA association, *Br. Med. J.* **2**:846–848.

Cudworth, A. G., Usher, N., and Woodrow, J. C., 1977, Factor B phenotypes in "juvenile onset" diabetes, *Diabetologia* **13**:388 (abstract).

Cudworth, A. G., Wolf, E., Spencer, K. M., Bodansky, H. J., Watson, B., Drummond, V., and Algar, V., 1981, The vital role of B lymphocyte alloantigens in determining susceptibility to Type 1 (insulin-dependent) diabetes, *Diabetologia* **21**:506 (abstract).

Daniels, C. A., Boros, T., Rapp, H. J., Snydermann, R., and Notkins, A. L., 1969, Neutralization of sensitized virus by fourth component of complement, *Science* **165**:508–509.

DeMouzon, A., Ohayon, E., Ducos, J., and Hauptmann, G., 1979, Bf and C4 markers for insulin-dependent diabetes mellitus in Basques, *Lancet* **2**:1364.

DeMouzon-Cambon, A., Ohayon, E., Hauptmann, G., Sevin, A., Abbal, M., Sommer, E., Vergnes, H., and Ducos, J., 1982, HLA-A,B,C, DR antigens, Bf, C4 and glyoxalase 1 (GLO) polymorphisms in French Basques with insulin-dependent diabetes mellitus (IDDM), *Tissue Antigens* **19**:366–379.

Dengbol, B., and Green, A., 1978, Diabetes mellitus among first- and second-degree relatives of early onset diabetics, *Ann. Hum. Genet.* **42**:25–47.

Deschamps, I., Lestradet, H., Marcelli-Barge, A., Benajam, A., Busson, M., and Dausset, J., 1979, Properdin factor B-alleles as markers for insulin-dependent diabetes, *Lancet* **2**:793.

Deschamps, I., Lestradet, H., Bonaiti, C., Schmid, M., Busson, M., Benajam, A., Marcelli-Barge, A., and Hors, J., 1980, HLA genotype studies in juvenile insulin-dependent diabetes, *Diabetologia* **19**:189–193.

Doniach, D., Cudworth, A. G., Khoury, E. L., and Bottazzo, G. F., 1982, Autoimmunity and the HLA-system in endocrine disease, in: *Recent Advances in Endocrinology and Metabolism*, vol. 2 (J. L. H. O'Riordan, ed.), pp. 99–132, Churchill Livingstone, Edinburgh.

Dornan, T. D., Bashir, H. V., and Moffitt, P., 1979, First Asia Oceania Histocompatibility Workshop (abstract).

Dornan, J., Allan, P., Noel, E. P., Larsen, B., and Farid, N. R., 1980, Properdin factor B(Bf) allele BfF1 specifies an HLA-B18 diabetogenic haplotype, *Diabetes* **29**:423–427.

Dornan, T. L., Ting, A., McPherson, C. K., Peckar, C. O., Mann, J. I., Turner, R. C., and Morris, P. J., 1982, Genetic susceptibiltiy to the development of retinopathy in insulin-dependent diabetics, *Diabetes* **31**:226–231.

Farid, N. R., and Bear, J. C., 1981, The human major histocompatibility complex and endocrine disease, *Endocr. Rev.* **2**:50–86.

Gamble, D. R., 1980, An epidemiological study of childhood diabetes affecting two or more siblings, *Diabetologia* **19**:341–344.

Gorsuch, A. N., Dean, B. M., Bottazzo, G. F., Listen, J., and Cudworth, A. G., 1980, Evidence that Type 1 diabetes and thyrogastric autoimmunity have different genetic determinants, *Br. Med. J.* **280**:145–147.

Gorsuch, A. N., Spencer, K. M., Lister, J., McNally, J. M., Dean, B. M., Bottazzo, G. F., and Cudworth, A. G., 1981, Evidence for a long prediabetic period in Type 1 (insulin-dependent) diabetes mellitus, *Lancet* 2:1363–1365.

Gorsuch, A. N., Spencer, K. M., Lister, J., Wolf, E., Bottazzo, G. F., and Cudworth, A. G., 1982a, Can future Type 1 diabetes be predicted: A study in families of affected children, *Diabetes* 31:862–866.

Gorsuch, A. N., Spencer, K. M., Wolf, E., and Cudworth, A. G., 1982b, HLA and family studies, in: *The Genetics of Diabetes Mellitus*, 2nd edition (J. Kobberling and R. B. Tattersall, eds.), pp. 42–53, Academic Press, London.

Hauptmann, G., 1980, C4 deficiency in early-onset insulin-dependent diabetes: A hypothesis, *Lancet* 1:1034.

Hodge, S. E., Anderson, C. E., Neiswanger, K., Field, L. L., Spence, M. A., Sparkes, R. S., Sparkes, M. C., Crist, M., Terasaki, P. I., Rimoin, D. L., and Rotter, J. I., 1981, Close genetic linkage between diabetes mellitus and Kidd blood group, *Lancet* 2:893–895.

Johnston, C., Pyke, D. A., Cudworth, A. G., and Wolf, E., 1982, Does the development of Type 1 (insulin-dependent) diabetes depend upon one or two alleles? Studies of HLA-DR3 and DR4 in identical twins, *Diabetologia* 22:388 (abstract).

Kirk, R. L., Rheophilus, J., Whitehouse, S., Court, J., and Zimmet, P., 1979a, Genetic susceptibility to diabetes mellitus: The distribution of properdin factor B (Bf) and glyoxylase (GLO) phenotypes, *Diabetes* 28:949–951.

Kirk, R. L., Serjeantson, S. W., Theophilus, J., Zimmet, P., Whitehouse, S., and Court, J. M., 1979b, Age relationship between insulin-dependent diabetes and rare alleles of properdin factor B, *Lancet* 2:537.

Köbberling, J., Bengsch, N., Bruggeboes, B., Schwarch, K., Tillil, H., and Weber, B., 1980, The chlorpropamide alcohol flush, *Diabetologia* 19:359–363.

Lachmann, P. J., and Hobart, M. J., 1978, Complement genetics in relation to HLA, *Br. Med. Bull.* 34:247–252.

Lamm, L. U., Buskjaer, L., Petersen, G. B., Hauge, M., and Svejgaard, A., 1980, Complement C2 and C4 and factor B allotypes in insulin dependent diabetes (IDD), in Denmark VIIIth International Histocompatibility Conference, Los Angeles (abstract).

Leddy, J. P., Simons, R. L., and Douglas, R. G., 1977, Effect of selective complement deficiency on the rate of neutralization of enveloped viruses by human sera, *J. Immunol.* 118:28–34.

Leslie, R. D. G., and Pyke, D. A., 1978, Chlorpropamide alcohol flushing: A dominant inherited trait associated with diabetes, *Br. Med. J.* 2:1519–1521.

Leslie, R. D. G., and Pyke, D. A., 1979, Letter to the Editor, *Diabetologia* 16:139.

Maeda, H., Takeuchi, F., Juji, T., Akanuma, Y., Kasuga, M., Lee, Y. S., Kosaka, K., and Tsai, S. H., 1980, HLA-DRW3 in juvenile onset diabetes mellitus in Chinese, *Tissue Antigens* 15:173–176.

McCann, V. J., Davis, R. E., Welborn, T. A., Constable, I. J., and Beale, D. G., 1981, Glyoxalase phenotypes in patients with diabetes mellitus, *Aust. N. Z. J. Med.* 11:380–382.

Moens, H., Payne, R., Carter, N. D., and Farid, N. R., 1980, Association of glyoxalase 1 allotypes with Graves' disease and diabetes mellitus, *Hum. Hered.* 30:62–64.

Nakao, Y., Matsumoto, H., Miyazaaki, T., Mizuno, N., Arima, N., Wakisaki, A., Okimoto, K., Akazaway, Tsuji, K., and Fugita, T., 1981, IgG heavy-chain (Gm) allotypes and immune response to insulin in insulin-requiring diabetes mellitus, *N. Engl. J. Med.* 304:407–409.

Neel, J. V., 1976, Diabetes mellitus: A geneticist's nightmare, in: *The Genetics of Diabetes Mellitus*, (W. Creutzfeldt, J. Köbberling, and J. V. Neel, eds.), pp. 1–11, Springer-Verlag, Berlin.

Nerup, J., Platz, P., Anderson, O. O., Christy, M., Lyngsoe, J., Poulsen, J. E., Ryder, L. P., Staub-Neilsen, L., Thomsen, M., and Svejgaard, A., 1974, HLA- antigens and diabetes mellitus, *Lancet* 2:864–866.

Owerbach, D., and Nerup, J., 1982, Restriction fragment length polymorphism of the insulin gene in diabetes mellitus, *Diabetes* 31:275–277.

Patterson, C. C., Smith, P. G., Mann, J. I., Thorogood, M., Heasman, M. A., and Clarke, J. A., 1981, Distribution of juvenile-onset diabetes cases in Scotland (1968–1976), *Diabetologia* 20:673 (abstract).

Pincus, G., and White, P., 1933, On the inheritance of diabetes mellitus. I. An analysis of 675 family histories, *Am. J. Med. Sci.* 186:1–19.

Platz, P., Thomsen, M., Svejgaard, A., Cudworth, A. G., Woodrow, J. C., and Nerup, J., 1978, More on genetics of diabetes mellitus, *N. Engl. J. Med.* **298**:1200–1201.

Platz, P., Jacobsen, B. K., Morling, N., Ryder, L. P., Svejgaard, A., Thomsen, M., Christy, M., Kromann, H., Benn, J., Nerup, J., Green, A., and Hauge, M., 1981, HLA-D and -DR antigens in genetic analysis of insulin dependent diabetes mellitus, *Diabetologia* **21**:108–115.

Raum, D., Alper, C. A., Stein, R., and Gabbay, K. H., 1979, Genetic markers for insulin-dependent diabetes mellitus, *Lancet* **1**:1208–1210.

Rittner, C., and Bertrams, J., 1981, On the significance of C2, C4 and factor B polymorphisms in disease, *Hum. Genet.* **56**:235–247.

Rodney, G. E., White, N., Frazer, T. E., Duquesnoy, R. J., and Santiage, J. V., 1979, HLA-DR specificities among black Americans with juvenile-onset diabetes, *N. Engl. J. Med.* **301**:810–812.

Rotter, J. I., and Rimoin, D. L., 1978, Heterogeneity in diabetes mellitus—update, 1978: Evidence for further genetic heterogeneity within juvenile-onset insulin-dependent diabetes mellitus, *Diabetes* **27**:599–608.

Rotter, J. I., and Rimoin, D. L., 1979, Diabetes mellitus: The search for genetic markers, *Diabetes Care* **2**:215–266.

Rubinstein, P., Suciu-Foca, N., Nicholson, J. F., Fotino, M., Molinaro, A., Harisiadis, L., Hardy, M. A., Reemtsma, K., and Allen, F. H., Jr., 1976, The HLA system in the families of patients with juvenile diabetes mellitus, *J. Exp. Med.* **143**:1277–1282.

Rubinstein, P., Ginsberg-Fellner, F., and Falk, C., 1981, Genetics of type 1 diabetes mellitus: A single, recessive predisposition gene mapping between HLA-B and GLO, *Am. J. Hum. Genet.* **33**:895–882.

Ryder, L. P., Andersen, E., and Svejgaard, A., 1979, *HLA and Disease Registry, Third Report*, Munskgaard, Copenhagen.

Schernthaner, G., 1980, Neue Aspekte in der Pathogenese und im Krankheitsverlauf des Typ-1-Diabetes Mellitus, *Wien. Klin. Wochenschr.* **114**(Suppl.):1–36.

Seignalet, J., Mirouze, J., Jaffiol, G., Selam, J. L., and Lapinski, H., 1975, HLA in Graves' disease and in diabetes mellitus, *Tissue Antigens* **6**:272–274.

Serjeantson, S. W., Ryan, D. P., Ram, P., and Zimmet, P., 1981, HLA and non-insulin dependent diabetes in Fiji Indians, *Med. J. Aust.* **1**:462–463.

Shaw, S., Kavathas, P., Pollack, M. S., Charmot, D., and Mawas, C., 1981, Family studies define a new histocompatibility locus, SB, between HLA-DR and GLO, *Nature* **293**:745–749.

Shenfield, G. M., McCann, V. J., and Tjokresetio, R., 1982, Acetylator status and diabetic neuropathy, *Diabetologia* **22**:441–444.

Simpson, N. E., 1962, The genetics of diabetes: A study of 233 families of juvenile diabetics, *Ann. Hum. Genet.* **26**:1–21.

Singal, D. P., and Blajchman, M. A., 1973, Histocompatibility (HL-A) antigens, lymphocytotoxic antibodies and tissue antibodies in patients with diabetes mellitus, *Diabetes* **22**:429–432.

Spencer, K. M., and Cudworth, A. G., 1982, Aetiology of insulin-dependent diabetes, in: *Diabetes in Epidemiological Perspective* (J. I. Mann, K. Puorala, and A. Teuscher, eds.), Churchill Livingstone, London.

Spielman, R. S., Baker, L., and Zmijewski, C. M., 1980, Gene dosage and susceptibility to insulin-dependent diabetes, *Ann. Hum. Genet.* **44**:13–150.

Suciu-Foca, N., O'Neill, G., and Rubenstein, P., 1980, Evidence for the existence of a possible Bf "null" allele, in: *Histocompatibility Testing 1980* (P. I. Terasaki, ed.), pp. 965–936, UCLA Tissue Typing Laboratory, Los Angeles, California.

Svejgaard, A., and Ryder, L. P., 1977, Associations between HLA and disease: Notes on methodology and a report from the HLA and Disease Registry, in: *HLA and Disease* (J. Dausset and A. Svejgaard, eds.), pp. 46–71, Munksgaard, Copenhagen.

Svejgaard, A., Platz, P., Ryder, L. P., Staub-Nielsen, L., and Thomsen, M., 1975, HL-A and disease associations: A survey, *Transplant. Rev.* **22**:3–43.

Svejgaard, A., Platz, P., and Ryder, L. P., 1980, Insulin-dependent diabetes mellitus, in: *Histocompatibility Testing 1980* (P. I. Terasaki, ed.), pp. 638–656, UCLA Tissue Typing Laboratory, Los Angeles, California.

Tattersall, R. B., 1974, Mild familial diabetes with dominant inheritance, *Q. J. Med.* **43:**339–357.

Tattersall, R. B., and Fajans, S. S., 1975, A difference between the inheritance of classical juvenile-onset and maturity-onset diabetes of young people, *Diabetes* **24:**44–53.

Teisberg, P., Olaisen, B., Nordhagen, R., Thorsby, E., and Geddedahl, T., 1980, A haemolytically nonactive C4 gene product, *Immunobiology,* **158:**91–95.

Thomas, D. J. B., Young, A., Gorsuch, A. N., Bottazzo, G. F., and Cudworth, A. G., 1982, Evidence for an association between rheumatoid arthritis and auto-immune endocrine disease, *Ann. Rheum. Dis.*

Thomsen, M., Platz, P., Anderson, O. O., Christy, M., Lyngsoe, J., Nerup, J., Rasmussen, K., Ryder, L. P., Staub-Nielsen, L., and Svejgaard, A., 1975, MLC typing in juvenile diabetes mellitus and idiopathic Addison's disease, *Transplant. Rev.* **22:**125–147.

Thomson, G., 1980, A two locus model for juvenile diabetes, *Ann. Hum. Genet.* **43:**383–398.

Thomson, G., and Bodmer, W. F., 1977, The genetic analysis of HLA and disease associations, in: *HLA and Disease* (J. Dausset and A. Svejgaard, eds.), pp. 84–93, Munksgaard, Copenhagen.

Thomson, G., and Bodmer, W., 1979, HLA haplotype association with disease, *Tissue Antigens* **13:**91–102.

Tokunaga, K., Omoto, K., Maeda, H., Juji, T., Ishiba, S., and Maruyama, H., 1981, Bf and C2 polymorphism in Japanese patients with juvenile onset diabetes mellitus: Existence of a variant Bf allele, *Tissue Antigens* **18:**356–368.

Tosi, R., Tanigaki, N., Gentis, D., Ferrara, G. B., and Pressman, D., 1978, Immunological dissection of human Ia molecules. *J. Exp. Med.* **148:**1592–1611.

Vague, P. H., Melis, C., Mercier, P., Vialettes, B., and Lassmann, V., 1978, The increased frequency of the Lewis negative blood group in a diabetic population, *Diabetologia* **15:**33–36.

Wakisaka, A., Aizawa, M., Mtsuura, N., Nakagawa, S., Nakayama, E., Itakura, K., Okuna, A., and Wagatsuma, Y., 1976, HLA and juvenile diabetes mellitus in the Japanese, *Lancet* **2:**970.

Walker, A., and Cudworth, A. G., 1980, Type 1 (insulin dependent) diabetic multiplex families: Mode of genetic transmission, *Diabetes* **29:**1036–1039.

Walsh, L. J., Wilson Cox, D., and Ehrlich, R. M., 1982, The HLA-B*18,BF*F1 in haplotype in Type 1 diabetes, *Am. J. Hum. Genet.* **11:**337–343.

Walton, C., Dyer, P. A., Klouda, P. T., Schofield, J. A., Harris, R., Mallick, N. P., and Oleesky, 1981, HLA and properdin factor B in diabetic nephropathy, *Diabetologia* **21:**515 (abstract).

West, K. M., 1978, Prevalence and incidence, in: *Epidemiology of Diabetes and its Vascular Complication,* Elsevier North Holland, New York.

Williams, R. C., Knowler, W. C., Butler, W. J., Pettitt, D. J., Lisse, J. R., Bennett, P. H., Mann, D. L., Johnson, A. H., and Terasaki, P. I., 1981, HLA-A2 and Type 2 (insulin independent) diabetes mellitus in Pima Indians: An association of allele frequency with age, *Diabetologia* **21:**460–463.

Wolf, E., Drummond, V., Savage, M., Dean, B., Bottazzo, G. F., Davidson, J. C., Chacra, A. R., and Cudworth, A. G., 1981a, HLA and islet cell antibodies in diabetics from the West Indies, Qatar and Brazil, *Diabetologia* **21:**80 (abstract).

Wolf, E., Marwick, J. R., Wells, L., Cudworth, A. G., 1981b, Complement factors Bf and C2 in Type 1 diabetes, *Diabetologia* **21:**80.

Wolf, E., Spencer, K. M., and Cudworth, A. G., 1982a, The genetic susceptibility to type 1 (insulin dependent) diabetes: Analysis of the HLA-DR association, *Diabetologia* in press.

Wolf, E., Cudworth, A. G., Markwick, J. R., Gorsuch, A. N., Spencer, K. M., and Bodansky, H. J., 1982b, The Bf system in diabetes—gene interaction or linkage disequilibrium? *Diabetologia* **22:**85–88.

Zimmet, P., 1982, Type 2 (non-insulin-dependent) diabetes—an epidemiological overview, *Diabetologia* **22:**399–411.

10

Virus and Insulin-Dependent Diabetes Mellitus

S. A. Huber and B. R. MacPherson

I. INTRODUCTION

The theory that viruses cause insulin-dependent diabetes mellitus (IDDM) has been advanced sporadically for more than a century. During the past decade this theory has attracted renewed interest following the description by Craighead and McLane (1968) of a murine model of IDDM induced by the M variant of encephalomyocarditis (EMC) virus. An intriguing aspect of this model, which recapitulates many of the metabolic and pathologic features of human IDDM, is that EMC viruses are picornaviruses closely related to certain human pathogens, specifically coxsackieviruses. Although there is little evidence to suggest that EMC viruses *per se* cause human diabetes, efforts to incriminate Coxsackieviruses in IDDM have met with considerable success. In this chapter, we will review the evidence linking viruses to the etiology of IDDM.

II. GENERAL ASPECTS OF INSULIN-DEPENDENT DIABETES MELLITUS

A. Epidemiological Studies

Several unique epidemiological characteristics of IDDM support the concept that infectious agents initiate this disorder. These characteristics include the age distribution, seasonality, family clustering, and temporal relationships between viral illnesses and diabetes cases. Typically IDDM is a disease occurring in children and adolescents with the vast majority of cases developing before the age of 40. Epidemiological surveys in Copenhagen (Christau *et al.*, 1977), Montreal (West *et al.*, 1979), and the United Kingdom (Bloom *et al.*, 1975) have demonstrated that the incidence of IDDM in-

S. A. Huber and B. R. MacPherson • Department of Pathology, University of Vermont, Burlington, Vermont 05405.

creases steadily after age 9 months, reaching a peak in children 10–12 years old. Following this peak the incidence of new cases drops sharply, forming a pleateau in late adolescence and young adulthood. Bloom *et al.* (1975), reviewing the records of more than 2000 cases in the United Kingdom, also observed a minor peak occurring at age 5. This observation was confirmed in both the Danish and Canadian reports. In some studies a slight male predominance was noted and the age distribution of new cases differed when boys and girls were compared. In particular, Bloom *et al.* found that cases in boys tended to occur in the younger (0–4 years) and older (10–15 years) age groups whereas cases in girls were clustered in the intermediate age range (5–10 years). Moreover, the peak incidence occurred 1–2 years earlier in girls in all three surveys. Although the explanation for these different patterns of susceptibility is unknown, it may be noteworthy that in experimental diabetes male mice are more susceptible than females to EMC virus-induced diabetes.

One of the most striking aspects of IDDM is the fact that the seasonal distribution of new cases is not uniform. The seasonality of IDDM was first noted in 1926 by Adams (1926) who stated:

> In taking the history of patients with acute diabetes, when the date of onset can be fixed
> with reasonable certainty, I was impressed by the fact that there are certain seasons of the year
> when the onset of the disease is more common.

Adams distinguished between adult- and juvenile-onset diabetes mellitus and observed that in the latter group nearly 85% of the cases occurred between August and April with a peak incidence in the autumn. Subsequently a number of investigators have confirmed and extended this observation. In an excellent, recent review of the epidemiological characteristics of IDDM, Gamble (1980b) noted that autumn and winter peaks in diabetes incidence have been observed in six different countries in both the northern and southern hemispheres. In an unpublished study involving 1000 IDDM cases occurring between 1964 and 1973 in Massachusetts, Gleason *et al.* (cited in Craighead, 1981) noted that the seasonal clustering of cases in the late summer and winter months was most apparent in younger patients whose disease began abruptly and who lacked a family history of diabetes. Cudworth *et al.* (1977) reported that cases occurring in patients with the HLA BW15 phenotype were clustered in the winter, but not the autumn peak. These observations are consistent with the possibility that infectious agents prevalent during these periods played a role in initiating disease and that the factors determining susceptibility are heterogeneous. Obviously, other environmental factors could also fluctuate with changing seasons, resulting in a coincidental relationship with infectious agents such as viruses. However, the importance of factors such as physical activity, dietary changes, thermal stress, etc., in the pathogenesis of diabetes is doubtful.

If a single virus were responsible for the bulk of diabetes cases, one would expect significant year-to-year variation in the incidence of IDDM corresponding to the prevalence of that virus in the population. Indeed Gundersen (1927) and Sultz *et al.* (1975) used such evidence to support the contention that mumps virus is an important etiologic factor in IDDM. However, most studies have found that the annual variation of IDDM is fairly small. Gamble (1980b), referring to cases registered by the British Diabetic

Association since 1972, noted that the seasonal periodicity and annual incidence were remarkably reproducible from year to year although variations within a limited range were observed. Similarly, in the reports from Copenhagen (Christau *et al.*, 1977) and Montreal (West *et al.*, 1979) only minor fluctuations from year to year were found. In the Massachusetts study (cited in Craighead, 1981), there was significant annual variation in new cases when the data from younger patients with abrupt onset disease were analyzed. However, this variability was not correlated with the prevalence of any particular infectious agent in the population. Since the latent period for patients with abrupt-onset disease is likely to be short, one would expect that the relationship between diabetes and a specific virus, if any, would be quite apparent in this group.

Alternatively, it might be supposed that many viruses are capable of triggering the onset of diabetes, obscuring any relationship which might exist with a single agent. For example, Gamble (1980b) points out that the annual incidence of acute respiratory infections is fairly constant despite the fact that several viruses cause this syndrome. Moreover, many investigators regard infectious illnesses as precipitating factors that merely unmask subclinical or unrecognized diabetes. Although it is true that intercurrent infections often increase the insulin requirements of diabetic patients, this does not explain the specific association between viral illnesses and diabetes nor the fact that the onset of symptoms usually occurs during convalescence.

Several investigators have commented upon the temporal relationship between infectious diseases and the onset of symptoms in IDDM. Reports of diabetes following mumps, measles, chickenpox, rubella, infectious mononucleosis, influenza, hepatitis, and various unidentified agents causing acute febrile illnesses have appeared in the medical literature for nearly a century. These reports are dealt with in the sections concerned with specific viruses. Several studies of a more general nature deserve comment here.

In 1949 Henry John, reviewing his personal experience with 500 cases of diabetes in children, concluded that infections played a role in causation of this disease. In his own series of patients nearly 35% gave a history of recent infection preceding the onset of symptoms attributible to diabetes. Although mumps was the most common illness cited, accounting for more than 25% of the infections, more than 20 clinical syndromes were included in his tabulation, the majority of which were viral illnesses.

Some reports have called attention to "outbreaks" of IDDM: clusters of cases occurring during a short time span in a geographically confined area. In 1958 Melin and Ursing reported one such "outbreak" occurring after a mumps epidemic in a small Swedish village. In this report 42 individuals contracted mumps following which 4 children developed diabetes. Although this remarkable association with a single rubella virus has not been repeated, many patients with IDDM report a history of viruslike illness preceding diabetes and objective evidence for a viral etiology has been obtained in some cases. Thus, Huff *et al.* (1974) investigated a cluster of 12 diabetes cases occurring during February and March, 1972, in Pinellas County, Florida. Most patients gave a history of antecedent illnesses such as upper respiratory infections, otitis media, influenzalike illness, or gastroenteritis occurring within the previous 6 weeks. A comprehensive serological evaluation revealed that eight of nine patients had elevated titers to at least one viral antigen, suggesting recent infection. Although the results of this study were inconclusive with regard to the role of viruses in the etiology of IDDM, the findings were compatible with the possibility that viral illnesses precipitated some cases.

In a recent prospective study, Cudworth *et al.* (1977) evaluated the role of environmental factors in 110 recently diagnosed diabetic patients. In this investigation 39% of these patients gave a history of antecedent illness. In nine subjects a viral etiology was confirmed. These included cases of varicella, measles, rubella, viral hepatitis, and influenza. The remaining subjects had febrile illnesses of unknown etiology. The onset of diabetic symptoms showed a typical seasonal distribution with most cases occurring in the autumn and winter months. Patients with HLA BW15 and coxsackievirus seroconverters were clustered in the winter peak (see Section III.C). The authors concluded that their evidence favored the hypothesis that viruses precipitated, rather than initiated, onset of diabetes.

Finally, in a retrospective study involving 1663 cases of IDDM in the United Kingdom, Gamble (1980a) identified 398 patients in whom diabetes was preceded by an acute febrile illness for which medical attention was sought. These illnesses included mumps, chickenpox, rubella, measles, and acute respiratory illnesses. Compared with the expected frequency of illness in the general population, only mumps infections were found in excess. However, since the viruses causing acute respiratory illnesses were not identified, the possibility of additional associations could not be excluded. An impressive feature of this study was the assortment of viral illnesses occurring within the month prior to the onset of symptoms, suggesting that infections with many viruses might act as a triggering event in diabetes induction.

B. Family Studies

Since family members share a limited gene pool, family studies, particularly studies in twins, provide a unique opportunity to examine environmental infuences in disease. The fact that concordant IDDM occurs in only 50% of identical twins indicates that environmental factors are of paramount importance in initiating diabetes (Nelson *et al.* 1975a). Exploring the possibility that common viruses might be such a factor, Nelson *et al.* (1975b) examined sera from 49 monozygotic twin pairs, 22 of whom were concordant for IDDM. Antibodies to mumps S and V antigens, cytomegalovirus, rubella, *M. pneumoniae* and coxsackie B virus types 1-5 were sought. Although antibodies to coxsackie B2, rubella virus, and *M. pneumoniae* were found more frequently in sera from discordant twins, the differences were small and comparisons between the groups failed to elicit evidence for a viral etiology in IDDM. Since many patients had had diabetes for years, however, age-related differences in susceptibility could have obscured the role of common viruses in promoting diabetes.

In family studies, the genetic relationships between family members must be taken into account. At the population level, IDDM is associated with HLA antigens B8, BW15 (Nerup *et al.*, 1974; Cudworth and Woodrow, 1975a, b), DRW3, and DRW4 (Garavoy *et al.*,1978; Rodey *et al.*, 1979). Segregation analysis of both multiplex (Cudworth and Woodrow, 1975a, b; Barbosa, *et al.*, 1977) and unselected families (Rubinstein *et al.*, 1977) with diabetic members has shown that the risk of concordant IDDM in siblings is markedly increased in individuals sharing one or both HLA haplotypes with the propositus. In fact, the frequency of concordant IDDM in HLA-identical siblings approaches that observed in identical twins. This observation led Rubinstein et al., (1977) to the conclusion that susceptibility to IDDM was inherited as a simple autosomal recessive characteristic linked to the major histocompatibility complex. Although this analysis has been disputed, evidence for the relationship between disease susceptibility and HLA-linked genes is overwhelming.

In view of the increased risk of IDDM in siblings, West and colleagues (1977) conducted a prospective serological study of 109 new IDM patients residing in Montreal and 72 sibling controls. Fourfold rises in antiviral antibody titers were found in many patients, particularly against coxsackieviruses (see Section III.C), whereas seroconversion was rarely encountered in controls even among HLA-identical siblings of the probands. These findings support the contention that virus infections may initiate diabetes in genetically susceptible individuals.

Familial clusters of cases, often occurring within days or weeks of each other, have been described in many series and case reports. Although often disease onset has been associated with evidence of acute febrile illnesses, seldom has a specific virus been identified. Exceptions to this generality include two case reports of mumps-related IDDM occurring nearly simultaneously in siblings (King, 1972; Messaritakis et al., 1971). In one instructive case in the Montreal study referred to above, one sibling developed IDDM 2 weeks after her HLA-identical brother. She exhibited a fourfold rise in antibody to coxsackie B4 virus, whereas her brother showed no serological evidence of recent virus infection. This observation emphasizes the fact that serological or virological evidence of infection must be proven before specific viruses can be incriminated as a cause of familial diabetes.

Since the risk of acquiring IDDM is sharply increased in HLA-identical siblings of diabetic children, careful prospective serological studies in HLA-typed families could provide valuable information regarding the relationship between virus infections and the initiation of diabetes. In one revealing study Gorsuch et al. (1981) determined HLA genotypes in 582 parents and siblings of 160 affected children and then tested these subjects for the presence of islet cell antibodies, (ICA). Sera from 7% of nondiabetic parents and 12% of siblings were positive for ICA. During the period of observation two parents and four siblings developed abrupt onset diabetes 3-30 months after being tested for ICA. All were positive for ICA from the outset and all shared either one or both HLA haplotypes with the propositus. Interestingly enough, half of the diabetic subjects had had upper respiratory infections within 2 weeks of disease onset. However, no attempt was made to identify the responsible virus. The authors interpreted their findings to mean that the prediabetic period is relatively long in IDDM and that the role of viruses is either nonspecific or the final insult in a cumulative process of B cell destruction.

C. Histopathological Features of IDDM

The histopathological features of the pancreas in IDDM have been well-described by LeCompte and Gepts (1977). Microscopically, the islets were reduced in size and number even very early in the disease. In cases of less than 6 months' duration a mononuclear cell infiltrate consisting largely of lymphocytes was usually found within and around the remaining islets. This lesion, originally termed "insulitis" by von Meyenburg in 1940, had been described in IDDM since the turn of the century, but was dismissed as a curiosity until LeCompte (1958) and Gepts (1965) demonstrated that patchy insulitis was remarkably common in diabetic pancreases if the interval between disease onset and death was short. Additional histopathological findings in early lesions included focal hyperplasia of the islets, islet cell regeneration, increased cytoplasmic RNA ("Kornchen"), and hydropic changes in the islet cells thought to represent accumulations of glycogen. Some residual islets consisted of serpentine cords of small cells with scant cytoplasm. Fibrosis and hyalinization of islets were noted in both acute and chronic cases. With disease of more than 6 months' duration insulitis disappeared and islets became progressively more difficult to locate.

The application of immunohistochemical techniques to the study of diabetic pancreases produced several interesting findings (Gepts and DeMey, 1978). Residual B cells, though markedly reduced in numbers, persisted in the majority of acute cases and in a surprisingly large number of cases of several years' duration. In some instances the distribution of insulitis in the pancreas correlated with the presence of residual insulin-containing beta cells. The majority of islets however, consisted of cells containing glucagon, somatostatin, or pancreatic polypeptide. In particular, the serpentine cords of cells found in chronic cases were often composed entirely of cells producing pancreatic polypeptide.

These histopathological findings, obviously, are nonspecific but could be consistent with a viral etiology. The fact that a small number of beta cells persist for years is difficult to reconcile with the theory that diabetes is caused by the cumulative effects of environmental toxins. Rather, this observation is more consistent with the possibility that islet cell injury occurs during childhood as a consequence of infectious diseases which diminish in frequency as immunity to a wide range of viruses is acquired.

III. INSULIN-DEPENDENT DIABETES MELLITUS AND VIRAL INFECTIONS

A. Mumps

1. Characteristics

Mumps virus is a paramyxovirus in the family Paramyxoviridae. The complete virion is spherical with an average diameter of approximately 200 nm. The helical nucleocapsid is enclosed within a trilaminar envelope, the external coat of which possesses both hemagglutinin and neuraminidase activity. The V (viral) antigen is associated with the envelope whereas the S (soluble) antigen is contained in the internal nucleocapsid. The tightly coiled ribonucleoprotein nucleocapsid consists of a linear, single strand of RNA.

Following infection, antibodies to both S and V antigens are detectable in the serum. Antibodies directed against S antigens decline rapidly whereas antibodies against V antigens persist for years. Therefore, rising titers against V antigens or the presence of antibodies against S antigens are indicative of recent infection. Delayed cutaneous hypersensitivity and T-cell-mediated immunity against virus-infected target cells can also be demonstrated during convalescence (Tsutsumi *et al.*, 1980) and may be important in protection of the host. Recovery from mumps results in durable, lifelong immunity.

2. Clinical Features

Mumps is an acute, highly contagious, self-limited disease which was major cause of morbidity in school age children prior to the widespread adoption of mumps immunization programs. The principal clinical manifestation of mumps is the familiar swelling of the salivary glands caused by infection of the acinar cells with concomitant inflammation and edema. Less frequently involvement of the nervous system, testes, and pancreas complicates mumps. Since the mortality in this disease is extremely low, little information is available regarding the pathology of mumps infection. In the few published reports of fatal cases, interstitial inflammation consisting mainly of mononuclear cells, cellular degeneration, and edema are generally observed in affected organs (Bostrom, 1968).

In unimmunized populations mumps occurs as an epidemic disease in the winter and early spring. Children aged 5–9 make up more than 50% of the cases. By the age of 16, 90% of individuals have circulating antibodies against mumps viral antigens indicating prior exposure (Centers for Disease Control, 1980). Subclinical disease occurs in 30% of individuals, a fact which has been confirmed experimentally (Henle *et al.*, 1948). Males and females are equally susceptible to infection.

The most common complication of mumps infection is encephalitis. Although more than half of mumps cases show pleocytosis in the cerebrospinal fluid, overt disease is observed in less than 1% (Marcy and Kibrick, 1977; Baum, and Litman, 1979). Nerve deafness may be a chronic sequela of CNS infection. Boys develop CNS disease three times as commonly as girls, but the age distribution of this complication resembles that of uncomplicated mumps. In contrast, mumps orchitis occurs primarily in postpubertal boys.

The association between mumps infection and acute pancreatitis is rare, but well documented (Farnam, 1922; Witte and Schanzer, 1968). Pancreatitis usually resolves without sequalae. In fatal cases the pancreas shows an interstitial and periductal mononuclear cell infiltrate (Bostrom, 1968). Although abnormalities in the pancreatic islets have been described, insulitis has not been observed (Lemoine and Lapasset, 1903; Limper and Miller, 1935). Remarkably, mumps virus has never been recovered from human pancreatic tissue.

3. Temporal Association of IDDM and Mumps Infection

The temporal relationship between mumps and IDDM has been the subject of numerous case reports. Although this association was noted by a Norwegian physician, J. Stang, in 1864 (cited by Gunderson, 1927), H. F. Harris (1899) was the first to report specific clinical details documenting the relationship between mumps infection and IDDM. Subsequently 25 additional cases have appeared in the medical literature (Table 1). In addition to individual case reports, epidemiological studies have included

Table 1.   Summary of Case Reports Linking Mumps Infection and Diabetes Mellitus

Reference	Age/sex	Serological confirmation of mumps infection	Interval between mumps and diabetes	Clinical features
Harris, 1899	42 y/M	—	1 month	Diabetes for 3 yrs at time of diagnosis
Barbieri, 1909	6 y/M	—	9 days	Diabetic symptoms accompanied by pancreatis; glycosuria disappeared 15 days later; patient recovered completely
Gilhespy and Holden, 1977	16 y/M	—	3–4 days	Abrupt onset of diabetes symptoms; patient also had tuberculosis; died 5 months after diagnosis; autopsy showed hyalinization and decreased numbers of islets
Patrick, 1924	8 y/F	—	2 weeks	Diabetes following uncomplicated mumps, patient died shortly after admission; no family history of diabetes
Cole, 1933, 1934	13 y/M	—	5 weeks	Abrupt onset of diabetes symptoms and diabetic coma; patient died shortly after admission; no family history of diabetes
	12 y/M	—	2 weeks	In addition to symptoms of diabetes patient had persistent abdominal pain associated with mumps; no family history of diabetes
	7 y/M	—	3 weeks	Mumps following "influenza"; onset of diabetes symptoms followed an 8-day history of abdominal pain; no family history of diabetes
Dick, 1934	13 y/F	—	1 month	Following "moderately severe" mumps patient developed marked weight loss and glycosuria; symptoms controlled with insulin
Kremer, 1947	15 y/M	—	6 weeks	Abrupt onset of diabetes symptoms controlled with insulin; no family history of diabetes
Melin and Urins, 1958	5 y/F	—	1 month	
	7 y/F	–	8 months	Diabetes following a mumps epidemic in a small Swedish village
	9 y/F	—	3 months	
	13 y/M	9 months		
Hinden, 1962	15 m/M	—	5 weeks	Diabetic coma on admission; 4 other siblings had mumps without sequelae; recovered with insulin therapy
Freeman, 1962	7 y/M	—	1 month	Polyuria, polydipsia, polyphagia after mumps; insulin therapy for 3 years at time of report: no family history of diabetes

King, 1962	7 y/F	—	0	Symptoms of diabetes concordant with mumps; diabetes diagnosed 4 months later; responded to insulin
	5 y/F	—	0	Sibling of patient above; developed mumps 2 weeks after her sister and simultaneously had symptoms of diabetes; diagnosis made at the same time as her sister. No family history of diabetes
McCrae, 1963	10 m/M	+	?	No parotitis; persistent diarrhea indicated possible pancreatitis; 2 siblings had mumps at the time of diagnosis; patient required insulin therapy
Kahana and Brant, 1967	10 m/M	+	?	Patient's mother had mumps 6 months previously; patient had frequent infections, but no clinical features of mumps; developed diabetic ketoacidosis 3 days after episodes of fever, vomiting and diarrhea; responded to insulin; no family history of diabetes
Messaritakis et al., 1971	6 y/F	+	2 months	4-week history of weight loss, thirst, and enuresis at time of diagnosis; required insulin
	8 y/M	+	2½ months	Sibling of patient above; developed symptoms of diabetes nearly simultaneously with her; required insulin; no family history of diabetes and both parents had normal results of glucose tolerance tests
Dacou-Voutetakis et al., 1974	4 y/M	—	10 days	Polyuria and polydipsia accompanied by abdominal pain and steatorrhea; required therapy with insulin and pancreatic extract; no family history
	11 y/F	—	20 days	Only abnormality at diagnosis was glycosuria; patient was insulinopenic; a paternal grandfather and uncle had elevated fasting blood sugar levels
Block et al., 1973	49 y/F	+	?	No clinical features of mumps; 2-week history of polyuria and polydipsia; diabetic ketoacidosis on admission controlled with insulin; laboratory evidence for pancreatitis; carbohydrate tolerance normal 8 months later and insulin therapy discontinued
Reddy and Crump, 1976	11 y/F	+	3 days	Fever, parotid swelling, and mild abdominal pain 3 days prior to development of excessive fluid intake and polyuria; other family members had mumps; responded to insulin therapy
Peig et al., 1981	6 y/M	+	20 days	Abrupt onset of diabetes symptoms 20 days after uncomplicated mumps; an HLA ½-identical sibling had mumps but did not develop diabetes; family history negative for diabetes

more than 50 cases of IDDM occurring within 6 months after mumps infection. Since many of these case reports appeared prior to the availability of serodiagnostic and virological methods for diagnosing mumps virus infection, only a few such cases have received laboratory confirmation.

Several individual reports are of special interest. In 1958 Melin and Ursing described four cases of IDDM occurring in a Swedish village of 550 people following a mumps epidemic. Forty children and two adults contracted mumps. Diabetes developed 1, 3, 8, and 9 months later in 3 girls aged 5, 7, and 9, and in one boy, aged 13. This remarkable occurrence has been cited as evidence for the existence of "wild strain" diabetogenic variants of mumps virus.

Two reports have documented the onset of nearly simultaneous IDDM following mumps in siblings (King, 1962; Messaritakis *et al.*, 1971). In both reports symptoms of IDDM developed within 8 weeks after mumps and in one serological evidence of recent mumps infection was obtained.

The clinical and epidemiological characteristics of IDDM occurring after mumps do not differ in any important respect from the majority of IDDM cases. There was a slight male predominance (15 : 11) in the reported cases. The mean age of onset was 8.0 years for boys and 7.9 for girls in those cases occurring in individuals under 40. The cases in boys tended to cluster in the 0–5 and 10–15 years age groups whereas cases in girls were more frequent in the 5–10 years age groups. Although mumps typically occurs in the winter and spring, there was no obvious seasonality in postmumps diabetes. In a few instances patients manifested symptoms or signs compatible with pancreatitis (Block *et al.*, 1973; Dacou-Voutetakis *et al.*, 1974), but in the majority of cases no such relationship was reported. Fatalities during the acute phase of the disease were rare and in no instance was mumps virus recovered from pancreatic tissue.

Characteristically postmumps diabetes occurred in patients lacking a family history of diabetes. The symptoms of diabetes developed abruptly, usually within 60 days after mumps. Serological proof of the diagnosis was obtained in a minority of cases, but the clinical features of the disease were sufficiently characteristic to permit reliable diagnosis in most instances. In two cases diabetes followed subclinical mumps proven serologically in patients exposed to siblings or parents with overt infection (McCrae, 1963; Kahana and Brant, 1967). There appeared to be no correlation between the severity of mumps and the development of IDDM.

During the past decade mumps immunization programs have been implemented in most areas of the United States. It might be anticipated that the frequency of IDDM cases would diminish as the practice of immunization became widespread if mumps was an important etiological agent initiating diabetes. No such diminution has been observed. However, as pointed out by Gamble (1980b), if mumps infection accounted for only a small proportion of diabetes cases, a reduction due to immunization could be missed.

Since mumps vaccine contains a live virus it is conceivable that immunization could result in an increased frequency of mumps-related diabetes. The coincidence of mumps immunization and the onset of IDDM has been reported in only one instance (Sinaniotis *et al.*, 1975). Thus, this theoretical possibility remains unsubstantiated.

4. Epidemiological Studies

In 1927, Gundersen, in a survey of 5951 Norwegian cases of diabetes mellitus, observed that the frequency of deaths due to diabetes in the 10–20 year age group coincided with the occurrence of mumps epidemics if allowance was made for a 2–4 year lag period.

These findings were extended by John in 1934. Reviewing his personal experience with 214 cases of diabetes in children, John noted that acute infections preceded the onset of diabetes in 21%. The most frequent infection reported in the series was mumps. In 1949 John updated and extended these observations. A history of antecedent infection was obtained in 164/500 (33%) cases. Mumps infection was reported in 37/164 (22%) instances. The majority of these infections occurred within 60 days prior to the onset of diabetes.

Additional evidence linking mumps infections to diabetes was developed by Sultz et al. (1975) in an epidemiological study involving children in Erie County, New York. Examining the incidence of childhood diabetes from 1946 to 1971, Sultz confirmed that fluctuations in incidence by season occurred reproducibly and that the incidence of new cases paralleled the occurrence of mumps epidemics with a lag phase of about 4 years. It was reported that mumps infection or exposure had preceded diabetes in 50% of these cases and that mumps vaccination had been performed in an additional 11%.

A recent epidemiological study performed by Gamble (1980a) provides further evidence for the involvement of mumps virus in some cases of diabetes. A questionnaire was sent to physicians registering new cases of childhood diabetes with the British Diabetic Association, inquiring about illnesses occurring in the 6 months prior to the development of diabetes. Information obtained from 1663 cases was compared with morbidity statistics for epidemic infections during the same period compiled by the Office of Population Censuses and Surveys. Mumps infection was reported as an antecedent illness in 25 cases, more than twice as frequently as expected. The majority of these infections occurred within 1 month of disease onset. Although many other viral and bacterial infections were reported in association with diabetes, none exceeded the expected frequency for the population. However, 658/1663 (39%) cases were associated with some antecedent illness in the 6 months preceding disease onset, in general agreement with the figure obtained by John several years previously. It was concluded that a small proportion of diabetes cases may result from recent mumps infection.

Attempts to link recent mumps infection to the onset of IDDM by applying seroepidemiological methods to both population and family studies have been uniformly unsuccessful. Cudworth et al. (1977) performed a prospective investigation of 110 newly diagnosed diabetes patients, searching for a viral etiology. In 41 cases a history of antecedent illness compatible with a virus infection was elicited and in 9 cases the etiologic agent was substantiated by clinical or laboratory evidence. Included among these cases were four instances of varicella and one each of measles, rubella, and viral hepatitis. Influenza B virus was isolated from one patient with clinical features of influenza infection and there was one case of congenital rubella. In no instance was clinical or serological evidence of acute infection with mumps virus obtained and there was no correlation between mumps antibody titers and HLA phenotypes, seasonal incidence, history of antecedent illness, or islet cell antibodies. In a retrospective study of identical twins concordant or discordant for diabetes, Nelson *et al.* (1975b) found that the vast majority of subjects in both groups possessed antibodies against mumps S or V antigens and there were no differences in the frequency or titers of these antibodies when the groups were compared. Since the interval between the onset of disease and the serological studies was several years in most cases, age-related differences in diabetes susceptibility could have obscured any relationship between infection and disease.

Since the frequency of concordant diabetes is increased in siblings sharing one or both HLA haplotypes with an affected member, it might be expected that differences in the frequency or titer of viral antibodies would be found in prospective studies of newly diagnosed patients. Recently West and colleagues (1981) reported the results of a prospective serological study involving 109 IDDM cases and 72 sibling controls. No differences in geometric mean titers against mumps antigens were found. When the patient and control groups were compared only one patient showed a fourfold rise in geometric mean titer, suggesting recent mumps infection. Collectively these results indicate that mumps virus is an unlikely cause of most diabetes cases. However, the possibility that mumps is responsible for some cases is neither proven nor disproven by these studies.

5. Virological and Histopathological Studies

The most convincing evidence that mumps virus is capable of infecting human beta cells is derived from studies by Prince and his colleagues (1978) who investigated the susceptibility of islet cells in tissue culture to virus infection. Islets isolated from human pancreatic tissue obtained at autopsy were cultured for 3-4 days, then infected with the ABC strain of mumps virus. At regular intervals insulin and virus-containing cells were simultaneously identified by immunofluorescence using a double-labeling technique. After 3 days more than 75% of both beta cells and non-beta cells contained mumps antigen. Virus titers increased to $10^{5.3}$ plaque-forming units 72 hr after virus inoculation. Although this report convincingly demonstrated that islet cells can be infected with mumps virus *in vitro,* the possibility that cultured beta cells differ from intact islets in susceptibility to infection must be acknowledged.

Support for the hypothesis that mumps virus infection is integrally related to IDDM would be advanced if mumps virus could be isolated from pancreatic tissue or localized to beta cells during acute infection. Despite the well-recognized association between mumps and pancreatitis and possibly IDDM, in no instance has mumps virus been recovered from the pancreas. Interestingly enough, in 1949 Weller and Craig attempted to recover the virus from a fatal case in which the pancreas was histologically normal. Mumps virus was isolated from the parotid gland and from either the pancreas or the ovary. However, a laboratory error precluded identifying the organ source with certainty and subsequent attempts to isolate the virus from pancreatic tissue were unsuccessful. Obviously, since fatal cases or mumps are extremely rare, opportunities for virological studies are limited. However, isolated reports of mumps fatalities continue to appear in the literature, and possibilities for such studies exist.

Similarly, very few reports documenting the pancreatic pathology in mumps have appeared and none have described the typical insulitis seen in early, acute IDDM reported by Gepts (1965). In 1968 Bostrom described the histological features in a fatal case of proven mumps myocarditis. Mononuclear cell infiltrates, interstitial edema, and epithelial cell degeneration were observed in the salivary glands, testes, and seminal vesicles. The pancreas showed similar changes, but the degree of pancreatic involvement was mild. Insulitis was not reported. These observations are generally in accord with autopsy findings in earlier reports in which the diagnosis of mumps was based on clinical findings alone. Advances in immunohistochemical identification of antigens in fixed, paraffin-embedded tissues raise the possibility that mumps antigen could be localized to beta cells using tissues from fatal cases but to date no such study has been performed.

6. Miscellaneous Studies

Finally there is one report in the literature in which islet cell antibodies were identified in sera from patients convalescing from mumps. Stimulated by the observation that one patient who had developed IDDM 3 weeks after mumps infection also had persistent islet cell antibodies, Helmke and his colleagues (1980) examined sera from 30 children with mumps confirmed serologically. Although several of these children had been hospitalized for mumps-related complications, none had had glycosuria or abnormal glucose tolerance tests. Fourteen sera were positve for islet cell antibodies. Sera from patients with other diseases including coxsackie, measles, rubella, influenza, and adenovirus infections were negative. There was no correlation between antibody titers against mumps antigens and titers of islet cell antibodies.

An attempt to confirm this intriguing observation was unsuccessful (Richens and Jones, 1981), but additional studies are warranted to clarify the relationship, if any, between mumps infection and islet cell antibodies.

B. Picornaviruses

1. Coxsackieviruses

a. Characteristics. Coxsackieviruses are enteroviruses in the Picornavirus family. These viruses range in size from 28 to 30 nm diameter and are comprised of a single-stranded RNA genome and an icosahedral protein capsid. They are divided into A and B subgroups of 24 and 6 serotypes respectively. The six coxsackie B viruses and coxsackievirus A_{19} share a common group antigen. Both A and B viruses replicate in the infected cell cytoplasm. Progeny virus particles are released by the virus directed lysis of the infected cell (Rekosh, 1977).

b. Clinicopathologic Characterization of Coxsackievirus Infection. Coxsackieviruses were first isolated in 1948 by Dalldorf (1950) in Coxsackie, New York, from the feces of two children with signs of clinical paralytic poliomyelitis. The viruses are very common in nature, and most individuals develop antibodies to at least one serogroup during their lifetime (Lerner *et al.*, 1975). The coxsackie group A viruses generally induce a milder disease characterized by diffuse myositis in the voluntary muscles. No association between coxsackie A viruses and IDDM has ever been reported (Ginsberg, 1980). Coxsackie B virus causes focal inflammation and necrosis of infected tissue. In the majority of the cases, coxsackie B virus infection is asymptomatic. In the remainder, the disease is generally mild and expressed as gastoenteritis and upper respiratory syndromes. Occasionally, the virus induces severe, life-threatening illnesses such as hepatitis, encephalitis, meningitis, myocarditis, and diabetes mellitus (Curnen, 1979; Ginsberg and Dulbecco, 1980). The same virus causes a broad spectrum of disorders ranging from subclinical infection to life-threatening disease in different individuals. It is not known what characteristics of the virus and the host determine the severity and the degree of tissue involvement. Several possibilities are the age and genetic constitution of the individual, the concentration of virus, and the metabolic state of the host.

Coxsackie B viruses have a high efficiency of infection. Approximately 80% of exposed individuals will seroconvert. The infection is most frequently spread within families and between individuals by fecal-oral contact, but can also be spread by nasal droplets and by insects such as flies and mosquitoes. Once the virus enters the host, the incubation period is 2–5 days. Primary virus replication occurs in the epithelial and paraepithelial lymphatic cells of the pharynx. At this time the host may be asymptomatic or may develop mild malaise, sore throat, and low-grade fever. Secondary sites of infection are the intestines and the respiratory tract. If a sufficient amount of virus is present, viremia may occur spreading the virus to a number of organs such as the pancreas, liver, skeletal muscles, heart, and nervous system (Curnen, 1979; Ginsberg and Dulbecco).

Antibodies to the specific serotype antigens and to the common coxsackie B virus group antigen arise within 1 week of infection. Peak antibody titers are generally observed by the 3rd week. Although these antibodies persist for years after the initial infection, the titers decrease rapidly after the first 2–3 months. The persistence of these antibodies undoubtedly confers long-lasting protection from reinfection with the same viral serotype (Davis *et al.*, 1969).

Severe forms of coxsackievirus infections are most prevelant in infants less than 12 months old. The mortality rate in this age group can reach 50%. Follow-up studies of infants contracting either coxsackieviral encephalitis or myocarditis indicate that permanent neurological and heart damage is not common. In contrast to the severe disease in neonatal life, coxsackievirus infections in early childhood are generally asymptomatic. After age 10, the disease may again become severe resulting in meningitis, hepatitis, myopericarditis, or diabetes mellitus but is rarely fatal (Woodruff, 1980).

There is evidence that some coxsackieviral diseases predominate in males. Sixty-six percent of clinical cases of coxsackie-B-virus-induced myocarditis occur in males. Shifts in hormone balances may also explain why pregnancy increases the susceptibility to and severity of picornavirus infections (Woodruff, 1980).

c. *Temporal Association of IDDM and Coxsackievirus Infection.* Although coxsackieviruses were described in 1948, Gamble *et al.* first associated these viruses with IDDM in 1969. Forty-five percent of diabetic patients with onset of symptoms of less than 3 months duration had elevated antibody titers to coxsackievirus B-4 compared to only 21% of control (nondiabetic) patients. In addition, the geometric mean antibody titers were inversely related to the duration of diabetes indicating recent infection. Similarly, in two studies (Wilson *et al.*, 1977; Ray *et al.*, 1980) a series of recently diagnosed IDDM patients, 10 of 16 had elevated antibody titers to coxsackie B viruses. Four of 17 of these patients had predominantly IgM antibody, indicating recent infection.

In 1974, Huff *et al.* reported a dramatic increase of new diabetes cases in Pinellas County, Florida. Twelve cases were reported in February and March of 1972, compared to a maximum of two cases reported in any month during the previous 4 years. Nine of the 12 new cases were studied. In eight, the patients had experienced a virus-like illness within the three months preceding hospitalization. One-third of the patients had elevated antibody titers to coxsackie B3 virus compared to 6% of control patients and 10% of the diabetic patients' family members. No information was given relative to a recent epidemic of coxsackievirus in the population.

Three series reporting seroepidemiological evidence of coxsackievirus infections in IDDM also demonstrated male dominance (Table 2). In the remainder of the studies, male/female ratios of individuals with IDDM and coxsackievirus antibody were either not reported, or, in one series, females predominated (West *et al.*, 1981). In the combined series, the ratio of males to females was approximately 1 : 1. Although no male dominance was demonstrated the number of patients in these studies are probably too few to draw statistically significant conclusions on the sex distribution of IDDM of suspected coxsackievirus etiology.

The seasonal incidence of coxsackievirus infections coincides remarkably well with the seasonal incidence of diabetes (Gamble and Taylor, 1969; Gamble *et al.*, 1973). In both cases, the frequency is greatest in the fall and winter months. The seasonality of IDDM is most evident in patients whose initial diabetic symptoms occurred between 0 and 19 years of age. Interestingly, in patients initially presenting with IDDM at 20–39 years of age, there are no significant and consistent seasonal differences. The optimal age of IDDM onset in cases of suspected coxsackievirus etiology varies from 4 to 19 years, but generally occurs in the 8– to 12-year age group. This is somewhat older than with mumps virus (7–8 years) but does not vary remarkably from the mean age of IDDM patients as a whole.

A number of investigators have been unable to obtain seroepidemiologic evidence for coxsackievirus infections in IDDM patients (Madden *et al.*, 1978; Nelson *et al.*, 1975b; Samantray *et al.*, 1977; Di Pietro *et al.*, 1979). In each case, there was no statistical difference in the number of IDDM patients positive for coxsackievirus antibodies compared to control groups. In two additional and separate series (Hierholzer and Farris, 1974; Dippe *et al.*, 1975) a total of 220 individuals were investigated who had contracted coxsackie B3 or B4 virus infections during a known epidemic. None of these individuals demonstrated alterations in glucose tolerance and did not develop overt diabetes over the 4- to 5-year period following infection.

Table 2. Summary of Seroepidemiological Evidence of Coxsackieviral Infections in IDDM

Reference	Number of patients with elevated antibody titers to coxsackievirus/total (percent)	Season of IDDM onset	Age at initial IDDM onset (yr)	Sex (M/F)	Virus serotype associated with IDDM
West et al., 1981	21/46 (46)	Autumn	0–19	NG[a]	Coxsackie B4 virus
Gamble et al., 1973	14/162 (70)	Winter	10–19	NG	Coxsackie B4 virus
Huff et al., 1974	8/9 (89)	Winter	4–13	5M/4F	Coxsackie B3 virus
Cudworth et al., 1977	25/110 (23)	Autumn–winter	11	65M/45F	Coxsackie B1–5 virus
Templeton et al., 1977	1	Autumn	11.5	M	Coxsackie B2 virus
Yoon et al., 1979	1	NG	10	M	Coxsackie B4 virus
Champsaur et al., 1980	1	NG	1.3	NG	Coxsackie B5 virus
El-Hagrassy et al., 1980	2/4 (50)	NG	6–11	NG	Coxsackie B1–5 virus
Ray et al., 1980	10/11 (91)	NG	8	7M/4F	Coxsackie B1–5 virus
Cited in Jenson et al., 1980	1	NG	5	F	Coxsackie B4 virus
West et al., 1980	31/109 (80)	Autumn–winter	1–16	13M/17F	Coxsackie B1–5 virus

[a]NG, not given.

d. Virological and Histopathological Studies. The best evidence that coxsackieviruses can cause IDDM comes from three cases in which the virus was directly isolated from children developing diabetic symptoms soon after coxsackie B viral infections. In the first case, a 10-year-old boy had developed ketoacidosis 3 days after the onset of a flu-like illness (Yoon *et al.*, 1979). At postmortem examination, the islets showed extensive mononuclear cell infiltration and necrosis. The patient had elevated antibody titers to coxsackie B4 virus, and the virus, which was isolated from the pancreas of the patient, induced diabeteslike symptoms in susceptible mice. In another case, a 5-year-old girl developed diabetes after open-heart surgery. She developed high antibody titers to coxsackie B4 virus and the virus was demonstrated in the islets of Langerhans (cited in Jensen *et al.*, 1980). A third child, 16 months of age, also developed diabetes within days of infection with a coxsackie B5 virus. The virus was isolated from the feces of the child and induced diabeteslike symptoms in mice (Champsaur *et al.*, 1980). Finally, in a related report, Jensen *et al.* (1980) reported that four of seven children with known fatal infections of coxsackie B viruses had islet lesions at autopsy. In three out of four of these cases, the infants showed inflammatory infiltrates in the islets, and all the infants had some islet cell degeneration. The incidence of islet lesions in fatal viral infections was greatest with coxsackie B and cytomegaloviruses (4 of 7 and 20 of 45, respectively). Only 2 of 45 fatal rubella infections affected the islets and no islet damage was seen in children infected with 11 other viruses including mumps, herpes simplex, and varicella zoster viruses.

2. Encephalomyocarditis Virus

Encephalomyocarditis (EMC) virus is an enterovirus in the Picornavirus family with morphological and physical characteristics resembling coxsackieviruses. EMC is closely related to Mengo, MM, Columbia SK, and Kissling viruses which can cause aspetic meningitis, encephalitis, and Guillain-Barré syndrome in humans. The prevalence of antibody to EMC virus in children (< 15 years) varies from 1.0% in England and Wales to 33.9% in New Hebrides. The prevalence in adults also varied from 3.2% in Ethiopia to 50.6% in New Hebrides. EMC infections were much more prevalent in the southern hemisphere (Tesh, 1978).

Encephalomyocarditis virus has been abundantly documented as causing diabeteslike disease in mice (Craighead and McLane, 1968; Craighead and Steinke, 1971), but little is known of its pathogenic capacity in humans. When serum from 41 patients from the Washington, D.C., area with IDDM of varying duration (< 1 month to > 1 year, mean time 2.68 years) were assayed for antibody to EMC virus, 5 (12%) showed slight elevations compared to 4 of 66 (6%) of nondiabetic controls. The limited number of patients in this study precludes the evaluation of these results for an association with the EMC virus group. EMC virus does not appear to be more likely to cause IDDM in geographical areas in which EMC virus infections in humans are more prevalent. In a study in Panama (Craighead, 1981) where EMC virus infections are common, no association was found between IDDM and elevated EMC virus antibody titers.

C. Rubella Virus

1. Characteristics

Rubella or german measles virus belongs to the Togaviridae family, genus *Rubivirus*. The virus particles are roughly spherical and 50–75 nm in diameter. They contain a single-stranded RNA of approximately 4.5×10^6 daltons in an electrondense core enclosed in an envelope covered with short projections on the surface. Replication takes place in the infected cell cytoplasm. The progeny viruses are released by budding from the cell surface. Generally rubella virus infections do not product noticeable cytopathic effects in tissue culture cell lines. In primary human amnionic cells, however, rounding of the cells, appearance of ameboid cells, and sloughing will occur 5–6 weeks after initial infection with the virus (Freeman, 1979; Ginsberg, 1980).

2. Clinicopathogenic Features

The incubation period for rubella infections is usually 14–21 days. Prior to the use of rubella vaccine, epidemics occurred every 6–9 years and approximately 80% of the population of the United States had antibody to the virus. Infections usually occurred in the spring (Nelson, 1979).

Humans are apparently the only known natural host. Spread of the virus occurs through oral droplets and in congenital rubella by transplacental transmission. In children, both sexes are equally at risk and the disease is most prevalent in the 5–14-year ago group. The disease in childhood is frequently mild. It is characterized mainly by a rash similar to that of rubeola and scarlet fever and is accompanied by enlargement of the postoccipital, retroauricular, and posterior cervical lymph nodes. In adults and older children, the disease may also involve the joints and cause purpura. Complications are rare in childhood rubella although neuritis, arthritis, and encephalitis have been described (Glasgow and Overall, 1979).

Rubella infection in early pregnancy was first recognized as a cause of congenital deformities in the offspring by Gregg in 1941. The mother acquires the infection through the respiratory tract and, after local virus replication, the virus is spread throughout the body. The placenta may be one target organ and may, in turn, serve as a source of the virus for the fetus. The incidence of infection in fetuses less than 8 weeks' of age exposed to material rubella is 50–80%. The incidence decreases to 10–20% in the second trimester and is relatively uncommon during the last trimester. Multiple organs can be involved. The virus can directly lyse infected cells, or can inhibit cell growth and cause chromosomal damage. Infection in the fetus is usually chronic. Virus can be isolated from the nasopharynx, urine, cerbrospinal fluid, stool, eye, bone marrow and peripheral leukocytes for periods as long as 12–18 months (Alford, 1976; Glasgow and Overall, 1979).

3. Association

There is no evidence that IDDM results from childhood infections of rubella virus. Seroepidemiologic studies of IDDM patients and nondiabetic identical twin siblings demonstrate identical antibody titers in both groups (Nelson *et al.*, 1975b). In a separate study of 43 patients with recent onset IDDM, no rise in antibody titers to rubella virus was noted (West *et al.*, 1981).

Although evidence is lacking for a rubella virus etiology in IDDM when the virus is contracted in childhood, there is an increasing association between congenital rubella (CR) infections and diabetes. Since Hay (1949) first described a case involving a child with CR and IDDM, 48 more cases have been described (Halvorson, 1977; Forest *et al.*, 1969; Forest *et al.*, 1971; Plotkin and Kaye, 1970; Johnson and Tudor, 1970; Cooper, 1975; Ziring, 1977; Patterson *et al.*, 1981; Smithells *et al.*, 1978; Floret *et al.*, 1980; Menser *et al.*, 1967; Menser *et al.*, 1974). Of this number, 13 had a known family history of diabetes. In the remainder, either no family history of the disease was known or none reported. The mothers most frequently contracted rubella infections in the first trimester of pregnancy as would be expected for CR. The patients were usually in the lower third percentile for height and/or weight and showed multiple and severe defects such as deafness, cardiovascular defects, cataracts, diabetic nephropathy, and diabetic retinopathy. Males were predominately affected (15 males compared to 9 females). The mean age of IDDM onset was 9.2 years (range, 18 months–28 years).

In one study, 45 CR patients were investigated. (Menser *et al.*, 1974). Of this number, 18 (40%) comprised of 10 males and 8 females developed overt or latent (abnormal glucose tolerance) IDDM. Half of the diabetic CR patients had HLA B8, an antigen frequently associated with IDDM. There was also an increase in HLA A1. This HLA type, while not associated with IDDM, is increased in patients with CR.

In one instance the virus was isolated from the children after birth. A boy with a family history of diabetes was born to a mother who contracted rubella during the first week of gestation (Plotkin and Kaye, 1970). The child had cardiovascular defects at birth. Rubella virus was isolated from a nasopharyngeal swab at age 2 months and his antibody titers increased from 1/16 to 1/32 between the 8th and 13th months. The child developed IDDM at 12 months of age. This and other studies (Menser *et al.*, 1974) demonstrate that diabetes may take a considerable time to develop after initial virus exposure. As stated earlier, rubella virus is not always cytopathic to infected cells but can result in chronic infection. In one instance, the virus was isolated from the urine of a 29-year-old woman with CR (Nelson, 1979). Chronic viral infections may result in accumulative beta cell damage, or deplete beta cell reserves so that subsequent infections or exposure to diabetogenic chemicals induce overt diabetes. That CR can predispose the patient for IDDM caused by another agent may be illustrated in another case reported by Plotkin and Kaye (1970). In this boy, no rubella virus was isolated and the child appeared normal at birth. The mother had contracted the infection at 13 weeks' gestation which was later than with most CR/IDDM patients. The patient first developed IDDM at 19 months of age, shortly after a respiratory illness. At that time, he was also shown to have an elevated antibody titer to rubella virus. The cause of the respiratory illness was not identified.

4. Virological and Histopathologic Studies

The studies described above suggest a relationship between CR and IDDM, but do not demonstrate that rubella virus can infect pancreatic tissue. Bunnell and Monif (1972) reported the autopsy findings from a girl with CR who died at 3½ months of age with congenital heart disease and bronchopneumonia. At autopsy, extensive lymphocytic infiltration in the interstitial and periglandular pancreatic tissue was found. The presence of the lymphocytic infiltrate suggested pancreatic infection. However, since no attempt was made to identify the virus, the histopathology provides only circumstantial evidence of rubella virus infection in the pancreas.

Despite the lack of direct evidence of rubella infection of human beta cells, it has been shown that tissues from CR patients contain the virus for extended periods. Rawls and colleagues (1965) attempted to establish tissue culture lines of autopsy material from 68 neonates dying with CR. The tissues used included thyroid, umbilicus, lung, bone marrow, and kidney. Eleven tissue culture lines were established, and 10 of the lines were shown to be infected with rubella. Chronically infected cells were not lysed, but showed morphological aberrations, pleomorphism, and growth inhibition (Rawls and Melnick, 1966).

D. Herpesviruses

Herpesviruses, a family of ubiquitous DNA viruses which includes cytomegalovirus, herpes simplex, varicella zoster, and Epstein–Barr virus, have been incriminated as pathogens in IDDM on rare occasions.

Several histopathological studies in adults and children with disseminated or congenital cytomegalovirus (CMV) infection have convincingly demonstrated islet cell lesions, including both typical intranuclear inclusions and mild insulitis. Jenson et al. (1980) reported islet cell damage in 20 of 45 cases of fatal cytomegalovirus infection and earlier reports by Smith and Vellios (1950) and Hultquist et al. (1973) described and illustrated similar lesions. However, the significance of CMV in initiating diabetes is doubtful, since only one case of IDDM has been reported, in a 13-month-old child with congenital cytomegalovirus infection (Ward et al., 1979). This association could well be coincidental. Similarly only one case of IDDM following infectious mononucleosis has been described (Burgess et al., 1974). Although the temporal relationship between diabetes onset and infection was impressive, the association was probably due to chance.

Chickenpox, caused by varicella zoster virus, has occasionally been associated with the onset of IDDM. In John's series, four cases of diabetes occurred within 30 days after typical chickenpox (John, 1949). Cudworth et al. (1977) documented four cases of chickenpox preceding diabetes in their prospective study. Finally, in Gamble's retrospective survey 18 cases of chickenpox were reported to have occurred in the 6 months prior to diabetes onset (Gamble, 1980). The frequency of chickenpox did not exceed expected values for the population, however. Some histopathological studies of fatal varicella zoster infections have reported islet cell lesions. In the study of fatal viral illnesses performed by Jenson et al. (1980) 5 of 14 patients with varicella zoster infection exhibited pancreatic pathology. In two instances islet cell damage was noted and in three cases interstitial pancreatitis was described.

E. Miscellaneous Viruses

In the various epidemiologic surveys cited previously an assortment of common viral illnesses such as measles, polio, influenza, and infectious hepatitis have occurred in the weeks and months prior to diabetes onset. However, evidence linking these viruses to IDDM is lacking. One report may be noteworthy. In 1974 Adi reported an increased frequency of diabetes mellitus associated with an epidemic of infectious hepatitis in eastern Nigeria. These patients ranged in age from 28 to 47 years and in each case the symptoms of diabetes disappeared in a few months. Unfortunately, the specific virus responsible for hepatitis in these patients was not identified and the relevance of this report to the relationship of viruses to IDDM is doubtful.

IV. MECHANISMS OF VIRUS-INDUCED BETA CELL INJURY

A. Virus-Mediated Cytolysis

There are several possible mechanisms of beta cell injury in IDDM having a viral etiology. The most obvious of these is direct virus-mediated destruction of infected cells. Although a number of viruses have been implicated in diabetes, RNA viruses predominate. These viruses can be divided into lytic, nonbudding viruses such as picornaviruses and budding viruses such as mumps and rubella viruses. To understand how viruses cause direct beta cell damage, it is important to understand their infection and replication cycles.

1. Picornaviruses

Picornaviruses are small viruses (28–30nm) composed of a single strand of RNA of 2.5×10^6 to 2.8×10^6 daltons. The icosahedral viral capsid which surrounds the RNA is comprised of four different polypeptides. These are designated VP 1, VP 2, VP 3, and VP 4 and have molecular weights ranging from 8×10^3 to 37×10^3. The earliest stage in the virus replication cycle is adsorption of the virus to a specific receptor on the cell surface. The host and cell range for susceptibility to infection by a specific virus is determined by these receptors. With the adsorption of the virus to the cell, the capsid apparently undergoes structural alteration with the loss of one of the virus proteins (VP 4). Any virus eluted from the cell at this point is no longer infectious.

After adsorption, the virus enters an eclipse period when no infectious virus and generally no virus-specific proteins or RNA are detectable. During this phase, the virus penetrates into the cytoplasm of the cell. The RNA is uncoated from the capsid and is replicated. Within 3–4 hr after infection, the virus RNA has succeeded in suppressing all host cell protein synethesis. At this time virus-specific protein and RNA synthesis in the cytoplasm of the host cell is maximal. The first cause of hypoinsulinemia in the infected individual may not be the lysis of the beta cell, but rather virus-directed suppression of insulin production.

The viral RNA acts as a messenger RNA and is translated from the 5′ end of the molecule into a single large protein with a molecular weight of $2–3 \times 10^5$ daltons. Cleavage of this macroprotein results in 12 smaller proteins. These proteins include the four structural (capsid) proteins, a 4×10^4-dalton protease for cleaving future macroproteins, and an RNA polymerase. Replication of the RNA begins when sufficient polymerase is formed. Transcription proceeds from the 3′ end of the molecule. The viral RNA (plus strand) is transcribed into complimentary minus strands. These minus strands may then be used as templates for the formation of progeny viral plus strands to be encapsulated into new virus particles (Joklik, 1980).

The assembly of the virus is presumed to proceed first by aggregation of the virus proteins into the capsid structure called the procapsid. RNA becomes incorporated into the procapsid and, following proteolytic cleavage of some of the capsid proteins, the infectious virus particle is fully formed.

The infectious virus particles remain in the cytoplasm forming intracytoplasmic crystals. Release of the virus from infected cells occurs with the rupture of the cell membrane. It is not clear how rupture of the membrane is effected, but this state is presumably under virus control, since the time of lysis varies between different picornaviruses (Rekosh, 1978; Ginsberg, 1980).

2. Mumps and Rubella Viruses

Paramyxo- and togaviruses are spherical, envelope-covered viruses containing a single strand of RNA of approximately 5×10^6 daltons. As with picornaviruses, the replicative cycle of these viruses begins with adsorption of the viruses to receptors on the mammalian cell surface. The envelope of the virus fuses with the plasma membrane of the cell releasing the viral nucleocapsid into the cell cytoplasm. When the RNA of the togaviruses is uncoated, approximately two-thirds of it is translated into four proteins ranging in molecular weight from 6 to 8.6×10^4. Two of these proteins comprise the RNA-polymerase. This enzyme causes the production of two types of messenger RNA: a 42S RNA which becomes the progeny viral RNA and a smaller 26S RNA. The smaller RNA is translated approximately three times faster than the larger molecule and codes for the structural proteins (Joklik et al., 1980).

Paramyxovirus RNA is transcribed into a series of short complimentary RNA molecules which are separately translated into six proteins. These proteins include three envelope proteins and three nucleocapsid proteins (Ginsberg and Dulbecco, 1980).

The envelope proteins of both toga- and paramyxoviruses are incorporated into the cell plasma membrane, replacing host proteins. The RNA progeny strands are bound by nucleocapsid proteins and migrate to the cell membrane where the viral envelope proteins are embedded. Adhesion of the nucleocapsid to the cytoplasmic side of the cell membrane causes the membrane to curve out. The viral envelope eventually encloses the nucleocapsid and the new virion is free of the cell. This process does not require the death of the cell, and may result in chronic infections. In these cases, thousands of virus particles can be released from the cell each hour for many hours (Ginsberg and Dulbecco, 1980).

Isolates of mumps (Prince et al., 1978), coxsackie B3 (Yoon et al., 1978) and reo, type 3 (Yoon et al., 1981) viruses have been shown to infect human beta cells in vitro. In each case, insulin concentrations in the cells decrease rapidly beginning 24 hr after infection and are inversely related to virus concentration.

In addition to the epidemiologic evidence of a viral etiology in IDDM, the best evidence that viruses can cause diabeteslike illness comes from animal studies. Although early investigators demonstrated that foot-and-mouth disease virus (FMDV) induced diabetes in cattle (Barboni and Manocchi, 1962), considerable progress in experimental virus-induced diabetes occurred only after Craighead and McLane (1969) developed a reliable murine model for the disease. Their model used inbred DBA/2 mice and the M strain of encephalomyocarditis (EMC-M) virus. Virus could be demonstrated in the beta cells in the islets of Langerhans after infection of susceptible strains of mice by either intraperitoneal or subcutaneous inoculation. The earliest signs of infection in the beta cells were degranulation and decreased insulin content. Peak virus concentrations were obtained in the islets on the 3rd day after infection. Virus concentrations rapidly decreased thereafter, but could occasionally persist for several weeks (Craighead, 1981). Mononuclear cells began to infiltrate the islets by the 3rd or 4th day. Inflammation was generally transient, disappearing after the 2nd week. Hyperglycemia appeared concomitantly with inflammation.

There are four possible results of EMC-M virus infection. Most (60–80%) of the animals develop moderate hyperglycemia lasting from 1 week to several months. Approximately 10–15% of the animals develop chronic hyperglycemia lasting 6 or more months, while smaller numbers of animals die from the severity of the infection. Finally, some animals do not show any beta cell damage (Rayfield and Seto, 1981). The amount of variability in the outcome of infection is remarkable since only highly inbred mice are used. However, these results are not unlike the discordance in IDDM between identical twins infected with coxsackie B viruses (Nelson et al., 1975b).

The variability in diabetes induction subsequent to infection may result from host, environmental and virus factors. Not all viruses or variants of the same virus will infect beta cells equally. Thus, while the E variant of encephalomyocarditis virus is highly neurotropic and causes rapid death in infected mice, the M variant of the same virus infects the heart and islet cells producing diseases such as myocarditis and insulitis (Craighead, 1966). Similarly, wild type viruses such as reovirus (Yoon et al., 1981) and coxsackie B viruses (Yoon et al., 1977) which either do not infect cells in vivo or produce little or no damage, may be made highly diabetogenic by repeated passage of the viruses in vitro in beta cell cultures (Yoon et al., 1977).

The mechanism by which the tropism of virus for selected tissue changes is not known. One possible explanation is that the original virus preparation represents a pool of diabetogenic and nondiabetogenic viruses. The nondiabetogenic virus may inhibit infection of the beta cells by the diabetogenic strain either by competitively binding to the virus receptors on the cell, or by causing an enhanced immune or interferon response by the host which more efficiently eliminates the viruses. Such an inhibitory virus was found in EMC-M virus pools by Yoon et al. (1980) Passage of the viruses in beta cells may preferentially select for the diabetogenic strain. An alternate explanation for changing virus tropisms is that in vitro passage of the nondiabetogenic virus selects for mutant and recombinant viruses with enhanced efficiency of binding to and replication in beta cells (Yoon et al., 1981).

Besides genetic variations in the virus, the diabetogenic capacity of a virus depends upon the genetic constitution of the host. EMC-M virus is diabetogenic in DBA/2 and SJL inbred mouse strains, but fails to induce diabetes in other strains (Craighead, 1974; Boucher et al., 1975; Yoon et al., 1976). The inability of the virus to cause diabetes in nonsusceptible mice could result from the lack of viral receptors on the beta cells. Evidence to support this hypothesis was reported by Chairez *et al.* (1978). Nearly 10 times more virus was found in susceptible beta cells than in nonsusceptible cells. In addition, up to twice as much virus attached to the susceptible cell surface. With significantly fewer viral receptors on the beta cell, infection of these cells with EMC-M virus and resulting beta cell lysis and degranulization is less apt to occur. Interestingly, fibroblasts derived from susceptible and nonsusceptible mice have equivalent numbers of EMC virus receptors.

Despite the work described above, other investigators have not been able to demonstrate differences in virus attachment to the beta cells from susceptible and nonsusceptible animals (Wilson *et al.*, 1980). These investigators indicated that even nonsusceptible mice will become diabetic after EMC virus infection if placed under metabolic stress such as obesity (D'Andrea *et al.*, 1981). In this case, the investigators concluded that beta cells from both susceptible and nonsusceptible animals are equally susceptible to infection but that host factors influence the severity of the disease. Similar conclusions were reached by DaFoe *et al.* (1980) in studies where islets from nonsusceptible mice were transplanted into susceptible recipients. When the recipients of transplanted ''resistant'' islets were infected, the beta cells became necrotic and the animals developed diabetes, illustrating the importance of host factors in determining diabetes susceptibility.

B. Immune Mechanisms of Injury

Replication of lytic viruses such as coxsackie B and EMC viruses in the beta cells undoubtedly results in cellular death. However, virus replication alone may not cause sufficient damage to prove IDDM. Viral infections generally induce mononuclear cell infiltrates in the affected tissues. Schmidt (1902) was the first to describe such an infiltrate in the pancreas of a diabetic patient. Since then, a number of studies have shown lymphocytic infiltrations in the islets of patients with recent onset diabetes (Warren, 1927; Perlman, 1961; Gepts, 1965; LeCompte, 1958; Junker *et al.*, 1977) as well as in individuals with known viral infections in the islets of the pancreas but no diabetes (Jenson *et al.*, 1980). The lymphoid cells in the islets may function in eliminating the virus and limiting cellular damage, therefore protecting rather than harming the beta cells. Alternatively, the lymphoid cells may become sensitized to beta cell surface antigens resulting in autoimmune destruction of the beta cells. IDDM is associated with autoimmune endocrine disorders such as pernicious anemia, Hashimoto's thyroiditis, chronic thyroiditis, and primary hypothyroidism with greater than expected incidence (Perlman, 1961; Battazzo and Lendrum, 1976; Irvine *et al.*, 1970; Nerup and Binder, 1973).

Evidence for an immune etiology in IDDM comes from both clinical and experimental systems. Lymphocytes from diabetic patients are significantly more adherent and cytolytic to human insulinoma cells and pancreas preparations *in vitro* than lymphocytes from nondiabetic individuals (Huang and McLaren, 1976; Richens *et al.*, 1976). However, the strongest evidence that lymphoid cells have an important role in the etiology of IDDM comes from animal models. T-lymphocyte-deficient mice (Buschard *et al.*, 1976) and mice immunosuppressed by treatment with irradiation

(Jansen *et al.*, 1977; Jansen *et al.*, 1979) fail to develop hyperglycemia following infection with EMC virus even though the virus is present in the islets.

T lymphocytes have a number of functions which may be involved in induction of IDDM-like disease in mice. First, T lymphocytes act as helper cells for IgG production. The antibody can either cause direct lysis of beta cells in the presence of complement, or cause lysis by antibody-dependent cell-mediated cytolysis in the presence of K cells (Kim *et al.*, 1980). Islet cell antibodies directed against a cytoplasmic antigen are characteristically found in the serum of IDDM patients at the time of diagnosis. These antibodies may be markers for susceptibility preceding the development of overt clinical manifestations. One report has described the occurrence of islet cell antibodies following mumps infection, but this observation has not been confirmed. Onodera *et al.* (1978) have described the formation of islet cell antibodies in inbred mice infected with reovirus type 1. In contrast to human ICA, these antibodies appeared to be directed against hormones such as insulin.

Since antibodies do not penetrate cells efficiently, it is unlikely that ICA produce beta cell cytotoxicity *in vitro*. However, Lernmark and his colleagues (1978) and Doberson *et al.* (1980) have demonstrated that sera from IDDM patients also contain antibodies which are cytolytic for rat beta cells in the presence of complement.

The relationship between the induction of beta cell antibodies and virus infections has not been explored. However, since similar antibodies are also identified in the sera of nondiabetic relatives, it is unlikely that islet cell surface antibodies alone are capable of causing IDDM.

A second function of T cells is cell-mediated cytolysis of virus-infected target cells (Huber *et al.*, 1980). These effector cells are either directly lytic or produce lymphokines which activate nonspecific cytolytic mechanisms (Walker *et al.*, 1976; Ruddle, 1979). Chemotactic, macrophage-activating and migration-inhibition factors may concentrate activated macrophages in the islets where phagocytosis and release of cytotoxic molecules could promote cytolysis of the beta cells (Fidler, 1975; Evans and Alexander, 1971; Pague *et al.*, 1978; Burch *et al.*, 1971).

T-cell-mediated antiviral cytotoxicity is HLA-restricted, providing hypothetical explanation for the skewed distribution of HLA antigens observed in IDDM. For example, McMichael (1978) has demonstrated that the activity of cytotoxic T cells developed in response to influenza virus infection varies considerably according to which histocompatibility antigens are shared by the effector and target cells. In these experiments, failure to lyse target cells was freqently observed when HLA A2, A3, and B44 were shared, whereas lysis was regularly demonstrated when B7 and B8 were matched. Experiments exploring the relevance of this phenonenon to immune-mediated destruction of virus-infected B cells have not been reported.

Natural killer (NK) cells activated by interferon or other immunoregulatory molecules could also be important in causing beta cell injury (Santoli and Koproski, 1979). The eradication of virus-infected targets by NK cells is not HLA-restricted (Huber *et al.*, 1981). However, several investigators have reported that cytotoxicity is least efficient when effector lymphocytes from donors possess HLA B7 (Santoli *et al.*, 1976). It is interesting that B7 is encountered infrequently in IDDM, but the connection, if any, between these observations is unknown and the significance of NK cell activity in diabetes is not defined.

V. CONCLUSIONS

Any unifying hypothesis concerning the etiology of IDDM must take into account the unique genetic, epidemiologic, and immunological characteristics of diabetes described earlier in this chapter. Genetic factors clearly play a pivotal role in determining susceptibility to diabetes. However, since discordance for diabetes in monozygotic twins is amply documented, environmental factors must also be crucial to disease expression.

Although toxins, hormonal imbalances, and abnormal metabolic responses to stress could all contribute to the development of overt diabetes, the hypothesis disease incidence, the close temporal relationship between acute febrile illnesses and symptomatic diabetes, and the morphological characteristics of the insular lesion are all compatible with a viral etiology.

In experimental mice the M variant of EMC virus causes a diabetic syndrome which closely resembles IDDM in humans. Although there is no evidence to suggest that EMC viruses *per se* are important pathogens in diabetes, this experimental model lends credence to the possibility that viruses can infect human beta cells *in vivo* and destroy them.

If viruses do cause IDDM, which virus is the culprit? As pointed out by Craighead (1975), the pancreas is susceptible to infection with an impressive variety of viruses. Quite possibly more than one virus is capable of triggering the sequence of events culminating in diabetes. Among the most likely candidates are mumps, rubella, and the coxsackieviruses. The evidence linking mumps virus to diabetes is circumstantial but, taken as a whole, quite persuasive. The well-documented temporal relationship between mumps infection and diabetes onset and the excessive number of mumps cases recorded in the 6 months prior to the development of diabetes support this hypothesis. Nonetheless, mumps alone could not possible account for more than a small proportion of diabetes cases even when subclinical infections are taken into consideration. Similarly, the increased frequency of diabetes in patients with congenital rubella indicates that these two entities are somehow related. However, there is no evidence to suggest that postnatal rubella infections are implicated in IDDM.

The best evidence that viruses have a causal relationship to the onset of IDDM is derived from investigations of coxsackie B virus infections. Symptomatic diabetes associated with serological evidence of recent coxsackie B virus infection has been documented on several occasions and in two cases coxsackie B4 virus has been localized to pancreatic tissue from diabetic patients. Moreover, injection of coxsackieviruses into susceptible mice produced a diabeteslike illness. Although some seroepidemiologic studies suggest that coxsackievirus infections could be implicated in as many as 60% of diabetes cases, conflicting data failing to show any such relationship have been reported as well. Additional prospective studies are necessary to determine the extent to which coxsackieviruses are implicated in IDDM.

Several difficulties hamper the interpretation of the studies reported to date. One of the most serious problems is that the IDDM patient population is undoubtedly heterogeneous. Different susceptibility factors such as HLA phenotypes, age, sex, season of disease onset, family history of diabetes, or autotoimmune polyendocrinopathy, to name a few, may be operative in subsets of patients whose disease results from entirely different pathogenetic mechanisms. Serological studies comparing geometric mean antibody titers in patients and controls are particularly subject to this sort of difficulty, since the majority of IDDM patients possess either B8, DRW3 or B15, DRW4. In view of the involvement of the major histocompatibility complex in immune responsiveness, it is not unlikely that hyperresponsiveness to some antigens could be associated with certain HLA phenotypes. If these phenotypes are overrepresented in the patient population, spurious associations with raised antiviral antibody titers could result. Clearly, more refined stratification of patients and controls must be employed to avoid these difficulties. Conceivably, prospective family studies involving nondiabetic HLA-typed first-degree relatives of IDDM patients could provide more meaningful information regarding the significance of viruses than that currently available.

Interpreting the studies to date is also hampered by the fact that the duration of the "latent" period between initial beta cell injury and the appearance of carbohydrate intolerance is imprecisely defined. If this time interval is measured in months or years (as suggested by the work of Cudworth *et al.*, 1977) or if IDDM is the end result of repetitive beta cell insults, it will be difficult to relate disease onset to a single cause in most cases. Furthermore, the development of IDDM may be influenced by poorly defined hormonal and metabolic responses to stress that are impossible to control.

A final pitfall stems from observations in experimental diabetes demonstrating that serologically identical viruses differ in their ability to cause diabetes. In fact, infection with nondiabetogenic variants of these viruses protects against diabetes induction. Whether diabetogenic variants of common human viruses exist in nature is unknown, but is certainly within the realm of possibility.

In view of these difficulties it is not surprising that the relationship between virus infections and diabetes mellitus remains poorly defined. During the past decade, however, advances in our understanding of the genetic factors influencing diabetes susceptibility, identification of candidate diabetogenic viruses, and characterization of the immunological abnormalities found in the pre- and postdiabetic state have provided important tools with which to determine more precisely the significance of viruses in diabetes. In 1927 Gunderson posed the question "Is diabetes of infectious origin?" For some individuals this question can be confidently answered in the affirmative. It remains for future studies to determine the frequency and mechanisms by which viral illnesses lead to the development of IDDM.

REFERENCES

Adams, S. F., 1926, The seasonal variation in the onset of acute diabetes: The age and sex factors in 1000 diabetic patients, *Arch. Intern Med.,* **37**:861–864.

Adi, F. C., 1974, Diabetes mellitus associated with epidemic of infectious hepatitis in Nigeria, *Br. Med. J.* **1**:183–185.

Alford, Jr., C. A., 1976, Rubella, in: *Infectious Diseases of the Fetus and Newborn Infant* (J. S. Remington and J. O. Klein, eds.), pp. 71–106, W. B. Saunders, Philadelphia.

Barbieri, V., 1909, Pancreatite subacuta e glicosuria secondairie a parotite epeidemica, *Gaz Osped.* **30:** 273, 1909.

Barboni, E., and Manocchi, I., 1962, Alterazionia pancreatiche in bovini con diabete mellito post-aftoso, *Arch. Vet. Ital.* **13:**477–489.

Barbosa, J., King, R., and Noreen, H. 1977, The histocompatibility system in juvenile, insulin-dependent diabetic multiplex kindreds, *J. Clin. Invest.* **60:**989–998.

Battazzo, G. F., Florino Christensen, A., and Doniach, A., 1974, Islet cell antibodies in diabetes mellitus with autoimmune polyendocrine deficiencies, *Lancet* **2:**1279–1283.

Baum, S. G. and Litman, M., 1979, Mumps virus, in: *Principles and Practice of Infectious Diseases* (G. L. Mandell, R. G. Douglas, and J. E. Bennett, eds.), pp. 1176–1185, John Wiley, New York.

Block, M. B., Berk, J. E., Fridhandler, L. S., Steiner, D. F., and Rubenstein, A. H., 1973, Diabetic ketoacidosis associated with mumps virus infection, *Ann. Intern. Med.* **78:**663–667.

Bloom, A., Hayes, T. M., and Gamble, D. R., 1975, Register of newly diagnosed diabetic children, *Br. Med. J.* **3:**580–583.

Bostrom, K., 1968, Pathoanatomical findings in a case of mumps with pancreatis, myocarditis, orchitis, epididymitis, and seminal vesiculitis, *Virchows Arch. Pathol. Anat.* **344:**111–117.

Boucher, D. W., Hayashi, K., Rosenthal, J., and Notkins, A. L., 1975, Virus induced diabetes mellitus. III. Influence of sex and strain of the host, *J. Infect. Dis.* **131:**462–466.

Bunnell, C. E., and Monif, G. R. G., 1972, Interstitial pancreatitis in the congenital rubella syndrome, *J. Pediatr.* **80:** 465–466.

Burgess, J. A., Kirkpatrick, K. L., and Menser, M. A., 1974, Fulminant onset of diabetes mellitus during an attack of infectious mononucleosis, *Med. J. Aust.* **2:**706–707.

Burch, G. E., Tsui, C-Y, Harb, J. M., and Colcolough, H. L., 1971, Pathologic findings in the pancreas of mice infected with coxsackievirus B4, *Arch. Intern. Med.* **128:**40–47.

Buschard, K., Rygaard, J., and Lund, E., 1976, The inability of diabetogenic virus to induce diabetes mellitus in athymic (nude) mice, *Acta Pathol. Microbiol. Scand.[C]* **84:**299–303.

Centers for Disease Control, 1980, Mumps vaccine: Recommendation of the Immunization Practices Advisory Committee, *Ann. Intern. Med.* **92:**803–804.

Chairez, R., Yoon, J.-W. and Notkins, A. L., 1978, Virus-induced diabetes mellitus. X. Attachment of encephalomyocarditis virus and permissiveness of cultured pancreatic B cells to infection, *Virology,* **85:**606–611.

Champsaur, H., Dussaux, E., Samolyk, D., Fabre, M., Bach, C. H., and Assan, R., 1980, Diabetes and coxsackie virus B5 infection, *Lancet* **1:**251.

Christau, B., Dromann, H., and Andersen, O. O., 1977, Incidence, seasonal, and geographical patterns of juvenile onset, insulin-dependent diabetes in Denmark, *Diabetologia,* **13:**281–284.

Cole, L., 1933, Pancreatitis in mumps, *Br. Med. J.* **1:**1080.

Cole, L., 1934, Diabetes mellitus in children, *Lancet* **1:947–950.**

Cooper, L. Z., 1975, *Infections of the Fetus and Newborn Infant,* Alan R. Liss, New York.

Craighead, J. E., 1966, Pathogenicity of the M and E variants of the encephalomyocarditis (EMC) virus. II. Lesions of the pancreas, parotid and lacrimal glands, *Am. J. Pathol.* **48:375–386.**

Craighead, J. E., and McLane, M. F. B., 1968, Diabetes mellitus. Induction in mice by encephalomyocarditis virus, *Science* **162:**913–914.

Craighead, J. E., and Steinke, J., 1971, Diabetes mellitus-like syndrome in mice infected with encephalomyocarditis virus, *Am. J. Pathol.* **63:**119–134.

Craighead, J. E. and Higgins, D. A., 1974, Genetic influences affecting the occurrence of a diabetes mellitus like disease in mice infected with the encephalomyocarditis virus, *Jr. Exp. Med.,* **139:**414–426.

Craighead, J. E., 1975, The role of viruses in the pathogenesis of pancreatic disease and diabetes mellitus, *Prog. Med. Virol.* **19:**161–214.

Cudworth, A. G., and Woodrow, J. C., 1975a, Evidence for HL-A-linked genes in "juvenile" diabetes mellitus, *Br. Med. J.* **3:**133–135.

Cudworth, A. G., and Woodrow, J. C., 1975b, HLA system and diabetes mellitus, *Diabetes* **24:**345–349.

Cudworth, A. G., White, G. B. B., Woodrow, J. C., Gambel, D. R., Lendrum, R., and Bloom, A., 1977, A etiology of juvenile-onset diabetes. A prospective study, *Lancet,* **1:**385–388.

Curnen, E. C., 1979, Enterovirus infections, in: *Textbook of Pediatrics* (W. E. Nelson, V. C. Vaughan III, R. J. McKay Jr., and R. E. Behrman, eds.), pp. 914–926, W. B. Saunders, Philadelphia.

Dacou-Voutetakis, C. D., Constantinidis, M., and Moschos, A., 1974, Diabetes mellitus following mumps, *Am. J. Dis. Child.* 127:890–891.

DaFoe, D. C., Naji, A., Plotkin, S. A., and Barker, C. F., 1980, Susceptibility to diabetogenic virus: Host versus pancreatic factors, *J. Surg. Res.* 28:338–347.

Daldorf, G., 1950, Coxackie viruses, *Bull. N. Y. Acad. Med.* 26:329–335.

D'Andrea, B. J., Wilson, G. L., and Craighead, J. E., 1981, Effect of genetic obesity in mice on the induction of diabetes by encephalomyocarditis virus, *Diabetes* 30:451–454.

Dick, J. S., 1934, Pancreatitis in mumps, *Br. Med. J.* 2:35.

Di Pietro, C., Del Guercia, M. J., Paolino, G. P., Barbi, M., Ferrante, P., and Chiumello, G., 1979, Type I diabetes and coxsackie virus infection, *Helv. Paediatr. Acta* 34:557–561.

Dippe, S. E., Miller, M., Bennett, P. H., and Maynard, J. E., 1975, Lack of causal association between coxsackie B-4 virus infection and diabetes, *Lancet* 1:1314–1317.

Doberson, M. J., Scharff, J. E., Ginsberg-Fellner, F., and Notkins, A. L., 1980, Cytotoxic autoantibodies to beta cells in the serum of patients with insulin-dependent diabetes mellitus, *N. Engl. J. Med.* 303:1493–1498.

El-Hagrassy, M. M. O., and Banatvala, J. E., 1980, Coxsackie B-virus specific IgM responses in patients with cardiac and other diseases, *Lancet* 2:1160–1162.

Evans, R. and Alexander, P. L., 1971, Rendering macrophages specifically cytotoxic by a factor released by immune lymphoid cells, *Transplantation* 12:227–229.

Farnam, L. W., 1922, Pancreatitis following mumps: Report of a case with operation, *Am. J. Med. Sci.* 163:859–870.

Fidler, I. J., 1975, Activation in vitro of mouse macrophages by syngeneic, allogeneic, or xenogeneic lymphocyte supernatants, *J. Natl. Cancer Inst.* 55:1159–1163.

Floret, D., Rosenberg, D., Hage, G. N., and Monnet, P., 1980, Hyperthyroidism, diabetes mellitus, and the congenital rubella syndrome, *Acta Paediatr. Scand.*, 69:259–261.

Forrest, J. M., Menser, M. A., and Harley, S. S, 1969, Diabetes mellitus and congenital rubella, *Pediatrics*, 44:445–446.

Forrest, J. M., Menser, M. A., and Burgess, J. A. 1971, High frequency of diabetes mellitus young adults with congenital rubella, *Lancet* 2:332–334.

Freeman, A. G., 1962, Mumps followed by diabetes, *Lancet* 2:96.

Freeman, B. A., 1979, *Textbook of Microbiology*, W. B. Saunders, Philadelphia.

Gamble, D. R., 1980a, Relation of antecedent illness to development of diabetes in children, *Br. Med. J.* 281:99–101.

Gamble, D. R., 1980b, The epidemiology of insulin dependent diabetes with reference to the relationship of virus infection to its etiology, *Epidemiol. Rev.*, 2:49–70.

Gamble, D. R., and Taylor, K. W., 1969, Seasonal incidence of diabetes mellitus, *Br. Med. J.*, 3:631–633.

Gamble, D. R., Kinsley, M. L., Fitzgerald, M. G., Bolton, R., and Taylor, D. W., 1969, Viral antibodies in diabetes mellitus, *Br. Med. J.* 3:627–630.

Gamble, D. R., Taylor, K. W., and Cumming, H., 1973, Coxsackie viruses and diabetes mellitus, *Br. Med. J.* 4:260–262.

Garavoy, M. R., Barbosa, J., Reddish, M., Martin, S., Norcen, H., Yunis, E. J., and Carpenter, C. B., 1978, HLA-DR antigens and unique serological reactions in juvenile-onset diabetes mellitus, *Transplant Proc.* 10:967–969.

Gepts, W., 1965, Pathologic anatomy of the pancreas in juvenile diabetes mellitus, *Diabetes* 14:619–633.

Gepts, W., and DeMey, J., 1978, Islet cell survival determined by morphology. An immunocytochemical study of the islets of Langerhans in juvenile diabetes mellitus, *Diabetes* 27:251–261.

Gilhespy, F. B., and Holden, H. S., 1917, Grave diabetes mellitus with pulmonary tuberculosis following mumps, *Br. Med. J.*, 2:115.

Ginsberg, H. S., 1969, Picornaviruses, in: *Microbiology* (Davis, B. D., Dulbecco, R., Eisen, H. N., Ginsberg, H. S., and Wood, W. B., eds.), pp. 1095–1118, Harper and Row, New York.

Ginsberg, H. S., and Dulbecco, R., 1980, Multiplication and genetics of animal viruses, in: *Microbiology*, 3rd edition (Davis, B. D., Dulbecco, R., Eisen, H. N., and Ginsberg, H. S., eds.), pp. 967–999, Harper and Row, Hagerstown, MD.

Glasgow, L. A., and Overall Jr., J. C., 1979, Infections, in: *Textbook of Pediatrics* (W. E. Nelson, V. C. Vaughan III, R. J. McKay Jr., and R. G. Behrman, eds.), pp. 483–485, W. B. Saunders, Philadelphia.

Gorsuch, A. N., Lister, J., Dean, B. M., Spencer, K. M., McNally, J. M., and Bottazzo, G. F., 1981, Evidence for along prediabetic period in type I (insulin-dependent) diabetes mellitus, *Lancet* **1**:1363–1365.

Gundersen, E., 1927, Is diabetes of infectious origin?, *J. Infec. Dis.*, **41**:197–202.

Halvorson, E. P., 1977, Diabetes mellitus and congenital rubella: Report of a case, *Mt. Sinai J. Med.* **44**:566–567.

Handwerger, B. S., Fernandes, G., and Brown, D. M., 1980, Immune and autoimmune aspects of diabetes mellitus, *Hum. Pathol.* **11**:338–352.

Harris, H. F., 1899, A case of diabetes mellitus quickly following mumps, *Boston Med. Surg. J.* **140**:465–469.

Hay, D. R., 1949, Studies in preventive hygiene from the Otago Medical School. I. The relation of maternal rubella to congenital deafness and other abnormalities in New Zealand, *N.Z. Med. J.* **48**:604–608.

Helmke, K., Otten, A., and Willerus, W., 1980, Islet cell antibodies in children with mumps infection, *Lancet* **2**:211–212.

Henle, G., Henle, W., Wendell, K. K., and Rosenberg, P., 1948, Isolation of mumps virus from human beings with induced apparent or inapparent infections, *J. Exp. Med.* **88**:223–232.

Hierholzer, J. C., and Farris, W. A., 1974, Follow-up of children infected in a Coxsackievirus B-3 and B-4 outbreak: No evidence of diabetes mellitus, *J. Infect. Dis.*, **129**:741–746.

Hinden, E., 1962, Mumps followed by diabetes, *Lancet* **1**:1381.

Huang, S. -W., and Maclaren, N. K., 1976, Insulin-dependent diabetes: A disease of autoaggression, *Science*, **192**:64–66.

Huber, S. A., Job, L. P., and Woodruff, J. F., 1980, Lysis of infected myofibers by Coxsackievirus B-3-immune T lymphocytes, *Am. J. Pathol.* **98**:681–694.

Huber, S. A., Job, L. P., and Woodruff, J. F., 1981, Sex-related differences in the pattern of Coxsackievirus B-3-induced immune spleen cell cytotoxicity against virus-infected myofibers, *Infect. Immun.* **32**:68–73.

Huff, J. C., Hierholzer, J. D., and Farris, W. A., 1974, An "outbreak" of juvenile diabetes mellitus: Consideration of a viral etiology, *Am. J. Epidemiol.* **100**:277–287.

Hulquist, G., Nordvall, S., and Sundstrom, C., 1973, Insulitis in cytomegalovirus infection in a newborn infant, *Ups. J. Med. Sci.* **78**:139–144.

Irvine, W. J., Clark, B. F., Scarth, L., Cullen, D. R., and Duncan, L. J. P., 1970, Thyroid and gastric autoimmunity in patients with diabetes mellitus, *Lancet* **2**:163–168.

Jansen, F. K., Muntefering, H., and Schmidt, W. A. K., 1977, Virus induced diabetes mellitus and the immune system. I. Suggestion that appearance of diabetes depends on immune reactions, *Diabetologia* **13**:545–549.

Jansen, F. K., Thurnezssen, O., and Muntefering, H., 1979, Virus induced diabetes and the immune system. II. Evidence for an immune pathogenesis of the acute phase of diabetes, *Biomedicine* **31**:1–2.

Jenson, A. B., Rosenberg, H. S., and Notkins, A. L., 1980, Pancreatic islet cell damage in children with fatal virus infections, *Lancet* **2**:354–358.

John, H. J., 1934, The diabetic child: Etiologic factors, *Ann. Intern. Med.* **8**:198–213.

John, H. J., 1949, Diabetes mellitus in children, *J. Pediatr.* **35**:723–744.

Johnson, G. M., and Tudor, R. B., 1980, Diabetes mellitus and congenital rubella infection, *Am. J. Dis. Child.* **120**:453–455.

Joklik, W. K., 1980, The virus multiplication cycle, in: *Zinsser Microbiology* (W. K. Joklik, H. Willet, and D. B. Amos, eds.), pp. 1040–1086, Appleton-Century-Crofts, New York.

Junker, K., Egeberg, J., Kromann, H., 1977, An autopsy study of the islets of Langerhans in acute-onset juvenile diabetes mellitus, *Acta Pathol. Microbiol. Scand. [A]* **85**:699–706.

Kahana, D., and Brant, M., 1967, Diabetes in an infant following inapparent mumps. *Clin. Pediatr.* **6**:124–125.

Kim, Y. B., Huh, N. D., Koren, H. S., and Amos, D. B., 1980, Natural killing (NK) and antibody-dependent cellular cytotoxicity (ADCC) in specific pathogen-free (SPF) miniature swine and germ free piglets. I. Comparison of NK and ADCC, *J. Immunol.* **125**:753–762.

King, R. C., 1962, Mumps followed by diabetes, *Lancet* **2**:1055.

Kremer, H. U., 1947, Juvenile diabetes as a sequel to mumps, *Am. J. Med.* **3**:257–258.

LeCompte, P. M., 1958, "Insulitis" in early juvenile diabetes, *Arch. Pathol.*, **66**:450–457.

LeCompte, P. M., and Gepts, W., 1977, The pathology of juvenile diabetes, in: *The Diabetic Pancreas* (B. W. Volk, and K. F. Wellmann, eds.), pp. 325–364, Plenum Press, New York.

Lemoine, L. G. H., and Lapassat, M. F., 1903, Un cas de pancreatite ourlienne avec autopsie, *Bull. Soc. Med. Hop., Paris* **24**:640–647.

Lerner, A. M., Wilson, F. M., and Reyes, M. P., 1975, Enteroviruses and the heart (with special emphasis upon the probable role of Coxsackieviruses, group B, types 1-5). I. Epidemiological and experimental studies, *Mod. Concepts Cardiovasc. Dis.* **44**:7–10.

Lernmark, A., Freedman, Z. R., Hofmann, C., Rubenstein, A. H., Steiner, D. F., Jackson, R. L., Winter, R. J., and Traisman, H. S., 1978, Islet cell surface antibodies in juvenile diabetes mellitus, *N. Engl. J. Med.* **299**:375–380.

Limper, M. A., and Miller, A. J., 1935, Diabetes mellitus with extensive gangrene in early infancy, *Am. J. Dis. Child.* **50**:1216–1230.

Madden, D. L., Fuccillo, D. A., Traub, R. G., Ley, A. C., Sever, J. L., and Beadle, E. L., 1978, Juvenile onset diabetes mellitus in pregnant women: Failure to associate with Coxsackie B1-6, mumps or respiratory syncytial virus infections, *J. Pediatr.* **92**:959–960.

Marcy, S. M., and Kibrick, S., 1977, Mumps, in: *Infectious Diseases,* 2nd ed., (P. D. Hoeprich, ed.), pp. 621–627, Harper and Row, Hagerstown, MD.

McCrae, W. M., 1963, Diabetes mellitus following mumps, *Lancet* **1**:1300–1301.

McMichael, A. J., 1978, HLA restriction of human cytotoxic T lymphocytes specific for influenza virus: Poor recognition of virus associated with HLA AZ, *J. Exp. Med.* **148**:1458–1467.

Melin, K., and Ursing, B., 1958, Diabetes mellitus som komplikation till parotitis epidemica, *Nord. Med.* **60**:1715–1716.

Menser, M. A., Dods, L., and Harley, J. D., 1967, A twenty-five year follow-up of congenital rubella, *Lancet* **2**:1347–1350.

Menser, M. A., Forrest, J. M., and Honeyman, M. C., 1974, Diabetes, HLA antigens and congenital rubella, *Lancet* **2**:1508–1509.

Messaritakis, J., Karabula, C., Kattamis, C., and Matserniotis, N., 1971, Diabetes following mumps in sibs, *Arch. Dis. Child.* **46**:561–562, 1971.

Nelson, P. G., Pyke, D. A., Cudworth, A. G., Woodrow, J. C., Batchelor, J. R., 1975a, Histocompatibility antigens in diabetic identical twins, *Lancet* **2**:193–194.

Nelson, P. G., Pyke, D. A., and Gamble, D. R., 1975b, Viruses and the etiology of diabetes: A study in identical twins, *Br. Med. J.* **4**:249–251.

Nerup, J., and Binder, C., 1973, Thyroid, gastric and adrenal autoimmunity in diabetes mellitus, *Acta Endocrinol.* **72**:279–286.

Nerup, J., Platz, P., Anderson, O. O., Christy, M., Lyngsoe, J., Poulson, J. E., Ryder, L. P., Thomsen, M., Staub Nielsen, L. S., and Svejgaard, A., 1974, HL-A antigens and diabetes mellitus, *Lancet* **2**:864–866, 1974.

Onodera, T., Jenson, A. B., Yoon, J. W., and Notkins, A. L., 1978, Virus induced diabetes mellitus. Reovirus infection of pancreatic B cells in mice, *Science* **201**:529–531.

Paque, R. E., Gauntt, C. J., Nealon, T. J., and Trousdale, M. P., 1978, Assessment of cell mediated hypersensitivity against Coxsackie virus B3 viral-induced myocarditis utilizing hypertonic extracts of cardiac tissue, *J. Immunol.* **120**:1672–1678.

Patrick, A., 1924, Acute diabetes following mumps, *Br. Med. J.* **2**:802.

Patterson, K., Chandra, R. S., and Bennett Jenson, A., 1981, Congenital rubella, insulitis, and diabetes mellitus in an infant, *Lancet* **1**:1048–1049.

Peig, M., Ercilla, G., Millan, M., Gomis, R., 1981, Post-mumps diabetes mellitus, *Lancet* **1**:1007.

Perlman, L. V., 1961, Familial incidence of diabetes in hyperthyroidism, *Ann. Intern. Med.* **55**:796–799.

Plotkin, S. A., and Kaye, R., 1970, Diabetes mellitus and congenital rubella, *Pediatrics* **46**:650–651.

Prince, G. A., Jenson, A. B., Billups, L. C., and Netkins, A. L., 1978, Infection of human pancreatic beta cell cultures with mumps virus, *Nature* **271**:158–161.

Rawls, W. E., Melnick, J. L., Rosenberg, H. S., and Bayatpoor, M., 1965, Spontaneous virus carrier cultures and postmortem isolation of virus from infants with congenital rubella, *Proc. Soc. Exp. Biol. Med.* **120**:623–626.

Rawls, W. E., and Melnick, J. L., 1966, Rubella virus carrier cultures derived from congenitally infected infants, *J. Exp. Med.* **123**:795–816.

Ray, C. G., Palmer, J. P., Grossley, J. R., and Williams, R. H., 1980, Coxsackievirus antibody responses in juvenile-onset diabetes mellitus, *Clin. Endocrinol.* **12**:375–378.

Rayfield, E. J., and Seto, Y., 1981, Viruses, in: *Handbook of Diabetes Mellitus*, Vol. I, *Etiology/Hormone Physiology* (M. Brownlee, ed.), pp. 95–120. Garland STPM Press, New York.

Reddy, C. M., and Crump, E. P., 1976, Diabetes mellitus following mumps, *J. Natl. Med. Assoc.* **68**:459–460.

Rekosh, D. M., 1978, The molecular biology of picornoviruses, in: *The Molecular Biology of Animal Viruses* (D. P. Nayak, ed.), pp. 63–110, Marcel Dekker, New York.

Richens, E. R., and Jones, W. G., 1981, Islet cell antibodies and mumps, *Lancet* **1**:507–508.

Richens, E. R., Ancil, R. J., and Hartog, M., 1976, Autoimmunity and viral infections in diabetes mellitus, *Clin. Exp. Immunol.* **23**:40–46.

Rodey, G. E., White, N., Frazer, T., Duquesnoy, R. J., and Santiago, J. V., 1979, HLA-DR specificities among black Americans with juvenile-onset diabetes, *N. Engl. J. Med.* **301**:810–812.

Rubinstein, P. Suciu-foca, N., Nicholson, J. F., 1977, Genetics of juvenile diabetes mellitus: A recessive gene closely linked to HLA D with 50 percent penetrance, *N. Engl. J. Med.* **297**:1036–1040.

Ruddle, N. H., 1979, Delayed hypersensitivity to soluble antigens in mice. II. Analysis in vitro, *Int. Arch. Allergy Appl. Immunol.* **58**:44–52.

Samantray, S. K., Christopher, S., Mukundan, P., and Johnson, S. C., 1977, Lack of relationship between viruses and human diabetes mellitus, *N.Z. J. Med.*, **7**:139–142.

Santoli, D., and Koprowski, H., 1979, Mechanisms of activation of human natural killer cells against tumor and virus-infected cells, *Immunol. Rev.* **44**:125–164.

Santoli, D., Trinchieri, G., Zmijewski, C., and Koprowski, H., 1976, HLA-related control of spontaneous and antibody-dependent cell-mediated cytotoxic activity in humans. *J. Immunol.*, **117**:765–772.

Schmidt, M. B., 1902, Über die Beziehung der Langerhanssche Inseln des Pankreas zum Diabetes Mellitus, *MMW* **49**:51–55.

Sinaniotis, C. A., Daskalopolou, E., Lapatsanis, P., Doxiadis, S., 1975, Diabetes mellitus after mumps vaccination, *Arch. Dis. Child.* **50**:749–750.

Smith, M. G., and Vellios, F., 1950, Inclusion disease or generalized salivary gland virus infection, *Arch. Pathol.* **50**:862–884.

Smithells, R. W., Sheppard, S., Marshall, W. C., and Peckham, C., 1978, Congenital rubella and diabetes mellitus, *Lancet* **1**:439.

Sultz, H. A., Hart, B. A., Zielezny, M., Schlesinger, E. R., 1975, Is mumps virus an etiologic factor in juvenile diabetes mellitus?, *J. Pediatr.* **86**:654–656.

Tesh, R. B., 1978, The prevalence of encephalomyocarditis virus neutralizing antibodies among various human populations, *Am. J. Trop. Med. Hyg.* **27**:144–149.

Tsutsumi, H., Chiba, Y., Abo, W., Chiba, S., and Nakao, T., 1980, T cell-mediated cytotoxic response to mumps virus in humans, *Infect. Immun.* **30**:129–134.

von Meyenburg, H., 1940, Uber "Insulitis" bei Diabetes, *Schweiz. Med. Wochenschr.* **21**:554.

Walker, S. M., Lee, S. C., and Lucas, Z. J., 1976, Cytotoxic activity of lymphocytes. VI. Heterogeneity of cytotoxins in supernatants of mitogen-activated lymphocytes, *J. Immunol.*, **116**:807–815.

Ward, K. P., Galloway, W. H., and Auchterlonie, I. A., 1979, Congenital cytomegalovirus infection and diabetes, *Lancet* **1**:497.

Warren, S., 1927, The pathology of diabetes in children, *JAMA,*: **88**:99–101.

Weller, T. H., and Craig, J. M., 1949, The isolation of mumps virus at autopsy, *Am. J. Pathol.* **25**:1105–1115.

West, R., Belmont, E., Colle, M. P., Crepeau, M. P., Wilkins, J., and Poirier, R., 1979, Epidemiologic survey of juvenile onset diabetes in Montreal, *Diabetes* **28**:690–693.

West, R., Colle, W. E., Belmonte, M. M., Tangle, A., Guttmann, R., Hynie, I., Thomas, D., Wilkins, J., Poirier, R., and Crepeau, M. P., 1981, Prospective study of insulin-dependent diabetes mellitus, *Diabetes* **30**:584–589.

Wilson, C., Connolly, J. H., and Thomson, D., 1977, Coxsackie B-2 virus infection and acute-onset diabetes in a child, *Br. Med. J.* **1:**1008.

Wilson, G. L., D'Andrea, B. J., Bellomo, S. C., and Craighead, J. C., 1980, Encephalomyocarditis virus infection of cultured murine pancreatic beta cells, *Nature* **285:** 112–113.

Witte, C. W., and Schanzer, B., 1968, Pancreatitis due to mumps, *JAMA* **203:**1068–1069.

Woodruff, J. F., 1980, Viral myocarditis: A review, *Am. J. Pathol.* **101:**425–484.

Yoon, J. W., Lesniak, M. A., Fussganger, R., and Notkins, A. L., 1976, Genetic differences in susceptibility of pancreatic cells to virus induced diabetes mellitus, *Nature* **264:**178–180.

Yoon, J.-W., Huang, S. W., MacLaren, N. K., Wheeler, C. J., Selvaggio, S. S., and Notkins, A. L., 1977, Antibody to encephalomyocarditis virus in juvenile diabetes, *N. Engl. J. Med.* **297:**1235–1236.

Yoon, J. W., Onodera, T., Jenson, A. B., and Notkins, A. B., 1978, Virus-induced diabetes mellitus. XI. Replication of Coxsackie B3 virus in human pancreatic beta cell cultures, *Diabetes* **27:**778–781.

Yoon, J. W., Austin, M., Onodera, T., and Notkins, A. L., 1979, Virus induced diabetes mellitus. Isolation of a virus from the pancreas of a child with diabetic ketoacidosis, *N. Engl. J. Med.* **300:**1173–1179.

Yoon, J. W., McClintock, P. R., Onodera, T., and Notkins, A. L., 1980, Virus-induced diabetes mellitus: XVIII. Inhibition by a nondiabetogenic variant of encephalomyocarditis virus, *J. Exp. Med.* **152:**878–892.

Yoon, J. W., Selvaggio, S., Onodera, T., Wheeler, J., and Jenson, A. B., 1981, Infection of cultured human pancreatic cells with reovirus type 3, *Diabetologia* **20:**462–467.

Ziring, P. R., 1977, Congenital rubella: The teenage years, *Pediatr. Ann.* **6:** 762–770.

11

Lymphocyte Response in Diabetes Mellitus

Sudhir Gupta

I. INTRODUCTION

During the past decade evidence has accumulated to suggest that the immune system plays an important role in the pathogenesis of insulin-dependent diabetes mellitus (Type I), which appears to be pathogenically a distinct disorder from insulin-independent diabetes (Type II). Studies in experimental animals have further suggested the role of lymphocytes and their subsets in the pathogenesis of Type I diabetes. It would be appropriate to discuss lymphocytes in general before discussing lymphocytes in diabetes mellitus.

Lymphocytes are major components of the immune system and play a critical role in various immune response. Rapid progress has been made in the recognition and definition of receptors/antigens on the surface of lymphocytes and in the understanding of their immunoregulatory and effector functions. It will become evident from this review that heterogeneous are the lymphocytes which make the immune system more and more complex. However, this complexity provides better understanding of various immune response in physiological states and their perturbations in disease states.

Lymphocytes are broadly categorized into two major subpopulations, T lymphocytes and B lymphocytes. T lymphocytes, which are processed under the inductive and differentiative influence of thymus, constitute the major (80%) pool of circulating lymphocytes and primarily home in the deep cortical area of lymph nodes and in the red pulp of the spleen. T cells are further subdivided into two major categories. Immunoregulatory T cells (suppressor and helpers) determine the tempo and magnitude of an immune response, whether of effector T cells or B cells. Effector T cells are responsible for the functions of cell-mediated immunity: defense against fungi, most viruses, and facultative intracellular bacteria; delayed cutaneous hypersensitivity;

Sudhir Gupta • Division of Basic and Clinical Immunology, Department of Medicine, University of California, Irvine, Irvine, California 92717.

graft-versus-host reaction, allograft rejection; and at least some forms of tumor immunity. B lymphocytes are thymus-independent and appear to differentiate and mature within the fetal liver and then in the bone marrow. B cells are the precursors of terminally differentiated plasma cells responsible for the synthesis and secretion of various classes of immunoglobulins and specific antibodies. B cells are comprised of approximately 10–15% of circulating blood lymphocytes. In the peripheral lymphoid tissues, B cells reside primarily in the far cortical area of lymph nodes, white pulp of the spleen, and in the tonsils. The immunoglobulins and specific antibodies provide the major mechanism of defense against encapsulated pyogenic bacteria and certain viruses.

Approximately 5–6% of peripheral blood lymphocytes do not meet the strict criteria of either T or B lymphocytes, and hence have been termed as "null" cells, "third population" cells, "K" cell, or "L" cells. The origin and lineage of this population of lymphoid cells remain unclear.

II. SURFACE MARKERS OF MAJOR SUBPOPULATIONS

During the process of differentiation and maturation T and B lymphocytes express a variety of differentiation antigens/receptors (Table 1).

It is beyond the scope of this review to discuss each of these markers in detail. They have recently been reviewed (Gupta and Good, 1979b, 1980, 1981b; Ross, 1979, Gupta et al., 1980a). The earliest identifiable cell of the B cell lineage is the pre-B cell. Pre-B cells first appear in the fetal liver at 5–7 weeks of gestation. They are characterized by the presence of intracytoplasmic μ heavy chain of IgM and lack of surface Ig. Among other receptors present on at least a subpopulation of pre-B cells are "DR" antigen and Epstein-Barr virus receptor. They also appear to contain high levels of terminal deoxynucleotidyl transferase activity, a marker that was assigned exclusively to pre-T cells and immature thymocytes. Pre-B cells are present in very small numbers (1%) in the bone marrow of young adults but are completely lacking in the peripheral blood. B lymphocytes are characterized by the presence of surface Ig, receptors for Ig Fc, mouse erythrocytes (MRBC), Epstein-Barr virus (EBV), complement components, and DR antigens. Among these surface Ig is the only reliable marker exclusively present on B cells. Surface IgM-bearing lymphocytes comprise most of the circulating B cells (10%). Only a minor population of B cells (<3–4%) in the circulating blood has surface IgG, IgA, or IgE.

Among the T-cell lineage, pre-T cells or early thymocytes are characterized by high terminal deoxynucleotidyl transferase (TdT) activity, receptors for peanut agglutinin and autologous erythrocytes, and presence of human thymus-derived lymphoid antigen (HTLA). Mature T cells are characterized by the presence for receptors of sheep erythrocytes (SRBC), presence of HTLA, and for Fc portions of various immunoglobulin isotypes (discussed below).

The so called "third-population" lymphoid cells lack surface Ig and receptors for SRBC but do process high-affinity receptors for IgG Fc. A subpopulation of this third population also appears to have receptors for complement components and EBV, and DR antigens.

Table 1. Markers of Human Lymphoid Cell Subpopulations

B-cell lineage	
Stem cell	? Alloantigen
Pre-B cells	Intracytoplasmic μ heavy chain
	EB virus receptor (subpopulation)
	DR antigen (subpopulation)
B cells	Surface immunoglobulin
	MRBC receptors
	Epstein–Barr virus receptor
	IgG Fc receptors
	IgM Fc receptors
	IgA Fc receptors
	IgE Fc receptors
	Complement component receptors
	DR antigen
T-cell lineage	
Stem cell	? Alloantigen
Pre-T cell	Terminal deoxynucleotidyl transferase (TdT)
	HTLA
	Peanut agglutinin
T cells	HTLA
	SRBC receptors
	IgG Fc receptors (Tγ)
	IgM Fc receptors (Tμ)
	IgA Fc receptors (Tα)
	IgE Fc receptors (Tε)
	IgD Fc receptors (Tδ)
Third-population "unclassified" lymphoid cells	
	IgG Fc receptors (high affinity)
	Complement component receptors
	Receptors for EBV (subpopulation)
	DR antigen (subpopulation)

III. FUNCTIONS OF MAJOR SUBPOPULATIONS

Cell separation techniques utilizing various markers have permitted the analysis of their function. Functions of T, B, and third population lymphoid cells are listed in Table 2. These functions have recently been reviewed (Gupta and Good, 1979b, 1980, 1981b; Gupta and Kapoor, 1980). T lymphocytes proliferate in response to soluble antigens, and in allogeneic and autologous mixed lymphocyte reaction (MLR). In contrast B lymphocytes stimulate in allogeneic and autologous MLR and proliferate in response to stimulus with Epstein-Barr virus. The third-population cells also stimulate in both allogeneic and autologous MLR.

Cell-mediated lympholysis (CML) is a function exclusive of T lymphocytes. All three major subpopulations are capable of mediating mitogen-induced cytotoxicity. B cells are devoid of antibody-dependent cytotoxicity (ADCC) and natural killer (NK) activity. "Third-population" cells and a subset of T cells with IgG Fc receptors (Tγ) contain almost wholly NK and ADCC activity. There is controversy regarding whether one or two distinct subsets perform NK and ADCC function.

Table 2. Functions of Human Lymphocyte Subpopulations[a]

Properties	T cells	B cells	Third-population lymphoid cells
Proliferative responses			
Antigens	+	−	−
Allogeneic cells (R)	+	−	−
Allogeneic cells (S)	−	+	+
Autologous cells (R)	+	−	+
Autologous cells (S)	−	+	+
Epstein-Barr virus	−	+	+S*
Cytotoxic responses			
Cell-mediated lympholysis	+	−	?
Antibody-dependent cytotoxicity	+S*	−	+
Natural killer activity	+S*	−	+
Mitogen-induced cytotoxicity	+	+	+
Lymphokine production			
Leukocyte migration inhibition factor	+	+	+
Macrophage migration inhibition factor	+	+	+
Blastogenic factor	+	+	+
Lymphotoxin (α)	+	+	+
Interferon	+	+	?
Antibody synthesis	−	+	+S*
Miscellaneous			
Precursors of B cells	−	−	+
Precursors of T cells	−	−	+
Precursors of granulocytes	−	−	+
Precursors of erythrocytes	−	−	+

[a]R, responder; S, stimulator; S*, subpopulation.

All three subsets of lymphoid cells appear to produce most of the lymphokines and therefore cannot be differentiated from one another based on lymphokine production. One exception is the production of T-cell growth factor (IL-2) produced by mature T cells but not by B lymphocytes.

Antibody and immunoglobulin synthesis is a function of B cells. Evidence suggests that a subpopulation of "third-population" cells, under appropriate experimental conditions, can be differentiated into immunoglobulin-synthesizing B lymphocytes.

"Third-population" lymphoid cells under appropriate conditions can be differentiated into mature erythrocytes, granulocytes, and T and B lymphocytes. Therefore, it can be concluded that "third-population" cells, although of lymphoid morphology, are the circulating committed stem cells for a number of cell lineages.

IV. HUMAN T-CELL SUBSETS DEFINED BY THE Fc RECEPTORS FOR IMMUNOGLOBULIN ISOTYPES

Human T lymphocytes have been shown to possess Fc receptors for IgM, (T_μ), IgG(T_γ), IgA(T_α), IgD(T_δ), or IgE(T_ϵ). T_μ and T_γ cells have been extensively studied and recently reviewed (Moretta et al., 1978; Gupta, 1978, 1981; Gupta and Good,

1978, 1979a, 1980, 1981a, b; Gupta and Kapoor, 1980). A detailed account is beyond the scope of this chapter. Characteristics of T_μ and T_γ cells are summarized in Table 3. These two subpopulations are distinct with regard to morphology, RNA content, locomotion property, electrophoretic mobility, cytotoxic activities, and immunoregulatory functions. T_μ cells have shown to contain spontaneous helper activity and precursors of concanavalin-A (Con A)-induced suppressor cells. In contrast, T_γ cells lack helper activity but suppress the B cell differentiation to plasma cells in the presence of pokeweed mitogen (PWM), by suppressing the helper activity of T_μ cells. Suppressor activity is contained within a subpopulation of T_γ cells that carry histamine (H_2 type) receptors (Rocklin et al., 1979). In contrast almost all NK and ADCC among T cells reside in a subpopulation of T_γ cells that lack histamine receptors (Gupta et al., 1980). Recently, it has been reported that a large population of T_γ cells reacts with a monoclonal antibody that is said to define monocytes and do not react with OKT5 monoclonal antibody that defines suppressor/cytotoxic T cells (Reinherz et

Table 3.   Characteristics of Human T-Cell Subpopulations[a]

Characteristics	$T\mu$ cells	$T\gamma$
B-cell differentiation	↑ s	↓
T-cell proliferation	?	↓ s
Natural killer activity	−	+s
Antibody-dependent cytotoxicity	−	+s
Blastogenic responses to:		
Phytohemagglutinin	+	−
Concanavalin A	+	+
Allogeneic cells	+	+
Mediator production		
Migration inhibition factor (LMIF)	+	−
Interferon	+	+
Adherence to nylon wool or glass	−	+s
Electrophoretic mobility	High	Low
Locomotor properties	+	−
Ia antigen	−	+
Histamine receptors	−	+s
Thymopoietin	−	↑
Sensitivity to:		
Corticosteroids	−	+
Irradiation	−	+
Pronase	+	+
Trypsin	+	−
Neuraminidase	+	−
RNA content	High	Low
Morphology		
Cytoplasmic nuclear ratio	Low	High
Golgi body	Few	Rich
Rough endoplasmic reticulum	Scanty	Abundant
Cytoplasmic granules	−	+
α-Nephthyl acetate esterase	+ Granular	−

[a]s, subpopulation; ↑, enhancement; ↓, inhibition.

al., 1980). Based on these observations these authors concluded that T_γ cells are not of T-cell lineage, rather they belong to monocyte–macrophage lineage. However it has been observed that this monoclonal antibody also reacts with neutrophils and "null" or "third-population" cells. A number of other monoclonal antibodies that define receptors for SRBC on T cells (true pan-T-cell antibodies) react with T_γ cells. A number of other characteristics, including their growth in IL-2, established that a majority of T_γ cells are of T-cell lineage and not of monocyte–macrophage lineage (Gupta *et al.*, 1980a; Gupta, 1981; Gupta and Good, 1981a).

V. MONOCLONAL-ANTIBODY-DEFINED LYMPHOCYTE SUBPOPULATIONS

The advent of hybridoma technology, whereby tumor clones can be generated to secrete desired monoclonal antibody, has provided a variety of monoclonal antibodies that define differentiation and maturation antigens. The lymphocyte subpopulation defined by a monoclonal antibody may not be as homogeneous with regards to its net function in healthy states as we might think. This would become evident in subsequent discussion especially of OKT4 monoclonal-antibody-defined T-cell subset. The cellular expression of various differentiation antigens and functional analysis of these subsets have been reviewed (Reinherz and Schlossman, 1980).

A. Differentiation Antigens on Cells of T-Cell Lineage

Several investigators have developed a number of monoclonal antibodies which are reactive with thymocytes and/or peripheral blood T cells. Among these, OKT series of monoclonal antibodies are the most extensively analyzed. The cellular expression of the antigens defined with these monoclonal antibodies is shown in Table 4. It is evident that the vast majority of human thymocytes react with many of these monoclonal antibodies, suggesting that a sizable proportion of thymocytes would bear multiple antigens. Using monoclonal antibodies and complement it was possible to define at least three major subpopulations of thymocytes. All thymocytes bear OKT10 antigen, the earliest thymocytes bear OKT9 and OKT10 or OKT10 antigen alone. However, OKT10 is not a thymus-specific marker but a general indicator for early cellular lineage of all cell types, including marrow B cells and thymus. OKT9 antibody is also not thymus-specific but a recognized transfer in receptor. The fraction of thymus-bearing OKT9 and OKT10 antigens is comprised of only 10% thymocytes. Further maturation of thymocytes results in the expression of OKT6 and simultaneous expression of OKT4, OKT5, and OKT8 antigens. This represents more than 70% of the thymocytes. With further maturation, thymocytes lose OKT6 antigen, acquire OKT3 antigen, and segregate into $OKT4^+$ and $OKT5^+/OKT8^+$ T-cell subsets. OKT6 antigen is also not thymus-specific because this antigen is expressed on Langerhans cells of the skin. When thymocytes are exported into the peripheral circulation, they lose OKT10 antigen. The exported $OKT1^+$, $OKT3^+$, $OKT4^+$, and $OKT1^+$, $OKT3^+$, $OKT8^+/OKT5^+$ subsets represent inducer/helper phenotype and suppressor/cytotoxic phenotype subsets, respectively.

Table 4. Monoclonal Antibodies to Human T-Cell Surface
Antigens

Monoclonal antibodies	Thymus	Percent peripheral blood	
		E+	E−
Anti T1	10	95–98	0
Anti T3	10	95–98	0
Anti T4 (inducer/helper)	75	60	0
Anti T5 (suppressor/cytotoxic)	80	20	0
Anti T8 (suppressor/cytotoxic)	80	30	0
Anti T6	70	0	0
Anti T9	10	0	0
Anti T10	95	5	10
Anti T11		100	0

More recently it has been demonstrated that activated T cells (activated with mitogens, antigens, or alloantigens) express Tac antigen defined with monoclonal antibody, anti-Tac (Uchiama et al., 1981a). Subsequent studies by the same group have shown that Tac antigen is a receptor for IL-2.

B. Functions of T-Cell Subsets

The functional characteristics of peripheral T-cell subsets are shown in Table 5. Both major populations (OKT4$^+$ and OKT5$^+$/OKT8$^+$) proliferate in response to Con A, soluable antigens, and alloantigens. Phytohemagglutinin-induced proliferation is predominantly seen in OKT4$^+$ population. In the autologous mixed lymphocyte reaction (AMLR) between T and non-T cells, OKT4$^+$ are the major responders (Damle et al., 1981), whereas in the T-T AMLR OKT8$^+$ T cells are the major responders (Damle and Gupta, 1982). Recently it has been shown that a major subpopulation of OKT4$^+$ T cells responds in AMLR and the remaining OKT4$^+$ subpopulation acts as helper (Reinherz et al., 1982). This observation demonstrates the heterogeneity of OKT4$^+$ T cells.

The most important difference among these subsets is in their immunoregulatory influence. OKT4$^+$ have been shown to be helpers for the response of T cells to mitogens and antigens and in the B-cell differentiation to immunoglobulin-producing plasma cells. But it has become evident that not all OKT4$^+$ cells are helper T cells, therefore enumeration of OKT4$^+$ cells might not correlate with in vitro helper function in disease states. Thomas et al. (1982), utilizing another monoclonal antibody (OKT17) have subdivided OKT4$^+$ into two subpopulations, a helper and a suppressor OKT4$^+$. We have also demonstrated that OKT4$^+$ cells contain precursors of Con-A-inducible suppressor cells (Damle and Gupta, 1982). OKT5$^+$/OKT8$^+$ are suppressors for the proliferative response of T cells and for the differentiation of B cells to plasma cells. This population also contain Con-A-inducible suppressor cells. Recently it has been shown that a subset of OKT8$^+$ T cells possesses histamine receptors and performs the suppressor function. The histamine-receptor-negative OKT8$^+$ population participates in cytotoxic function. This also shows heterogeneity of OKT8$^+$ T cells.

Table 5. Immunologic Functions of T-Cell Subsets
Defined with Monoclonal Antibodies

Functions	OKT4+	OKT8+
Proliferative response		
Soluble antigens	+	−
Con A	+	+
PHA	+	±
Allogeneic MLC	±	+
Autologous MLC	+S[a]	−
Interleukin 2 production	+	±
Cytotoxicity (CML)	−	+
Regulatory functions		
Helper		
T–T interaction	+	−
T–B interaction	+	−
T–macrophage	+	−
Suppressor		
T–T interaction	−	+
T–B interaction	−	+

[a]S = Subpopulation.

Because of this functional heterogeneity within OKT4$^+$ and OKT5$^+$/OKT8$^+$ T cells subsets, data from the quantitative analysis of these subsets in disease states should be carefully interpreted especially in relation to their immunoregulatory functions. At this stage it would be appropriate to define OKT4$^+$ and OKT5$^+$/OKT8$^+$ T cells as helper/inducer "phenotype" and suppressor/cytotoxic "phenotype," respectively.

C. B-Cell Subsets

Two groups of investigators have developed monoclonal antibodies that define differentiation antigens on B lymphocytes. Nadler et al. (1981a,b) named them as B1 and B2 and Zola (1980) has termed them FMC1 and FMC7. B1 and FMC1 antigens are present early in B-cell differentiation whereas B2 and FMC7 antigens are present on mature B cells. It is not known if antibodies of B series and FMC series define the same antigens.

D. Natural Killer (NK) Cells

NK activity was originally demonstrated in "third-population" lymphoid cells and then also in T_γ cells. There have been numerous efforts to find cell surface marker or characteristics exclusive to NK cells. These cells have capacity to lyse various target cells in the absence of antibody and without prior sensitization. NK cells appear to be important in immune surveillance against tumor, resistance against viruses, and in hematopoietic allograft rejection. Morphologically they are large granular lymphocytes with high cytoplasm/nucleus ratio, pale cytoplasm, and slightly eccentric reniform nucleus with 6–12 azurophilic granulses in their cytoplasm (Timonen et al., 1979). Recently two monoclonal antibodies have developed that react exclusively with large granular lymphocytes. HNK1 antigen is present on almost all NK cells (Abo and Balch, 1981). Anti-HNK1 antibody does not react with any other cells in the blood or a panel of tumor cell lines. Another monoclonal antibody, NK8, reacts with a subpopulation (33%) of large granular cells, but not other cell types in the peripheral blood or a panel of cell lines representing the T, B, myeloid, or erythroid lineage (Nieminen *et al.*, 1982). It appears that HNK1 marks all large granular lymphocytes whereas NK8 is specific only for those large granular lymphocytes capable of binding to target cells. Large granular lymphocytes are OKT10$^+$, approximately 50% react with OKM1, and about 25% with OKT8 monoclonal antibodies (Ortaldo *et al.*, 1981).

VI. INSULIN RECEPTORS

Gavin *et al.* (1972), using monoiodoinsulin, demonstrated specific binding sites on all leukocytes, erythrocytes, and cultured fibroblasts. It is interesting that the cultured tumor lymphocytes and the isolated normal lymphocytes have very similar apparent binding constants, specificities, and kinetics of binding but about a 10-fold difference in the calculated number of sites per cells. However, this could be due to cultured lymphocytes having 10 times more surface area than normal resting lymphocytes. Krug *et al.* (1972) failed to demonstrate insulin binding to peripheral blood lymphocytes passed over tightly packed nylon wool column. However such a procedure would deplete B cells and monocytes that could have receptors for insulin. Schwartz *et al.* (1975) reported insulin receptor on human monocytes rather than on lymphocytes. Gozes *et al.* (1981) failed to demonstrate cryptic insulin receptors on resting lymphocytes in contrast to the presence of cryptic receptors in liver and fat cell membranes.

Helderman and Strom (1978) demonstrated presence of insulin receptors on rat T cells activated *in vivo* by allogeneic skin graft or graft-versus-host disease and *in vitro* by MLR, Con A, and PHA. B lymphocytes activated with lipopolysaccharide also demonstrated insulin receptors. These investigators concluded that insulin receptors appear to be a universal marker of activated T and B cells. Helderman *et al.* (1979) have demonstrated that insulin-receptor-bearing cells are Ly 2$^+$3$^+$ and could also be induced on Ly 1$^+$ T cells. It appears likely, therefore, that insulin could play an important physiological role in various immune responses. Helderman and Raskin (1980) examined insulin receptors on PHA-activated T cells from patients with juvenile-onset diabetes mellitus, adult-onset diabetes mellitus, and healthy controls. The specific insulin binding was comparable between juvenile-onset diabetes and control groups. In contrast, binding was reduced in adult-onset diabetics and obese subjects. Insulin receptor affinity was normal but the receptor numbers were decreased.

VII. MORPHOLOGY OF LYMPHOID TISSUES IN DIABETES

Souadjian *et al.* (1970) examined thymuses in patients who died with the diagnosis of diabetes. These included 17 patients with juvenile-onset diabetes (Group A) and 34 with adult-onset diabetes mellitus (Group B). Patients in Group A were further divided into those who had died between 0 and 15 years (Group A1, 9 patients) and those who had died between the ages 18 and 35 (Group A2, 8 patients). The thymic medulla were measured for number of Hassall's corpuscles, average diameter of Hassall's corpuscles, diameter of largest corpuscles, number of lymphocytes, and number of epithelial cells. The number of Hassall's corpuscles per unit area of the size of the largest corpuscles were significantly increased in patients with juvenile onset diabetes. No significant difference was observed in patients with adult-onset diabetes. The epithelial cells were significantly smaller in juvenile diabetes mellitus. In pancreatectomized rats, thymus shows a significant reduction in weight and cellularity, splenic size is normal, but there is a pronounced depletion of perifollicular mantal of small lymphocytes. Germinal centers, in contrast, are well developed (Fabris and Piantanelli, 1977).

VIII. LYMPHOCYTE SUBPOPULATIONS IN DIABETES

Selam et al. (1979) studied circulating lymphocyte subpopulations in 39 patients with Type I diabetes (14 well-controlled and 25 poorly controlled) and compared them with lymphocyte subsets in 50 age- and sex-matched healthy controls. Although in the two groups of diabetes the mean age was comparable, male/female ratio was different (in the poorly controlled group it was 22:3 whereas in the well-controlled group it was 8:6). The criterion for well-controlled diabetes was mean blood glucose levels. The absolute lymphocyte count in the patient and healthy control group was comparable. The proportion and absolute number of "total" T cells as determined by rosette formation with SRBC (E-RFC) was significantly decreased in Type I diabetes. The poorly controlled diabetics had significantly lower proportion of E-RFC than those with well-controlled diabetes. This is in agreement with the results reported by Cattaneo et al. (1976). Muller et al. (1980) also reported "minor" decrease in absolute number of total T cells, however they gave no statistical analysis of their data. In contrast, others have reported normal proportion of total E-RFC in Type I diabetes mellitus (Gupta et al., 1981, 1982; Hann et al., 1976; Bersani et al., 1981; MacCuish et al., 1974b). The reason for such discrepancy is not known. The difference in technique and selection of patients (age, sex, etc.) however, could be responsible. Total T cells, as determined by heteroantiserum defining human T lymphocyte surface antigen (HTLA; Selam et al., 1979) or with monoclonal antibody OKT3 (Mascart-Lemone et al., 1982) and 3A1 (Jackson et al., 1982) in patients with Type I diabetes were comparable to healthy control group. Salam et al. (1979) reported normal numbers and proportions of "active" E-RFC, that detect a subset of T cells in Type I diabetics irrespective of control of their diabetes. Muller et al. (1980) reported minor differences in absolute numbers and proportions of "high-affinity" E-RFC in Type I diabetes. Analysis of T-cell subsets as defined with monoclonal antibodies has also resulted in controversial data. The proportion of OKT4$^+$ (inducer/helper phenotype) cells in Type I diabetes is reported to be normal (Jackson et al., 1982; Gupta et al., 1982) or decreased (Mascart-Lemone et al., 1982). The proportion of OKT8$^+$ T cells (suppressor/cytotoxic phenotype) is normal (Jackson et al., 1982; Mascart-Lemone et al., 1982) or decreased (Gupta et al., 1982). Therefore ratios of OKT4$^+$/OKT8$^+$ T cells in Type I diabetes are reported to be normal (Jackson et al., 1982), increased (Gupta et al., 1982) or decreased (Mascart-Lemone et al., 1982). Gupta et al. (1982) reported data on individual patients, whereas

Jackson *et al.* (1982) and Mascart-Lemone *et al.* (1982) lumped the data in groups. No correlation, however, was observed between changes in T cell subsets and duration of disease, control of diabetes or insulin-treatment (Gupta *et al.*, 1982; Mascart-Lemone *et al.*, 1982). Jackson *et al.* (1982) also reported increase in the number and proportion of "activated" Ia-bearing T cells, as defined with monoclonal antibodies, in Type I diabetes mellitus. Increased Ia-bearing T cells were found in early onset of Type I diabetes and not in long-term Type I diabetes. This observation could reflect the activation of immune system in general. However, significance of this observation is not clear. We have also reported a relative deficiency of T cells with IgG Fc receptor (T_γ) in a subgroup of patients with Type I diabetes (Gupta *et al.*, 1981a).

B lymphocytes in patients with Type I diabetes mellitus have been studied, using surface immunoglobulins and complement–receptor (erythrocyte–antibody–complement complexes, EAC). EAC^+ cells were found to be normal (Stratton *et al.*, 1977; MacCuish *et al.*, 1974b) or decreased (Selam *et al.*, 1979). Selam *et al.* (1979) reported comparable EAC^+ cells in well-controlled diabetics and controls; however a significantly decreased proportion of EAC^+ cells was observed in poorly controlled diabetics when compared to healthy controls. The values of EAC^+ cells in healthy controls reported by these investigators were significantly different, which could explain the different results in their studies. It should be pointed out however, that C3 receptor is not the best marker for B cells, because not all B cells have C3 receptors and not all the cells with C3 receptors are B cells: C3 receptor is also present on a subset of "third-population" lymphoid cells. B cells defined with surface Ig are normal in patients with Type I diabetes (MacCuish *et al.*, 1974b; Selam *et al.*, 1979; Hahn *et al.*, 1976). Hahn *et al.* (1976) observed the proportion of surface IgG^+ B cells in control and patient groups to be higher than surface IgM^+ B cells. This appears to be due to majority of "third-population" cells with cytophilic IgG detected in their assay as B cells. Bersani *et al.* (1981) observed significantly increased proportion of B lymphocytes in the islet-cell-antibody-positive group of Type I diabetes when compared to healthy group. This difference was observed for both surface IgG- and surface IgM-positive B cells between the islet-cell-antibody-positive group and healthy control group and not between islet-cell-antibody-negative group and control group. Surface IgA-positive B cells were increased in both islet-cell-antibody-positive and -negative groups. These authors suggested that, like persistence of autoantibodies and/or islet cell antibody, increased levels of B cells could be a markers for Type IB (possible autoimmune pathogenesis) diabetes mellitus.

The results of T-cell, T-cell-subset, and B-cell analyses have been shown to be independent of metabolic status of patient (good vs. poor control of diabetes, duration of disease, or insulin treatment) (Gupta *et al.*, 1981b, 1982; Cattaneo *et al.*, 1976; MacCuish *et al.*, 1974b; Mascart-Lemone *et al.*, 1982), although this observation is based on indirect evidence. Selam *et al.* (1979) examined the influence of metabolism disturbance on lymphocyte subsets. Eight patients with poorly controlled diabetes were examined before and immediately following a period of optimal blood glucose control by means of an external artificial pancreas. They demonstrated normalization of ERFC and EARFC (FcIgG receptor on B cells, third-population cells, and T_γ cells) following good control of diabetes. These authors concluded that the decreased in E-RFC T cells and EA+ cells is due to metabolic abnormality. It should be stressed, however, that these influences could be due to the inhibitory effect of glucose on binding of indicator cells to lymphocytes, because the number of T lymphocytes defined with HTLA remained normal. Furthermore, they did not examine the effect of good control on B cells. Cattaneo *et al.* (1976) reported a normal proportion of T cells in Type II diabetes.

IX. BLASTOGENIC RESPONSE IN DIABETES

A. Response to Mitogens

Fabris and Piantenelli (1977) reported depressed cell-mediated immunity, as expressed by prolonged allograft skin-graft rejection and blastogenic response to phytohemagglutinin (PHA) or to alloantigens, in rats with experimentally induced diabetes when compared to age-matched sham-treated controls. Brody and Merlie (1970) reported depressed mitogenic response of lymphocytes from patients with diabetes mellitus, when stimulated with PHA. In this study, however, patients were not divided into Type I or Type II diabetes. Ragab *et al.* (1972) failed to demonstrate any abnormality in PHA or *Candida albicans* antigen-induced blastogenic response in lymphocytes from patients with unclassified diabetes mellitus. Delepesse *et al.* (1974) reported depressed proliferative response to PHA in 29 patients with insulin-dependent diabetes when compared to age-matched control. The depressed PHA response correlated with the severity of diabetes. Insulin-independent (Type II) diabetics had a significantly better PHA response than Type I patients, but significantly lower than the controls. Glassman and Bennett (1980) also reported depressed PHA response in Type II diabetes. MacCuish *et al.* (1974b) studied PHA response in 40 well-controlled and 40 poorly controlled Type I diabetics and 40 matched normal subjects. Proliferative response to three different concentrations of PHA was similar in well-controlled diabetics and healthy normals. The proliferative response to all three concentrations of PHA was, however, significantly depressed in poorly controlled diabetics compared to the matched healthy normal subjects. These observations would suggest that this defect in Type I diabetes is due to inadequately corrected metabolic disturbances rather than an inherent immunological abnormality. Selam *et al.* (1979) also examined proliferative response to PHA, Con-A, and PWM in 39 Type I diabetics. No significant difference was observed between patient and control groups. When data were analyzed according to control of diabetes, a significantly increased response was observed in well-controlled diabetics compared to healthy controls. No difference was observed between poorly controlled and healthy subjects, a finding in contrast to that reported by MacCuish *et al.* (1974b).

As expected, a significant difference in PHA response was observed between poorly and well-controlled diabetics, but this is not a evidence of poor proliferative response in poorly controlled diabetics because response was comparable to healthy subjects. Proliferative response to Con A was comparable in both well-controlled and poorly controlled diabetics when each was compared with normal subjects. A significantly depressed Con A response was observed in poorly controlled diabetics as compared to well-controlled diabetics but this was because of moderate but not significantly increased proliferation to Con A in well-controlled diabetics compared to healthy group.

No depression of proliferative response to PHA or Con A was observed in either poorly or well-controlled Type I diabetics when compared to healthy controls. The response to PWM was, however, depressed in poorly controlled diabetics when compared to control healthy group or well-controlled diabetics. When eight poorly controlled diabetics were reexamined following good control by external artificial pancreas a significant increase (over the baseline response comparable to healthy controls) in PHA response was observed. However, no significant improvement was observed in proliferative response to Con A or PWM (the latter being lower than in controls). These investigators concluded that the defect in mitogen response was due to metabolic abnormality. This appears to be an overinterpretation of their data, because PHA responses that were comparable to healthy controls increased, whereas PWM responses that were depressed when compared to healthy controls did not improve following good control of diabetes. Therefore, these abnormalities could not be simply due to metabolic disturbances.

Helderman (1981) reported that insulin augments intermediary metabolism of activated rat T cells above the mitogen-stimulated level. This could suggest that insulin would have a classic physiological role in the activated lymphocytes.

B. Response to Alloantigens and Autoantigens

Very limited information is available regarding allogeneic mixed lymphocyte reaction (MLR) and autologous MLR (AMLR) in patients with Type I diabetes mellitus. Delepesse et al. (1974) showed that five of nine patients demonstrated deficient MLR, though the mean proliferative responsee of diabetic group was comparable to control group. We have recently examined AMLR and MLR in patients with Type I diabetes (Gupta et al., 1983). None of these patients were newly diagnosed cases. The AMLR was deficient in 6 of 20 patients with Type I diabetes when compared with the age- and sex-matched simultaneously studied healthy controls, although the mean peak proliferative response in the AMLR for the patient group was not significantly different from that of control. The peak response in both patient and control group was observed on day 6. In the allogeneic MLR, T cells from patients responded normally, however non-T-cells from patients were poor stimulators against responder T cells from healthy controls. Because both helper and suppressor functions are generated in the AMLR, an abnormality of the AMLR in Type I diabetes further supports an abnormal immune regulation that might be important in the pathogenesis and autoimmune manifestations of Type I diabetes. Since in the AMLR several subsets of T, B, and macrophages, and biologically active molecules interact, to determine the cellular/molecular basis of deficient AMLR in Type I diabetics, studies of identical or matched siblings are required.

X. IMMUNE RESPONSE TO PANCREATIC ANTIGENS

Lymphocytic infiltration in and around the islets of Langerhans is characteristic of Type I diabetes of short duration (Gepts, 1965). The subtypes of lymphocytes in these infiltrates and their significance remain unclear. However, their presence in the pancreas could suggest cell-mediated immune response to pancreatic antigens. Nerup *et al.* (1971) studied organ-specific cellular hypersensitivity against porcine pancreatic components in 22 diabetics by means of the leukocyte migration test. A fraction III prepared from pooled porcine pancreatic gland in which atrophy of the exocrine tissue was induced by ligation of the pancreatic duct, was used as an antigen. Twelve of 22 patients (55%) had migration index below 0.70 in comparison with only 1 of 18 control subjects. Inhibition of the leukocyte migration was not induced by porcine or bovine insulin or by liver or kidney preparations. Therefore reaction to pancreatic fraction III must be considered organ-specific: the reactivity appears to be directed against some cytoplasmic antigenic component(s) of the atrophic pancreatic gland. Four of six patients with low migration indices demonstrated classical delayed-type hypersensitivity when intercutaneous injection of same preparation was given. Nerup *et al.* (1974) subsequently studied 112 diabetics for antipancreatic cellular immunity. These patients were divided into three groups: Group A included 48 patients with untreated Type I diabetes or insulin-treated for less than 1 year, Group B was comprised of 38 patients with Type I diabetes treated with insulin for more than 1 year, and Group C included 26 patients with Type II diabetes. Forty-five volunteers served as controls. Specific migration inhibition was induced by fetal calf pancreas extract in 31 of 112 diabetics (28%) studied. Abnormal migration indices were found equally frequent in male and female patients. No correlation was found with the presence of insulin antibodies. When data were analyzed according to subgroups, cellular immunity to pancreatic antigens was found predominantly in Type I diabetes of short duration.

Richens *et al.* (1973) also reported positive results of leukocyte migration test to rat liver mitochondria in 72% of insulin-dependent diabetics, 46% non-insulin-dependent diabetics, and 11% in the control group. The reaction appears to be specific to liver mitochondria since comparable preparations of rat kidney and rat adrenal gland did not induce inhibition. The reaction also appears to be species nonspecific since human liver mitochondria also elicited positive leukocyte migration. No significant difference was found for abnormal migration test results between Type I patients with short duration or with a longer duration. MacCuish *et al.* (1974a) examined leukocyte migration inhibition test results in 101 diabetics and 50 healthy controls, using human pancreatic extract as an antigen. Seventeen of 31 insulin-dependent diabetics demonstrated positive migration inhibition as compared to only 4 of 27 young controls. In contrast, leukocyte migration test results were essentially normal in older diabetics treated with oral hypoglycemic agents or with diet. The rat liver mitochondria as antigen failed to induce migration inhibition. This observation is in contradiction to the observation of Richens *et al.* (1973).

Cell-mediated immunity in Type I diabetes was also investigated by Boitard *et al.* (1981). They demonstrated that lymphocytes from patients with Type I diabetes suppress insulin release from isolated mice islet cells.

XI. CELL-MEDIATED IMMUNITY TO INSULIN

Faulk *et al.* (1975) examined cell-mediated immunity to insulin and its fragments in 35 insulin-treated diabetics. The age range was 21–77 years and duration of disease was

1–30 years. Twenty-five randomly selected nondiabetic controls were used. Cell-mediated immunity was measured by skin tests and blastogenic response. Twenty-two (60%) patients gave a positive blastogenic response to insulin or its isolated polypeptide fragments. Twenty-one patients responded to intact molecule, 16 reacted to B chain, and 8 reactions to A chain. These data suggested that intact molecules are the most immunogenic. None of the controls gave positive blastogenic response to intact molecule or its fragments. Many patients produced positive skin tests: most of these were immediate reactions to either the intact molecule or to B chain. Three patients responded to a classic delayed hypersensitivity reaction with intact insulin only. MacCuish *et al.* (1975) studied lymphocyte transformation to bovine and porcine insulin and fragments in 50 established Type I diabetes mellitus with no evidence of insulin allergy, 10 newly diagnosed diabetes (5 untreated), and 30 nondiabetic controls. Fifteen well-established and five newly diagnosed (three untreated and two insulin-treated for less than 3 weeks) showed significant lymphocyte transformation as compared to positive response in only one control.

The responses to porcine insulin were almost identical. Twenty established, six newly diagnosed diabetics, and two controls showed significant positive lymphocyte transformation. A chain of either insulin was almost without effect (one subject showed positive response); in contrast the B chain of bovine insulin induced significant transformation in 14 (67%) of 21 patients tested. In some patients B chain was more potent stimulus than intact insulin. These studies suggest that B chain is the major antigenic site for the cell-mediated immune response, whereas A chain is major antigenic site for the antibody response.

XII. SERUM IMMUNOGLOBULINS AND SPECIFIC ANTIBODY RESPONSE

The literature on serum immunoglobulin levels and specific antibody response in Type I diabetes mellitus is limited. Farid and Anderson (1973) reported mildly elevated serum IgA and mildly decreased IgG levels in insulin-dependent diabetics. Serum IgM and C3 levels were normal. We have examined levels of serum Ig in 25 patients with Type I diabetes (Gupta *et al.*, 1982). All patients were receiving insulin. The duration of diabetes ranged from 0.5 to 11 years. Age range was 6–19 years. No significant difference in the levels of IgM, IgG, or IgA was observed between patient and control groups. Two patients had significantly low levels of IgA (28 and 24 mg/dl, compared to 90–450 mg/dl for the controls). Smith *et al.* (1978), using less than 10 mg/dl of serum IgA levels as the criterion for IgA deficiency, reported 9 of 366 patients with juvenile-onset insulin-dependent diabetics as IgA-deficient; in contrast, none of 421 patients with adult-onset insulin-dependent diabetes had IgA deficiency. This study demonstrates an increased prevalence of IgA deficiency in juvenile-onset insulin-dependent diabetes.

Antibody formation following *in vivo* immunization has been reported to be normal in human diabetics (Lipscomb *et al.*, 1959), in alloxan-induced diabetic mice (Dolkart *et al.*, 1977), and in pancreatectomized rats (Fabris and Piantanelli, 1977). The latter investigators did not find any quantitative alteration in the number of antibody-producing cells in the spleen or the circulating antibody titers against SRBC, brucella antigen, or bovine serum albumin. Ludwig *et al.* (1976) reported that the percentage of juvenile-onset diabetics with agglutinin to *E. coli* and staphylococcal antigens is significantly lower and the percentage of diabetics without antibodies to pertussis and diphtheria toxoid is increased when compared to controls.

XIII. IMMUNOREGULATION

The presence of a variety of autoantibodies and antipancreatic cell-mediated response strongly suggests that abnormal immunoregulation could play an important role in the pathogenesis of Type I diabetes. Horowitz *et al.* (1977) reported deficient Con-A-inducible suppressor cell activity against allogeneic MLC in six of nine patients with insulin-dependent diabetes. No correlation was observed between deficient suppressor cell activity and age, sex, duration of diabetes, or control of the disease. Buschard *et al.* (1980) studied Con-A-induced suppressor cell activity in Type I diabetics against proliferative response of allogeneic lymphocytes to Con A. They observed deficient suppressor cell activity in newly diagnosed patients only but normal suppressor cell activity in patients with disease duration of 2–8 months or 5–8 years. This is in contrast to the observation of deficient Con-A-inducible suppressor cell activity in Type I diabetics irrespective of duration of disease (Lederman *et al.*, 1981; Gupta *et al.*, 1981; Fairchild *et al.*, 1982). Gupta *et al.* (1981) and Lederman *et al.* (1981) used a system almost identical to that used by Buschard *et al.* (1980).

The difference in the results could be due to patient population. Gupta *et al.* (1981) and Lederman *et al.* (1981) used patients in their teens, whereas Buschard *et al.* (1980) used patients in their 20s. Slater *et al.* (1980) reported increased Con-A-inducible suppressor cell activity in Type I diabetics. However, their data are difficult to interpret because the mean suppression in the control group was only 6%. Fairchild *et al.* (1982) also reported deficiency of antigen-specific (islet cell homogenates) suppressor cell activity in Type I diabetics. Suppressor cell activity was reported to be normal in Type II diabetes (Lederman *et al.*, 1981; Fairchild *et al.*, 1982). Metabolic control of diabetes appears not to influence suppressor cell activity (Gupta *et al.*, 1981; Lederman *et al.*, 1981; Buschard *et al.*, 1982; Fairchild *et al.*, 1982). Gupta *et al.* (1982) observed a direct correlation between deficiency of Con-A-inducible suppressor cell activity and the deficiency in the proportion of OKT8$^+$ (suppressor/cytotoxic phenotype) T cells.

Deficiency of suppressor cell function in Type I diabetes could be responsible for the expression of autoimmunity and increased cytotoxicity against pancreatic beta cells.

XIV. CYTOTOXIC RESPONSE

Huang and Maclaren (1976) examined lymphocytes from 23 patients with insulin-dependent diabetes mellitus for cytoadherence and cytotoxicity against insulinoma cells. The mean percentage of cytoadherence of lymphocytes from insulin-dependent diabetes was four to five times greater than that from healthy controls. Eighteen of 23 patients showed more than 10% cytoadherence as compared to none of the 12 controls.

The cytotoxicity as estimated by eosin exclusion was also significantly greater by lymphocytes from patients than controls. The mean cytotoxicity with patients lymphocytes was 24% as compared to 9% by lymphocyte from controls. Fifteen of 23 patients demonstrated 21% cytotoxicity as compared to none in 12 controls. Using patients' serum (containing antiinsulinoma antibody) and fractionated T and non-T cells, it was demonstrated that T-cell-mediated cytotoxicity, antibody dependent cytotoxicity (ADCC), or both T-cell-mediated and antibody-dependent cytotoxicities were present. These studies lead the authors to suggest that lymphocyte and not antibodies are the primary aggressors in the process of pancreatic B cell autoaggression.

Pozzilli *et al.* (1974) and Sensi *et al.* (1981) reported increased proportion of low-affinity E-RFC and increased ADCC in patients with Type I diabetes. Eight of 16 patients and 7 of 11 nondiabetic siblings with positive islet cell antibody had increased low-affinity ERFC. ADCC in the newly diagnosed patient group was comparable to the control group, however nondiabetic healthy siblings with islet cell antibodies had increased ADCC activity. These authors, however, did not give data on individual subjects. When data were analyzed according to increased low-affinity ERFC, patients as well as healthy siblings had increased ADCC, whereas patients and healthy siblings with normal proportion of low-affinity ERFC had normal ADCC.

The role of insulin in modulation of lymphocyte mediated cytotoxicity and ADCC has been examined. Storm *et al.* (1975) have demonstrated that physiological concentrations of insulin enhance the cytotoxic function of alloimmune splenic lymphocytes from lewis rats. This influence was observed on effector lymphocytes and not on target cells. The effect of insulin closely resembled the action of cholinomimetics, guanosine $3',5'$-monophosphate (cGMP). Since both insulin and cholinomimetics elevate intracellular concentrations of cGMP, a common mode of action was suggested. More recently Helderman *et al.* (1979) reported that the cytotoxic cells and insulin-receptor-positive cells were predominantly $Ly2^+3^+$ but $Ly1^+$ cells could also be induced to bear insulin receptor using density gradient centrifugation. Cytotoxic T cells generated in MLC and insulin-receptor-bearing T cells were enriched in the same fraction. Gelfand *et al.* (1982) reported that at low effector-to-target-cell ratios, the addition of insulin resulted in a dose-dependent reduction of erythrocyte target cell lysis but not of tumor target cells. In patients with insulin resistance and lipodystrophy, insulin failed to inhibit ADCC. The authors suggested that this may serve as a reliable and simple assay for the demonstration of altered insulin receptors or for the detection of antiinsulin receptors antibodies.

In the past decade the theory that viruses causes Type I diabetes has attracted new interest following the description of a murine model of Type I diabetes induced by the M variant of encephalomyocarditis virus (Chapter 3).

There is increasing evidence that natural killer (NK) cells, the large granular lymphocytes, play an important role in resistance against viruses. The significance of NK cells in Type I diabetes mellitus is not well defined. Recently we have studied NK and ADCC in a small sample of previously treated Type I diabetics. No significant difference was observed in either ADCC or NK activity when compared to controls (Gupta and Fernandes, unpublished observations). However, small sample size and lack of newly diagnosed patients precludes any definitive conclusions from this study.

XV. SUMMARY

In this chapter I have reviewed lymphocyte subpopulations and their functions in healthy states and in patients with diabetes mellitus. There is strong evidence to suggest that abnormal immunoregulatory functions exist in Type I diabetes, however the cellular and molecular bases of such a defect are unclear. The data on lymphocyte subpopulation, including those defined with monoclonal antibodies, are conflicting. Carefully planned and properly interpreted results of various studies do not support the theory that metabolic abnormalities account for most of immunological changes observed in Type I diabetes. Studies are required to examine *in vivo* effect of insulin on certain immune functions by studying newly diagnosed untreated patients and following them after insulin treatment. It is very likely that at least some immune functions will be modified by the administration of insulin in the light of the fact that patients with Type I diabetes have increased proportion of circulating activated T cells and activated T cells have shown to express insulin receptors. Furthermore, studies are required to examine the subpopulations of lymphocytes in the pancreatic infiltrates in Type I diabetes in order to understand their role in the B cell destruction.

REFERENCES

Abo, T., and Balch, C. M., 1981, A differentiation antigen of human NK and K cells identified by a monoclonal antibody (HNK1) *J. Immunol.* **127**:1024–1029.

Bersani, G., Zanco, P., Padovan, D., and Betterle, C., 1981, Lymphocyte subpopulations in insulin-dependent diabetics with or without serum islet-cell autoantibodies, *Diabetologia* **20**:47–50.

Boitard, C., Debray-Sachs, M., Pouplard, A., Assan, R., and Hamburger, J., 1981, Lymphocytes from diabetics suppress insulin release in vitro, *Diabetologia* **21**:41–46.

Brody, J. I., and Merlie, K., 1970, Metabolic and biosynthetic features of lymphocytes from patients with diabetes mellitus: Similarities to lymphocytes in chronic lymphocytic leukemia, *Br. J. Haematol.* **19**:193–201.

Buschard, K., Madsbad, S., and Rygaard, J., 1980, Depressed suppressor cell activity in patients with newly diagnosed insulin-dependent diabetes mellitus, *Clin. Exp. Immunol.* **41**:25–32.

Buschard, K., Madsbad, S., Krarup, T., and Rygaard, J., 1982, Glycaemic control and suppressor cell activity in patients with insulin-dependent diabetes mellitus, *Clin. Exp. Immunol.* **48**:189–195.

Cattaneo, R., Saibene, V., and Pozza, G., 1976, Peripheral T-lymphocytes in juvenile-onset diabetics (JOD) and in maturity-onset diabetics (MOD), *Diabetes* **25**:223–226.

Damle, N. K., Hansen, J. A., Good, R. A., and Gupta, S., 1981, Monoclonal antibody analysis of human T lymphocyte subpopulations exhibiting autologous mixed lymphocyte reaction, *Proc. Natl. Acad. Sci. (USA)* **78**:5096–5099.

Damle, N. K., and Gupta, S., 1982, Autologous mixed lymphocyte reaction in man. V. Functionally and phenotypically distinct human T-cell subpopulations responding to non-T and activated T cells in AMLR, *Scand. J. Immunol.* **16**:59–68.

Delepesse, J., Duchateau, J., Bastenie, P. A., Lauvaux, J. P., Collet, H., and Govaerts, A., 1974, Cell-mediated immunity in diabetes mellitus, *Clin. Exp. Immunol.* **18**:461–467.

Dolkart, R. E., Halpern, B., and Perlman, J., 1971, Comparison and antibody responses in normal and alloxan diabetic mice, *Diabetes* **20**:162–167.

Fabris, N., and Piantanelli, L., 1977, Differential effect of pancreatectomy on humoral and cell-mediated immune response, *Clin. Exp. Immunol.* **28**:315–325.

Fairchild, R. S., Kyner, J. L., and Abdon, N. I., 1982, Specific immunoregulation abnormality in insulin dependent diabetes mellitus, *J. Lab. Clin. Med.* **99**:175–185.

Farid, N. R., and Anderson, J., 1973, Immunoglobulins and complement in diabetes mellitus, *Lancet* **2**:92.

Faulk, W. P., Girard, J. P., and Welscher, H. D., 1975, Cell-mediated immunity to insulin and its polypeptide chains in insulin-treated diabetics, *Int. Arch. Allergy Appl. Immunol.* **48**:364–371.

Gavin, J. R., Roth, J., Jen, P., and Freychet, P., 1972, Insulin receptors in human circulating cells and fibroblasts, *Proc. Natl. Acad. Sci. (USA)* **69**:747–751.

Gelfand, E. W., Ipp, M. M., and Riordan, J. R., 1982, Insulin modulation of antibody-dependent cytotoxicity and the detection of anti-receptor antibodies, *J. Lab. Clin. Med.* **99**:39–45.

Gepts, W., 1965, Pathologic anatomy of the pancreas in juvenile diabetes mellitus. *Diabetes* **14**:619–633.

Glassman, A. B., and Bennett, C. E., 1980, B and T lymphocytes: Quantitation, Function, and clinical applicability, *Ann. Clin. Lab. Sci.* **8**:455–462.

Gozes, Y., Carusso, J., and Strom, T. B., 1981, The absence of cryptic insulin receptors on resting lymphocytes, *Diabetes* **30**:314–316.

Gupta, S., 1978, Functionally distinct subpopulations of human T lymphocytes. A brief review, *Clin, Bull.* **8**:100–107.

Gupta, S., 1981, Human T cell subpopulations with receptors for immunoglobulin isotypes, *Clin. Immunol. Newsletter* **2**:51–57.

Gupta, S., and Good, R. A., 1978, Human T cell subsets in health and disease, in: *Human Lymphocyte Differentiation: Its Application to Cancer* (B. Serrou and S. Rosenfeld, eds.), pp. 367–374, North-Holland Biomedical Press, Amsterdam.

Gupta, S., and Good, R. A., 1979b, Lymphocytes—1979, *Henry Ford Hosp. Med. J.* **27**:224–235.

Gupta, S., and Good, R. A., 1979a, Human T lymphocytes as defined by Fc receptors, *Thymus* **1**:135–149.

Gupta, S., and Good, R. A., 1980, Markers of human lymphocyte subpopulations in primary immunodeficiency and lymphoproliferative disorders, *Semin. Hematol.* **17**:1–29.

Gupta, S., and Good, R. A., 1981a, Subpopulations of human T lymphocytes. Laboratory and clinical studies, *Immunol. Rev.* **56**:89–114.

Gupta, S., and Good, R. A., 1981b, Clinical significance of human lymphocyte subpopulations, in: *Contemporary Hematology* (A. S. Gordon, R. D. Silber, and J. LoBue, eds.), pp. 153–226, Plenum Press, New York.

Gupta, S., and Kapoor, N., 1980, Lymphocyte subpopulations; surface, intracellular, enzymatic markers and functions, in: *Infections Complicating the Abnormal Host* (M. H. Grieco, ed.), pp. 84–128, Yorke Medical Books, New York.

Gupta, S., Winchester, R. J., and Good, R. A., 1980a, General orientation of human lymphocyte subpopulations, in: *Clinical Immunobiology*, vol. 4 (F. H. Bach and R. A. Good, eds)., pp. 1–31 Academic Press, New York.

Gupta, S., Fernandes, G., Rocklin, R., and Good, R. A., 1980, Histamine receptors on human T cell subsets, in: *International Symposium on New Trends in Human Immunology and Cancer Immunology* (B. Serrou and C. Rosenfeld, eds.), pp. 36–47, Doin Editier, Paris.

Gupta, S., Fikrig, S. M., Damle, N. K., Khanna, S., and Orti, E., 1981, Abnormal immunoregulatory function in patients with insulin-dependent diabetes mellitus, *Human Lymphocyte Differentiation* **1**:197–202.

Gupta, S., Fikrig, S. M., Khanna, S., and Orti, E., 1982, Deficiency of suppressor T cells in insulin-dependent diabetes mellitus. An analysis with monoclonal antibodies, *Immunol. Lett.* **4**:289–294.

Gupta, S., Fikrig, S., and Orti, E., 1983, Autologous mixed lymphocyte reaction in man. VI. Deficiency of autologous mixed lymphocyte reaction in type I (insulin-dependent) diabetes mellitus, *J. Lab. Clin. Med.* **11**:59–62.

Hann, S., Kaye, R., and Falkner, B., 1976, Subpopulations of peripheral lymphocytes in juvenile diabetes, *Diabetes* **25**:101–103.

Helderman, J. H., 1981, Role of insulin in the intermediary metabolism of the activated thymic-derived lymphocyte, *J. Clin. Invest.* **67**:1636–1642.

Helderman, J. H., and Raskin, P., 1980, The T lymphocyte insulin receptor in diabetes and obesity. An intrinsic binding defect, *Diabetes* **29**:551–557.

Helderman, J. H., and Strom, T. B., 1978, Specific insulin binding site on T and B lymphocytes as a marker of cell activation, *Nature* **274**:62–63.

Helderman, J. H., Strom, T. B., and Dupuy-D'Angeac, A., 1979, A close relationship between cytotoxic T lymphocytes generated in the mixed lymphocyte culture and insulin-receptor bearing lymphocytes. Enrichment by density gradient centrifugation, *Cell Immunol.* **46**:247–258.

Horowitz, S. D., Borcherding, W., and Bargman, G. J., 1977, Suppressor T cell function in diabetes mellitus, *Lancet* **2**:1291.

Huang, S-W., and MacLaren, N. K.,1976, Insulin-dependent diabetes: A disease of autoaggression, *Science* **193**:64–66.

Jackson, R. A., Morris, M. A., Haynes, B. F., and Eisenbarth, G. S., 1982,1 Increased circulating Ia-antigen-bearing T cells in type I diabetes mellitus, *N. Engl. J. Med.* **306**:785–788.

Krug, U., Krug, F., and Cuatrecasas, P., 1972, Emergence of insulin receptors on human lymphocytes during *in vitro* transformation, *Proc. Natl. Acad. Sci. (USA)* **69**:2604–2608.

Lederman, M. M., Ellner, J., and Rodman, H. M., 1981, Defective suppressor cell generation in juvenile onset diabetes, *J. Immunol.* **127**:2051–2055.

Lipscomb, H., Dodson, H. L., and Green, J. A., 1959, Infection in the diabetic. *South Med. J.* **52**:16–23.

Ludwig, H., Erbl, M., Schernthaner, G., Erd, W., and Maye, W. R., 1976, Humoral immunodeficiency to bacterial antigens in patients with juvenile onset diabetes mellitus, *Diabetologia* **12**:259–262.

MacCuish, A. C., Jordan, J., Campbell, C. J., Duncan, L. P. J., and Irvine, W. J., 1974a, Cell-mediated immunity to immunity to human pancreas in diabetes mellitus, *Diabetes* **23**:693–697.

MacCuish, A. C., Urbaniak, S. J., Campbell, C. J., Duncan, L. P. J., and Irvine, W. J., 1974b, Physohemagglutinin transformation and circulating lymphocyte subpopulations in insulin-dependent diabetic patients, *Diabetes* **23**:708–712.

MacCuish, A. C., Jordan, J., Campbell, C. J., Duncan, L. P. J., and Irvine, W., J., 1975, Cell-mediated immunity in diabetes mellitus. Lymphocyte transformation by insulin and insulin fragments in insulin-treated and newly-diagnosed diabetics, *Diabetes* **24**:36–43.

Mascart-Lemone, F., Delespesse, G., Dorchy, H., Lemiere, B., and Servais, G., 1982, Characterization of immunoregulatory T lymphocytes in insulin-dependent diabetic children by means of monoclonal antibodies, *Clin. Exp. Immunol.* **47**:296–300.

Moretta, L., Ferrarini, M., and Cooper, M. D., 1978, Characterization of human T cell subpopulations as defined by specific receptors for immunoglobulins, *Contemp. Top. Immunobiol.*, **8**:19–53.

Nadler, L. M., Stashenko, P., Hardy, R., van Agthoven, A., Terhorst, C., and Schlossman, S. F., 1981a, Characterization of a human B cell-specific antigen (B2) distinct from B1, *J. Immunol.* **126**:1941–1947.

Nadler, L. M., Ritz, J., Hardy, R., Pesando, J. M., and Schlossman, S. F., 1981b, A unique cell surface antigen identifying lymphoid malignancies of C cell origin, *J. Clin. Invest.* **67**:134–140.

Nerup, J., Andersen, O. O., Bendixen, G., Egeberg, J., and Poulsen, J. E., 1971, Antipancreatic cellular hypersensitivity in diabetes mellitus, *Diabetes* **20**:424–427.

Nerup, J., Andersen, O. O., Bendixen, G., Egeberg, J., Gunnarsson, R., Kromann, H., and Poulsen, J. E., 1974, Cell-mediated immunity in diabetes mellitus, *Proc. R. Soc. Med.* **67**:506–513.

Nieminen, P., Paasivuo, R., and Saksela, E., 1982, Effect of a monoclonal anti-large granular lymphocyte antibody on the human NK activity, *J. Immunol.* **128**:1097–1101.

Ortaldo, J. R., Sharrow, S. O., Timonen, T., and Herberman, R. B., 1981, Determination of surface antigens on highly purified NK cells by flow cytometry with monoclonal antibodies, *J. Immunol.* **127**:2401–2409.

Pozzilli, P., Sensi, M., Gorsuch, A., Bottazzo, G. F., and Cudworth, A. G., 1979, Evidence for raised K-cell levels in type I diabetes, *Lancet* **2**:173–175.

Ragab, A. H., Hazlett, B., and Cowan, D. H., 1972, Response of peripheral blood lymphocytes from patients with diabetes mellitus to phytohemaggutinin and candida albicans antigen, *Diabetes* **21**:906–907.

Reinherz, E. L., and Schlossman, S. F., 1980, The differentiation and function of human T lymphocytes, *Cell* **19**:821–827.

Reinherz, E. L., Moretta, L., Roper, M., Breard, J. M., Mingari, M. C., Cooper, M. D., and Schlossman, S. F., 1980, Human T lymphocyte subpopulations defined by Fc receptors and monoclonal antibodies. A comparison, *J. Exp. Med.* **151**:969–976.

Reinherz, E. L., Morimoto, C., Fitzgerald, K. A., Hussey, R. E., Daley, J. F., and Schlossman, S. F., 1982, Heterogeneity of human OKT4 + cells defined by a monoclonal antibody that delineates two functional subpopulations, *J. Immunol.* **128**:463–468.

Richens, E. R., Ancill, R. J., Gough, K. R., and Harbog, M., 1973, Cellular hypersensitivity to mitochondrial antigens in diabetes mellitus, *Clin. Exp. Immunol.* **13**:1–7.

Rocklin, R. E., Beard, J., Gupta, S., Good, R. A., and Melman, K., 1979, Characterization of the human blood lymphocytes that produce a histamine-induced suppressor factor (HSF), *Cell Immunol.* **51**:226–237.

Ross, G. D., 1979, Identification of human lymphocyte subpopulations by surface marker analysis, *Blood* **53**:799–811.

Schwartz, R. H., Bianco, A. R., Handbuerger, B. S., and Kahn, R., 1975, Demonstration that monocytes rather than lymphocytes are the insulin-binding cells in preparation of human peripheral blood mononuclear leukocytes: Implications for studies of insulin-resistant states in man, *Proc. Natl. Acad. Sci. (USA)* **72**:474–478.

Selam, J. L., Clot, J., Andary, M., and Mirouze, J., 1979, Circulating lymphocyte subpopulations in juvenile insulin-dependent diabetes, *Diabetologia* **16**:35–40.

Sensi, M., Pozzilli, P., Gorsuch, A. N., Bottazo, G. F., and Cudworth, A. G., 1981, Increased killer cell activity in insulin-dependent (type I) diabetes mellitus, *Diabetologia* **20**:106–109.

Slater, L. M., Murray, S. L., Kershnar, A., and Mosher, M. A., 1980, Immunological suppressor cell activity in insulin-dependent diabetes, *J. Clin. Lab. Immunol.* **3**:105–109.

Smith, W. I., Rabin, B. S., Huellmantel, A., Thiel, D. H. V., and Drash, A., 1978, Immunopathology of juvenile-onset diabetes mellitus. I. IgA deficiency and juvenile diabetes, *Diabetes* **27**:1092–1097.

Souadjian, J. V., Molnar, G. D., Silverstein, M. N., and Titus, J. L., 1970, Morphologic studies of the thymus in acromegaly, diabetes mellitus and Cushing's syndrome, *Metabolism* **19**:401–405.

Stratton, J. A., Nies, K. M., Louie, J. S., and Sperling, M. A., 1970, Cellular immunity in juvenile diabetes mellitus, *Diabetes* **15**:101.

Strom, T. B., Bear, R. A., and Carpenter, C. B., 1975, Insulin-induced augmentation of lymphocyte-mediated cytotoxicity, *Science* **187**:1206–1208.

Thomas, Y., Rogozinski, L., Irigoyen, O. H., Shen, H. H., Talle, M. A., Goldstein, G., and Chess, L., 1982, Functional analysis of human T cell subsets defined by monoclonal antibodies. V. Suppressor cells within the activated OKT4 + population belong to a distinct subset, *J. Immunol.* **128**:1386–1390.

Timonen, T., Ranki, A., Saskela, E., and Hayry, P., 1979, Fractionation, morphological and functional characterization of effector cells responsible for human natural killer activity against cell-line targets, *Cell Immunol.* **48**:121–132.

Uchiama, T., Nelson, D. L., Fleisher, T. A., and Waldmann, T. A., 1981a, A monoclonal antibody (anti-Tac) reactive with activated and functionally mature human T cells. II. Expression of Tac antigen on activated cytotoxic killer T cells, suppressor cells and one of two types of helper T cells, *J. Immunol.* **126**:1398–1403.

Uchiama, T., Broder, S., and Waldman, T. A., 1981b, A monoclonal antibody (anti-Tac) reactive with activated and functionally mature human T cells. I. Production of anti-Tac monoclonal antibody and distribution of Tac (+) cells, *J. Immunol.* **126**:1393–1397.

Zola, H., 1980, Monoclonal antibodies against human cell membrane antigen. A review, *Pathology* **12**:539.

12

Autoimmunity

Jørn Nerup, Åke Lernmark, and Joanne Scott

I. INSULITIS

Early in this century several authors found the typical pathological lesion in patients dying from untreated ketotic diabetes mellitus to be mononuclear infiltration in and around the islets of Langerhans (Opie, 1901; Schmidt, 1902; Herbert, 1911). This lesion—later called *insulitis* (von Meyenburg, 1940)—was thought to be rather specific for ketosis-prone diabetes mellitus, but was occasionally seen in endocrine disorders, such as idiopathic Addison's disease (Guttman, 1930). The existence of insulitis was rediscovered by Gepts in the 1960s (Gepts, 1965) and was further characterized as a lymphocytic infiltration occurring together with a selective loss of B cells. Thus, in analogy with, for instance, the chronic atrophic lymphocytic thyroiditis and the chronic atrophic lymphocytic adrenalitis seen in primary myxedema and idiopathic Addison's disease, respectively, the lesion in young patients with insulin-dependent diabetes mellitus (IDDM) of recent onset might be characterized as a chronic, atrophic lymphocytic insulitis in which the B cell is the only endocrine cell type in the islet to disappear (Fig. 1).

Against the background of the general interest in autoimmune endocrinopathies, the paper by Gepts (1965) triggered widespread interest and the researchers began to look for evidence of autoimmunity against specific determinants of the endocrine pancreas in patients with diabetes mellitus. Until recently, insulitis was thought to be rare, occurring only in the early stages of clinically manifest IDDM.

Except for the case of Addison's disease mentioned above, insulitis has not been described in nondiabetics or in non-insulin-dependent diabetes mellitus (NIDDM) patients, and it is not known if it occurs in the prediabetic phase of IDDM. It is interesting, however, that destruction of B cells together with acute and chronic inflammatory

Jørn Nerup • Steno Memorial Hospital, DK-2820 Gentofte, Denmark. Åke Lernmark and Joanne Scott • Hagedorn Research Laboratory, DK-2820 Gentofte, Denmark.

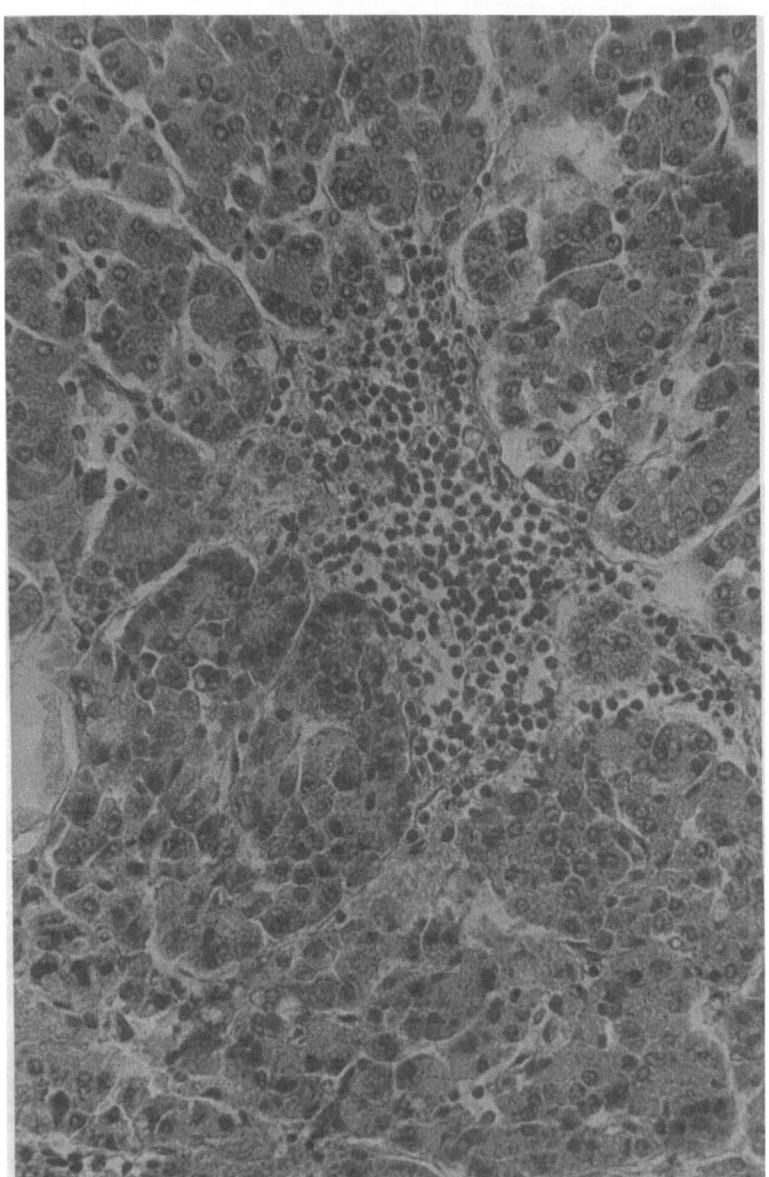

Figure 1. Islet of Langerhans with infiltration by mononuclear cells from a child dying from untreated diabetic ketoacidosis (courtesy of Dr. J. Egeberg, Institute of Anatomy B, University of Copenhagen).

infiltrates in the islets were found in about half the infants dying with fulminant coxsackie B virus infections (Jenson *et al.*, 1980).

The exact nature of the infiltrating cells in insulitis remains to be clarified. Morphologically they have the features of small lymphocytes. Plasma cells are very rarely, if ever, present. Studies applying cell-surface markers specific for lymphocytic subpopulations have not been published. To clarify if the cellular infiltrates in the islets of Langerhans are of pathogenetic importance it will be of great interest to identify the type(s) of lymphoid cells capable of infiltrating the islets. The recognition of B-cells by host lymphoid cells could require specific receptors for B cell-membrane-specific self- or neoantigen(s) to allow the cellular infiltrate to build up.

Insulitis is associated with young age of onset and short duration of IDDM and is seen only in islets still containing B cells (Gepts and Le Compte, 1981). Signs of regeneration/neoformation of islet cells, either from existing islets or *de novo* from duct epithelial cells, have been described, suggesting that the B cell loss in IDDM reflects a disturbed balance between renewal and destruction of B cells. Thus, IDDM may become manifest only when B cell regeneration cannot compensate for destruction, either because regeneration capacity is reduced by inheritance and exhausted by single or repeated injuries to the endocrine pancreas or because regeneration cannot catch up with continuous cell destruction.

II. CLINICAL AND IMMUNOLOGICAL ASSOCIATIONS OF IDDM WITH AUTOIMMUNE ENDOCRINOPATHIES

IDDM occurs more frequently than should be expected by change alone in clinical assocation with autoimmune endocrinopathies, such as idiopathic Addison's disease, Graves' disease, primary myxedema, Hashimoto's thyroiditis, hypergonadotropic hypogonadism (female), idiopathic hypoparathyroidism, and pernicious anemia. The prevalence of IDDM in idiopathic Addison's disease is 30–50 times higher than that of the background population (Nerup, 1974) and a similar increase is seen of IDDM in autoimmune thyroid disorders. The opposite situation (an increased prevalence of the autoimmune endocrinopathies in IDDM) is less well documented, but estimates suggest a four- to five-fold increase over the prevalence in the background population. The prevalence of subclinical primary thyroid failure in IDDM was recently reported to be close to 12%, with the overall prevalence of both clinically unrecognized and recognized thyroid disease about 20% (Gray *et al.*, 1980). Thyroglobulin, thyroid microsomal, and/or gastric parietal cell autoantibodies were more frequent among IDDM patients (Nerup and Binder, 1973; MacCuish and Irvine, 1975; Christy *et al.*, 1977). The overall prevalence was reported to be 23–29% with higher prevalence among female (32–39%) than male (16–19%) patients (Irvine *et al.*, 1970, 1977a,b; Lendrum *et al.*, 1976). The prevalence of these thyrogastric antibodies was found to increase with age both in the control population and among IDDM-patients (Irvine *et al.*, 1970, 1977a; Lendrum *et al.*, 1976). The prevalence of thyrogastric antibodies in IDDM was increased in patients who had had diabetes for more than 3 years, especially in patients with islet cell cytoplasmic antibodies (Bottazzo *et al.*, 1978a). In newly diagnosed IDDM children or young adults, the prevalence of thyroid microsomal, thyroglobulin, or gastric parietal cell antibodies did not differ from controls (Lernmark *et al.*, 1981a; Dorchy *et al.*, 1981) and no association was found between islet cell cytoplasmic antibodies and other organ-specific autoantibodies in young IDDM patients without overt endocrine disease (Lendrum *et al.*, 1976). In other studies, it was found that among islet-cell-antibody-negative IDDM children 11% had thyrogastric antibodies compared to 2–4% among controls (Bottazzo *et al.*, 1978b) and that such patients more often expressed HLA-B8 or DR3 (Bottazzo *et al.*, 1978b; Irvine *et al.*, 1977a) or HLA-B15 (Rodger *et al.*, 1980). Adrenal antibodies were demonstrated in some IDDM patients with normal adrenal function (Nerup *et al.*, 1973). Recently, thyroid-stimulating immunoglobulins were demonstrated in a small series of euthyroid IDDM patients (Schenthaner *et al.*, 1980). These antibodies, however, did not correlate well with the presence of HLA-DR3.

Furthermore, Bottazzo *et al.* (1982) have reported in IDDM the occurrence of autoantibodies to endocrine cells in the gut and the anterior pituitary. Such antibodies were also demonstrable in first-degree relatives of IDDM patients, particularly in relatives who later became diabetic.

Thus, clinical and subclinical disease as well as an increased prevalence of autoantibodies to endocrine cells link IDDM to the family of autoimmune endocrinopathies. At the present time an explanation for this is lacking.

III. RELATION TO OTHER AUTOIMMUNE PHENOMENA

Autoantibodies unrelated to endocrine organs (mitochondrial, smooth muscle, hepatic microsomal, salivary glands, and reticulin antibodies) are found with prevalence in IDDM similar to controls (MacCuish *et al.*, 1975; Dorchy *et al.*, 1981).

It might be of interest that autoantibodies have been observed, especially in recently diagnosed patients, against single-stranded DNA, double-stranded RNA from reovirus (but not from statolon virus) as well as to synthetic double-stranded RNA such as polyadrenylic–polyurifylic acid and polyinosinic–polyctidylic acid (Huang and MacLaren, 1978). In accord with the observations that unaffected relatives of diabetics seem to possess an increased prevalence of islet cell antibodies and other autoantibodies, the antibodies to nucleic acids were also more frequent in first-degree relatives (Huang *et al.*, 1981). The presence of nucleic acid antibodies did not correlate with any particular HLA type. However, since certain RNA viruses may be diabetogenic in humans (Craighead, 1978; Notkins, 1977), it is of particular interest that the prevalence against reovirus double-stranded DNA was increased. Mice infected with reovirus were recently found to develop a number of autoantibodies including growth hormone and insulin autoantibodies (Onodera *et al.*, 1981).

The pathogenic importance of autoantibodies against peripheral lymphocytes is not known, but it cannot be excluded that such antibodies in complement- or cell-mediated cytotoxic reactions may be responsible for removal of a specific lymphocyte subpopulation. Lymphocytotoxic antibodies were recently described in patients with IDDM of short duration (Serjeantson *et al.*, 1981). The antibodies did not correlate with islet cell cytoplasmic antibodies but were more frequent among individuals with HLA B8 or B18 phenotype. Although total T cell number seems not to be affected in

IDDM in humans (Bersani *et al.*, 1981; Muller *et al.*, 1980), it was reported that the BB rat, a Wistar rat strain, which spontaneously develops IDDM along with insulitis (Nakhooda *et al.*, 1977), has a major T cell lymphocytopenia independent of the development of diabetes (Jackson *et al.*, 1981).

Since T-suppressor lymphocytes seem to be decreased in number in IDDM patients of recent onset (Lederman *et al.*, 1981), it is tempting to speculate that lymphocytotoxic antibodies directed against this particular subset of T lymphocytes—possibly induced by a viral infection of the immune system—might be of pathogenic or even etiologic importance in IDDM. Studies to analyze the specificity, prevalence, temporal occurrence, and relation to HLA-DR determinants of relevance for IDDM of these lymphocytotoxic antibodies should certainly be initiated.

IV. ANTIPANCREATIC CELL-MEDIATED AUTOIMMUNITY (APCI)

The first direct experimental evidence for the existence of autoaggressive immune reactions against antigenic determinants of the endocrine pancreas in IDDM patients was provided by Nerup and co-workers in 1971. Using the leukocyte migration inhibition test (LMT), it was demonstrated that circulating leukocytes of IDDM patients showed inhibited migration in the presence of porcine pancreas homogenates (Nerup *et al.*, 1974). This phenomenon was later confirmed by other laboratories (Table 1), using human pancreas homogenates as antigen, while another involved the use of insulinoma extracts (MacCuish *et al.*, 1974b; Irvine *et al.*, 1976). The migration inhibition was most frequent in newly diagnosed diabetic patients and tended to fade away with increasing duration of the disease, possibly reflecting the loss of the islet cell antigen. It was also shown that intracutaneous injection or porcine pancreatic homogenate in patients with positive leukocyte migration inhibition had a delayed hypersensitivity skin reaction to that antigen (Nerup *et al.*, 1971). This observation strengthened the validity of the *in vitro* migration inhibition test as an indication of *in vivo* cell-mediated immunity toward the pancreas. It has been shown that the LMT is dependent on the migration and sensitization of T lymphocytes and is thus a valid measure of cell-mediated immunity. The presence of APCI did not correlate well with the occurrence of islet cell antibodies (Christy *et al.*, 1976) but did show increased frequency in HLA B8- and B15-positive diabetics.

Table 1.   Leukocyte Migration Inhibition Studies in Diabetes Mellitus

Antigen	Percentage of patients showing migration inhibition
Duct-ligated porcine pancreas (fraction prepared by differential centrifugation)	65 (IDDM only)
Homogenate of fetal calf pancreas	28 (All types of diabetic patients)
Homogenate of human pancreas	29 (All types of diabetic patients)
Extract, human insulinoma	50 (IDDM only)
Homogenate human pancreas	54 (IDDM only)

Since cell-mediated autoimmune reactions are perhaps more likely to have primary target cell-damaging effect than circulating antibodies, it is surprising that the literature on APCI is scarce. One report has shown that lymphocytes were able to suppress insulin release induced by glucose plus theophylline from cocultured mouse islets (Boitard *et al.*, 1981). No convincing information is available for studies of the possible effect of specifically reactive cytotoxic T lymphocytes from IDDM patients on human β cells. Such studies are urgently needed.

Passive Transfer

In vivo studies of the interaction between specifically sensitized lymphoid cells from IDDM patients and the intact cells of the islets of Langerhans were made possible by the discovery of the athymic nude mouse which lacks T-cell-dependent immune mechanisms. Theoretically, the transfer of lymphocytes from LMT-positive patients would cause insulitis and impaired glucose tolerance or diabetes in the recipients. This experimental approach to study diabetes has turned out to be controversial.

Peripheral lymphocytes from each of six patients with newly diagnosed IDDM were transplanted intraperitoneally in athymic nude mice (Buschard *et al.*, 1978). During the 30-day follow-up period, blood glucose concentrations to about 260 mg/dl were observed in some of the mice in the experimental group, compared with about 110 mg/dl in control mice which received lymphocytes from nondiabetic subjects. The pancreatic morphology of the recipients was not investigated. Several laboratories have not been able to confirm this study (Lipsick *et al.*, 1979; Thurneyssen *et al.*, 1979; Serra *et al.*, 1979; Neufeld *et al.*, 1979).

Both insulitis and diabetes can be induced in mice by treatment with low-dosage streptozotocin (Like and Rossini, 1976). A successful transfer of hyperglycemia from streptozotocin-treated mice to normal syngeneic and congenic recipients by means of lymphocytes has been reported (Buschard and Rygaard, 1977, 1979). Although insulitis has been transferred by lymphocytes in other laboratories no hyperglycemia was observed in the recipient mice (Kiesel *et al.*, 1980, 1981). Insulitis has also been transferred from spontaneously diabetic rats (''BB'' Wistar) to athymic nude mice (Nakhooda *et al.*, 1981). In the latter study, transfer of lymphocytes from the diabetic rats resulted in insulitis in 38% of the recipient mice, with 13% of the islets affected. The demonstration that insulitis can be produced in healthy recipients following transfer of lymphocytes from an affected individual provides suggestive evidence for cell-mediated immune mechanisms being involved in the pathogenesis of IDDM. Eisenbarth *et al.* (personal communication) have found increased levels of circulating HLA DR-positive T cells in IDDM. T cells are thought to express DR antigen only on activated T cells (Altevogt *et al.*, 1980). The function(s) of HLA DR + T cells and their relationship to IDDM remains to be determined.

V. ISLET CELL ANTIBODIES

A variety of antibodies reacting with antigenic components of the endocrine pancreas have been described (Table 2). This classification of islet cell antibodies is based mainly on the way by which they are demonstrated. Until identification and characteri-

Table 2. Humoral Immune Phenomena in IDDM: Approximate Prevalence (0/0) at Time of Diagnosis

Islet cell cytoplasmic antibodies	80–90
Islet cell surface antibodies	70–80
Immunoprecipitating antibodies	80
Organ-specific autoantibodies (e.g., thyroid, gastric, adrenal)	30
Immune complexes	50
Complement-dependent cytotoxicity	50–70
Antibody-dependent cellular cytotoxicity	Unknown (probably <10)
Somatostatin cell antibodies	Unknown (probably <1)
Glucagon cell antibodies	Unknown (probably <1)
Gastric inhibitory peptide cell antibodies	Unknown (probably <1)

zation of the antigens has been carried out, it is not possible to prove that the antibodies listed in Table 2 are different.

A. Islet Cell Cytoplasmic Antibodies

Antibodies reacting with cells of the endocrine pancreas were first demonstrated by Bottazzo et al. (1974) in patients with polyendocrine diseases. Antibodies were demonstrated on frozen sections of fresh human pancreas from individuals of blood group 0 as antigen by an immunofluorescence test. This finding was soon confirmed (MacCuish et al., 1974a). These antibodies, called islet cell cytoplasmic antibodies (ICA), react with all endocrine islet cells and show cross-species reactivity. Methods for ICA determination using Bouin- or formalin-fixed paraffin-embedded blood group 0 pancreas have been developed (Doberson et al., 1979; Sewell et al., 1980) and it has been claimed that more brilliant fluorescence and higher titers result from this technique. In our laboratory (Marner et al., 1982) consistent results with this modification of ICA determination could not be obtained. In contrast to other organ-specific antoantibodies in other endocrine diseases, ICA are always of the IgG class but show IgG subclass restriction with IgG3 occurring very rarely (Bottazzo et al., 1982).

The antigen with which ICA reacts remains to be identified and characterized, but that its subcellular localization is in the "microsomal" fraction of the cytoplasm has been suggested. It is also suggested that this antigen, through fusion with the cell membrane during exocytosis of secretory granular, might also be present at the cell surface (Bottazzo et al., 1982).

Islet cell cytoplasmic antibodies are detected in the serum of 0.1–1.0% of the background population and in about 15–30% of IDDM patients, irrespective of the length of their disease (Irvine et al., 1977a; Lendrum et al., 1976; Bottazzo et al., 1978). At the time of onset of insulin-dependent diabetes the immunofluorescent reaction is detected in about 80–90% of the patients (Irvine et al., 1977a; Lendrum et al., 1976; Lernmark et al., 1981a) (Table 2). The antibodies tend to disappear within a year after onset; however, persistent ICAs are observed in patients wiht concomitant endocrine autoimmune disease (Irvine et al., 1977a; Bottazzo et al., 1974). Patients with persistent ICAs seemed to carry the HLA antigen B8 more often than antibody-negative patients (Irvine et al., 1977a, 1978; Bottazzo et al., 1978; Christy et al.,

1976, 1977). In another study, however, such a correlation was not observed, but HLA B15-positive patients were associated with cell-mediated immune reactions to pancreatic antigens and with the presence of organ-specific autoantibodies (Richens et al., 1979). ICAs were, however, found to be more frequent among patients with different autoimmune endocrine disorders without diabetes (Irvine et al., 1977a; Del Prete et al., 1977). In the normal population the prevalance (Irvine et al., 1977a; Bottazzo et al., 1978; Rodger et al., 1980) of ICAs varies between 0.01 and 1%, and among the first-degree relatives of IDDM patients the prevalence was reported to be as high as 4–10% (Irvine et al., 1977a; Bottazzo et al., 1978; Gorsuch et al., 1981). In accordance with the experience in other autoimmune disorders where the levels of autoantibodies reflect disease activity, attempts have been made to test whether ICAs in a healthy individual are of predictive value.

In a large series of first-degree relatives of IDDM probands (Bottazzo et al., 1982) ICA was found in 6.2% of whom one-sixth became insulin-dependent diabetics 4–36 months after the first detection of ICA. It is of interest to note that these individuals shared at least one, and in half the cases, two, HLA-haplotypes with the diabetic proband. Thus, it is quite possible that ICA may be considered a signal of an islet cell destructive process and that its demonstration could be taken as a predictive marker of developing IDDM. Furthermore, ICAs have been demonstrated in patients treated with oral hypoglycemic agents who later require insulin (Irvine et al., 1979) and in some patients with onset of IDDM preceded by viral infections (Helmke et al., 1980).

When the immunofluorescence test was extended to involve a sandwich technique with normal human serum as the source of complement and fluorescent antihuman C-3 conjugates to detect bound complement, approximately 55% of ICA-positive sera were capable of fixing complement (Bottazzo et al., 1980, 1981). It was claimed that these complement-fixing ICA were closely related to the onset of diabetes and therefore would reflect damage of pancreatic islet cells (Bottazzo et al., 1980). This may well be the case. However, any assessment of risk for a given individual will be dependent on the ability to determine accurately the presence of antibodies during a follow-up period. This is of particular importance since temporary islet cell antibodies were found in healthy individuals, children with recent virus infections, as well as in newly diagnosed patients.

ICA, perhaps complement-fixing ICA to an even greater extent, might be important markers of islet cell destruction. It is surprising, however, that so little information about assay variability within and between laboratories is available. Comparisons between numbers for prevalence and titer given in different papers should be carried out with great caution. An interobserver variation of 12–16% was recently reported (Marner et al., 1982). The same authors report an assay sensitivity, that is, number of positive samples read as positive, varying between 40 and 98%. The main determinants for poor sensitivity were long ischemia time and greater age of the pancreatic tissue donor. The establishment of generally accepted standardized assay procedures and the development of a quantitative assay for ICA would be of great interest.

A pathogenetic role (i.e., interference with cell function) of ICA or complement-fixing ICA is not described. In IDDM only the cells are destroyed and ICA reacts with all the endocrine cell-types of the islets. Transplacental passage of ICA has been reported, but was not shown to be associated with abnormalities of fetal growth, congenital malformation, cord blood insulin levels, or neonatal complications (Tingle *et al.*, 1979).

Antibodies reacting with D cells (somatostatin-producing) and A cells (glucagon-producing) of the islets have been described (Bottazzo *et al.*, 1982) in diabetics as have antibodies to cells in the gut producing gastric inhibitory peptide (GiP). No clinically significant role can be ascribed to these antibodies today.

B. Islet Cell Surface Antibodies

Living cells are impermeable to antibodies which will bind only to antigens presented on the cell surface. Antibodies reacting with the surface of islet cells—were demonstrated by indirect immunofluorescence technique on dispersed islet cells from mice and rats (Lernmark *et al.*, 1978a). Their occurrence was soon confirmed and demonstrated also by the use of other assay systems (Table 2), but using islet cell suspensions from rodents. ICSA were detected using human insulinoma cells (MacLaren *et al.*, 1975), but these experiments are difficult to interpret since this particular cell line did not produce insulin. Recently, however, surface staining of living human fetal islet cells cultured for 6–8 days in monolayers has been demonstrated (Pujol-Borrell *et al.*, 1982). The stained cells were shown to contain insulin. Quantitative analyses by the fluorescence-activated cell sorter (Van de Winkel *et al.*, 1981) demonstrated that ICSA in sera from IDDM patients bind mainly to the cells.

So far, studies of assay reproducibility, precision, and their relation to HLA determinations are also lacking in relation to ICSA. However, the use of defined standardized suspension of islet cells (Lernmark *et al.*, 1978a) or cell lines (Eisenbarth *et al.*, 1981a) and protein A—specifically reacting with immunoglobulin (Lernark *et al.*, 1980)—have made more precise and quantitative assays possible.

ICSA were demonstrated in an indirect immunofluorensce test with dispersed islet cells from rat or mouse pancreatic islets in 2–4% control subjects and in approximately 30% of patients with IDDM (Lernmark *et al.*, 1978a, 1981a; Freedman *et al.*, 1979). Prior to the initiation of insulin therapy nearly 70% of IDDM children of young adults had surface antibodies and the prevalence diminished with increasing duration of the disease (Lernmark *et al.*, 1981a). The assays for ICSA and ICA in the same sera did not yield concordant results. In fact, the antibodies were found independently of each other or in combination and with various patterns of persistence (Lernmark *et al.*, 1981a).

Since ICSA bind to the surface of living islet cells, it is possible to study the possible inference of autoantibodies with B cell function.

Using perfused islet cells it has been shown that immunoglobulin from ICSA-containing sera from IDDM inhibit proinsulin synthesis (Lernmark *et al.*, 1979) as well as glucose-induced insulin release from rat islet cells (Lernmark *et al.*, unpublished observation). These experiments hae led to speculations that some ICSA may recognize a cell surface determinant (antigen) representing a receptor protein for the glucose signal to insulin production in the B cell.

C. Complement-Dependent Cytotoxic Antibodies

Lysis of target cells occurs if antibodies bound to cell surfaces, are recognized by components of the complement system. Several attempts have been made to test whether sera from IDDM patients could affect cell function in whole islets from rats. However, since the isolated islet represents a dense parenchyma of cells, often surrounded by a capsule, antibodies would have to diffuse through the extracellular space to reach individual cells. Methods were therefore developed to prepare single-cell suspensions from isolated pancreatic islets (Lernmark, 1974). In our early attempts to detect islet cell surface antibodies, it was observed that whole serum from humans as well as from other species induced a prompt release of insulin, blocked K^+ accumulation increased the release of ^{51}Cr from mislabelled B cells (Lernmark et al., 1978b). These effects were prevented by heating (50°C or 56°C for 30 min to inactivate complement), and an extended series of experiments demonstrated that dispersed islet cells from mice can activate complement via the alternative pathway (Idahl et al., 1980). This phenomenon is not unique to islet cells and should be taken into account when mechanisms of cell damage are considered.

Sera from IDDM patients, or immunoglobulins prepared from such sera, appear capable of mediating a complement-dependent cytotoxic reaction against rat islet cells (Soderstrum et al., 1979, Doberson et al., 1980), rat insulinoma cells (Eisenbarth et al., 1981a; Kende et al., 1981), or from dispersed human islet cells (Soderstrum, W. K., personal communication). In the cytotoxicity assay the cells were labeled with radioactive chromium and the release of radioactivity was taken as an index of viability after the addition of controlled preparations of complement. About 30% of IDDM patients had cytotoxic antibodies (Eisenbarth et al., 1981a; Kende et al., 1981), but the prevalence increased among newly diagnosed subjects. Cytotoxic islet cell antibodies were detected in sera from patients with islet cell surface antibodies, but not in diabetic sera with islet cell cytoplasmic antibodies alone (Doberson et al., 1980). In a double-fluorescence technique combining a vital stain with fluorescent hormone antibodies it was found that islet-cell-surface-positive sera lysed more than 80% of the cells stained with insulin antibodies while only 4–12% of the cells stained with glucagon, somatostatin, or pancreatic polypeptide (PP) were lysed (Doberson et al., 1981). The pathogenic importance of complement-dependent cytotoxic antibodies remains doubtful since they were found in 25% of nondiabetic first-degree relatives to IDDM probands (Doberson et al., 1980), a figure which is far beyond the number of relatives who will eventually develop IDDM themselves.

It is also unclear to what extent islet cell surface antibodies and macromolecules of the complement system are able to transverse the capillary cells and basement membranes within the islets. Glucose-induced insulin release from an isolated mouse pancreas perfused with complement was not blocked by immunoglobulin prepared from a patient with islet cell surface antibodies (Lernmark et al., 1981b). In contrast, in column-perfused dispersed rat islet cells, islet cell surface antibodies, and complement induced a block in glucose-induced insulin release (Kanatsuna et al., 1981).

The islet cell antibodies need to be characterized in terms of immunoglobulin class, reactivity with human islet cells, as well as their prevalence in newly diagnosed patients and relatives.

D. Antibody-Dependent Cellular Cytotoxicity

Immune cytotoxic T cells, macrophages, granulocytes, natural killer (NK), and killer cells (K cells) mediating antibody-dependent cell-mediated cytotoxicity (ADCC) can react against target cells (e.g., tumor cells and cells expressing altered self-antigens on their surface) (Herberman 1981). An ADCC assay is normally carried out with ^{51}Cr-labeled target cells (e.g., dispersed pancreatic B cells) that have been exposed to antibodies directed against these cells. Cells with receptors for the Fc-portion of an antibody molecule are added and rapid lysis of the target cells can occur. ADCC against rat pancreatic islet cells was found in one hour of 14 newly diagnosed IDDM patients (Soderstrum, W. K., personal communication). Increased levels of K cells have been found in early diabetes (Sensi et al., 1981). Further investigations will be needed to determine whether this observation is relevant to IDDM. It should also be pointed out that in vivo correlation to the in vitro ADCC reaction remains to be identified.

VI. CIRCULATING IMMUNE COMPLEXES

Immune complexes are formed by the binding of one or more antibody molecules to one or more antigen molecules. Such a complex would be formed either within a tissue or in the circulation with a soluble antigen. Since immune complexes can cause inflammatory reactions in tissues it is relevant to ask whether islet cell antibodies may form immune complexes with tissue antigens or whether circulating immune complexes may be deposited within the islets.

Immune complexes have been detected in approximately 50% of newly diagnosed IDDM patients but only in 6% of controls (Irvine et al., 1977b; Delespesse et al., 1980). The occurrence of circulating immune complexes has been found associated with the occurrence of late diabetic complications (DiMario et al., 1980; Virella et al., 1981). In diabetic patients, insulin–insulin antibody immune complexes have been identified, but complexes consisting of other and more pathogenetically relevant antigens and antibodies remain to be demonstrated. Recently, methods to identify hitherto unknown antigenic components of immune complexes have been developed (Theofilopoulos et al., 1978).

Removal of immune complexes appears to be dependent on the Fc-receptor function of tissue macrophages (Wiggins and Cochrane, 1981) and it was recently reported that individuals with HLA B8/DR3 have defective Fc-receptor functions (Lawley et al., 1981). It may be of significance in this respect that both IDDM patients and their siblings, HLA-identical or not, have increased immunofluorescent staining for IgG in extracellular membranes (Barbosa et al., 1980).

Immunoprecipitating Antibodies

The ability of islet cell antib. dies to form immune complexes with islet antigens has been investigated in immunoprecipitation experiments (Lernmark and Baekkeskov, 1981). Pancreatic islets were isolated from cadaver kidney donors, labeled biosynthetically with radioactive amino acids, and solubilized in detergents. The solubilized, radioactively labeled islet cell proteins were then incubated with sera from newly diagnosed diabetic children and healthy controls. Immune complexes were isolated and analyzed by gel electrophoresis combined with autoradiography to detect labeled antigens. The diabetic sera were found to contain antibodies against at least two proteins (mol. wt. approx. 64,000 and 38,000) present in normal human islets. These results indicate that islet cell antibodies may form immune complexes and that it should be possible to isolate and characterize target antigens.

VII. MONOCLONAL ANTIBODIES

In studies of islet cell antibodies, methods of lymphocyte hybridoma preparation and cellular cloning (Kohler and Milstein, 1975) have recently been introduced. The hybridomas produce one antibody type only, so-called monoclonal antibodies. A number of monoclonal-antibody-secreting hybridomas have been produced after immunizing mice with rat insulinoma cells and fusion with mouse myeloma cells (Eisenbarth, 1981). Several insulinoma-cell-specific clones were obtained along with antibodies which cross-reacted with other cell types as well. The antigens remain to be identified, but indirect evidence suggested that gangliosides and glycolipids were important.

The development of human myeloma cell lines (Olsson and Kaplan, 1980) has made it possible to fuse such cells with lymphocytes from diabetic patients (Eisenbarth *et al.*, 1981b,c). One hybridoma culture, B6, produced an IgM antibody which bound to the cytoplasma of islet cells in sections of frozen human pancreas. This experiment demonstrates that B lymphocytes expressing the gene for an islet cell antibody can circulate in the blood of a diabetic patient. This technique should make it possible to produce highly specific reagents to probe and isolate those antigens involved in the self-recognition phenomena in IDDM. Furthermore, treatment of experimental animals with monoclonal antibodies may teach us important lessons about the possible mechanisms through which spontaneously occurring antibodies are damaging to tissues, for example, induction of myasthenia gravis by a monoclonal acetylcholine receptor antibody (Lennon and Lambert, 1980).

VIII. CONCLUSIONS AND CLINICAL PERSPECTIVES

Research performed during the 1970s has provided considerable evidence to demonstrate the existence of islet-specific *autoimmune phenomena* in IDDM. Data to suggest that autoimmune phenomena might in fact be damaging to B cells, that is, an *autoimmune mechanism* of pathogenic importance, are beginning to emerge. The immune system seems to be able to recognize B-cell-specific antigens, but the evidence that specific B-cell-cytotoxic T lymphocytes exist is still very scarce and much more work is needed in this area.

The presence of islet cell antibodies is a feature of newly diagnosed IDDM. However, the predictive value of islet cell antibodies is still ambiguous. Antibodies reactive with the islet cell surface have the ability to mediate complement-dependent cytotoxicity *in vitro*. The cytotoxic effect results in an inability of the B cells to release insulin. However, a major problem in evaluating the clinical significance of these observations is that, so far, information about the effect of islet cell antibodies and/or sensitized lymphoid cells from IDDM patients is derived only from experiments using target B cells from other species. Obviously, if we want to learn about human IDDM, future studies should evaluate the effects of human sera and lymphoid cells on human B cells.

The identification, isolation, purification, and production of the B-cell-specific antigens involved should now be possible. Recombinant DNA technology will make possible production of large quantities of B-cell-specific membrane antigen, which will lead to sensitive, accurate, and quantitative assays for islet cell antibodies and the occurrence of specifically reactive lymphoid cells. Thus, diagnosis of a continuing possible B-cell-cytotoxic process in individuals at high genetic risk for IDDM is a realistic possibility in the not-too-distant future. Such assays will be necessary to monitor effects of future therapeutic measures as well.

Provided that the autoimmune phenomena are shown to be of pathogenetic importance in IDDM, early detection of such B-cell-damaging processes in the prediabetic phase of the disease will offer interesting possibilities for immunological intervention. The possibility of generating immortalized clones of either T lymphocytes or cells producing monoclonal antibodies will provide a source of highly specific reagents an' will be of potential importance to both diagnosis and therapy.

REFERENCES

Altevogt, P., Fohlman, J., Kurmick, J. T., Peterson, P., and Wigzel, H., 1980, Biochemical comparison of HLA-DR molecules derived from autologous human T and B lymphoblasts, *Eur. J. Immunol.* **10**:908.

Barbosa, J., Cohem, R. A., Chavers, B., Michael, A. F., Steffes, M., Hoogwerf, B., Szalapski, E., and Mauer, M., 1980, Muscle extra-cellular membrane immunofluorescence and HLA as possible markers of prediabetes, *Lancet,* **2**:330.

Bersani, G., Zanco, P., Padovan, D., and Betterle, C., 1981, Lymphocyte subpopulations in insulin-dependent diabetics with and without serum islet cell auto-antibodies, *Diabetologia* **20**:47.

Boitard, C., Debray-Sachs, M., Pouplard, A., Assan, R., and Hamburger, J., 1981, Lymphocytes from diabetes suppress insulin release *in vitro, Diabetologia* **21**:41.

Bottazzo, G. F., 1982, Minkowski lecture, 18th Annual Meeting of the European Association for the Study of Diabetes Mellitus, Budapest.

Bottazzo, G. F., Florin-Christensen, A., and Doniach, D., 1974, Islet cell antibodies in diabetes mellitus with autoimmune polyendocrine deficiencies, *Lancet,* **21**:41.

Bottazzo, G. F., Cudworth, A. G., Moul, D. J., Doniach, D., and Festenstein, H., 1978a, Evidence for a primary autoimmune type of diabetes mellitus, *Br. Med. J.* **2**:1253.

Bottazzo, G. F., Mann, J. I., Thorogood, M., Baum, J. D., and Doniach, D., 1978b, Autoimmunity in juvenile diabetes and their families, *Br. Med. J.* **1**:165.

Bottazzo, G. F., Dean, B. M., Gorsuch, A. N., Cudworth, A. G., and Doniach, D., 1980, Complement-fixing islet-cell antibodies in Type I diabetes: possible monitors of active cell damage, *Lancet,* **1**:668.

Bottazzo, G. F., Pujol-Borrell, R., and Doniach, D., 1981, Humoral and cellular immunity in diabetes mellitus, *Clin. Immunol. Allergy* **1**:139.

Bottazzo, G. F., Mirakian, R., Dean, B. M., McNally, J. M., and Doniach, D., 1982, How immunology helps to define heterogeneity in diabetes mellitus, in: *Genetics of Diabetes Mellitus* (J. Kobberling and R. Tattersall, eds.), p. 79. Serono Symp. No. 147.

Buschard, K., and Rygaard, J., 1977, Passive transfer of streptozotocin induced diabetes mellitus in mice, *Acta. Pathol. Microbiol. Scand.[C]* **85**:469.

Buschard, K., and Rygaard, J., 1979, T-lymphocytes transfer streptozotocin-induced diabetes in mice, *Acta Pathol. Microbiol. Scand.[C]* **86**:277.

Buschard, K., Madsbad, S., and Rygaard, J., 1978, Passive transfer of diabetes mellitus from man to mouse, *Lancet,* **1**:908.

Christy, M., Nerup, J., Bottazzo, G. F., Doniach, D., Platz, P., Svejgaard, A., Ryder, L. P., and Thomsen, M., 1976, Association between HLA-B8 autoimmunity in juvenile diabetes mellitus, *Lancet,***2**:142.

Christy, M., Deckert, T., and Nerup, J., 1977, Immunity and autoimmunity in diabetes mellitus, *Clin. Endocrinol. Metab.* **6**:305.

Craighead, J. E., 1978, Current views on the etiology of insulin-dependent diabetes mellitus, *New Engl. J. Med.* **299**:1439.

Delespesse, G., Gausset, Ph. Sarfati, M., Dubi-Rucquoy, M., Debisschop, M. J., and van Haelst, L., 1980, Circulating immune complexes in old people and in diabetics: Correlation with autoantibodies, *Clin. Exp. Immunol.* **40**:96.

Del Prete, G. F., Betterle, C., Padovan, D., Erle, G., Toffolo, A., and Borsahi, G., 1977, Incidence and significance of islet-cell antibodies in different types of diabetes mellitus, *Diabetes* **26**:909.

DiMario, U., Iavicoli, M., and Andreani, D., 1980, Circulating immune complexes in diabetes, *Diabetologia* **19**:89.

Doberson, M. F., Bell, A. M., Jenson, A. B., and Notkins, A. L., 1979, Detection of autibodies to islet cells and insulin with paraffin-embedded pancreas as antigen. *Lancet* **2**:1078.

Doberson, M. J., Scharff, J. E., Ginsberg-Fellner, F., and Notkins, A. L., 1980, Cytotoxic autoantibodies to beta-cells in the serum of patients with insulin-dpeendent diabetes mellitus, *N. Engl. J. Med.* **303**:1493.

Doberson, M. J., Ginsberg-Fellner, F., and Notkins, A. L., 1981, Insulinoma target cells for measurement of cytotoxic autoantibodies in patients with insulin-dependent diabetes mellitus (IDDM), *Diabetes* **30**(Suppl. 1):65A.

Dorchy, H., Lemiere, B., Toussaint, D., and Gausset, P., 1981, Anticorps anti-cellules des ilots de Langerhans et specifiques d'organes chez les jeunes diabetiques, *Nouv. Presse Med.* **10**:2795.

Eisenbarth, G. S., 1981, Monoclonal antibodies to islets, T-lymphocyte and neuronal cell surface differentiation antigens, in: *Monoclonal Antibodies in Endocrine Research* (R. Ellows and G. S. Eisenbarth, eds.), p. 33, Raven Press, New York.

Eisenbarth, G. S., Morris, M. A., and Scearce, R. M., 1981a, Cytotoxic antibodies to cloned rat islet cells in serum of patients with diabetes mellitus, *J. Clin. Invest.* **67:403.**

Eisenbarth, G. S., Linnenbach, A., Jackson, R., and Croce, C., 1981b, Antibody Bb: A human monoclonal anti-islet antibody, *Clin. Res.* **29**:404A.

Eisenbarth, G. S., Oie, Gazder, A., Chick, W., Schultz, J. A., and Scearce, R. M., 1981c, Production of monoclonal antibodies reacting with rat islet cell membrane antigens, *Diabetes* **30**:226.

Freedman, Z. R., Feed, C. M., Irvine, W. J., Lernmark, A., Rubenstein, A. H., Steeiner, D. F., and Huen, A., 1979, Islet-cell cytoplasmic and cell-surface antibodies in diabetes mellitus, *Trans. Assoc. Am. Physicians* **96**:64.

Gepts, W., 1965, Pathologic anatomy of the pancreas in juvenile diabetes mellitus, *Diabetes* **14**:619.

Gepts, W., and LeCompte, P. M., 1981, the pancreatic islets in diabetes, *Am. J. Med.* **70**:105.

Gorsuch, A. N., Spencer, K. M., Lister, J., McNally, J. M., Dean, B. M., Bottazzo, G. F., and Cudworth, A. G., 1981, The natural history of Type I (insulin-dependent) diabetes mellitus: Evidence for a long pre-diabetic period, *Lancet* **2**:1363.

Gray, R. S., Borsey, D. Q., Seth, J., Herd, R., Brown, N. S., and Clarke, B. F., 1980, Prevalence of subclinical thyroid failure in insulin-dependent diabetes, *J. Clin. Endocrinol. Metab.* **50**:1034.

Guttman, P. H., 1930, Addison's disease. A statistical analysis of 566 cases and a study of the pathology, *Arch. Pathol.* **10**:742.

Helmke, K., Otten, A., and Willems, W., 1980, Islet cell antibodies in children with mumps infection, *Lancet* **2**:211.

Herberman, R., 1981, Natural killer cells and cells mediating antibody-dependent cytotoxicity against tumor cells, in: *Clinical Immunobiology.* (F. H. Bach, and R. A. Good, eds.), p. 73.

Herbert, K. A., (1911), Studien uber die pathologischen-anatomischen Grundlage des Diabetes mellitus, *Virchows Arch. Pathol. Anat.* **204**:175.

Huang, S.-W., and MacLaren, N. K. (1978) Antibodies to nucleic acids in juvenile-onset diabetes, *Diabetes* **27**:1105.

Huang, S.-W., Hallquist Haedt, L., Rich, S., and Barbosa, J., 1981, Prevalence of antibodies to nucleic acids in insulin-dependent diabetes and their relatives, *Diabetes* **30**:873.

Idahl, L.-A., Sehlin, J., Taljedal, I.-B., Thornell, L.-E., 1980, Cytotoxic activation of complement by mouse pancreatic islet cells, *Diabetes* **29**:636.

Irvine, W. J., Clarke, B. F., Scarth, L., Cullen, D. R., and Duncan, L. J. P., 1970, Thyroid and gastric autoimmunity in patients with diabetes mellitus, *Lancet* **2**:163.

Irvine, W. J., MacCuish, A. C., Campbell, C. J., and Duncan, L. J. P., 1976, Organ-specific cell-mediated autoimmunity in diabetes mellitus, *Acta Endocrinol. (Kbh.)* **83**(Suppl. 205):65.

Irvine, W. J., McCallum, C. J., Gray, R. S., Campbell, G. J., Duncan, L. J. P., Farquhar, J. W., Vaughan, H., and Morris, P. J., 1977a, Pancreatic islet cell antibodies in diabetes mellitus correlated with the duration and type of diabetes, coexistent autoimmune disease, and HLA-type, *Diabetes* **26**:138.

Irvine, W. J., Al Khateeb, S. F., Di Mario, U., Feck, C. M., Gray, R. S., Edmond, B., and Duncan, L. J. P., 1977b, Soluble immune complexes in the sera of newly diagnosed insulin-dependent diabetics and in treated diabetics, *Clin. Exp. Immunol.* **30**:16.

Irvine, W. J., Di Mario, U., Feck, C. M., Gray, R. S., Ting, A., Morris, P. J., and Duncan, L. J. P., 1978, Autoimmunity and HLA antigens in insulin-dependent (Type I) diabetes, *J. Clin. Lab. Immunol.* **1**:107.

Irvine, W. J., Sawers, J. S. A., Feck, C. M., Prescott, R. J., and Duncan, L. J. P., 1979, The value of islet cell antibody in predicting secondary failure of oral hypoglycemic agent therapy in diabetes mellitus, *J. Clin. Lab. Immunol.* **2**:23.

Jackson, R., Rassi, N., Crump, T., Haynes, B., and Eisenbarth, G. S., 1981, The BB diabetic rat: Profound T-cell lymphocytopenia, *Diabetes* **30**:887.

Jenson, A. B., Rosenberg, H. S., and Notkins, A. L., 1980, Pancreatic islet-cell damage in children with fatal viral infections, *Lancet* **2**:354.

Kanatsuna, T., Lernmark, A., Rubenstein, A. J., and Steiner, D. F., 1981, Block in insulin release from column-perfused pancreatic B cells induced by islet cell surface antibodies and complement, *Diabetes* **30**:231.

Kende, M., Dobersen, M. J., Ginsberg-Fellner, F., and Notkins, A. L., 1981, Insulinoma target cells for measurement of cytotoxic autoantibodies in patients with insulin-dependent diabetes mellitus, *Diabetes* **30**(Suppl. 1):65A.

Kiesel, U., Freytag, G., Biener, J., and Kolb, H., 1980, Transfer of experimental autoimmune insulitis by spleen cells in mice. *Diabetologia* **19**:516.

Kiesel, U., Kolb, H., and Freytag, G., 1981, Strain dependency of the transfer of experimental immune insulitis in mice, *Clin. Exp. Immunol.* **43**:430.

Kohler, G., and Milstein, C., 1975, Continuous cultures of fused cells secreting antibody of predefined specificity, *Nature* **256**:495.

Lawley, T. J., Hall, R. P., Fauci, A. S., Katz, S. I., Hambuerger, M. I., and Frank, M. M., 1981, Defective Fc-receptor functions associated with the HLA-B8/DRw3 haplotype, *N. Engl. J. Med.* **304**:185.

Lederman, M. M., Ellner, J. J., and Rodman, H. M., 1981, Immunoregulatory defects in insulin dependent diabetes, *Diabetes* **30**(Suppl. 1):66A.

Lendrum, R., Walker, G. J., Cudworth, A. G., Theophanides, C., Pyke, D. A., Bloom, A., and Gamble, D. R., 1976, Islet-cell antibodies in diabetes mellitus, *Lancet* **2**:1273.

Lennon, V. A., and Lambert, E. J., 1980, Myasthenia gravis induced by monoclonal antibodies to acetylcholine receptors, *Nature* **285**:238.

Lernmark, A., 1974, The preparation of, and studies on, free cell suspensions from mouse pancreatic islets, *Diabetologia* **10**:431.

Lernmark, A., and Baekkeskov, S., 1981c, Islet cell antibodies—theoretical and practical implications, *Diabetologia* **21**, 431.

Lernmark, A., Freedman, Z. R., Hofmann, C., Rubenstein, A. H., Steiner, D. F., Jackson, R. L., Winter, R. J., and Traisman, H. S. 1978a, Islet cell surface antibodies in juvenile diabetes mellitus, *N. Engl. J. Med.* **299**:375.

Lernmark, A., Sehlin, J., Taljedal, I.-B., Kromann, H., and Nerup, J., 1978b, Possible toxic effects of normal and diabetic patient serum on pancreatic B-cells, *Diabetologia* **14**:25.

Lernmark, A., Kanatsuma, T., Rubenstein, A. H., and Steiner, D. F., 1979, Detection and possible functional influence of antibodies directed against the pancreatic islet cell surface, *Adv. Exp. Med. Biol.* **119:**157.

Lernmark, A., Kanatsuna, T., Patzelt, C., Diakoumis, K., Carroll, R., Rubenstein, A. H., and Steiner, D. F., 1980, Antibodies directed against the pancreatic islet cells plasma membrane, *Diabetologia* **19:**445.

Lernmark, A., Hagglof, B., Freedman, Z. R., irvine, W. J., Ludvigsson, J., and Holmgren, G., (1981a), A prospective analysis of antibodies reactive with pancreatic islet cells in insulin-dependent diabetic children, *Diabetologia* **20:**471.

Lernmark, A., Bonnevie-Nielsen, V., Baekkeskov, S., Dyrberg, T., Kanatsuna, T., and Scott, J., 1981b, Islet cell antibodies, in: *Ethiology and Pathogenesis of Insulin-Dependent Diabetes Mellitus* (J. M. Martin, R. M. Ehrlich, and F. J. Holland, eds.), p. 61, Raven Press, New York.

Like, A. A., and Rossini, A. A., 1976, Streptozotocin-induced pancreatic insulitis: New model of diabetes mellitus, *Science* **193:**415.

Lipsick, J., Beattie, G., Osler, A. G., and Kaplan, N. O., 1979, Passive transfer of lymphocytes from diabetic man to athymic mouse, *Lancet* **1:**1290.

MacCuish, A. C., and Irvine, W. J., 1975, Autoimmunological aspects of diabetes mellitus, *Clin. Endocrinol. Metab.* **4:**435.

MacCuish, A. C., Jordan, M., Campbell, C. J., Duncan, L. J. P., and Irvine, W. J., 1974a, Antibodies to islet-cells in insulin-dependent diabetics with coexistent autoimmune disease, *Lancet* **2:**1529.

MacCuish, A. C., Jordan, J., Campbell, C. J., Duncan, L. J. P., and Irvine, W. J., 1974b, Cell-mediated immunity to human pancreas in diabetes mellitus, *Diabetes* **23:**693.

MacLaren, N. K., Huang, S. W., and Fogh, J., 1975, Antibody to cultured human insulinoma cells in insulin-dependent diabetes, *Lancet* **1:**997.

Marner, B., Lernmark, A., Nerup, J., Molenaar, J. L., Bruining, G. J., and Tuk, C. W., 1983, Quantitative analysis of islet cell antibodies on sections of human pancreas, *Diabetologia*, in press.

Muller, R., Kolb, H., Juschak, D., Joerghens, D., and Gries, F. A., 1980, Analysis of T-lymphocyte subpopulations in juvenile-onset diabetics, *Clin. Exp. Immunol.* **39:**130.

Nakhooda, A. F., Like, A. A., Chappel, C. I., Myrray, F. T., and Marliss, E. B., 1977, The spontaneously diabetic Wistar rat: Metabolic and morphologic studies, *Diabetes* **26:**100.

Nakhooda, A. F., Sima, A. A. F., and Marliss, E. B., 1981, Passive transfer of insulitis from the spontaneously diabetic "BB" rat to the nude mouse, *Diabetes* **30**(Suppl. 1):66A.

Nerup, J., 1974, The clinical and immunological association of diabetes mellitus and Addison's disease, in: *Immunity and Autoimmunity in Diabetes Mellitus* (P. A. Bastenie, and W. Gepts, eds.), p. 149, Excerpta Medica, Amsterdam.

Nerup, J., and Binder, C., 1973, Thyroid gastric and adrenal autoimmunity in diabetes mellitus, *Acta Endocrinol.* **72:**279.

Nerup, J., Andersen, O. O., Bendixen, G., Egeberg, J., and Poulsen, J. E., 1971, Antipancreatic cellular hypersensitivity in diabetes mellitus, *Diabetes* **20:**424.

Nerup, J., Andersen, O. O., Bendixen, G., Egeberg, J., Gunnarson, R., Kromann, H., and Poulsen, J. E., 1974, Cell-mediated immunity in diabetes mellitus, *Proc. R. Soc. Med.* **67:**506.

Neufeld, M., McLaughlin, J., MacLaren, N. K., Rosenbloom, E., and Donelly, W., 1979, Failure to transfer diabetes mellitus from man to mouse, *N. Engl. J. Med.* **301:**665.

Notkins, A. L., 1977, Virus-induced diabetes mellitus, *Arch. Virol.* **54:**1.

Olsson, L., and Kaplan, H. S., 1980, Human-human hydridomas producing monoclonal antibodies of predefined specificity, *Proc. Natl. Acad. Sci. (USA)* **77:**5429.

Onodera, T., Toniolo, A., Ray, U. R., Jenson, A. B., Knazek, R. A., and Notkins, A. L., 1981, Virus-induced diabetes mellitus. XX. Polyendocrinopathy and autoimmunity, *J. Exp. Med.* **153:**1457.

Opie, E. L., 1901, The relation of diabetes mellitus to lesions of the pancreas, *J. Exp. Med.* **5:**527.

Pujol-Borrell, R., Khoury, E. L., and Bottazzo, G. F., 1982, Islet cell surface antibodies in Type I (insulin-dependent) diabetes mellitus: Use of human fetal pancreatic cultures as substrate, *Diabetologia* **22:**89.

Richens, E. R., Quilley, J., and Hartog, M., 1979, Immunological features of juvenile onset diabetic patients correlated to HLA type, *Clin. Exp. Immunol.* **36:**198.

Rodger, B., Wittingham, S., Martin, F. I. R., Hawkins, B. R., Hawkins, R. L., and Welborn, T. A., 1980, A population survey of pancreatic islet cell antibodies, *Clin. Exp. Immunol.* **89:**125.

Schernthaner, G., Schleusener, H., Mayr, W. R., Kotulla, P., Ludwig, H., and Wenzel, B., 1980, TSH-displacing auto-antibodies in type 1 diabetes mellitus, in: *Thyroid Research VIII, Proceedings of the 8th International Thyroid Congress* (C. Stockigt, S. Nagataki, eds.), p. 685, Australian Academy of Science, Canberra.

Schmidt, M. B., 1902, Uber die Beziehung der Langerhans'schen Inseln des Pancreas zum Diabetes mellitus, *Muench Med. Wochenschr.* **49:**51.

Sensi, M., Pozzilli, P., Gorsuch, A. N., Bottazzo, G. F., and Cudworth, A. G., 1981, Increased killer cell activity in insulin-dependent (Type 1) diabetes mellitus, *Diabetologia* **20:**106.

Serjeantson, S., Theophilus, J., Zimmet, P., Court, J., Crossley, J. R., and Elliot, R. B., 1981, Lymphocytotoxic antibodies and histocompatibility antigens in juvenile-onset diabetes mellitus, *Diabetes* **30:**26.

Serra, A. S., Farndon, J. R., Shenton, B. K., and Johnson, I. D. A., 1979, Passive transfer system of lymphocytes from diabetic man to athymic mouse, *Lancet* **1:**1292.

Sewell, M., Smith, D. I., Willox, A., and Barnes, C. A., 1980, Demonstration of islet-cell antibodies, *Lancet* **1:**102.

Soderstrum, W. K., Freedman, Z. R., and Lernmark, A., 1979, Complement-dependent cytotoxic islet cell surface antibodies in insulin-dependent diabetes, *Diabetes* **28:**397.

Theofilopoulos, A. N., Eisenberg, T. A., and Dixon, F. J., 1978, Isolation of circulating immune complexes using Raji cells. Separation of antigens from immune complexes and production of antiserum, *J. Clin. Invest.* **61:**1570.

Thurneyssen, O., Jansen, F. K., Vialettes, B., Vague, P., Selam, J. L., and Mirouze, J., 1979, Passive transfer of lymphocytes from diabetic man to athymic mouse, *Lancet* **1:**1291.

Tingle, A. J., Lim, G., Wright, V. J., Dimmick, J. E., and Hunt, J. A., 1979, Transplacental passage of islet cell antibody in infants of diabetic mothers, *Pediatr. Res.* **13:**1323.

Van de Winkel, M., Smets, G., Gepts, W., and Pipeleers, D. G., 1981, Identification of islet cells binding to circulating cell-surface antibodies of diabetic patients, *Diabetologia* **21:**338.

Virella, G., Wohltmann, H., Sagel, J., Lopes-Virella, M. F. L., Kilpatrick, M., Philips, C., and Colwell, J., 1981, Soluble immune complexes in patients with diabetes mellitus: Detection and pathological significance, *Diabetologia* **21:**184.

von Meyenburg, H., 1940, Uber "Insulitis" bei Diabetes, *Schweiz. Med. Wochenschr.* **21:**554.

Wiggins, R. C., and Cochrane, C. G., 1981, Immune-complex-mediated biological effects, *N. Engl. J. Med.* **304:**518.

13

Phagocytic Cell Functions in Diabetes Mellitus

Michael E. Miller

I. INTRODUCTION

The mechanisms by which the patient with diabetes mellitus demonstrates increased susceptibility to infections have aroused much interest. Consideration of possible defects has been divided into two major areas. In the first, potential abnormalities of the T- and/or B-cell system and their effects upon immunological functions in the diabetic patient have been probed. These studies are extensive and are reviewed elsewhere in this text (Chapter 11). The second group of studies has concerned a different component of the host defense system; the phagocytic cell lines. Although more contemporary in terms of active investigation, a sizable literature now exists through which investigators have implicated primary granulocyte dysfunctions as (a) major contributing factor(s) to infection in the diabetic host (Bagade, 1976). In this chapter, I will review the evidence for possible phagocytic dysfunction as a primary or major secondary cause of infections in the diabetic patient. These studies will then be summarized with reference to the limitations of *in vitro* assays of phagocyte function.

II. INFECTIONS

Before proceeding with a discussion of phagocyte function in the diabetic patient, it would be worthwhile to review the evidence for increased susceptibility to infections in such patients. A common assumption held by many clinicians is that diabetic patients have a generalized, increased susceptibility to infection compared with nondiabetic patients. When we review the literature in support of this hypothesis, however, we find

Michael E. Miller • Department of Pediatrics, University of California at Davis, Sacramento, California 95817.

that the available supporting data are less than overwhelming. Robbins and Tucker (1944) studies the autopsy results from 307 patients with diabetes mellitus and compared them with similar findings in 2800 nondiabetic patients. Pulmonary infections and most other serious systemic infections occurred with equal frequency in both groups. Only two infections occurred with significantly greater frequency in the diabetic patients: pyelonephritis and infection of the extremities. Pell and D'Alonzo (1970) compared the incidence of infections between a large group of diabetic patients and normal controls for 10 years. Infection was not an important cause of death in either group. Utilizing a somewhat different approach, Cohn and co-workers (1964) studied 143 cases of postoperative staphylococcal wound infections. They were unable to correlate increased risk of this infection with diabetes mellitus.

An extensive study of 662 diabetic employees of the DuPont Company demonstrates this point (Pell and D'Alonzo, 1967). The number of infectious illnesses causing absence from work was not statistically different from age-matched and job-matched nondiabetic controls. Duration of disability of 10 or more days was seen in 27.7% of those with diabetes and in only 14.8% of controls ($p > 0.01$). While there is little evidence, therefore, for a primary increase in susceptibility to infections among diabetic subjects, further complications of the disease such as the vascular impairment, neuropathy, and hypoglycemia associated with diabetes mellitus may cause certain infections to be of longer duration and severity. Peripheral vascular disease is a well-recognized complication of long-standing diabetes and increases the risk of infections in patients. This association is hardly surprising, since increased local circulation is a primary component of normal host defenses to infections. One might, therefore, expect that infection occurring in an extremity where vascular supply is comprised would be exaggerated. Data of Vejlsgaard (1965) support this conclusion. This study demonstrated a signficant correlation between the incidence of urinary tract infections and the presence of generalized vascular disease in persons with diabetes. The association was independent of duration of disease, presence of neurogenic bladder, or nephropathy.

Neuropathy may predispose the diabetic subject to infection in several ways. First, bladder dysfunction is present even in many asymptomatic cases of diabetes mellitus (Ellenberg and Weber, 1967). The neurogenic bladder with residual urine permits multiplication of organisms within the bladder. Iatrogenic infection may be a further complication when urinary retention in the patient leads to instrumentation. A significant sensory deficit of the extremities, which occurs in many patients with diabetes mellitus, may result in failure to recognize minor trauma, thereby permitting the development of significant infection before the patient recognizes the problem.

Hypoglycemia is generally believed to influence the growth of microorganisms, but even this observation has not been well documented (Edwards *et al.*, 1979). Robson and Heggers (1969) used plasma with varying amounts of added glucose and noted that gram-positive organisms grew well in relatively high glucose concentrations, while gram-negative organisms grew poorly. Sheldon and Bauer (1962) studied the role of predisposing factors in experimental infections in rabbits and mice rendered hyperglycemic. There was little difference noted in the extent of induced infection in animals made hyperglycemic by intravenous insion of glucose compared with controls.

In summary, then, there is little evidence that uncomplicated diabetes mellitus has a primary, significant association with increased susceptibility to infections. Some evidence, however, suggest that diabetes, along with one or more of its common complications (vasculitis, neuropathy, and/or hyperglycemia) may predispose the host to more frequent and extensive infections. Even in such situations, however, it appears that the increased susceptibility to infections is limited to selected body systems. We will now consider some of the unique aspects of infection in these sites in patients with diabetes mellitus.

A. Urinary Tract Infections

As we have already noted, the frequency of urinary tract infections is increased in patients with diabetes mellitus in whom there is associated vascular disease or neuropathy. In patients with well-controlled diabetes and in children, the incidence of urinary tract infection is no greater than that in age-matched controls (Huvos and Rocha, 1959; Pometta et al., 1967). Thus, we again note that the complications of the disease are superimposed upon the primary abnormality before the increased susceptibility to infections occurs.

By contrast, pyelonephritis occurs with greater frequency among diabetic patients, apparently independent of secondary complications. In studies by Baldwin and Root (1940), Edmondson et al., (1947), and Warren et al. (1966), as many as 20% of diabetic patients showed histological evidence of pyelonephritis at autopsy. Robbins and Tucker (1944) found acute pyelonephritis at autopsy in 6.8% of diabetic subjects, compared with an incidence of only 1.6% in nondiabetic subjects. This difference was partially explained by the obstruction to flow of normal urine in association with neurogenic bladder, although the incidence of neurogenic bladders in patients demonstrating pyelonephritis in their study was not reported.

In experimental animals, it is well-recognized that obstruction of the lower urinary tract enhances the development of pyelonephritis. Comparative studies of the incidence of *clinical* pyelonephritis in diabetic and nondiabetic subjects are, however, not available. Such correlations, therefore, depend upon the histological diagnosis of pyelonephritis. It has recently been theorized that these pathologic diagnoses may not reflect chronic infection, but represent disease modified by noninfectious factors. It therefore remains unclear whether pyelonephritis secondary to acute persistent infection by a microorganism occurs more frequently in diabetic than in nondiabetic persons (Halverstadt et al., 1966).

Several other disorders of the urinary tract which may be associated with infection are seen in greater frequency in diabetic subjects than in normals. Renal papillary necrosis (Lauler et al., 1960) occurs with high incidence in diabetic persons. These authors suggested that the presence of small vessel disease superimposed on renal infections may account for this association.

Cystitis emphysematosa also occurs with increased frequency in patients with diabetes mellitus (Bailey, 1961). This condition is characterized by the presence of gas vesicles in the bladder wall is associated with infection by coliform organisms in patients with glycosuria. The disease generally follows a benign clinical course and is sometimes associated with a history of pneumaturia. Definitive diagnosis, however, is made radiographically.

B. Tuberculosis

In retrospective studies, Muller and Higgins (1963) found no increased incidence of diabetes among patients with proven diagnoses of tuberculosis. They found diabetes in 4.2% of 118 adult patients in a tuberculosis sanitarium compared with an incidence of only 2.9% of diabetes among adults in a nearby geographic region. Despite equal incidence of tuberculosis among diabetic subjects, as in normals, there is some evidence that the clinical course and morbidity of the disease are more severe in the diabetic patient. Thus, the American Thoracic Society includes patients with diabetes in their list of patients who are considered immunosuppressed enough to require isoniazid for a positive PPD (purified protein derivative) reaction (American Thoracic Society, 1974). Younger and Hadley (1971) describe diabetic tuberculosis as a fulminant, exudative, rapidly progressive disease associated with significant caseation and a toxic downhill course. The incidence of advanced tuberculosis and lower lobe disease is also increased in diabetes (Weaver, 1974).

With the advent of newer forms of antituberculous drug therapy, marked reductions in the death rate from tuberculosis among diabetic subjects have been noted. In the 1960s the death rate fell from the 1920s level of 5.5% to 3.0%. It is notable, however, that this rate was still higher than the death rate in the general population in persons with tuberculosis.

The explanation for this increased morbidity and mortality in the diabetic subject is unclear. While partial explanation may lie in the several phagocytic dysfunctions I will shortly discuss, other nonspecific factors may also play a role. Long (1930) noted that forced feedings of glycerol to rats increased their suspectibility to tuberculosis. Since glycerol is known to enhance the growth of tubercle bacilli, increased levels of glycerol from the metabolism of fat in diabetic subjects may contribute to the increased morbidity. Dubon (1953) showed that addition of dihydroxyacetone or beta-hydroxybutyric acid enhanced *in vitro* growth of both mycobacteria and staphylococci. The study was carried out in an acidic medium, thereby approximating the conditions encountered in inflammatory areas and in the intracellular environment of leukocytes after phagocytosis.

C. Fungal Infections

Mucocutaneous candidiasis occurs relatively frequently in diabetic patients. It is particularly frequent in diabetic women with prolonged glycosuria complicated by pruritus vulvae. This condition is obviously seen more frequently in patients with poorly controlled diabetes. Knight and Fletcher (1971) have shown a direct correlation between glucose concentrations in saliva and the *in vitro* growth of *Candida* species. This correlation probably explains the increased incidence of mucocutaneous candidal infections in the poorly controlled diabetic subject.

Another complication of infection by *Candida* organisms is intertrigo. The frequency of this infection is probably no greater than that in normal subjects, but once it occurs in a poorly controlled diabetic subject, its eradication may be difficult.

Mucormycosis is a rare and extremely severe disease in patients with diabetic ketoacidosis. When it occurs, it is extremely difficult to treat and often proves fatal. Infecting organisms invade through nasal passages and cause severe necrosis and black-pus formation. Cerebral involvement occurs in approximately two-thirds of the infected subjects. Sequelae of such involvement include proptosis, ophthalmoplegia, headache, and signs of diffuse cerebrovascular involvement. Although the disease is usually fatal, treatment consisting of correction of the acidosis, surgical drainage when possible, and amphotericin B is sometimes effective. Sheldon and Bauer (1959, 1962) compared the possible potentiating effects of acidosis and hyperglycemia in the pathogenesis of mucormycosis in diabetic animals. Studying rabbits with acute alloxan diabetes, they found diminished polymorphonuclear leukocyte migration and increased growth of fungus. Normal rabbits made hyperglycemic by an infusion of glucose were no different from nondiabetic controls in their response to mucormycosis infection. Thus, hyperglycemia *per se* was not a significant contributing factor to increased morbidity. Acidosis, by contrast, seemed to play an important role. Control of the metabolic status of the diabetic patient is thus important in the prevention and control of mucormycosis. The significance of diminished neutrophil migration will be considered in more detail below.

D. Cutaneous Infections

Several studies have demonstrated that insulin-using diabetic patients have increased carrier rates of *Staphylococcus aureus* on their skin and mucous membranes (Smith *et al.*, 1966; Tuajon *et al.*, 1975). This finding, along with the fact that such patients break the skin barrier daily by injection of insulin, has led to the supposition that staphylococcal infections of the skin occur more frequently in subjects with diabetes mellitus. There is, however, no clinical evidence to support this increased frequency. In fact, in at least one retrospective study (Johnson, 1970), diabetes mellitus was observed only rarely among patients with recurrent furunculosis.

E. Osteomyelitis

Ostemyelitis is frequently associated with diabetes mellitus, particularly in those patients whose disease is complicated by neuropathy and/or vascular disease. In studies at the Joslin Clinic over a 7-year period, 408 of 415 cases of osteomyelitis occurring in diabetic subjects involved an extremity and all but one were due to extension from local infection (Younger and Hadley, 1971).

F. Nonclostridial Gas Gangrene

Another infection which occurs commonly in diabetic patients is nonclostridial gas gangrene. In a study of diabetic patients admitted with orthopedic vascular problems,

Bessman and Wagner (1975) found that 17% of 268 patients had nonclostridal-gas-containing infections. Only 0.3% (one patient) had clostridial gangrene. Patients with nonclostridial gas gangrene had mixed infections with gram-negative rods and enterococci. It is critically important to determine the nonclostridial nature of such infections, because the treatment for clostridial gas gangrene involved aggressive surgical management, frequently including amputation.

Bessman and Wagner (1975) noted that 41 of their 48 patients with nonclostridial gas gangrene received below-knee or more distal amputations with only one patient requiring above-knee amputation. Above-the-knee amputation would, of course, be the rule rather than the exception in clostridial gas gangrene infections.

G. Malignant Pseudomonas External Otitis

Malignant external otitis is an uncommon infection at best, but most of the reported cases have been in subjects with diabetes mellitus (Zaky et al., 1976). It begins insidiously but is soon characterized by an extensive and painful purulent discharge leading to a polypoid mass of granulation tissue. The infection is associated with high morbidity and mortality following necrosis of the external auditory canal. The explanation for increased frequency of this infection in subjects with diabetes mellitus is unclear.

In summary, I have reviewed the more common infections which occur in patients with diabetes mellitus. For the most part, the well-managed, uncomplicated diabetic subject is probably at no increased risk for occurrence of most bacterial and fungal infections. As pointed out by Hill et al. (1974), however, "when infections do occur in diabetic patients, they tend to be protracted and severe." I shall now review the available data on phyagocytic dysfunctions as they occur in juvenile onset (Type I) and adult onset diabetes (Type II) patients under good or poor control. In the discussion that follows, I will attempt to correlate these findings (wherever possible) with the data just reviewed on the frequency and types of infectious organisms likely to be present in the patient with diabetes mellitus.

III. PHAGOCYTIC ACTIVITIES

In describing the phagocytic defects identified in patients with diabetes mellitus and the interpretation of their clinical significance, it is first necessary to briefly review the mechanisms involved in the three major activities of circulating and sessile phagocytes: movement, ingestion, and intracelluar killing. A comprehensive review of these activities is outside the scope of this chapter.

A. Normal Movement of Phagocytes

A prerequisite for effective participation in host defense mechasims by phagocytes is their ability to move from the bone marrow and other storage sites of the body. It is now obvious that this process requires active movement on the part of phagocytic cells. In 1962, Steven Boyden developed an in vitro assay to study movement of neutrophils (PMNs). This provided a major advance in our ability to study clinically significant dysfunctions of phagocyte movement. Prior to this development, it was believed that little, if any, biological significance resulted from the movement of phagocyte cells. The Boyden assay, the prototype of all filter techniques, consists of measuring the movement of cells through a small-pored filter towards a chemotactically active gradient. A variety of stimuli can be utilized in generating this gradient. The most common sources are derived by activation of complement following exposure of fresh serum to endotoxin or antigen antibody complexes. Other substances which have chemotactic activity include serum factors, coagulation-derived factors, bacterial metabolites, secretory products of sensitized lymphocytes and PMNs, denatured proteins, and synthetic chemotactic factors such as the N-formylmethionyl peptides (Gallin and Quie, 1978; Ackerman and Douglas, 1979). Various endogenously produced deriviities of arachidonic acid are also chemotatic for PMNS (Goetzl and Sun, 1979).

Although the precise sequence by which PMN movement is triggered has not yet been delineated, a number of important steps are involved in the process. Initially, a brief but rapid membrane depolarization occurs. This is associated with calcium and/or sodium influx and is followed by a prolonged period of hyperpolarization and increased potassium permeability (Gallin *et al.*, 1978). Subsequent events include: increased levels of cyclic guanosine monophosphate (cGMP) (Hill, 1978), lysosomal enzyme release (Becker and Showell, 1974), increased glycolysis and hexose monophosphate shunt activity (Goetzl and Austen, 1974), cell swelling (Becker, 1976), increased numbers of microtubules (Stossel, 1978), and probable actuation of contractile proteins (Boxer *et al.*, 1978).

Information on the specific mechanisms of cell movement derived via the filter technique is somewhat limited. Consequently, other assays have been developed to permit observations of single and/or small numbers of cells during movement. These include direct visualization (Wilkinson and Allan, 1978), visual assay systems (Zigmond, 1978) in which cells are observed under phase microscopy on a bridge across which a chemotactic gradient has been established, assays of deformability of PMNs by the technique of cell elastimetry (Miller and Myers, 1975); and cinemicrography and videotape analysis of PMNs subjected to a chemotactic gradient (Cheung *et al.*, 1982).

B. Normal Phagocytosis

Following the arrival of phagocytes at the site of foreign particle or microbial presence, ingestion or phagocytosis takes place. Particulate matter (phagocytosis) or soluble materials (pinocytosis) are ingested in two distinct steps: recognition and ingestion. The recognition phase involves specific receptors of the cell membrane. A number of receptors of the PMN membrane have been identified, including a receptor for the Fc fragments of immunoglobulin molecules and for several activation products of complement (C3b and C5a) (Henson, 1976). It is presumed that these receptors act in increasing the efficiency of the ingestion process by fixing opsonized particles to the cell surface.

The second phase of the phagocytic process is the actual ingestion which follows the adherence. Many of the same cellular functions and activities involved in movement of phagocytes are involved in ingestion. Indeed, some investigators believe that the two activities are part of the same overall process, although there is not unanimous agreement on this point. Ingestion involves the flow of cytoplasmic hyaline pseudopods around the ingested particle (Stossel, 1975; Wilkinson, 1976). The contractile protein system is presumably involved in the formation of these pseudopods (Stossel, 1975; Stossel and Hartwig, 1976). A phagosome is formed by the pseudopod surrounding and fusing with the attached particle. This internalized phagosome is then merged with by lysosomes and degranulation occurs with ultimate discharge of lysosomal contents into the phagosome, that is, phagolysosome.

C. Normal Bactericidal Activity

One ingested, a microbe is subjected to a sophisticated array of biochemical processes available to the human PMN in killing or disposing of ingested materials. There is an obvious association of bactericidal activity of PMNs with oxidative activity, although the precise relationships are not known.

Following contact with the PMN membrane by a foreign particle, a sequence of metabolic events is activated, known as the "respiratory burst." This includes increased oxygen consumption, oxidation of glucose via the hexomonophosphate shunt, and the generation of hydrogen perioxide (Johnston and Newman, 1977).

During this metabolic activation, a number of potentially bactericidal products are generated. The activation of the sequence is presumably resultant upon a membrane-bound or associated enzyme. Oxidases such as NADH, NADPH, or glutathione peroxidase are particularly likely candidates. Activation of the oxidase(es) results in the transfer of a single electron to oxygen, thereby forming an unstable radical known as superoxide anion. Hydrogen perioxide is formed by two superoxide radicals when they spontaneously interact. The continuing reaction between hydrogen perioxide and superoxide yields free hydroxyl radical, a potent oxidizing agent. Transfer of energy from superoxide to an unstable excited species called singlet oxygen may result in a burst of energy which can be measured as emitted light in the assay of chemiluminescence. "Extra" electrons from superoxide anions may be transferred and account for the NBT dye reduction effect.

Each of the oxidation products—superoxide anion, hydrogen peroxide, hydroxyl radicals, and singlet oxygen—is a potent bactericidal agent. Although the precise role each plays in the bactericidal process of various microorganisms has not been determined, it is presumed that this group of agents has clinical significance. In additon to these metabolic products, microbicidal activities result from the release of PMN lysosomal materials including myeloperoxidase, lysozyme, phagocytin, and other cationic proteins.

IV. DISORDERS OF MOVEMENT

Studies of movement of neutrophils have revealed apparent deficiencies in patients with both adult- and juvenile-onset diabetes. These studies have utilized the filter technique of study of neutrophil movement (Boyden, 1962). As pointed out in the brief review of the mechanisms of cell movement, the filter technique is dependent upon multiple factors and may not reveal the true nature of a particular phagocytic activity. In adult subjects, Mowat and Baum (1971) demonstrated defects in filter movement of neutrophils in whole blood. They further observed that the addition of insulin *in vitro* improved phagocytic movement. Miller and Baker (1972) and Hill *et al.* (1974) studied neutrophil movement in patients with juvenile-onset diabetes mellitus. Similar results to those reported by Mowat and Baum were observed in both of these studies with reference to the PMNs. In addition, Miller and Baker demonstrated a deficiency in the generation of chemotactically active materials from plasma or serum of diabetic children. Preliminary studies failed to reveal the basis for this deficiency in the generation of humoral activity. The significance of the *in vitro* insulin studies is controversial. Although, as noted, *in vitro* improvement of phagocyte movement has been observed upon the addition of insulin, no relationship between *in vivo* insulin levels and abnormality of neutrophil chemotaxis has been demonstrated.

Among the factors that influence results obtained in the filter chemotactic assay is the ability of PMNs to adhere to the surface of the filter. In other words, if neutrophils are poorly adherent, they may detach from the lower surface of the filter, thereby yielding a falsely low level of chemotactic responsiveness when one counts the number of cells per high-powered field on the lower surface of the filter. Humbert and co-workers (1976) evaluated neutrophil chemotaxis in a large group of diabetic children utilizing a system designed to evaluate adherence of cells to the surface of the filter. In these studies, three different chemotactic attractants were utilized. When the chemotactic mediator was either sterile filtrate from a 4-day culture of *Escherichia coli*, or human plasma which had been activated for 35 min with bovinve albumin/antialbumin complexes, no deficiency in cellular neutrophil chemotaxis was found and there was no abnormal detachment of neutrophils from the lower surface of the filter. With a chemotactic mediator derived from plasma which has been activated for 5 min with albumin/antialbumin complexes, chemotaxis was also normal, but neutrophils adhered poorly to the filters. The authors concluded that no basic or directional locomotion defect exists in neutrophils of children with diabetes mellitus, but that under certain circumstances the adhesive properties of diabetic neutrophils may be impaired. An alternative hypothesis also considered by the authors was that an excessively high rate of cell locomotion (increased chemokinesis) could account for the apparent chemotactic defect. This possibility was ruled out by the demonstration of identical random filter migration in diabetic and control neutrophils. This study was consistent with the data of Bagdade and Steward (1976) who demonstrated impaired granulocyte adherence in patients with diabetes mellitus under poor metabolic control.

Viollier and co-workers (1979) have studied *in vivo* mobilization of neutrophils by the utilization of skin chambers. They found that mobilization of neutrophils was markedly decreased in diabetic subjects compared with normal individuals. This impaired mobilization was apparently independent of the state of metabolic control. It should be noted that such studies do not rule out the suggestion of impaired adherence as an important factor in experimental movement data, since adherence may also be a factor affecting mobilization of PMNs *in vivo*.

V. DISORDERS OF PHAGOCYTOSIS

Many investigations of phagcytosis in blood or isolated cellular elements of patients with diabetes mellitus have been reported. In general, such studies have yielded highly inconsistent results and have failed to reveal a primary defect in phagocytosis in the diabetic subject. One of the more convincing of these studies was that of Drachman and co-workers (1966) in which the phagocytic capabilities of polymorphonuclear leukocytes were studies in rats rendered chronically diabetic. In their system, these workers attempted to mimic several conditions frequently found in diabetes, including high levels of glucose and small volumes of inflammatory exudate in which the neutrophils would be attempting to phagocytose bacteria. They found that both the *in vivo* and *in vitro* phagocytic activities of neutrophils were adversely affected by high levels of glucose. The authors contended that their system was clinically significant because it mimicked the conditions found in the diabetic subject. A major criticism of these studies was that the levels of glucose necessary to achieve phagocytic inhibition *in vitro* were well in excess of those realistically encountered in a patient with diabetes. In answer to this criticism, the authors emphasized that glucose levels in an inflammatory exudate or abscess area may significantly exceed levels found in the periopheral blood. The clinical significance of these studies remains controversial. With the advent of newer techniques which are at least as sensitive and critical as the system utilized by Drachman and co-workers, studies of phagocytic function have not confirmed this data. One possible interpretation of the studies of Drachman and co-workers is that the ultimate phagocytic value being measured is affected by chemotactic activity. As discussed above, some evidence suggests chemotactic deficiencies in patients with diabetes. If so, these defects might explain the apparent defects reported in phagocytic function.

The kinetics of the phagocytic process may also be a factor in determining the effectiveness of this mechanism of host defense. Nolan and co-workers (1978) assayed the engulfment and intracellular killing of *S. aureus* 502A by neutrophils of 17 diabetic patients with fasting hyperglycemia. In phagocytosis, neutrophils from the diabetic subjects engulfed a smaller proportion of a 10^6 inoculum of bacteria after 20 min of incubation *in vitro*. The diabetic neutrophils ingested $56.8 \pm 9.4\%$ of the bacterial incolum, while neutrophils from normal subjects ingested $72.4 \pm 3.6\%$ (mean $\pm$ S.E. of 10 patients + paired controls.) These data were significant by Student's t test, $p > 0.05$. In contrast to this difference at 20 min, however, after 60 min of incubation, no differences were noted between the percentage of inoculum ingested by neutrophils from diabetic subjects and those from normal individuals.

It thus appears that phagocytic defects present in the diabetic subject require fairly extreme conditions in order to be of clinical significance.

VI. DISORDERS OF BACTERICIDAL ACTIVITY

Investigations of the bactericidal activity of phagocytes from patients with diabetes mellitus have yielded conflicting results. Marble and co-workers (1938), Richardson (1942), Bybee and Rogers (1964), and Crosby and Allison (1966) found normal bactericidal activities. These early studies failed, however, to take into account a number of aspects of experimental design considered by later investigators. First, these studies generally tested only qualitatively the killing ability of neutrophils using a single low ratio of bacteria per neutrophil. Second, they failed to evaluate the bactericidal effectiveness of neutrophils from diabetic and nondiabetic subjects during bacterial infection. Finally, the state of metabolic control was usually not probed in a critical manner. More recent studies which have taken some of these factors into account seem to support the presence of a primary defect in bactericidal activity of diabetic PMNs with a clear dependency upon metabolic control.

Tan and co-workers (1975) studied killing by neutrophils from 31 nonketoacidotic patients with diabetes mellitus. In their study group, 21 patients were infection-free at the time of study and 10 patients had a history of recurrent infections with bacterial organisms. The organism used for their studies was *S. aureus* 502A. When compared with bactericidal activity of PMNs from 25 normal individuals, bactericidal activities of the diabetic PMN towared ingested staphylococci were significantly decreased. In 17 of 31 diabetic patients studied, PMN killing was greater than 2 standard deviations less than the control mean. The authors also studied phagocytosis by the lysostaphin assay technique. Of the 31 diabetic patients studied, 11 had PMNs which phagocytized poorly. Of these 11, three also had decreased bactericidal activities leading to a combined defect. The phagocyte abnormalities were not corrected by the addition of normal serum or by suspension in serum with normal blood glucose levels. In attempting to correlate the neutrophil dysfunctions with clinical history of recurrent infections, the authors found that 5 of the 10 patients with recurrent infections and 12 of the 21 patients without recurrent infections had neutrophil dysfunctions. All three patients with defective bactericidal activity and phagocytosis had severe bacterial infections. Whether this small number is adequate to prove the case remains to be seen.

Nolan *et al.* (1978) assayed intracellular killing of the same organism, *S. aureus* 502A. As in the above study, they found an intracellular killing defect of *Staphylococcus* in diabetic PMNs and correlated the finding with metabolic control. Thus, PMNs from six of seven patients which were retested when the subjects were under good metabolic control showed improved functional activity. As noted in the section on phagocytosis, the authors also studied phagocytosis and concluded that a combined phagocytic and bactericidal defect was a significant contributor to infections in the diabetic subject. Both functions improved with metabolic control in their assay system.

Similar results were obtained by Viollier and Senn (1979). They found decreased killing of *E. coli* by diabetic PMNs which improved upon normalization of metabolic state. Thus, unlike the situation with phagocytic and movement activities, most of the bactericidal studies have demonstrated an effect of metabolic control upon function of diabetic PMNs.

The study of Repine and co-workers (1980) extended these results and provided more evidence of the metabolic relationship to bactericidal function of neutrophils from patients with diabetes mellitus. First, these authors noted that neutrophils from diabetic patients failed to increase their bactericidal activity in response to infection to the same degree as neutrophils from nondiabetic subjects. The difference between the diabetic and normal PMNs was more pronounced the poorer the metabolic control. The defect was pronounced with plasma glucose levels greater than 130 mg/100 ml, but was also present in plasma glucose levels less than 130 mg/ml in diabetic subjects. Further, killing of *S. aureus* by neutrophils from poorly controlled, uninfected diabetic subjects was less than the killing by neutrophils from normal subjects or from diabetic subjects under good metabolic control. Two patients were studied while undergoing controlled insulin withdrawal. During this period, their neutrophils developed a bactericidal defect which was corrected *in vivo* by reinstitution of insulin therapy. Incubation of their PMNs with insulin *in vitro* also improved bactericidal activities. The authors concluded that defective neutrophil bactericidal activity may contribute to the presumed increased susceptibility to bacterial infections in diabetes.

VII. SUMMARY AND SPECULATIONS

This review of phagocytic functions in patients with diabetes mellitus has emphasized the inconsistency and difficulty of interpreting presently available data. If a significant primary phagocyte dysfunction is present, then it is hard to explain the relatively good resistance mustered against most bacterial organisms by the dieabetic patient. On the other hand, as more experience with phagocyte dysfunctions has been gained, it has become apparent that subtle and mild predisposition to infection often characterizes this group of clinical disorders.

In attempting to interpret the available data, it is my impression that the most convincing studies address the areas of bactericidal defects and their worsening in states of poor metabolic control. The data on phagcytosis and movement have been inconcsistent and have not considered a number of variables of the experimental assay or the patient's clinical condition. In a recent study, for example, Murphy and Miller (1977) found that neutrophil function in juvenile diabetes mellitus may be entirely normal prior to the institution of insulin therapy. Following insulin administration, sometimes within as little as 12–24 hr, highly significant decreases were found in both cellular and humoral chemotaxis. In subsequent studies, Murphy and Miller (unpublished observations) found that normal neutrophils incubated in the presence of insulin showed decreases in both chemotactic responsiveness and deformability.

The more recent studies of bactericidal activity, by contrast, have consistently suggested a significant defect of phagocytic killing which is worsened in states of poor metabolic control. Although such studies are convincing, they still fail to explain the clinical spectrum of organ systems and infections seen in the usual diabetic subject. Finally, it should be noted that the degree of secondary complicating factors, such as vascular disesase or neuropathy, may be exceedingly difficult to determine in a particular patient. One might assume that the patient with poor metabolic control is a better candidate for such complicating factors, but this is only speculation.

REFERENCES

Ackerman, S. K., and Douglas, S. D., 1979, Pepstatin A—a human leukocyte chemoattractant, *Clin. Immunol. Immunopathol.* **14**:244–250.

American Thoracic Society, Statement on preventive therapy of tuberculosis infection, *Am. Rev. Respir. Dis.* **110**:371–374.

Bagdade, J. D., 1976, Phagocytic and microbicidal function in diabetes mellitus, *Acta Endocrinol. (Copenh.)* **83**(Suppl. 205):27–33.

Bagdade, J. D., and Steward, M., 1976, Host defense in diabetes mellitus: *Impaired granulocyte adherence in poorly controlled diabetic patients (abstract,)* Clin. Res. 24:112A.

Bailey, H., 1961, Cystitis emphysematosa: 19 cases with intraluminal and interstitial collections of gas, AJR 86:850–862.

Baldwin, A. D., and Root, H. F., 1940, Infections of upper urinary tract in diabetic patients, N. Engl. J. Med. 223:244–250.

Becker, E. L., 1976, Some interrelations among chemotaxis, lysosomal enzyme secretion and phagocytosis by neutrophils, in: Molecular and Biological Aspects of the Acute Allergic Reaction (S. G. O. Johanson, K. Strandberg, and B. Uvnas, eds.), pp. 353–370, Plenum Press, New York.

Becker, E. L., and Showell, H. J., 1974, The ability of chemotactic factors to induce lysosomal enzyme release. II. The mechanism of release, J. Immunol. 112:2055–2062.

Bessman, A. N., and Wagner, W., 1975, Nonclostridial gas gangrene, JAMA 233:958–963.

Boxer, L. A, Hedley-Whyte, E. T., and Stossel, T. P., 1974, Neutrophil actin dysfunction and abnormal neutrophil behavior, N. Engl. J. Med. 291:1093–1099.

Boyden, S., 1962, Chemotactic effect of mixtures of antibody and antigen on polymorphonuclear leukocytes, J. Exp. Med. 115:453–466.

Bybee, J. D., and Rogers, D. E., 1964, The phagocytic activity of polymorphonuclear leukocytes obtained from patients with diabetes mellitus, J. Lab. Clin. Med. :64:1–13.

Cheung, A. T. W, Miller, M. E., and Keller, S. R., 1982, Movement of human polymorphonuclear leukocytes: A videotape analysis, J. Reticuloendothel. Soc., :31193–205, 1982.

Cohn, L. S., Fekety, F. R., and Cluff, L. E., Studies on the epidemiology of staphylococcal infection. VI. Infections in the surgical patient, Ann. Surg. 159:321, 1964.

Crosby, B., and Allison, F., Jr., 1966, Phagocytic and bactericidal capacity of polymorphonuclear leukocytes recovered from venous blood of human beings, Proc. Soc. Exp. Biol. Med. 123:+660–664.

Drachman, R. H., Root, R. K., and Wood, W. B., Jr., 1966, Studies on the effect of experimental nonketotic diabetes mellitus on antibacterial defense. I. Demonstration of a defect in phagocytosis, J. Exp. Med. 124:227–240.

Dubos, R. J., 1953, Effect of ketone bodies and other metabolites on the survival and multiplication of staphylococci and tubercle bacilli, J. Exp. Med. 98:145–155.

Edmondson, H. A., Martin, H. E., and Evans, N., 1947, Necrosis of renal papillae and acute pyelonephritis in diabetes mellitus, Arch. Intern. Med.79:148–175.

Edwards, J. E., Jr., Tillman, D. B., Miller, M. E., and Pitchon, H. E., 1979, Infection and diabetes mellitus–Teaching Conference, Harbor-University of California, Los Angeles, Medical Center, Torrance, and VA Wadsworth Medical Center, Los Angeles (Specialty Conference). West J. Med. 130:515–521.

Ellenberg, M., and Weber, H., 1967, Incipient asymptomatic diabetic bladder, Diabetes 16:331–335.

Esmann, V., 1972, The diabetic leukocyte, Enzyme 13:32–55.

Gallin, J. I., and Quie, P. G. (eds.), 1978, Leukocyte Chemotaxis: Methods, Physiology, and Clinical Implications, Raven Press, New York.

Gallin, J. E., Gallin, E. K., Mallech, H. L., and Cramer, E. B., 1978, Structural and ionic events during leukocyte chemotaxis, in: Leukocyte Chemotaxis (J. I. Gallin and P. G. Quie, eds.), pp. 123–141, Raven Press, New York.

Goetzl, E. J., and Austen, K. F., 1974, Stimulation of human neutrophil leukocyte aerobic glucose metabolism by purified chemotatic factors, J. Clin. 53:591–599.

Goetzl, E. J., and Sun, F. F., 1979, Generation of unique monohydroxyeicosatetraenoic acids from arachinoid acid by human neutrophils, J. Exp. Med. 150:406–411.

Halverstadt, D. B., Leadbetter, G. W., Jr., and Field, R. A., 1966, Pyelonephritis in the diabetic. Correlation of open renal biospsies and bacteriologic studies, JAMA 195:827–829.

Henson, P. M., 1976, Membrane receptors on neutrophils, Immunol. Commun. 5:757–775.

Hill, H. R., 1978, Cyclic nucleotides as modulators of leukocyte chemotaxis, in: Leukocyte Chemotasis (J. I. Gallin and P. G. Quie, eds.), pp. 179–193, Raven Press, New York.

Hill, H. R., Sauls, H. S., Dettlof, J. L., and Quie, P. G., 1974, Impaired leukotactic responsiveness in patients with juvenile diabetes mellitus, Clin. Immunol. Immunopathol. 2:395–403.

Humbert, J. R., Hambridge, K. M., Moore, L. L., Lindstrom, S. A., and Martinez, B., 1976, Absence of neutrophil chemotactic defect in diabetes, Clin. Res. 24:180A.

Huvos, A., and Rocha, H., 1959, Frequency of bacteriuria patients with diabetes mellitus, N. Engl. J. Med. 261:1213–1216.

Johnson, J. E., 1970, Infection in diabetes, in: *Diabetes Mellitus: Theory and Practice,* (M. Ellenberg and H. Rifkin, eds.), p. 739, McGraw-Hill, New York.

Johnston, R. B., Jr. and Newman, S. L., 1977, Chronic granulomatous disease, *Pediat. Clin. North Am.* **24:**365–376.

Knight, L. and Fletcher, J., 1971, Growth of *Candida albicans* in saliva: Stimulation by glucose associated with antibotics, corticosteroids, and diabetes mellitus, *J. Infect. Dis.* **123:**371–377.

Lauler, D. P., Schreiner, G. E., and David, A., 1960, Renal medullary necrosis, *Am. J. Med.* **29:**132–156.

Long, E. R., 1930, A chemical view of the pathogenesis of tuberculosis, *Am. Rev. Tubercul.* **22:**467–490.

Marble, A., White, H. J., and Fernald, A. T., 1938, The nature of the lowered resistance to infection in diabetes mellitus, *J. Clin. Invest.* **17:**423–430.

Miller, M. E., and Baker, L., 1972, Leukocyte functions in juvenile diabetes mellitus: Humoral and cellular aspects, *J. Pediatr.* **81:**979–982.

Miller, M. E., and Myers, K. A., 1975, Cellular deformability of the human peripheral blood polymorphonuclear leukocyte: Method of study, normal variation and effects of physical and chemical alterations, *J. Reticuloendothel. Soc.* **18:**337–345.

Mowat, A., and Baum, J., 1971, Chemotaxis of polymorphonuclear leukocytes from patients with diabetes mellitus, *N. Engl. J. Med.* **284:**621–627.

Muller, L. M., and Higgins, G. K., 1963, Incidence of undiscovered adult diabetes in a tuberculosis sanitarium, *Canad. Med. Assoc. J.* **88:**424–425.

Murphy, S., and Miller, M. E., 1977, Impaired movement and deformability of neutrophils from patients with juvenile diabetes mellitus. An insulin induced defect? *Pediatr. Res.* **11** (No. 4):520 (abstract).

Nolan, C. M., Beaty, H. N., and Bagdade, J. D, 2978, Further characterization of the impaired bactericidal function of granulocytes in patients with poorly controlled diabetes, *Diabetes* **27:**889–894.

Pell, S., and D'Alonzo, C. A., 1967, Sickness absenteeism in employed diabetics, *Am. J. Public Health* **57:**253–260.

Pell, S., and D'Alonzo, C. A., 1970, Factors associated with long-term survival of diabetics, *JAMA* **214:**1833–1840.

Pometta, D., Rees, S. B., Younger, D., and Kass, E. H., 1967, Asymptomatic bacteriuria in dieabetes' mellitus, *N. Engl. J. Med.* **276:**1118–1121.

Repine, J. E., Clawson, C. C., and Goetz, F. C., 1980, Bactericidal function of neutrophils from patients with acute bacterial infections and from diabetes, *J. Infect. Dis.* **142**(No. 6):869–875.

Richardson, R., 1942, Immunity in diabetes. IV. Measurements of phagocytic activity in diabetes mellitus. *Am. J. Med. Sci.* **204:**29–35.

Robbins, S. L., and Tucker, A. W., Jr., 1944, The cause of death in diabetes: A report of 307 autopsied cases, *N. Engl. J. Med.* **231:**865–868.

Robson, M. D., and Heggers, J. R., 1969, Effect of hyperglycemia on survival of bacteria, *Surg. Forum* **20:**56–57.

Sheldon, W. H., and Bauer, H., 1959, The development of acute inflammatory response to experimental mucormycosis in normal and diabetic rabbits, *J. Exp. Med.* **110:**845–852.

Sheldon, W. H., and Bauer, H., 1962, The role of predisposing factors in experimental fungal infections, *Lab. Invest.* **11:**1184–1191.

Smith, J. A., O'Connor, J. J. and Willis, A. T., 1966, Nasal carriage of *Staphylococcus aureus* in diabetes mellitus, *Lancet* **2:**766–666.

Stossel, T. P., 1975, Phagocytosis: Recognition and ingestion, *Semin. Hermatol.* **12:**83–116.

Stossel, T. P., 1978, The mechanism of leukocyte locomotion, in: *Leukocyte Chemotaxis* (J. I. Gallin and P. G. Quie, eds.), pp. 143–160, Raven Press, New York.

Stossel, T. P., and Hartwig, J. H., 1976, Interaction of actin, myosin, and a new actin-binding protein of rabbit pulmonary macrophage. II. Role in cytoplasmic movement and phagocytosis, *J. Cell Biol.* **68:**602–619.

Tan, J. S., Anderson, J. L., Watanakunakorn, C., and Phair, J. P., 1975, Neutrophil dysfunction in diabetes mellitus, *J. Lab. Clin. Med.* **85:**26–33.

Tuajon, C. U., Perez, A., Kishaba, T., and Sheagren, J. N., 1975, Staphylococcus aureus among insulin-injecting diabetic patients, *JAMA* **231:**1272.

Vejlsgaard, R., 1965, Significant bacteriuria in relation to vascular disease of diabetics of long duration, in: *Progress in Pyelonephritis* (E. H. Kass, ed.), pp. 492–500, F. A. Davis, Philadelphia.

Viollier, A. F., and Senn, H. J., 1979, Granulozytäre Infektabwehr bei Diabetes Mellitus unter besonderer Berücksichtigung der Bakterizidie, *Schweiz. Med. Wochenschr.* **109**:1896.

Warren, S., Le Compte, P. M., and Legg, M. A., 1966, *The Pathology of Diabetes Mellitus,* 4th Edition, Lea and Febiger, Philadelphia.

Weaver, R. A., 1974, Unusual radiographic presentation of pulmonary tuberculosis in diabetic patients, *Am. Rev. Respir. Dis.* **109**:162–163.

Wilkinson, P. C., 1976, Recognition and response in mononuclear and granular phagocytes, *Clin. Exp. Immunol.* **25**:355–366.

Wilkinson, P. C., and Allan, R. B., 1978, Assay systems for measuring leukocyte locomotion: an overview, in: *Leukocyte Chemotaxis* (J. I. Gallin and P. G. Quie, eds.), pp. 1–24. Raven Press, New York.

Younger, D., and Hadley, W. B., 1971, Infection and diabetes, in: *Joslin's Diabetes Mellitus* (A. Marble and P. White, eds.), p. 628, Lea and Febiger, Philadelphia.

Zaky, D. A., Bentley, D. W., Lowy, K., Betts, R. F., and Douglas, R. G., 1976, Malignant external otitis: A severe form of otitis in diabetic patients, *Am J. Med.* **61**:298–302.

Zigmond, S. H., 1978, A new visual assay of leukocyte chemotaxis, in: *Leukocyte Chemotaxis* (J. I. Gallin and P. G. Quie, eds), pp. 57–66, Raven Press, New York.

14

Circulating Immune Complexes

Dinesh Kumar

I. INTRODUCTION

Antigens, self or foreign, induce an immune response leading to production of specific antibodies that interact with the inciting antigens and may form antigen–antibody (immune) complexes. An immune response is normally developed as a defense mechanism which eliminates and neutralizes the undesirable antigens. In addition, immune complexes have a regulatory role in both the cellular and humoral immune responses by virtue of their capacity to interreact with Fc and complement receptor-bearing lymphocytes and macrophages. The formation of the immune complexes under certain circumstances could be pathogenic, resulting in disease states.

Since the recognition of circulating insulin–insulin-antibody complexes by Berson and co-workers in 1956, attempts have been made to associate such complexes with the diabetic complications (Andersen, 1976). With the development of laboratory techniques of detecting immune complexes (Barnett *et al.*, 1979) a new approach to investigate the role of immune complexes in the pathogenesis of various diseases became available. During the past 5 years, those techniques have also been applied to explore the role of immune complexes in the pathogenesis of diabetes mellitus and its long-term sequelae particularly nephropathy and angiopathy (Di Mario *et al.*, 1980). In this chapter I will present those features of diabetes mellitus in common with the other immune complex diseases, and our current knowledge concerning the circulating immune complexes in diabetes mellitus.

II. DETERMINANTS OF CIRCULATING IMMUNE COMPLEXES

The subject of immune complexes and their role in diseases has attracted a significant attention in the past decade, and has recently been reviewed (Theofilopoulos and

Dinesh Kumar • Division of Diabetes and Clinical Nutrition, University of Southern California School of Medicine, Los Angeles, California 90033.

Dixon, 1979; Barnett *et al.*, 1979; Inman and Day, 1981; Wiggins and Cochrane, 1981; Williams, 1981). Before I discuss immune complexes and diabetes, it will be appropriate to discuss various general characteristics of immune complexes. The antigen and antibody reactions can occur in circulation (Cochrane and Koffler, 1973), in interstitial fluids (Clagett *et al.*, 1974) or within tissues (Theofilopoulos and Dixon, 1979). The formation, composition, concentration, and fate of immune complexes in circulation depend on a number of factors including characteristics of antibodies, antigen, and status of host reticuloendothelial system (Table 1). The immunoglobulin class of antibodies, their valence and avidity for the specific antigen, their ability to bind to cellular Fc receptors, and to activate complement system appear to be important. Equally significant is the nature of the antigen itself. Monovalent antigens produce complexes that generally fail to form lattice, do not bind complement, and remain in circulation for a long period. Polyvalent antigens form immune complexes of varying composition depending on the molar concentrations of antigen and antibodies. In antigen excess, the size of soluble complexes vary inversely with the amount of antigen (Arend *et al.*, 1972). Immune complexes formed in the antibody excess are large and insoluble, and are rapidly phagocytosed. However, such complexes react with complement. The complexes of intermediate size seem to have most pathologic potential as they are cleared slowly, react with complement compounds, and can activate both the classic and alternative complement pathways (Gotze and Muller-Eberhard, 1976; Austen, 1974; Spiegelberg, 1974; Osler and Sandberg, 1973; Gigli, 1976; Rodrick *et al.*, 1978; Porter and Reid, 1978).

Immune complexes are removed from circulation by phagocytes, both circulating leukocytes and reticuloendothelial system (Theofilopoulos and Dixon, 1979). This process requires participation of complement and Fc receptors. An overwhelming load of immune complexes can saturate the receptor sites resulting in deficient phagocytic activity and delayed clearance of complexes (Haakenstad and Mannik, 1974).

Tissue damage is due to a local antigen and antibody reaction or to the deposition of circulating immune complexes. In acute experimental serum sickness of the rabbit, a

Table 1. Factors Influencing the Size, Composition, Fate, and Biological Activities of Circulating Immune Complexes

Antigen
  Molecular weight
  Valence
  Physiochemical properties
  Steric distribution of antigentic determinants
  Availability
Antibodies
  Immunoglobulin class and subclass
  Affinity
  Valence
  Concentration
  Complement activation properties
Complement system
State of phagocytic system

model of immune complex disease, a leukocyte-dependent and complement-independent mechanism initiates the deposition of immune complexes in tissues (Henson and Cochrane, 1971). There is degranulation of basophils sensitized with IgE antibody and antigen. Subsequent release of other mediators such as vasoactive amines from platelets (Henson and Oades, 1976), anaphylatoxins C3a and C5a produced by complement activation increase vascular permeability. Immune complexes deposited along the vascular basement membrane evoke an inflammatory reaction involving neutrophils. The lysosomal enzymes released from neutrophils cause local damage (Theofilopoulos and Dixon, 1979). Histologically, deposits of antigen, antibodies and complement components can be identified.

In addition to the activation of complement system, immune complexes interact with a variety of cells including lymphocytes, macrophages, eosinophils, neutrophils, platelets, basophils, erythrocytes, and tumor cells via their surface receptors. Interaction with T and B lymphocytes could modulate the cellular and humoral immune responses. The antibody production has been suppressed through a number of mechanisms. Theofilopoulos and Dixon (1979) summarized seven such mechanisms where immune complexes block directly B-cell activities or cause suppression through activation of suppressor T cells or by inducing T cells to produce immunoregulatory molecules. On the other hand, an enhancement of the immune response can be observed especially by the immune complexes formed in an antigen excess. Antigen complexed with antibody has a higher affinity for lymphocytes (Revoltella et al., 1975) and macrophages and can be easily localized in the lymphoid follicles.

Immune complexes may affect other cellular immune reactions. Inhibition of cell-mediated cytolytic reactions and enhancement of antibody-dependent cellular cytoxicity (ADCC) have been demonstrated in neoplastic cells (Hellstrom and Hellstrom, 1974; Baldwin and Robins, 1976). The ADCC is involved also in elimination of viral infections and in autoimmune diseases (Theofilopoulous and Dixon, 1979).

III. METHODS OF DETECTION

There are two general approaches to the detection of circulating immune complexes. Antigen-specific methods are used when the antigen is known and available in a suitable form, for example, bacterial and viral antigens. Because the nature of the involved antigen is generally not known, detection of immune complexes is frequently performed by indirect methods using physicochemical and immunological properties. The physicochemical methods are based on size separation, diminished solubility at 4°C, and differential solubility in solutions such as polyethylene glycol. The polyethylene glycol precipitation is also used to isolate immune complexes for further analysis of the involved components. Immunological methods are based on complement-binding (C1q) and -activation, immunoglobulin content, and on interaction of immune complexes with the cell-surface receptors for complement components or the Fc region of IgG (Barnett et al., 1979). Fluid phase (Digeon et al., 1977) and solid-phase (Hay et al., 1978) C1q binding assays are used most frequently. These assays, however, do not detect those complexes which do not bind C1q. Furthermore, they can give false-positive results due to aggregates of immunoglobulins. The microcomplement test provides presumptive evidence of the presence of immune complexes by assessing the consumption of a standard amount of added complement to a preheated, decomplemented sample. False-positive results are frequent due to the formation of IgG aggregates during heating. The conglutinin assay (Casali *et al.*, 1977) detects immune complexes that contain complement products, particularly C3. Several cellular techniques have been described but the Raji cell assay is the most popular of all. Raji cells derived from Burkitt's lymphoma have C3b receptors and therefore bind C3b containing immune complexes. The cell bound complexes are subsequently quantitated by an antiimmunoglobulin (Theofilopoulous *et al.*, 1976). This assay is sensitive, but may give false positive results due to the presence of antilymphocyte antibodies in some conditions, for example, systemic lupus erythematosus. Other cellular techniques have similar problems (Theofilopolous and Dixon, 1979).

Among various detection techniques, the solid-phase C1q and polyethylene glycol precipitation assays correlate well with each other (Barnett *et al.*, 1979). The results of other assays correlate poorly when same sera are tested in the same or separate laboratories (Lambert *et al.*, 1978). The difference between assays is due to the fact that each assay is based on a different principle and measures a certain type of immune complexes. The interlaboratory differences are disturbing and may be largely due to variations in sensitivity of the techniques. These facts indicate limitations and caution required in the interpretation of given data.

IV. EVIDENCE OF CIRCULATING IMMUNE COMPLEXES IN DIABETES MELLITUS

In 1977, Irvine and co-workers, using the Raji cell assay, reported detectable levels of immune complexes in 7 of 13 newly diagnosed Type I diabetics and in 17 of 32 established Type I cases. Subsequently, they extended their study by increasing the number of newly diagnosed cases to 110, and using two different assay techniques: C1q binding and Raji cell systems (Irvine *et al.*, 1978a). Circulating immune complexes were found in 39% of all the cases by C1q assay, and in 50% of 52 cases tested by Raji cell assay. Both these percentages were significantly higher than the percentage positivity in age–sex matched nondiabetic controls. Charlesworth *et al.* (1979) observed an increased sensitivity of Raji cell assay compared to C1q test. Immune complexes were found in 11 (31%) insulin-treated diabetics by the Raji cell assay, and none had positive results of the C1q test.

Using $[^{125}I]$C1q-binding test, Kumar and Quismorio (1978) found evidence of circulating immune complexes in 6 of 30 newly diagnosed and 45 of 175 established diabetic patients. Using a similar detection technique, Schernthaner and co-workers (1979) reported circulating immune complexes in 33 (23%) of 145 diabetic patients. Since C1q-binding and Raji cell assays are antigen-nonspecific, other detection techniques have also been utilized (Di Mario *et al.*, 1980; Virella *et al.*, 1981). Virella *et al.* (1981) compared results of four different antigen-nonspecific tests: direct nephelometry, C1q-binding, determinations of polyethylene glycol precipitable IgG (PEG-IgG) and C4 (PEG-C4), and an antigen-specific assay which measured insulin-antibody-containing complexes. Positive results were found in 42 (33%) of 127 cases by Clq test, in 29 (25%) of 110 cases by the direct nephelometry, in 33 (26%) of 143 cases by PEG-C4 assay, and in 40 (27%) of 148 cases by PEG-IgG technique. Insulin–insulin-antibody complexes were found in 75 (57%) of 139 cases tested. Sixteen percent of the total cases had three or more positive results in the five tests used. Regardless of the assay system utilized, it seems well-established that there is an increased incidence of the circulating immune complexes in diabetic patients.

In order to evaluate the relationship between the duration of diabetes and the levels of circulating immune complexes, Irvine et al. (1978a) evaluated a group of newly diagnosed insulin-dependent diabetics (Type I). It was observed that the circulating immune complexes disappeared within few months of diagnosis and only 3 out of 37 cases had detectable levels of circulating immune complexes at the end of 1 year. Other investigators reported a slightly higher incidence of circulating immune complexes in diabetics with longer duration of disease (Kumar and Quismorio, 1978; Schernthaner et al., 1979). The apparent discrepancy between the results of Irvine et al. (1978a) and others is most likely due to the fact that insulin therapy induces antibodies which form circulating complexes. The complexes detected at the onset of diabetes must be different than those found several months later.

Delespesse et al. (1980) studied 189 nondiabetic controls and observed increasing incidence of circulating immune complexes with aging. Such phenomenon was not seen in the insulin-dependent diabetic patients; young diabetic patients (age < 30 years) had 57% incidence of immune complexes, which was significantly higher than the age-matched controls. Among older patients (> 30 years old), immune complexes were detected in 10 of 38 cases and the percentage positivity was not different from controls.

An increased incidence of circulating immune complexes in diabetes could represent production of some specific antibodies induced by exogenous or endogenous antigens. Alternatively, it may be due to a defect in clearance mechanisms. Certain HLA markers, particularly HLA B8 and DRw3, are associated with defective Fc receptor functions (Lawley et al., 1981). Bartolotti (1981) proposed that similar defects may be present in Type I diabetics, where increased frequencies of HLA B8 and DRw3 are seen. Impaired phagocytic activity has been recently demonstrated in diabetics who had evidence of circulating immune complexes (Iavicoli et al., 1982). The injected collidal material was removed slowly.

Generally immune complex diseases are associated with decreased complement levels in blood. Charlesworth et al. (1979) determined levels of C1, C4, C3, factor B, and C5 and found no differences between diabetics and nondiabetics. In fact a moderate increase rather than decrease in complement level has been reported in diabetics (Klein, 1973).

V. NATURE OF IMMUNE COMPLEXES

The characterization of antigens and antibodies involved in the circulating immune complexes and in pathologic lesions is required to elucidate the pathologic role of immune complexes. Using radiolabeled or fluorescein-conjugated insulin preparations, insulin–insulin-antibody complexes have been identified in plasma and in glomerular lesions. The possibility of other antigens (Oldstone and Dixon, 1971) and antibodies exists but definite evidence is lacking.

A. Insulin–Insulin-Antibody Complexes

Jayarao and co-workers (1974) investigated insulin-treated diabetics and confirmed previous observations of Berson and co-workers (1956) that such cases had circulating insulin–insulin-antibodies complexes. Folling (1976) prepared immune complexes *in vitro* by adding increasing amounts of insulin to an antiinsulin guinea pig serum, and showed that three classes of complexes were formed depending upon the molar ratio of insulin and antibodies. In the equivalence state, large complexes were seen which had complement-binding properties. When sera of insulin-treated diabetics was incubated with [^{125}I]insulin to allow exchange between labeled and antibody-bound insulin and subsequently subjected to ultracentrifugation, Folling (1976) found high-molecular-weight complexes that contained [^{125}I]insulin. Recent investigations of Kilpatrick and Virella (1980) confirmed the presence of insulin antibodies in circulating immune complexes. Kumar *et al.* (1979) observed an increased incidence of C1q binding in insulin-resistant cases, who also had high titers of insulin antibodies. Serum samples were treated with 3% polyethylene glycol and precipitated proteins were analyzed for immunoglobulin and antiinsulin antibody contents. The precipitated proteins contained immunoglobulin IgG (0.49 ± 0.07% of total serum IgG), and [^{125}I]insulin-binding IgG (8.2 ± 1.4% of total circulating insulin antibodies) in 42 [^{125}I]C1q positive sera tested. Insulin antibodies were of IgG class (Kumar *et al.*, 1979; Virella *et al.*, 1981) and antiinsulin IgM antibodies could not be demonstrated.

Circulating insulin antibodies react with exogenous insulin and form insulin–insulin-antibody complexes. Since the levels of complexes depend on the relative concentrations of antigens and antibody, this author studied effect of increasing circulating insulin levels. Intravenous infusion of insulin caused an increase in C1q-binding complexes in three insulin-resistant cases. The [^{125}I]C1q binding increased from 33.2 ± 12% to 43.6 ± 13% in 2 hr of insulin infusion (Kumar, unpublished results). A possible involvement of insulin antibodies in immune complexes was also reported by Irvine *et al.* (1977).

In contrast to the above data, one report suggested that insulin antibodies were not involved in immune complexes. Bodansky *et al.* (1982) failed to find insulin antibodies in 2% polyethylene-glycol-precipitated fractions of sera from 18 diabetics. Since it is very likely that 2% polyethylene glycol did not precipitate immune complexes of low-molecular-weight, therefore their negative results could be misleading. On the basis of all available data it is reasonable to conclude that insulin antibodies are involved in the circulating immune complexes.

Insulin-treated diabetics develop detectable levels of circulating antiinsulin IgE. Such antibodies have been demonstrated in patients with insulin allergy (Kumar, 1977; Kahn and Rosenthal, 1979) as well as in patients who did not have any allergic symptoms (Kumar, 1977). However, there is no evidence to suggest that these antibodies form circulating immune complexes.

Commercial insulin preparations derived from porcine and bovine pancreas contain variable amounts of contaminant proteins including proinsulin and insulin aggregates (Root *et al.*, 1972). In comparison to insulin, proinsulin is a larger molecule with multiple antigenic determinants and has marked species variations. It is a potent immunogen and induces antibody formation in diabetic patients (Kumar and Miller, 1973). Although involvement of proinsulin antibodies in immune complexes has not been investigated, it is very likely that these antibodies make higher-molecular-weight complexes which could induce tissue damage. Results of Wehner's (1976) experiments favor such a possibility. Guinea pigs and rabbits immunized with commercial insulin (contaminated with proinsulin and proinsulinlike proteins) developed proliferation of mesangial cells and thickening of mesangium matrix in 3 months. On the other hand, animals immunized with highly purified insulin showed no significant changes in glomeruli.

B. Idiotypic Antibodies

The variable region of immunoglobulin may induce an immune response resulting in the production of idiotypic antibodies. Jerne (1974) suggests that an idiotypic network controls the concentrations of immunoglobulins within the body. Circulating immune complexes containing antiimmunoglobulins have been induced in experimental animals (Rose and Lambert, 1980). There is preliminary evidence to suggest the presence of idiotypic antibodies against insulin antibodies in sera of insulin-treated diabetics (Kumar *et al.*, 1981), and these antibodies may be associated with the circulating immune complexes in insulin-treated diabetic patients.

C. Immune Complexes and Islet Cell Antibodies

Irvine *et al.* (1977) found islet cell antibodies in six of seven sera which were positive for immune complexes. They suggested that some antigens derived from islet cells were involved in the immune complexes. A significant correlation between islet cell antibodies and circulating immune complexes was observed by Delespesse *et al.* (1980). Eight of their 18 immune-complex-positive cases had islet-cell antibodies. However, circulating immune complexes were not analyzed to ascertain the presence of islet cell antigens or antibodies. Kumar *et al.* (1979) investigated 47 Type I diabetic patients, and observed that only 7 (15%) cases had both islet cell cytoplasmic antibodies and [^{125}I]C1q binding. Bodansky *et al.* (1982) precipitated circulating immune complexes by 2% polyethylene glycol, and analyzed the precipitated serum proteins. Islet cell antibodies, either classic or complement-fixing type, were not found in the precipitates in any of 18 cases investigated. Thus, there is insufficient evidence to support the involvement of islet cell antibodies in circulating immune complexes. However, such antibodies produce complement-dependent cytotoxicity and therefore could cause a local immune injury to the islets of Langerhans (Kanatsuna *et al.*, 1982).

D. Organ-Specific Antibodies

Could there be other organ-specific antibodies involved in immune complexes? Delespesse *et al.* (1980) found some evidence of autoantibodies in 17 (94%) of 18 immune-complex-positive diabetic cases. In contrast, Bodansky *et al.* (1982) failed to detect any antibodies to gastric parietal cell, thyroglobulin, and thyroid microsome, or antinuclear antibodies in circulating immune complexes in diabetics. In view of these conflicting reports this issue remains unsettled.

Our knowledge of the nature and composition of circulating immune complexes in diabetic patients is very limited. Future progress in analytical technqiues for the isolation of immune complexes will allow us to define their precise composition and will certainly help in understanding their role in pathogenesis and progression of diabetic syndromes.

VI. ROLE OF IMMUNE COMPLEXES IN DIABETIC COMPLICATIONS

Immune complexes contribute significantly to pathogenesis of glomerular, vascular, and connective tissue lesions in several human diseases (Cochrane and Koffler, 1973). It has been shown that immune complexes can initiate platelet aggregation and release of vasoactive amines which cause an increased vascular permeability (Henson and Spiegelberg, 1973). Observations of Rothberger *et al.* (1977) suggest that soluble antigen–antibody complexes stimulate production of leukocyte procoagulant, which has tissue-thromboplastin-like properties, and may contribute to intravascular thrombosis and deposition of fibrin–fibrinogen. Mathews *et al.* (1974) proposed that immune mechanisms may contribute to the development of atherosclerosis. Deposits of IgG have been demonstrated in medial layers of affected vessel (Lattime and Strausser, 1977). Fust *et al.* (1977) found circulating immune complexes in 52 (69%) of 75 patients with atherosclerosis, cerebral arterial disease, or arteriosclerosis obliterans. Immune complexes can leak into the vessel wall and deposit on subendothelial basement membrane. Deposits of immune complexes have been demonstrated on limiting basement membranes of renal glomeruli, arteries, and choroid plexi (Wilson and Dixon, 1974).

There is a rapid progression of atherosclerosis in diabetic individuals. In addition, there is microangiopathy, which involves retina, glomeruli and other organs including skin. Although the nature and etiology of vascular lesions are not clearly known, it is tempting to consider an immune mechanism which may either initiate or enhance the pathological processes.

A. Diabetic Retinopathy

Several observations suggest that immune complexes may have some role in the pathogenesis of diabetic micro- and macroangiopathy. Deposits of IgG and C3 complement have been found in kidneys and dermal vessels (Gallo, 1970; Beregi, 1973; Urizer *et al.*, 1969, Larsson, 1967). The endothelial lining and basement membrane of retinal vessels may contain insulin-binding substances (Werner and Larsen, 1969). Vascular permeability of retinal capillaries can be increased by infusing high-molecular-weight complexes in rabbits, or by infusing antigen, bovine IgG in immunized rabbits (Howes and McKay, 1975). Since the extravasation of fluorescein dye is the earliest manifestation of retinal angiopathy in diabetes, a possible involvement of circulating immune complexes in the pathogenesis of retinal microangiopathy has been considered. Irvine and co-workers (1978b) and others (Andreani *et al.*, 1982) found a positive association between immune complexes detected by C1q-binding assay as well as by Raji cell assay and microangiopathy. The investigations of Bodansky et al. (1982) have confirmed this association. These authors found a higher prevalence (53%) of raised levels of circulating immune complexes in subjects with retinopathy than in subjects without retinopathy (31%). The presence of circulating immune complexes in these patients does not help in determining whether they are cause or effect. Until the nature of complexes is defined or their presence demonstrated in the lesions, their role in pathogenesis of diabetic retinopathy remains unproven.

B. Diabetic Nephropathy

A possible role of immune complexes in the pathogenesis of diabetic glomerulosclerosis has been considered for a long time. Immunoglobulin (Gallo, 1970) and complements (Urizer et al., 1969) deposits had been described in diabetic kidneys, but proper identification and nature of these deposits remained doubtful. Binding of fluorescein-labeled insulin to renal tissue in diabetic glomerulosclerosis (Farrant and Sheddon, 1965) suggested a direct involvement of antiinsulin antibodies in those lesions. However, an immune etiology of glomerular lesion has remained unlikely because such lesions were found in some patients who had not been treated with exogenous insulin and the linear and nodular lesions of diabetic glomerulosclerosis did not fix heterologous complement. Recent studies on the immune complexes provide some additional support to the concept of immune-complex-mediated damage of glomeruli. Andreani et al. (1982) and Virella et al. (1982) observed a higher incidence of circulating immune complexes in diabetic patients with nephropathy. Meade et al. (1981) described the presence of IgG, IgM, C3 deposits in the glomeruli of diabetic mice (db/db mutants of C57BL/KsJ and C57BL/6J). The former (db/bb C57BL/KsJ) had severe hyperglycemia while the latter (db/db C57BL/6J) mutants were mildly hyperglycemic. Insulin deposits were seen occasionally, and immunoglobulins eluted from the lesions had an antiinsulin activity. Since animals had not received exogenous insulin, these experiments are of significant interest and suggest that endogenous insulin may be involved in immune reactions. Although no antiglomerular antibodies have been reported either in blood or glomerular lesions, it is likely that some immune complexes are deposited in glomeruli and thus contribute to the progression of diabetic nephropathy.

C. Necrobiosis Lipoidica

Some diabetic patients develop an unusual skin condition characterized by asymptomatic, slightly depressed plaques often occurring along the anterior aspect of legs. Histological appearance of these lesions resembles rhematoid arthritis nodules or lesions of erythema annulare. There is thickening and hyalinization of collagen which is surrounded by histiocytes, lymphocytes, epithelial cells, and occasional giant cells. Blood vessels have thickened walls (Bauer and Levan, 1970). Immunofluorescence of skin biopsy specimens showed deposits of IgM in vessel walls in 6 (50%) of 12 cases. IgM, C3, and fibrinogen were found at the dermal–epidermal junction (Ullman and Dahl, 1977). However, no investigations of the circulating immune complexes in these cases have been performed.

D. Lipoatrophy

Some diabetic patients develop lipoatrophy at the insulin injection sites. Biopsy specimens of these lesions indicate that it is caused by deposition of immune complexes in dermal vessels, and at the dermoepidermal junction (Reeves *et al.*, 1980). As expected, all patients also had antiinsulin antibodies in their blood. These atrophic lesions respond to treatment with highly purified insulin preparations, and also to locate steroid therapy (Kumar *et al.*, 1977), which again suggests the role of immune mechanisms. Any association between the lipoatrophy and circulating immune complexes remains speculative because such complexes have not been investigated.

E. Insulitis

Hultquist and Olding (1981) reported eosinophilic cell infiltrates in the pancreas of infants of diabetic mothers. Infiltration was most marked in the close vicinity of the largest islets, and appeared to be related to the B cell nuclear size. Since passive administration of insulin antibodies caused eosinophilic infiltrates in pancreas of experimental animals (Lacy and Wright, 1965; Kloppel *et al.*, 1971), Hultquist and Olding (1981) proposed that a similar mechanism could be responsible in those infants. Maternal insulin antibodies enter fetal circulation through placenta, and perhaps induce some immune reaction in the pancreas. Eosinophils may serve a phagocytic purpose to remove some antigen–antibody complexes (Sabesin, 1963).

VII. IMMUNE COMPLEXES AND METABOLIC CONTROL

Insulin antibodies could increase the need for the exogenous insulin due to their interaction with antibodies (Berson *et al.*, 1956). Most insulin–insulin-antibody complexes are removed by the reticuloendothelial system (Frikke *et al.*, 1974) but some stay in circulation and dissociate to release free insulin (Kurtz *et al.*, 1977). The free insulin may have biological functions. This phenomenon depends on the characteristics of insulin antibodies (Kumar, D., Rhodes, J., and Parameswaran, unpublished findings) and causes prolongation of biological activity of exogenous (Dixon *et al.*, 1975) and endogenous insulin (Anderson *et al.*, 1978).

Since most insulin antibodies induce a conformational change in insulin molecule, the antibody-bound molecules generally do not react with insulin receptors. Conversely, Shechter *et al.* (1979) observed that an antiporcine insulin IgG, purified from a guinea pig antiserum, enhanced insulin binding to liver membrane and to cultured fibroblasts but not to adipocytes. That antibody increased insulin's bioactivity on fibroblasts. When a monovalent Fab fragment was tested, no enhancement in the insulin binding or bioactivity was seen. Kahn *et al.* (1978) observed that bivalent antibody-bound insulin facilitated insulin receptor aggregation, and as the antibody concentration was increased a progressive reduction in receptor-bound insulin became apparent, indicating a competition. Thus characteristics as well as concentration of insulin antibodies determine overall metabolic effects.

The quality of insulin used in treatment of diabetes has been improved in the past decade. Highly purified porcine insulin is less antigenic in humans (Root *et al.*, 1972), and generally induces low titers of insulin antibodies. It is likely that the titers of circulating insulin–insulin-antibody complexes will be reduced when the purified porcine insulin is used (Charlesworth *et al.*, 1979). What effect such therapy would have on other circulating complexes remains to be seen.

VIII. SUMMARY

An increased incidence of circulating immune complexes is found in diabetic patients. There is some association between microangiopathy (retinopathy and nephropathy) and circulating immune complexes. Analysis of the isolated immune complexes revealed presence of antiinsulin antibodies especially in insulin-treated patients. It has been suggested that anti-islet-cell and other autoantibodies are also involved.

Association of circulating immune complexes with microangiopathy and the immune deposits in glomeruli and in dermal vessels supports an immune mechanism in the pathogenesis of diabetic vascular complications. Since a proper identification of the immune components of circulating complexes and tissue deposits is unestablished, it is difficult to ascribe a specific role to the circulating immune complexes. Future improvements in analytic techniques for the isolation and identification of immune components will elucidate the role of circulating immune complexes in the pathogenesis of diabetes and associated vascular complications.

REFERENCES

Andersen, O. O., 1976, Anti-insulin antibodies and late diabetic complications, *Acta Endocrinol. (Kbh.)* **83**:329–340.

Anderson, J. H., Blackard, W. G., Goldman, J., and Rubenstein, A. H., 1978, Diabetes and hypoglycemia due to insulin antibodies, *Am. J. Med.* **64**:868–873.

Andreani, D., Di Mario, U., Galfo, C., Ventriglia, L., and Iavicoli, M., 1982, Circulating immune complexes in diabetics with severe microangiopathy, evaluation by two different methods, *Acta Endocrinol. (Kbh.)* **99**:239–244.

Arend, W. P., Teller, D. C., and Mannik, M., 1972, Molecular composition and sedimentation characteristics of soluble antigen-antibody complexes, *Biochemistry* **11**:4063–4072.

Austen, K. F., 1974, Symposium on the immunobiology of complement, *Transplant. Proc.* **6**:1–88.

Baldwin, R. W., and Robins, R. A., 1976, Factors interfering with immunological rejection of tumors, *Br. Med. Bull.* **32**:118–123.

Barnett, E. V., Knutson, D. W., Abrass, C. K., Chia, D. S., Young, L. S., and Liebling, M. R., 1979, Circulating immune complexes, their immunochemistry, detection and importance, *Ann. Intern. Med.* **91**:430–440.

Bartolotti, S. R., 1981, Defective Fc-receptor functions with the HLA-b8/DRw3 haplotype, *N. Engl. J. Med.* **305**:346.

Bauer, M., and Levan, N. E., 1970, Diabetic dermangiopathy, a spectrum including pigmented pretibial patches and necrobiosis lipoidica diabeticorum, *Br. J. Dermatol.* **83**:528–535.

Beregi, E., 1973, Immunopathologic study of renal changes of diabetic individuals, *Int. Urol. Nephro.* **5**:179–186.

Berson, S. A., Yalow, R. S., Bauman, A., Rothchild, A., and Newerly, K., 1956, Insulin-I^{131} metabolism in human subjects, demonstration of insulin binding globulin in circulation of insulin treated subjects, *J. Clin. Invest.* **35**:170–190.

Bodansky, H. J., Wolf, E., Cudworth, A. G., Dean, B. M., Nineham, L. J., Buttazzo, G. F., Mathews, J.

A., Kurtz, A. B., and Kohner, E. M., 1982, Genetic and immunologic factors in microvascular disease in type 1 insulin-dependent diabetes, *Diabetes* **31**:70–74.

Casali, P., Bossus, A., Carpentier, N. A., and Lambert, P. H., 1977, Solid phase enzyme immunoassay or radioimmunoassay for the detection of immune complexes based on their recognition by conglutinin:conglutinin-binding test. A comparative study with[125]I labelled C1q binding and Raji-cell RIA tests, *Clin. Exp. Immunol* **29**:342–354.

Charlesworth, J. A., Campbell, L. V., Quin, J., Lazarus, L., and Macdonald, G. J., 1979, Immune complexes in diabetes mellitus, *Aust. N.Z. J. Med.* **9**:370–373.

Clagett, J. H., Wilson, C. B., and Weigle, W. O., 1974, Intersitial immune complex thyroiditis in mice, the role of autoantibody to thyroglobulin, *J. Exp. Med.* **140**:1439–1456.

Cochrane, C. G., and Koffler, D., 1973, Immune complex disease in experimental animals and man, *Adv. Immunol.* **16**:186–264.

Delespesse, G., Gausset, P. H., Sarfati, M., Dubi-Rucquoy, M., Dibesschop, M. J., and Van Haelst, L., 1980, Circulating immune complexes in old and in diabetics: correlation with autoantibodies, *Clin. Exp. Immunol.* **40**:96–102.

Digeon, M., Laver, M., Rixa, J., and Bach, J. F., 1977, Detection of circulating immune complexes in human sera by simplified assays with polyethylene glycol, *J. Immunol. Methods* **16**:165–183.

Di Mario, U., Iavicoli, M., and Andreani, D., 1980, Circulating immune complexes in diabetes, *Diabetologia* **19**:89–92.

Dixon, K., Exon, P. D., and Malins, J. M., 1975, Insulin antibodies and control of diabetes, *Q. J. Med.* **44**:543–553.

Farrant, P. C., and Sheddon, W. I. H., 1965, Observations on the uptake of insulin conjugated with fluorescein isothiocyanate by diabetic kidney tissue, *Diabetes* **14**:274–278.

Folling, I., 1976, Insulin-anti-insulin complexes, *Acta Endocrinol.* (Kbh.) **83**(Suppl. 205):199–209.

Frikke, M. J., Gingerich, R. L., Stranahan, P. D., Carter, G., Bauman, A. K., Greider, M. H., Wright, P. H., and Lacy, P. E., 1974, Distribution of injected insulin and insulin-antibody complexes in normal and insulin-immunized animals, *Diabetologia* **10**:345–351.

Fust, G., Szekley, J., and Gero, S., 1977, Circulating immune complexes in vascular diseases, *Lancet* **1**:193–194.

Gallo, G. R., 1970, Elution studies in kidneys with linear deposition of immunoglobulin in glomeruli, *Am. J. Pathol.* **61**:377–385.

Gigli, I., 1976, Immunochemistry and immunobiology of complement system, *J. Invest. Dermatol.* **67**:346–353.

Gotze, O., and Muller-Eberhard, H. J., 1976, The alternative pathway of complement activation, *Adv. Immunol.* **24**:1–35.

Haakenstad, A. O., and Mannik, M., 1974, Saturation of the reticuloendothelial system with soluble immune complexes, *J. Immunol.* **112**:1939–1948.

Hay, F. C., Nineham, L J., and Roitt, I. M., 1976, Routine assay for the detection of immune complexes of known immunoglobulin class using a solid phase C1q, *Clin. Exp. Immunol.* **24**:396–400.

Hellstrom, K. E., and Hellstrom, I., 1974, Lymphocyte mediated cytotoxicity and blocking serum activity to tumor antigens, *Adv. Immunol.* **18**:209–277.

Henson, P. M., and Cochrane, C. G., 1971, Acute immune complex disease in rabbits. The role of complement and of a leukocyte-dependent release of vasoactive amines from platelets, *J. Exp. Med.* **133**:54–571.

Henson, P. M., and Oades, Z. G., 1976, Activation of platelets by platelets-activating factor (PAF) derived from IgE-sensitized basophils. II The role of serine proteases, cyclic nucleotides, and contractile elements in PAF-induced secretion, *J. Exp. Med.* **143**:953–968.

Henson, P. M., and Spiegelberg, H. L., 1973, Release of serotinin from human platelets induced by aggregated immunoglobulins of different classes and subclasses *J. Clin. Invest.* **52**:1282–1288.

Howes, E. L., and McKay, D. G., 1975, Circulating immune complexes. Effects on ocular vascular permeability in the rabbit, *Arch. Ophthalmol.* **93**:365–370.

Hultquist, G. T., and Olding, L. B., 1981, Endocrine pathology of infants of diabetic mothers, *Acta Endocrinol. (Kbh.)* **97**(Suppl. 241):1–202.

Iavicoli, M., Di Mario, U., Pozzilli, P., Canalese, J., Vetriglia, L., Galfo, C., and Andreani, D., 1982, Impaired phagocytic function and increased immune complexes in diabetics with severe microangiopathy, *Diabetes* **31**:7–11.

Inman, R. D., and Day, N. K., 1981, Immunologic and clinical aspects of immune complex diseases, *Am. J. Med.* **70**:1097–1106.

Irvine, W. J., Al-Khateeb, S. F., Di Mario, U., Feek, C. M., Gray, R. S., Edmond, B., and Duncan, L. J. P., 1977, Soluble immune complexes in the sera of newly diagnosed insulin-dependent diabetics and in treated diabetics, *Clin. Exp. Immunol.* **30**:16–21.

Irvine, W. J., Di Mario, U., Guy, K., Feek, C. M., Gray, R. S., and Duncan, L. J. P., 1978a, Immune complexes in newly diagnosed insulin dependent (type 1) diabetics, *J. Clin. Lab. Immunol.* **1**:183–186.

Irvine, W. J., Di Mario, U., Guy, K., Iavicoli, M., Pozzilli, P., Lumbroso, B., and Andreani, D., 1978b, Immune complexes and diabetic microangiopathy, *J. Clin. Lab. Immunol.* **1**:187–191.

Jayarao, K., Faulk, W. P., Karam, J. H., Grodsky, G. M., and Forsham, P. H., 1974, Evidence in support of the concept of immune-complex disease in insulin-treated diabetics, in: *Immunity and Autoimmunity in Diabetes Mellitus* (P. A. Bastenie and W. Gepts, eds.), pp. 255–263, Excerpta Medica, Amsterdam.

Jerne, N. K., 1974, Towards a network theory of immune system, *Ann. Immunol.* **125**:373–389.

Kahn, C. R., and Rosenthal, A. J., 1979, Immunolgoic reactions to insulin: Insulin allergy, insulin resistance, and autoimmune insulin syndrome, *Diabetes Care* **2**:283–295.

Kahn, C. R., Baird, K. L., Jarret, D. B., and Flier, J., 1978, Direct demonstration that receptor crosslinking or aggregation is important in insulin action, *Proc. Natl. Acad. Sci. USA* **75**:4209–4213.

Kanatsuna, T., Freedman, Z. R., Rubenstein, A. H., and Lernmark, A., 1982, Effects of islet cell surface antibodies and complement on the release of insulin and chromium from perifused B cells, *Clin. Exp. Immunol.* **47**:85–92.

Kilpatrick, J. M., and Virella, G., 1980, Isolation and characterization of soluble insulin-anti-insulin immune complexes formed in vitro and in vivo in sera from patients with diabetes mellitus, *Clin. Exp. Immunol.* **40**:445–452.

Klein, V. G., 1973, Quantitative immunological determination of plasma proteins in diabetic microangiopathy. *Wein. Klin. Wochenschr.* **85**:192–194.

Kloppel, G., Altenahr, E., and Freytag, G., 1971, Electronemicroskopische untersuchugen zur experimentellen insulitis nach injection von anti-insulin serum, *Virchows Arch. Pathol. Anat.* **354**:324–335.

Kumar, D., 1977, Anti-insulin IgE in diabetics, *J. Clin. Endocrinol. Metab.* **45**:1159–1164.

Kumar, D., and Miller, L., 1973, Proinsulin specific antibodies in huamn sera, *Diabetes* **22**:361–366.

Kumar, D., and Quismorio, Jr., F. P., 1978, Immune complexes in diabetic patients, *Diabetes* **27**:222.

Kumar, D., Miller, L. V., and Mehtalia, S. D., 1977, Use of dexamethasone in treatment of insulin lipoatrophy, *Diabetes* **26**:296–299.

Kumar, D., Rhodes, J., and Miller, A., 1981, Idiotypic antibodies against insulin antibodies in circulating immune complexes, *Diabetes* **30**(Suppl. 1):94A.

Kumar, D., Zeidler, A., and Quismorio, Jr., F. P., 1979, Circulating immune complexes, islet-cell and insulin antibodies, *Diabetes* **28**:378.

Kurtz, A. B., Mustaffa, B. E., Dagget, P. R., and Nabarro, J. D. N., 1977, Effects of insulin antibodies on free and total plasma insulin, *Lancet* **2**:56–58.

Lacy, P. E., and Wright, P. H., 1965, Allergic interstitial pancreatitis in rats injected with guinea pig anti-insulin serum, *Diabetes* **14**:634–642.

Lambert, P. H., Dixon, F. J., Zubler, R. H., Agnello, V., Cambiaso, C., Casali, P., Clarke, J., Cowdery, J. S., McDuffie, F. C., Hay, F. C., Maclennan, I. C. M., Masson, P., Muller-Eberhard, H. J., Penthinen, K., Smith, M., Tappeiner, G., Theofilopoulos, A. N., and Verroust, P., 1978, A WHO collaborative study for the evaluation of eighteen methods for detecting immune complexes in serum, *J. Clin. Lab. Immunol.* **1**:1–15.

Larsson, O., 1967, Studies of small vessels in patients with diabetes. A clinical histological and immunohistochemical study of diabetic and non-diabetic subjects with special reference to the occurrence of various plasma proteins in the dermal vessel walls, *Acta Med. Scand. [Suppl.]* **480**:5–65.

Lattime, E. C., and Strausser, H. R., 1977, Atherosclerosis. Is stress-induced immune suppression a risk factor? *Science* **198**:302–303.

Lawley, T. J., Hall, R. P., Fauci, A. S., Katz, S. I., Hamberger, M. I., and Frank, M. M., 1981, Defective Fc-receptor functions associated with the HLA-B8/DRw3 haplotypes: Studies in patients with dermatitis herpetiformis and normal subjects, *N. Engl. J. Med.* **304:**185–192.

Mathews, J. D., Whittingham, S., and Mackay, I. R., 1974, Autoimmune mechanisms in human vascular disease, *Lancet* **2:**1423–1427.

Meade, C. J., Brandon, D. R., Smith, W., Simmonds, R. G., Harris, S., and Sowter, C., 1981, the relationship between hyperglycemia and renal immune complex deposition in mice with inherited diabetes, *Clin. Exp. Immunol.* **43:**109–120.

Muller-Eberhard, H. J., 1975, Complement, *Annu. Rev. Biochem.* **44:**697–724.

Oldstone, M., and Dixon, F., 1971, Immune complex disease in chronic viral infections, *J. Exp. Med. (Suppl)* **134:**32s–39s.

Osler, A. G., and Sandberg, A. L., 1973, Alternate complement pathways, *Prog. Allergy* **17:**51–92.

Porter, R. R., and Reid, K. B. M., 1978, The biochemistry of complement, *Nature* **275:**699–704.

Reeves, W. G., Allen, B. R., and Tattersall, R. B., 1980, Insulin-induced lipoatrophy, evidence for an immune pathogenesis, *Br. Med. J.* **280:**1500–1503.

Revoltella, R., Pediconi, M., Bertolini, L., and Bosman, C., 1975, In vitro immune response by murine bone marrow cells stimulated against soluble immune complexes, *Cell. Immunol.* **20:**117–132.

Rodrick, M., Allan, R., and Isliker, H., 1978, Activation of the classical and alternative pathways of complement fixation by immune complexes containing normal and tryptophan-modified immunoglobulin G, *J. Immunol. Methods* **22:**211–218.

Root, M., Chance, R. E., and Galloway, J. A., 1972, Immunogenicity of insulin, *Diabetes,* **21:**657–660.

Rose, L. M., and Lambert, P. H., 1980, The natural occurrence of circulating idiotype anti-idiotype complexes during a secondary immune response to phosphorylcholine, *Clin. Immunol. Immunopathol.* **15:**481–492.

Rothberger, H., Zimmerman, T. S., Spiegelberg, H. L., and Vaughn, J. H., 1977, Leukocyte procoagulant activity. Enhancement of production in vitro by IgG and antigen-antibody complexes, *J. Clin. Invest.* **59:**549–557.

Sabesin, S. M., 1963, A function of the eosinophil: Phagocytosis of antigen–antibody complexes, *Proc. Soc. Exp. Biol. Med.* **112:**667–670.

Schernthaner, G., Ludwig, H., Tappeiner, G., Mayr, W. R., 1979, Circulating immune complexes (CIC), IgG-insulin antibodies (I-ab), islet-cell antibodies (ICA) and HLA antigens in insulin-dependent diabetics, *Diabetes* **28:**378.

Shechter, Y., Chang, K-J, Jacobs, S., and Cuatrecasas, P., 1979, Modulation of binding and bioactivity of insulin by anti-insulin antibody: Relation to possible role of receptor self-aggregation in hormone action, *Proc. Natl. Acad. Sci. USA* **76:**2720–2724.

Spiegelberg, H. L., 1974, Biological activities of immunoglobulins of different classes and subclasses,*o Adv. Immunol.* **19:**259–294.

Theofilopoulos, A. N., and Dixon, F. J., 1979, The biology and detection of immune complexes, *Adv. Immunol.* **28:**89–220.

Theofilopoulos, A. N., Wilson, C. B., and Dixon, F. J., 1976, The Raaji cell radioimmune assay for detecting immune complexes in human sera, *J. Clin. Invest.* **57:**169–182.

Ullman, S., and Dahl, M., 1977, Necrobiosis lipoidica, An immunofluorescence study. *Arch. Dermatol.* **113:**1671–1673.

Urizer, R. E., Schwartz, A., Top, F., and Vernier, R. L., 1969, The nephrotic syndrome in children with diabetes mellitus of recent onset, *N. Engl. J. Med.* **281:**173–181.

Virella, G., Wohltmann, H., Sagel, J., Lopes-Virella, M. F. L., Kilpatrick, M. Phillips, C., and Colwell, J., 1981, Soluble immune complexes in patients with diabetes mellitus, detection and pathological significance, *Diabetologia* **21:**184–191.

Wehner, H., 1976, The influence of insulin and insulin antibodies on the glomerular structure, *Acta Endocrinol. (Kbh)* **83**(Suppl. 205):241–253.

Werner, A. U., and Larsen, H. W., 1969, Immunohistological studies on human diabetic and non-diabetic eyes. I Fluorescent labelling of insulin and insulin-antibodies, *Acta. Ophthalmol. (Kbh.)* **47:**935–937.

Wiggins, R. C., and Cochrane, C. G., 1981, Immune-complex-mediated biologic effects, *N. Engl. J. Med.* **304:**518–520.
Williams, R. C., 1981, Immune complexes in huamn diseases, *Annu. Rev. Med.* **32:**13–28.
Wilson, C. B., and Dixon, F. J., 1974, Diagnosis of immunopathologic renal disease, *Kidney Int.* **5:**389–401.

15

Insulin Hypersensitivity: Pathogenesis, Diagnosis, and Management

Roy Patterson, Leslie C. Grammer, and Peter Y. Chen

I. INTRODUCTION

Hypersensitivity to insulin has received considerable attention in the medical literature for several reasons. One of these is the high incidence of diabetes mellitus; another is the requirement that some cases of diabetes must be treated with the insulin to which they are allergic. In contrast to many drugs which cause allergic reactions, insulin is a complete protein suitable for the application of sensitive and sophisticated immunological measurements. Finally, the fine structure of the insulin molecule has been thoroughly studied and highly purified insulins of different species and even synthesized insulins have been available for *in vitro* or *in vivo* immunological studies. This chapter will review the problems of insulin hypersensitivity with emphasis on the practical management of clinical problems.

II. CLASSIFICATION

The classification of an immunological reaction to a drug that may cause more than one type of reaction is best done using the classification of Gell and Coombs (1969).

Type I reactions are immediate-type, anaphylactic-type reactions to insulin. These are IgE-mediated and result in local or systemic reactions. Most allergic reactions to insulin are of this type.

Roy Patterson, Leslie C. Grammer, and Peter Y. Chen • Section of Allergy–Immunology, Department of Medicine, Northwestern University Medical School, Chicago, Illinois 60611.

Type II reactions are cytotoxic reactions that occur when an antibody is directed against a cell-surface antigen or against a hapten fixed to a cell, resulting in destruction of that cell. We are not aware of any evidence for this type of reaction causing insulin hypersensitivity.

Type III reactions are antigen–antibody complex reactions resulting in complement fixation and leukocyte attraction with resultant inflammatory response. The classic Type III reaction is serum sickness due to the administration of foreign serum and such a reaction is possible with insulin therapy. The major immunological reactants in Type III reactions are usually antibodies of the IgG class and these antibodies may also result in immunological insulin resistance (Chapter 8).

Type IV reactions are lymphocyte-mediated reactions. Such reactions have been described using *in vitro* stimulation of lymphocytes of patients treated with insulin and may be involved in some local reactions in humans treated with insulin (Faulk *et al.*, 1975). Local reactions of this type due to zinc have been reported (Feinglos and Jegasothy, 1979). The classification of allergic reactions to insulin is summarized in Table 1 using the Gell and Coombs type of classification.

III. LOCAL REACTIONS TO INSULIN

A. Cutaneous

These reactions result from purposeful skin testing with insulin or from insulin on the shaft of the needle used for injection. The insulin reactions are of the immediate type with a wheal and flare reactions present within 30 min. This type of reaction was the major experimental method of analysis of allergic antibody against insulin until *in vitro* IgE antibody assays became available. Biphasic reactions are immediate-type reactions followed by a persistent reaction or recurrence of a later reaction. The immediate-type reactions are classic IgE-mediated, wheal and flare reactions. The late-phase reactions have been suggested as being due to Arthus-type mechanisms on the basis of histological appearance (de Shazo *et al.*, 1977). Studies using the immediate-type, IgE-mediated skin test reaction to insulin have demonstrated that positive skin tests are

Table 1.   Summary of Allergic Reactions to Insulin Using the Gell and Coombs (1969) Classification

Type I. Immediate-type
  Mediated by IgE antibody; most common reaction
  Local reactions
    Immediate-type
    Biphasic (immediate and late reactions)
  Generalized reactions: anaphylaxis
Type III. Serum sickness type
  Mediated by IgG antibody
  Very rare
Type IV. Delayed type, lymphocyte-mediated
  Late local reactions

common in insulin-treated patients. For example Arkins *et al.* (1962) found positive reactions in more than 50% of insulin-treated diabetics and Lieberman (1971) found positive skin tests in 40% of patients treated with insulin. These studies were done in patients with no systemic or other clinical allergic reactions to insulin, and thus the positive skin tests had no clinical relevance. The results emphasize that a single skin test cannot help establish a clinical diagnosis of insulin allergy since the skin tests are positive in such a high proportion of insulin-treated diabetics with no problem of clinical allergy to insulin. The skin tests may be used to compare different degrees of sensitivity to different insulins in the same patient. For example, a patient who has had a generalized reaction to a mixture of beef and pork insulin can be tested with serial dilutions of separate beef and separate pork insulins. For example, 10^{-2}, 10^{-3}, 10^{-4}, 10^{-5}, 10^{-6}, and 10^{-7} dilutions of beef and pork insulin can be used for testing. After injection of insulin the results are recorded and the end point is the highest dilution of insulin giving a positive immediate-type skin reaction. For example, a patient reacting to a 10^{-7} dilution of beef insulin and a 10^{-4} dilution of pork insulin would be more sensitive to beef insulin, and therapy with pork insulin might be most appropriate. The IgE antibody mediating these reactions can be demonstrated by passive transfer of allergic antibody to normal human skin. This is done by injecting 0.1 ml of allergic serum intracutaneously into normal human skin and then testing with insulin at the serum injection site in 48 hr. A positive wheal and flare skin reaction due to the transfer of allergic antibody occurs at the injection site. This reaction is called the Prausnitz-Küstner reaction and the test was an important method of studying allergic antibody against insulin until the development of *in vitro* assays for IgE antibody. As stated earlier skin tests have little or no value in diagnosing allergy and rarely are skin titrations to insulin necessary for selection of insulin for therapeutic use.

B. Subcutaneous

These reactions are a clinical problem in occasional patients. The reactions are immediate-type, IgE-mediated reactions occurring subcutaneously at the site of the therapeutic injection of insulin. Because the reaction is deeper in tissue, the swelling is more diffuse than it would be at a cutaneous skin test reaction site. The subcutaneous reaction will have swelling and erythema, and may be painful or pruritic. Such reactions usually occur during the first few weeks of newly initiated insulin therapy. They almost always subside and disappear with continued insulin therapy and thus are no significant clinical problem. Usually simply reassuring the patient that no major problem exists and that the reactions will subside is sufficient management of these local reactions. Occasionally the reactions are sufficiently severe to cause significant discomfort. When this occurs the reactions can be suppressed with an antihistamine such as chlorpheniramine, 4 mg four times daily, until the reactions subside spontaneously. In more severe cases, it may be necessary to divide the dose of insulin between two or even three sites to reduce the size of the local reactions until spontaneous remission occurs. Rarely it might be necessary to consider changing to a more purified preparation of a single insulin, usually pork (Davidson *et al.*, 1974). Biphasic subcutaneous reactions may occur at the subcutaneous injection site. These are early immediate-type which may persist or may be followed by a second, later-onset, reaction. Management similar to that for the other subcutaneous reactions described above is recommended. The biphasic reactions will also subside with continued insulin therapy.

IV. GENERALIZED, IMMEDIATE-TYPE IgE-MEDIATED REACTIONS

These reactions have justifiably resulted in far more concern than the local reactions because of their systemic nature and potential seriousness. It is possible that such reactions to insulin may progress to anaphylactic shock although we are unaware of any recent fatality from anaphylaxis.

A. Clinical Manifestation

These are the same as any anaphylactic-type reaction in humans. Generalized pruritus, urticaria, angioedema, erythema, asthma, and hypotension can occur in any sequence. The most serious manifestations of laryngeal edema and shock may immediately precede death but, as stated above, are extremely uncommon.

The incidence of the generalized reactions to insulin is low. In the allergy consultation service of our large medical center we see approximately one case per year. Clear epidemiologic data appear unavailable but the incidence of generalized reactions in our experience has appeared to decline, perhaps because of increased purity of insulin. Many physicians dealing either with diabetes or allergy have not seen such generalized reactions and the first case of insulin allergy seen may become one of confused urgency while a physician experienced with the problem is sought. As we shall describe, the management is in general not difficult.

In almost all cases we observed (Mattson et al., 1975), there was interrupted insulin therapy. The typical history involves a patient thought to require insulin initially. Insulin therapy was started and then stopped. Subsequently, after months or years insulin therapy was resumed because of clear medical indication. After insulin therapy is reinstituted, there are usually several days of treatment without allergic reactions, followed by immediate-type local reactions which increase on successive days. Then a systemic or generalized reaction occurs with the symptoms described above. The generalized reaction is accompanied by a large local reaction at the insulin injection site. Usually the only manifestations are urticaria, angioedema, or both (Mattson et al., 1975).

B. Differential Diagnosis

The diagnosis is usually not difficult because of the typical course described above. Confusion may occur in the patient who is receiving multiple drugs but the presence or absence of a large local reaction at the insulin injection site makes the diagnosis quite simple. Thus the presence of generalized urticaria and a large local reaction at the site of insulin injection can be considered to be insulin allergy. Occasionally insulin allergy is inappropriately confused with adult-onset idiopathic urticaria and angioedema. The latter problem may occur in a patient with diabetes treated with insulin. If it occurs coincidentally with the initation of insulin therapy, insulin is almost certain to be suspected as the cause of the urticaria. Because insulin allergy will be accompanied by local reactions at the injection site and idiopathic urticaria will not, the differential diagnosis is usually simple. As described above in the discussion of cutaneous reactions there may be positive skin tests to insulin in up to 50% of asymptomatic insulin-treated diabetics so skin testing must be interpreted with caution: A positive skin test is not confirmatory, but an appropriately done negative skin test excludes insulin allergy.

C. Symptomatic Management

Drug therapy for the acute reaction is similar to management of any acute allergic drug reaction and depends on the severity of the reaction. Thus, in mild cases oral antihistamines such as chlorpheniramine 4 mg four times daily may suffice. Epinephrine, 0.3 ml 1 : 1000 subcutaneously, will reduce the acute symptoms. Prednisone, 30–50 mg stat and then daily may be necessary for severe reactions. Usually 1–3 days of therapy is sufficient for control of symptoms.

D. Insulin Therapy

Often the patient must be managed by a physician who has not had experience with a similar case because the low incidence of reactions results in limited experience with the problem. Certain principles are important. If management is cautious, the outcome will be satisfactory. We have not found any patient who could not safely and continuously use insulin. The physician first should determine the necessity for insulin therapy, receiving expert consultation when necessary. The problem must be explained to the patient, including the potential risk of even serious anaphylaxis with administration of further insulin. An allergist is best qualified to supervise the administration of insulin but such a subspecialist might not be available. The theoretical aspect and immunologic mechanism of insulin desensitization will be reviewed later. The practical aspects follow.

E. Continued Insulin Therapy

The decision to terminate insulin therapy following a systemic reaction is often made inappropriately because of a lack of experience with the problem. Immediately after treatment of the allergic symptoms the next determination is whether further insulin therapy is essential based on the nature of the patient's diabetes. If insulin is required, it must be continued without interruption in therapy. Thus insulin should be given the day after the onset of the allergic insulin reaction. The principle for this approach is that a patient who has had a generalized reaction to a dose of an allergen can receive a smaller dose of that allergen without a generalized reaction a short time (days) later, but the risk increases the longer the interval becomes. The next daily dose of insulin can be one-third of that causing the reaction or, for extreme caution, one-sixth of the dose. The procedure is best done in the hospital, and emergency therapy for anaphylaxis must be immediately available. A hypothetical case could involve a patient having successively larger local reactions at the site of injection of 30 U intermediate-acting insulin given daily and then having a generalized reacton with urticaria and angioedema. The patient would be treated symptomatically for the reaction as described above. The problem would be explained to the patient and the next daily dose of the same preparation of insulin would be reduced to 10 U. The insulin dose would be increased by 5 U on successive days. After following this regimen, the previously used 30 U, or an even higher dose, could be given. Rarely, the desired single dosage might result in repeat episodes of generalized urticaria and the patient might have to be managed with divided doses. For example, in the case described above, 25 U in the morning and 5 U in the afternoon would likely be tolerated with no systemic allergic reaction.

F. Antiallergic Therapy during Continued Insulin or Desensitization Therapy

We do not advise continuous antihistamine or corticosteroid therapy during these procedures. The principle is that it is difficult to treat a systemic allergic reaction occurring during antiallergic therapy, since the patient is already receiving the very drugs one would use to suppress the reaction. Thus it is preferable to have a margin of safety by determining the dosages which result in large local reactions or mild generalized reactions which can be treated with antiallergic therapy and future insulin dose reduction.

G. Insulin Desensitization

When a patient has had a generalized allergic allergic reaction to insulin therapy which is required for management of diabetes and there is an interval of weeks, months, or years since the last insulin therapy, insulin desensitization is required. This is accomplished by first determining the need for insulin and explaining the risk of anaphylaxis to the patient. The desensitization procedure should be carried out in the hospital with preparation for emergency treatment of anaphylaxis. The immunological mechanisms of desensitization will be discussed below. The clinical principle of desensitization therapy in allergy to insulin is simply that there is a dosage of insulin sufficiently low not to induce an anaphylactic reaction. That dosage is given and when no reaction occurs there is an increase in the dosage, based on clinical experience until either a large local, mild systemic, or therapeutic level of insulin is reached. If large local or mild systemic reactions occur the dosage is reduced to the previous dosage which did not cause a significant reaction and again slowly increased. Using this regimen, we have successfully desensitized all cases in which insulin was required for management of diabetes. Since our last report (Mattson *et al.*, 1975) we have desensitized several subsequent patients and neither we nor various colleagues with whom we have reviewed the problem have been unable successfully to desensitize a patient. Further, none of the patients have had recurrences of the problem of insulin allergy unless it was discontinued and resumed nor has any patient required chronic antihistamine or corticosteroid therapy for insulin allergy. A practical insulin desensitization regimen is shown in Table 2.

V. INSULIN AS AN ANTIGEN

The immunology of insulin may be reviewed in relation to IgE antibodies against insulin preparations resulting in immediate-type reactions and IgG antibodies against insulin preparations resulting in serum sickness or insulin resistance. These are outlined in

Table 2. Representative Insulin Desensitization Schedule[a]

Day[b]	Time	Units of insulin	Preparation of insulin
1	Morning	0.0001	Regular
	Noon	0.001	Regular
	Afternoon	0.01	Regular
2	Morning	0.1	Regular
	Noon	1.0	Regular
	Afternoon	2.0	Intermediate-acting
3	Morning	4.0	Intermediate-acting
	Noon	8	Intermediate-acting
	Afternoon	10	Intermediate-acting
4	Morning	15	Intermediate-acting
	Noon	15	Intermediate-acting
5	Morning	20	Intermediate-acting
	Noon	20 or less	Intermediate-acting

[a]Initial insulin preparation: Regular beef–pork. Intermediate-acting insulin preparation: NPH or Lente beef–pork. Route of administration: Subcutaneous. Rate of administration: In emergency for ketoacidosis, every 10 min. For nonemergency cases, the regimen below is satisfactory.
[b]Subsequent to day 5, the morning dose is increased by 5 U to the therapeutic dosage; any lesser dose may be given later in the day for diabetic management.

Table 3. Only IgG antibodies against the insulin molecule can be associated with insulin resistance because antibodies against contaminants (unless there is cross-reactivity) could not result in insulin resistance and IgE antibodies against insulin are not present in sufficient amounts to cause insulin resistance.

Early in the use of insulin, most allergic reactions were thought to be due to noninsulin contaminants and it is likely that this was true. As insulin preparations of increased purity became available, allergic reactions to insulin continued to occur. When sophisticated immunoassays became available and the structure of insulin was understood, more attention was directed toward the insulin molecule itself as an antigen causing allergic reactions and insulin resistance.

Table 3. Antigen Materials (Proven or Presumptive) in Insulin Preparations

Material	Example	Characteristics	Possible reactions
Heterologous insulin	Beef insulin	Foreign protein	IgE and IgG-mediated allergic reactions; IgG-mediated insulin resistance
Altered heterologous insulin	Beef insulin	Foreign protein plus new antigenic determinants	Same as above
Protein contaminants in insulin	Noninsulin beef proteins	Foreign proteins	IgE- and IgG-mediated allergic reactions
Nonprotein additives	Zinc	Nonprotein antigens	Incriminated in late skin reactions

A. Noninsulin Protein Contaminants

Although noninsulin protein contaminants have been incriminated as a cause of allergic reactions to insulin there are only limited studies in support of this. In a study of quantitative cutaneous reactions to various insulins in a group of insulin-treated diabetics in 1971, it was shown that about half of the skin-reactive patients reacted to noninsulin pork and beef proteins, suggesting that the patients receiving beef and pork insulins had been sensitized to these noninsulin heterologous proteins (Fig. 1) (Lieberman *et al.*, 1971). Further, the least skin reactivity to the various insulins tested was against chromatographically purified beef and human insulins, further suggesting that some cutaneous reactivity is against noninsulin heterologous proteins (Lieberman *et al.*, 1971). However, in the same study, five patients had had systemic allergic reactions to beef and pork insulin and none of these patients had skin reactivity to noninsulin beef and pork proteins although they reacted to beef, pork, and human insulins. This was considered evidence for reactivity against the insulin molecule itself (Lieberman *et al.*, 1971).

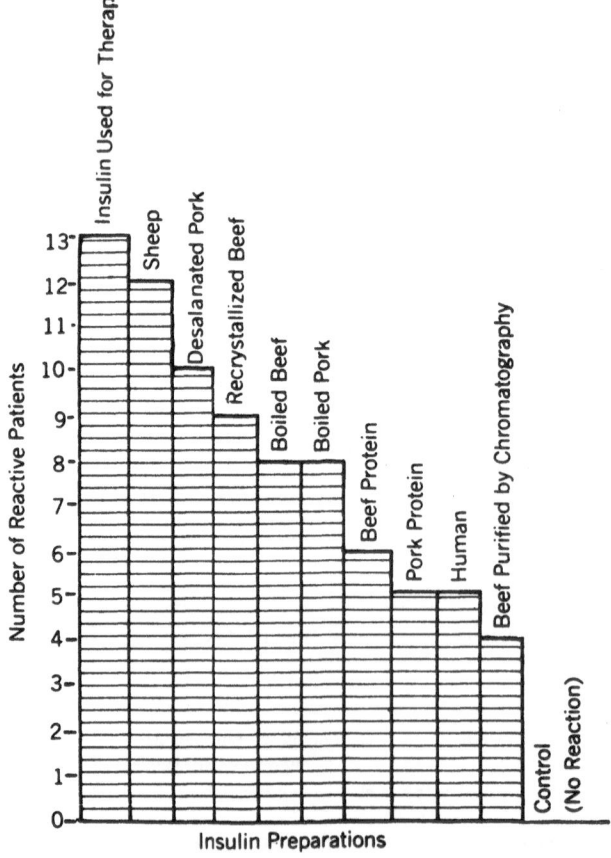

Figure 1. Results of direct intradermal tests with 10 varieties of insulin in 13 diabetic patients, showing skin reactivity to insulin. No subject showed systemic reactivity.

B. Antigenicity of Native Insulins

Insulin is a polypeptide with an α and β chain. Beef insulin differs from human insulin by three amino acids while pork insulin differs by only one amino acid. This greater difference between human and beef insulins has been cited as an explanation for lesser antigenicity of pork insulin as compared to beef insulin. Although this may have some relevance to antigenic differences between beef and pork insulins it has also been demonstrated that human antibodies are directed against different conformations of the insulin molecules dependent upon their secondary and tertiary structure (Patterson et al., 1973b). With the limited sera available the insulins from various animal species have been studied and incomplete cross-reactivity exists (Patterson et al., 1973b).

C. Antigenicity of Altered Insulins

Homologous or autologous proteins may be altered structurally by a variety or procedures so that they become antigenic for members of the same species. This was shown definitively with insulin by demonstrating that a patient allergic to foreign insulins also reacted to his own insulin after it was extracted by the acid–alcohol procedure (Patterson et al., 1969). We have seen two patients with systemic allergic reactions to animal insulins who have immediate cutaneous reactivity to human (recombinant DNA) insulin.

In summary, antibody responses to proteins in insulin solutions may be directed against noninsulin, heterologous protein contaminants, the heterologous native insulin molecule, or the altered insulin molecule. In the allergic reaction any or all of these may be responsible for the reaction in the individual patient. Determining which type of antigen is the cause of the allergic reaction to insulin is a major research undertaking. Thus the approach for insulin desensitization described above is regarded as practical, safe, and inexpensive and has proven successful in the management of patients who have had allergic reactions to insulin. The concept that allergic reactions to insulins were due only to protein contaminants and that highly purified insulins would solve the problem is not consistent with the antigenicity of insulin either native or altered forms. This position is supported by a report of human anaphylaxis to highly purified monocomponent insulin (Goldman et al., 1976) and by a report of the antigenicity of monocomponent pork insulin (Yue and Turtle, 1975).

In contrast to allergic reactions to insulin preparations where reactivity may be against protein contaminants, in IgG-mediated insulin resistance the IgG antibody must be directed against the insulin molecule. It has been reported that antibody levels against insulin decline with use of highly purified insulin with the suggestion that contaminants may in some way stimulate antibody response against insulin (Kurtz et al., 1980).

D. Mechanism of Desensitization

The allergic antibody responsible for the insulin allergy in those cases where the immunoglobulin class has been demonstrated has been shown to be IgE (Patterson et al., 1973a). In patients in whom insulin desensitization is not carried out, the IgE antibody against insulin may persist for months or years. This can be demonstrated by persistent high levels of IgE antibody shown by in vitro or in vivo techniques (Fig. 2).

During insulin desensitization the total serum IgE level and IgE antibody level

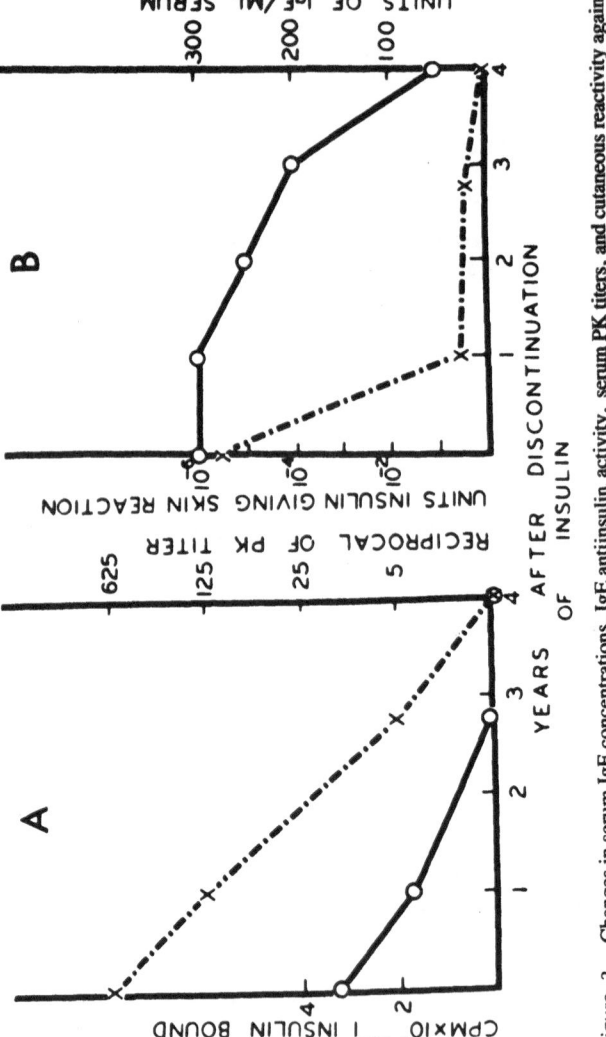

Figure 2. Changes in serum IgE concentrations, IgE antiinsulin activity, serum PK titers, and cutaneous reactivity against insulin in a patient after an allergic reaction to insulin and discontinuation of insulin therapy. (A) [^{125}I]bovine insulin bound by serum IgE, o———o; Prausnitz-Küstner (PK) titer against insulin, x · · · · · x. (B) Serum IgE concentration, x · · · · · x; direct cutaneous titer to skin testing with insulin, o———o.

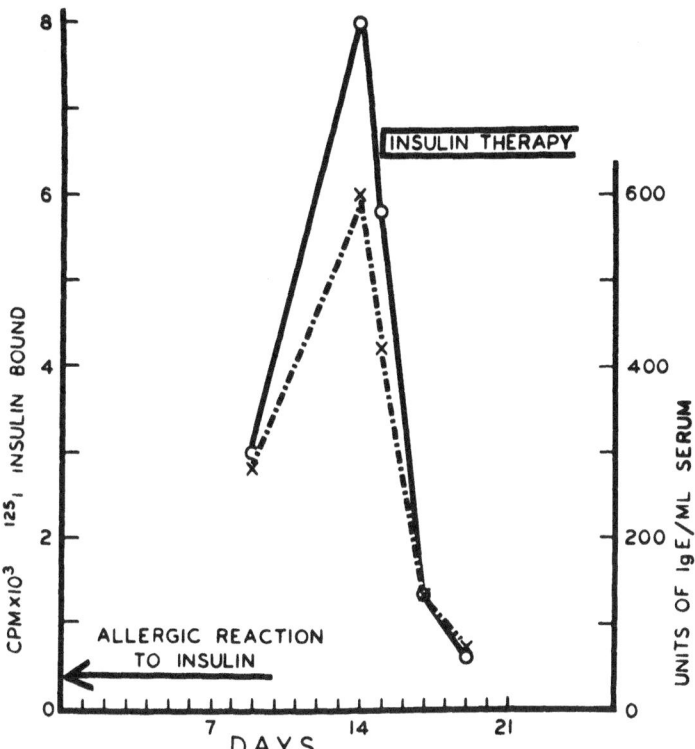

Figure 3. Changes in serum IgE concentration and IgE antiinsulin activity in a patient after a systemic allergic reaction to insulin and rapid insulin desensitization. Serum IgE concentration, ×·····×; [^{125}I]insulin bound by serum IgE, ○———○.

against insulin may first rise but then decline rapidly (Fig. 3) or may decline with no rise (Fig. 4). We interpret these results to show that during progressive insulin desensitization the IgE antibodies against insulin are neutralized by the insulin administration and continued IgE antibody production does not occur, resulting in resolution of the clinical allergy. It has been suggested that IgG antibodies, serving as blocking antibodies, may result from insulin desensitization and be the protective mechanism permitting insulin therapy in the previously allergic patient. This has been suggested in part, because IgG-mediated immunological insulin resistance may follow insulin desensitization (Patterson *et al.*, 1973a). It is possible that such IgG antibodies may contribute to protection of the desensitized patient but the more likely explanation for successful desensitization is the decline in IgE antibodies.

E. Allergic Reactions to Nonprotein Materials

Delayed-type cutaneous reactivity and peripheral blood lymphocyte reactivity to zinc have been reported in patients with cutaneous reactivity to insulin (Feinglos and Jegasothy, 1979).

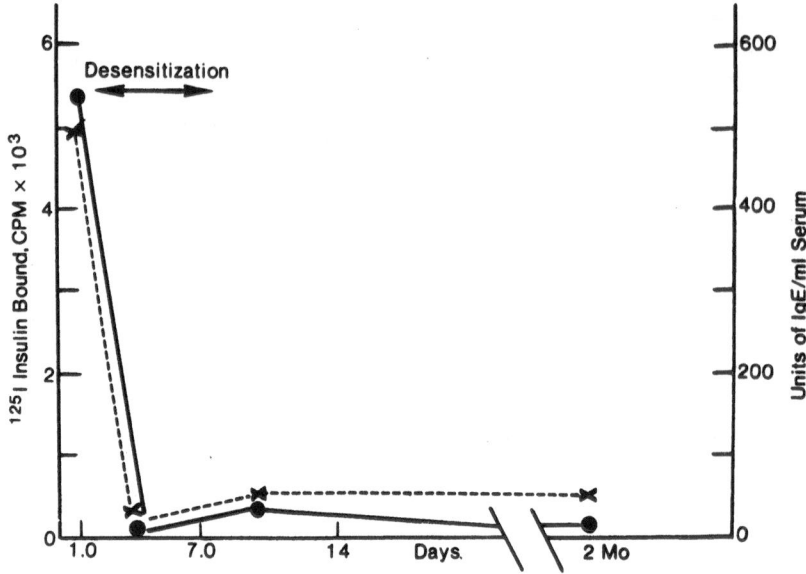

Figure 4. Rapid decline in IgE antiinsulin binding following desensitization. Counts per minute (CPM) of
^{125}I-labeled insulin bound by 1 ml serum (o————o); serum IgE concentration (× · · · · · ×).

F. Mechanism of Serum Sickness

A case of lymphadenopathy associated with insulin resistance in retrospect is considered to be consistent with a serum sickness type of reaction. This is Patient A described
by Patterson *et al.* (1973b). The patient had lymphadenopathy and IgG antibodies
against insulin. Both the symptoms and the insulin requirement declined with
prednisone therapy (Fig. 5). In this case, insulin–IgG-antiinsulin complexes could be
demonstrated in the serum (Patterson *et al.*, 1973b). Thus the mechanism of
antigen–antibody complex damage could be implicated. Furthermore, IgG antibody
was produced *in vitro* tissue culture using lymph node cells from this patient.

G. Immunological Insulin Resistance

This topic is covered in a preceding chapter (Chapter 8) and is mentioned here only to
cite our experience briefly. In contrast to a series of about 30 cases of insulin allergy we
have seen only five cases of insulin resistance. Three of these were studied in detail and
IgG antibody shown to be responsible (Patterson *et al.*, 1973b). In our clinical experience, patients with a high insulin requirement for whom the question of immunological
insulin resistance was raised almost always had a different reason for high insulin requirement. In those patients where the insulin resistance was immunologically based
(Patterson *et al.*, 1973b), IgG antibodies were responsible. The immunological insulin-
resistant cases we have seen have responded to moderate- to low-dose prednisone therapy. When we evaluate a potential case of immunological insulin resistance and the

immunological explanation for the high insulin requirement appears possible, we recommend a trial of modest dose prednisone therapy (30 mg daily). If immunological insulin resistance is present, a rapid decline in insulin requirement may be expected and lower-dosage alternate-day prednisone maintenance therapy used as long as necessary. Some caution is required with the initial use of prednisone in such cases as the insulin requirement may decline rapidly with prednisone (Fig. 5) and hypoglycemia may occur unless the physician is alert to this possibility and decreases insulin dosage rapidly in response to declining blood sugars.

VI. SUMMARY

True immunological reactions to insulin are uncommon and do not create significant clinical problems. The local IgE-mediated reactions are most common and almost always subside spontaneously. Generalized, IgE-mediated immediate-type reactions are the most significant allergic problems but are managed successfully by temporary reduction in dosage of insulin or by insulin desensitization. The other immunological reactions—insulin resistance and IgG-mediated serum sickness—are even more rare and respond to prednisone therapy.

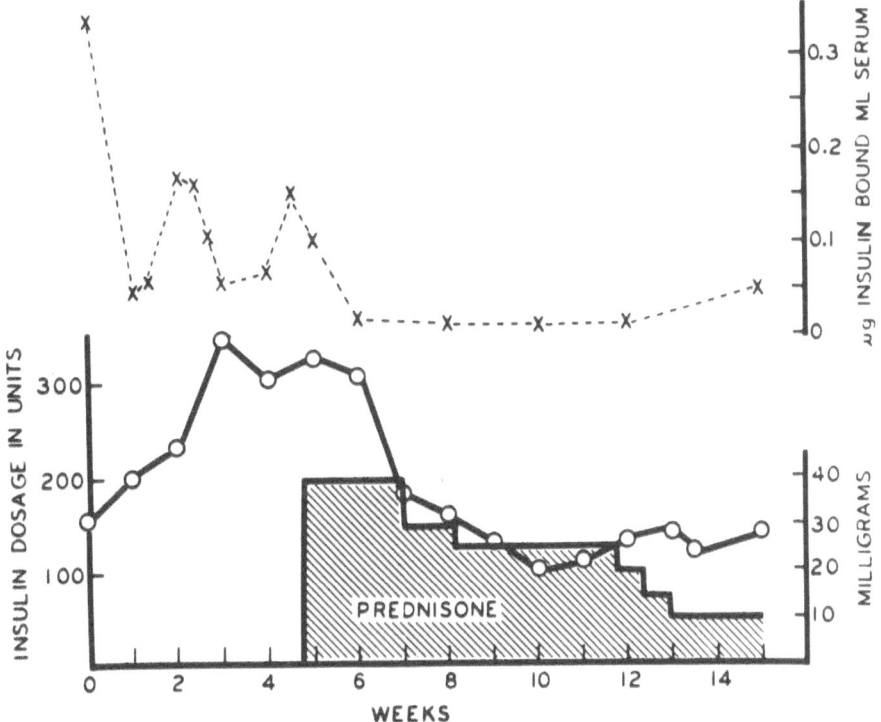

Figure 5. Insulin requirements and serum insulin binding of a patient with insulin resistance before and during treatment with prednisone.

ACKNOWLEDGMENTS.   This work was supported by the Ernest S. Bazley Trust.

REFERENCES

Arkins, J. A., Engbring, N. H., and Lennon, E. J., 1962, The incidence of skin reactivity to insulin in diabetic patients, *J. Allergy* **33**:69–72.

Davidson, J. A., Galloway, J. A., Petersen, b. H., Wentworth, S. M., and Crabtree, R. E., 1974, Use of purified insulin in insulin allergy, *Diabetes* **23**(Suppl. 1):352.

deShazo, R. D., Levinson, A. I., Boehm, T., Evans, R., III, and Ward, G., 1977, Severe persistent biphasic local (immediate and late) skin reactions to insulin, *J. Allergy Clin. Immunol.* **59**:161–164.

Faulk, W. P., Girard, J. P., and Welscher, H. D., 1975, Cell mediated immunity to insulin and its polypeptide chains in insulin-treated diabetes, *Int. Arch. Allergy Appl. Immunol.* **48**:364–371.

Feinglos, M. N., and Jegasothy, B. V., 1979, "Insulin" allergy due to zinc, *Lancet* **1**:122–124.

Gell, P. G. H., and Coombs, R. R. A., (eds.), 1969, *Clinical Aspects of Immunology,* 2nd edition, FA Davis, Philadelphia.

Goldman, R. A., Lewis, A. E., and Rose, L. I., 1976, Anaphylactoid reactions to single-component pork insulin, *JAMA* **236**:1148–1149.

Kurtz, A. B., Matthews, J. A., Mustaffa, B. E., Daggett, P. R., and Nabarro, J. D. N., 1980, Decrease of antibodies to insulin, proinsulin, and contaminating hormones after changing treatment from conventional beef to purified pork insulin, *Diabetologia* **18**:147–150.

Lieberman, P., Patterson, R., Metz, R., and Lucena, A., 1971, Allergic reactions to insulin, *JAMA* **215**:1106–1112.

Mattson, J. R., Patterson, R., and Roberts, M., 1975, Insulin therapy in patients with systemic insulin allergy, *Arch. Intern. Med.* **135**:815–821.

Patterson, R., Lucena, G., Metz, R., and Roberts, M., 1969, Reaginic antibody against insulin: Demonstration of antigenic distinction between native and extracted insulin, *J. Immunol.* **103**:1061–1071.

Patterson, R., Mellies, C. J., and Roberts, M., 1973a, Immunologic reactions against insulin: IgE anti-insulin, insulin allergy and combined IgE and IgG immunologic insulin resistance, *J. Immunol.* **110**:1135–1145.

Patterson, R., O'Rourke, J., Roberts, M., and Suszko, I., 1973b, Immunologic reactions against insulin: IgG anti insulin and insulin reactions, *J. Immunol.* **110**:1126–1134.

Yue, D. K., and Turtle, J. R., 1975, Antigenicity of "monocomponent" pork insulin in diabetic subjects, *Diabetes* **24**:625–632.

Index